Neurology in Clinical Practice

Neurology in Clinical Practice

Editor: Steven Graham

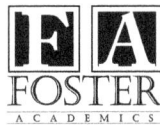

FA
FOSTER
ACADEMICS

www.fosteracademics.com

www.fosteracademics.com

FA FOSTER
ACADEMICS

Cataloging-in-Publication Data

Neurology in clinical practice / edited by Steven Graham.
    p. cm.
Includes bibliographical references and index.
ISBN 978-1-63242-718-2
1. Neurology. 2. Nervous system. 3. Nervous system--Diseases. I. Graham, Steven.
RC346 .N48 2019
616.8--dc23

Foster Academics,
118-35 Queens Blvd., Suite 400,
Forest Hills, NY 11375, USA

ISBN 978-1-63242-718-2 (Hardback)

Contents

Preface

This book has been an outcome of determined endeavour from a group of educationists in the field. The primary objective was to involve a broad spectrum of professionals from diverse cultural background involved in the field for developing new researches. The book not only targets students but also scholars pursuing higher research for further enhancement of the theoretical and practical applications of the subject.

Neurology is a branch of medicine concerned with the disorders of the nervous system. The diagnosis and treatment of the conditions of the peripheral and central nervous systems, their coverings, blood vessels and all effector tissues is under the scope of this science. Some of such conditions are stroke, dementia, Parkinson's disease, Tourette's syndrome, Alzheimer's disease, multiple sclerosis, etc. A comprehensive medical history in combination with a physical examination helps to evaluate nervous system health. The assessment of the cognitive function, motor strength, reflexes, sensation, coordination and gait is done through a neurological examination. Imaging techniques such as magnetic resonance imaging, computed axial tomography and ultrasonography of the blood vessels of the head and neck are used for further evaluation. Depending on the evaluation, a treatment strategy involving surgery, medications or physical therapy is devised. This book brings forth some of the most innovative concepts and elucidates the unexplored aspects of neurology. The objective of this book is to give a general view of the different neurological conditions and their management strategies. The extensive content of this book provides the readers with a thorough understanding of the subject.

It was an honour to edit such a profound book and also a challenging task to compile and examine all the relevant data for accuracy and originality. I wish to acknowledge the efforts of the contributors for submitting such brilliant and diverse chapters in the field and for endlessly working for the completion of the book. Last, but not the least; I thank my family for being a constant source of support in all my research endeavours.

Editor

Association of white matter hyperintensities with migraine features and prognosis

Hui Xie[1], Qiang Zhang[1,2], Kang Huo[1], Rui Liu[1], Zhi-Jie Jian[1], Yi-Tong Bian[3], Guo-Liang Li[4], Dan Zhu[1], Li-Hui Zhang[1], Jian Yang[3] and Guo-Gang Luo[1*]

Abstract

Background: White matter hyperintensities (WMHs) are frequently detected in migraine patients. However, their significance and correlation to migraine disease burden remain unclear. This study aims to examine the correlation of WMHs with migraine features and explore the relationship between WMHs and migraine prognosis.

Methods: A total of 69 migraineurs underwent MRI scans to evaluate WMHs. Migraine features were compared between patients with and without WMHs. After an average follow-up period of 3 years, these patients were divided into two groups, according to the reduction of headache frequency: improved and non-improved groups. The percentage and degree of WMHs were compared between these two groups.

Results: A total of 24 patients (34.8%) had WMHs. Patients with WMHs were significantly older (39.0 ± 7.9 vs. 30.6 ± 10.4 years, $P < 0.001$) and had a longer disease duration (median: 180.0 vs. 84.0 months, $P = 0.013$). Furthermore, 33 patients completed the follow up period (15 patients improved and 18 patients did not improve). Patients in the non-improved group had a higher frequency of WMHs (55.6% vs. 13.3%, $P = 0.027$) and median WMHs score (1.0 vs. 0.0, $P = 0.030$).

Conclusions: WMHs can predict unfavorable migraine prognosis. Furthermore, WMHs may have a closer association with age than migraine features.

Keywords: Migraine, White matter hyperintensities, Clinical significance, Prognosis

Background

Migraine is a chronic debilitating headache characterized by recurrent moderate-to-severe headache attacks and autonomic nervous system related-symptoms [1]. Globally, migraine affects approximately 15% of the general population, and it preferentially affects females [2]. Migraine can be regarded as a risk factor associated with white matter hyperintensities (WMHs) [3], which are hyper-intense brain lesions in T2-weighted and Fluid-Attenuated Inversion Recovery (FLAIR) images [4]. Accumulating evidence documented the high incidence of WMHs in patients with migraine [3, 5]. However, the exact correlation between WMHs and the clinical features of migraine remain

unclear. A population-based CAMERA study suggested the increased risk of WMHs in migraine patients with higher attack frequencies (≥1 attack per month), compared with patients with lower attack frequencies (< 1 attack per month) [3]. Trauninger et al. demonstrated that both disease duration and attack frequency were associated with WMHs in migraine patients [6]. On the other hand, Toghae et al. observed an association between WMHs and the age and migraine duration of patients, but not with attack frequency [7]. Recent studies have reported that WMHs are associated with the age of patients, and not with disease burden (disease duration and attack frequency) [8, 9]. Therefore, additional studies are required to gain insight into the exact correlation between WMHs and the features of migraine.

Larger or confluent WMHs are usually observed in cerebrovascular diseases and cognitive decline cases [10,

* Correspondence: lguogang@163.com
[1]Department of Neurology, The First Affiliated Hospital of Xi'an Jiaotong University, No. 277 Yanta West Road, Xi'an 710061, Shaanxi, China
Full list of author information is available at the end of the article

11]. However, WMHs associated with migraine tend to be punctate and mild [10]. Nevertheless, studies that have investigated the clinical implication of WMHs are scarce. Longitudinal population-based studies have previously indicated that WMHs in migraine are not associated with stroke or the decline in cognitive function [10, 12]. However, migraine has a variable short- or long-term prognosis. Some patients achieve complete or partial remission, while others experience persistent or even progressive attacks [13]. Recently, Eggers proposed that WMHs might be caused by multiple microemboli, which are induced by platelet aggregation abnormalities usually observed in migraine patients [14]. This supports the notion that WMHs may reflect an abnormal internal environment in patients. Therefore, the present study aimed to investigate the prognostic value of WMHs in migraine patients. To this end, the T1- and T2-weighted, as well as the T2-weighted FLAIR, magnetic resonance imaging (MRI) data obtained from migraine patients were analyzed to describe the imaging characteristics of WMHs. Furthermore, the association between WMHs and the clinical features of migraine were investigated, and the relationship between WMHs and migraine prognosis were examined.

Methods
Patients
A total of 69 migraine patients (52 females and 17 males, average age: 33.6 years old) were consecutively recruited from the Headache Clinic of the Department of Neurology, The First Affiliated Hospital of Xi'an Jiaotong University from February 2012 to November 2016. Inclusion criteria included: (1) patients with migraine who fulfilled the International Classification of Headache disorders (ICHD)-3 (β) criteria [1]), and (2) age between 12 and 55 years old. Exclusion criteria: (1) patients with major neurological diseases, (2) patients with major systemic diseases, (3) patients with thyroid diseases, (4) pregnant and/or lactating patients, and (5) patients with claustrophobia. The present study was approved by the Ethics Committee of the First Affiliated Hospital of Xi'an Jiaotong University (XJTU1AF2015 LSK-159), and an informed written consent was obtained from each patient. For minor patients (< 16), the written consent form was obtained from the accompanying parents.

Demographic characteristics and clinical features
All enrolled patients were required to complete a standard questionnaire to collect basic clinical information at the Headache Clinic. This questionnaire assessed the demographic characteristics, past history, family history and features of migraine, and any accompanying symptoms and self-rating depression scale (SDS). Migraine features include disease duration, attack frequency, attack duration

and the visual analogue scale (VAS) score. In addition, the questionnaire also investigated the history of smoking, hypertension, diabetes, oral contraceptive use, past vascular events, heart diseases, tumors, intracranial organic diseases and other medical conditions.

Image data acquisition and evaluation of WMHs
All participants underwent MRI scans at the Department of Radiology, The First Affiliated Hospital of Xi'an Jiaotong University, using a 3.0 T GE Discovery MR scanner and a standard 8-channel phase array head coil. High-resolution structural images were acquired using a three-dimensional T1-weighted sequence with the following parameters: TR, 10.276 ms; TE, 4.9 ms; matrix, 256 × 256; section-thickness, 1 mm; FOV, 256 mm. T2-weighted images were acquired with the following parameters: TR, 6000 ms; TE, 104.4 ms; matrix, 385 × 384; section-thickness, 5 mm; FOV, 240 mm. FLAIR images were acquired with the following parameters: TR, 9102 ms; TE, 168.7 ms; matrix, 288 × 224; section-thickness, 5 mm; FOV, 240 mm.

WMHs were visible as hyperintense lesions on FLAIR images, and as isointense or slightly hypointense lesions on T1-weighted images. MRI scans were assessed for the number and features of WMHs, including the appearance, number, size and anatomical location. All MRI scans were reviewed by an experienced neurologist and neuroradiologist. The degree of WMHs was assessed using the Scheltens visual rating scale [15]. Briefly, WMHs were separately graded in each of the following locations: frontal lobes, temporal lobes, parietal lobes and occipital lobes. WMHs were graded as follows: 0 (no lesions), 1 (hyperintensity < 3 mm and $n \leq 5$), 2 (hyperintensity < 3 mm and $n \geq 6$), 3 (hyperintensity 4–10 mm and $n \leq 5$), 4 (hyperintensity 4–10 mm and $n \geq 6$), 5 (hyperintensity ≥11 mm and $n \geq 1$), and 6 (confluent). The sum of scores from each location was considered as the final score [15, 16]. According to WMH, migraine patients were divided into two groups: non-WMH group (complete absence of WMHs or WMHs score = 0) and WMH group (presence of WMHs or WMHs score ≥ 1). Next, the features of WMHs and its correlation to the clinical variables were analyzed. Finally, a retrospective follow-up study was conducted to analyze the association of WMHs and migraine prognosis.

Patient follow-up
In December 2016, patients who were enrolled in the study for a mean period of > 24 months ($n = 45$) were recruited for a follow up visit. A total of five patients were excluded due to percutaneous closure of the patent foramen ovale, and another seven patients dropped out from the follow up study. The study flow chart is illustrated in Fig. 1.

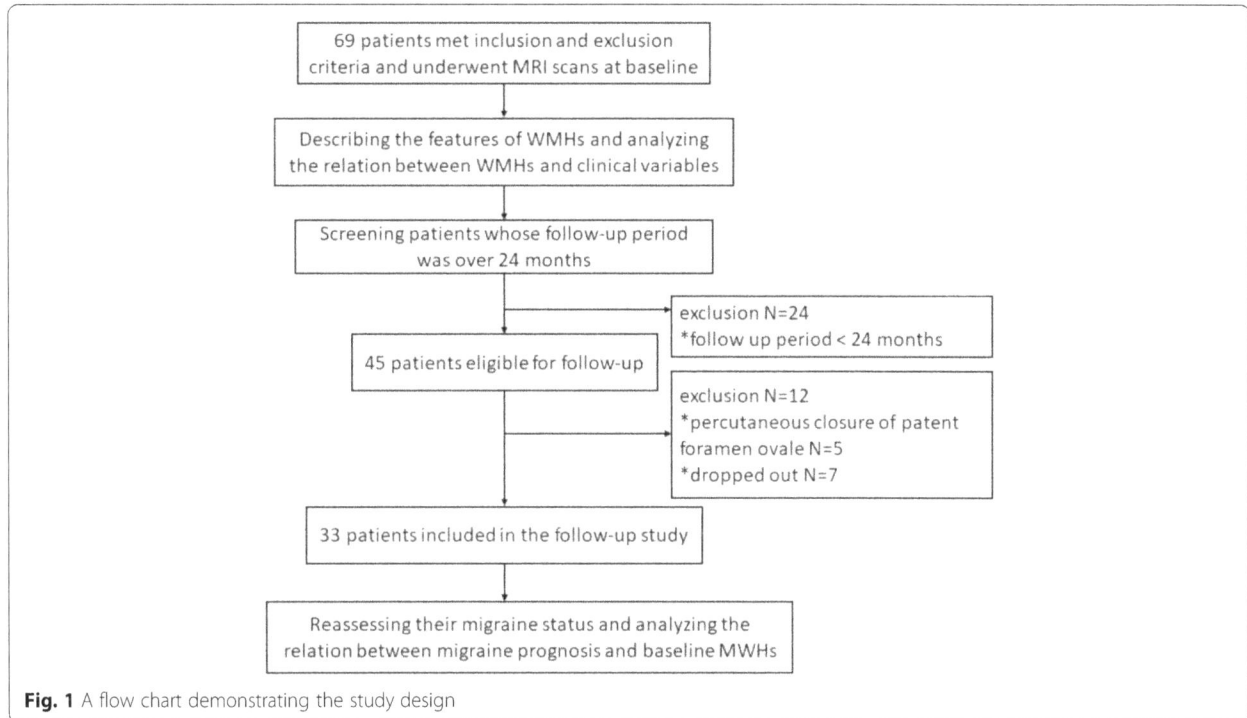

Fig. 1 A flow chart demonstrating the study design

A total of 33 patients were re-interviewed to assess their migraine status and determine the present headache attack frequency per month. Patients were divided into improved and non-improved groups based on the mean percentage of attack frequency calculated from the 3 months that preceded the follow-up appointment. The outcome was defined as improved if the attack frequency decreased by more than 50% compared to that of baseline. On the other hand, if the attack frequency failed to decrease by more than 50% at follow up, the patient was considered to be non-improved. Next, the outcome was further classified into four categories including complete remission, partial remission, persistence and progression. Complete remission was defined as zero migraine attacks in the 3 months that preceded the follow-up. Partial remission was defined as the reduction of migraine frequency by more than 50%. Persistence group had the change of migraine frequency hovering around the 50%. Progression was defined as the increase of migraine frequency by more than 50%. It is worth mentioning that despite our efforts, most of the patients who were followed up denied to undergo a follow-up MRI scan.

Therapeutic regimen

The usage of medication during the follow-up period was recorded. Migraine patients were administered with migraine prophylactic medications (including calcium channel blockers, anticonvulsants, or β-blockers) or non-steroidal anti-inflammatory drugs, according to the recommendation of physicians.

Statistical analysis

Demographic and clinical characteristics were tabulated using descriptive statistics, including percentages, quartiles (non-normal data) and means (normal data). Chi-square test and Fisher's exact probability test were used to test for differences in categorical data. Student's t-test was used to compare the means of normally distributed variables. Non-parametric tests were used for non-normally distributed data. A correlation analysis between WMHs and patient prognosis was performed using Spearman correlation. Further, logistic regression was conducted to evaluate contributing factors to migraine prognosis. Statistical analyses were performed using the SPSS 23.0 software. A P-value < 0.05 was considered statistically significant.

Results

Demographic characteristics and migraine features

A total of 69 patients with an average age 33.6 years old (range: 14–54 years old) were enrolled in the present study. Among these patients, 52 patients (75.4%) were females. The demographic characteristics and clinical features of migraine are summarized in Table 1. Furthermore, 19 patients (27.5%) presented with aura including visual aura ($n = 16$), visual and sensory aura ($n = 2$), and brainstem aura ($n = 1$). Five patients were presented with chronic migraine, while the remaining patients were episodic. Moreover, a total of eight patients (11.6%) were smokers, and another five patients (7.2%) were hypertensive, but none of the enrolled patients were diabetic.

Table 1 Comparison of clinical characteristics between the non-WMH group and WMH group

	Non-WMH group ($n = 45$)	WMH group ($n = 24$)	P-value
Age (year, mean ± SD)	30.6 ± 10.4	39.0 ± 7.9	< 0.001*
Gender			0.592
Female, n (%)	33 (73.3%)	19 (79.2%)	
Male, n (%)	12 (26.7%)	5 (20.8%)	
BMI (kg/m², mean ± SD)	20.7 ± 2.9	21.8 ± 2.2	0.127
Hypertension, n (%)	2 (4.4%)	3 (12.5%)	0.458
Smoking, n (%)	5 (11.1%)	3 (12.5%)	1.000
Oral contraceptive use, n (%)	1 (2.9%)	1 (5.3%)	1.000
Headache characteristics			
Aura, n (%)	14 (31.1%)	5 (20.8%)	0.363
Disease duration (month, quartile)	84.0 (42.0, 198.0)	180.0 (75.0, 297.0)	0.013*
Attack frequency (day/month, quartile)	3.0 (2.0, 7.0)	4.0 (2.0, 10.0)	0.465
Attack duration (hour, quartile)	5.0 (3.0, 10.0)	9.5 (4.0, 24.0)	0.172
Visual analogue scale, mean ± SD	7.0 ± 1.9	7.8 ± 1.5	0.080
Accompany symptoms			
Nausea, n (%)	37 (84.1%)	21 (87.5%)	0.983
Vomiting, n (%)	28 (63.6%)	15 (62.5%)	0.926
Photophobia, n (%)	32 (72.7%)	18 (75.0%)	0.839
Phonophobia, n (%)	33 (75.0%)	18 (75.0%)	1.000
Dizziness, n (%)	21 (47.7%)	13 (54.2%)	0.612
Family history of migraine, n (%)	26 (57.8%)	11 (45.8%)	0.343
SDS scores (quartile)	42 (36, 56)	44.5 (37.3, 56.8)	0.653

*A significance level, $P < 0.05$; *SD* standard deviation, *BMI* body mass index

Next, WMHs were investigated through T2-weighted and FLAIR MRI scans. According to WMH, migraine patients were divided into two groups: non-WMH group (complete absence of WMHs or WMH score = 0) and WMH group (the presence of WMHs or a WMH score of ≥1) (Table 1). Among these 69 migraine patients, a total of 24 patients (34.8%, 19 females and five males) presented with WMHs. Furthermore, there was a significant difference in age between the WMH and non-WMH groups. Patients in the WMH group were significantly older compared to patients in the non-WMH group (39.0 ± 7.9 years vs. 30.6 ± 10.4 years; $P = 0.000$). Among the disease burden related variables, disease duration was significantly higher in the WMH group than in the non-WMH group (median: 180 months vs. 84 months; $P = 0.013$). Furthermore, a moderate positive correlation was observed between age and disease duration ($r = 0.589$, $P < 0.001$), which indicate a possible confounding effect of age in the association between disease duration and WMHs. A scatter plot was preformed to show the changing trend of disease duration with age. The trend was similar between the improved group and non-improved group

(Fig. 2). No significant difference was observed in the presence of aura between these two groups. It is worth mentioning that the exclusion of hypertension or smoking status (12 cases) did not affect the data analyses between these two groups.

Features of WMHs

In the WMH group ($n = 24$), most lesions were punctuate (22 patients), and two patients presented with confluent lesions (Fig. 3b and c). Among patients with WMHs, a total of 171 lesions were detected. WMHs were significantly higher in the frontal lobes (74.9%), followed by the parietal lobes (21.6%) (Fig. 4a). Furthermore, it was observed that WMHs in migraine patients were generally mild, most lesions (94.7%) were < 5 mm (Fig. 4b), and the average number of lesions per patient was generally small, with a median number of 2.5 (range: 1–52) (Fig. 4c). According to the Scheltens scale, the WMH scores of patients were low, with a median score of 2.5 (range: 0–10) (Fig. 4d). Furthermore, the difference in numbers and scores between males and females with WMHs was not statistically significant.

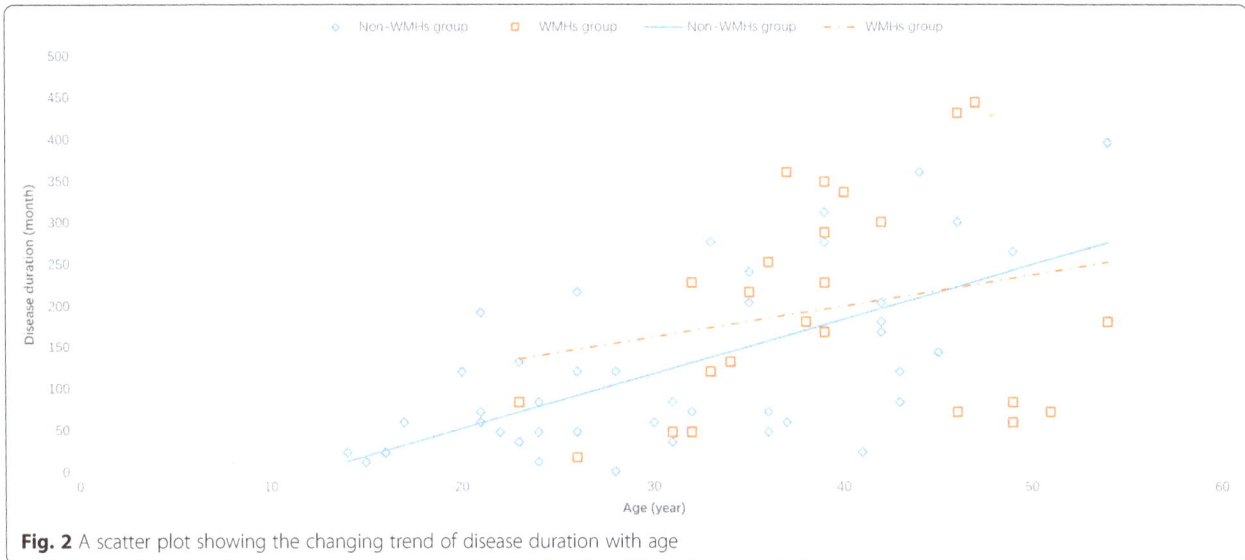

Fig. 2 A scatter plot showing the changing trend of disease duration with age

Correlation between WMHs and migraine prognosis

A total of 33 patients were followed up in the present study (Fig. 1). The average follow-up period was 3 years, which ranged within 2–4 years. Among these 33 re-assessed patients, 15 patients (45.5%) were assigned to the improved group while 18 patients (54.5%) were assigned to the non-improved group. Specifically, 4 patients (12.1%) achieved complete remission and they were free of migraine attacks for more than 1 year. Eleven patients (33.3%) achieved partial remission. Fourteen patients (42.4%) were in persistence group. Four patients (12.1%) were in the progression group. The four patients attaining complete remission were 30, 34, 39 and 41 years old at follow-up, excluding the potential effect of menopausal state. Differences in age, gender, or BMI between the improved and non-improved groups were not statistically significant. None of our patients had hypertension or diabetes. Among the headache characteristics, aura was more frequent in the improved group (60.0% vs. 11.1%, $P = 0.008$) (Table 2).

Among the 18 patients in the non-improved group, 10 patients had one or more WMHs, while WMHs were detected in only two of 15 patients in the improved group, and the difference was statistically significant ($P = 0.027$, Table 3). Furthermore, patients in the non-improved group had a significantly higher median WMHs score compared to patients in the improved group ($P = 0.030$).

Next, we examined the impact of prophylactic treatments on the migraine outcome. We compared the rate of regular prophylactic treatment between the improved and non-improved groups administered for more than 3 months regardless of drug classes or doses. Our results demonstrated the absence of significant difference between both patient groups (Table 2). It is worth mentioning that none of the patients reported the use triptans.

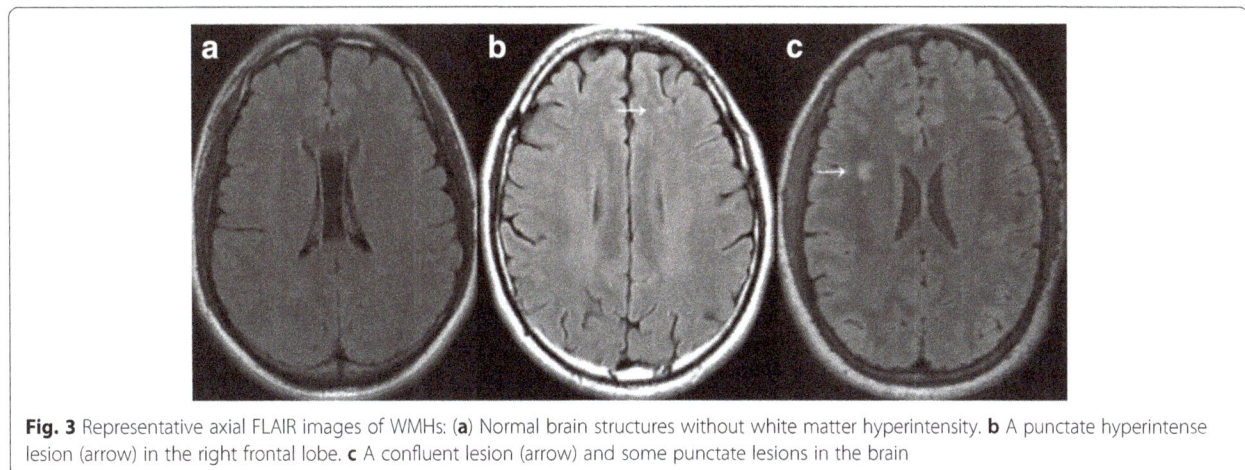

Fig. 3 Representative axial FLAIR images of WMHs: (**a**) Normal brain structures without white matter hyperintensity. **b** A punctate hyperintense lesion (arrow) in the right frontal lobe. **c** A confluent lesion (arrow) and some punctate lesions in the brain

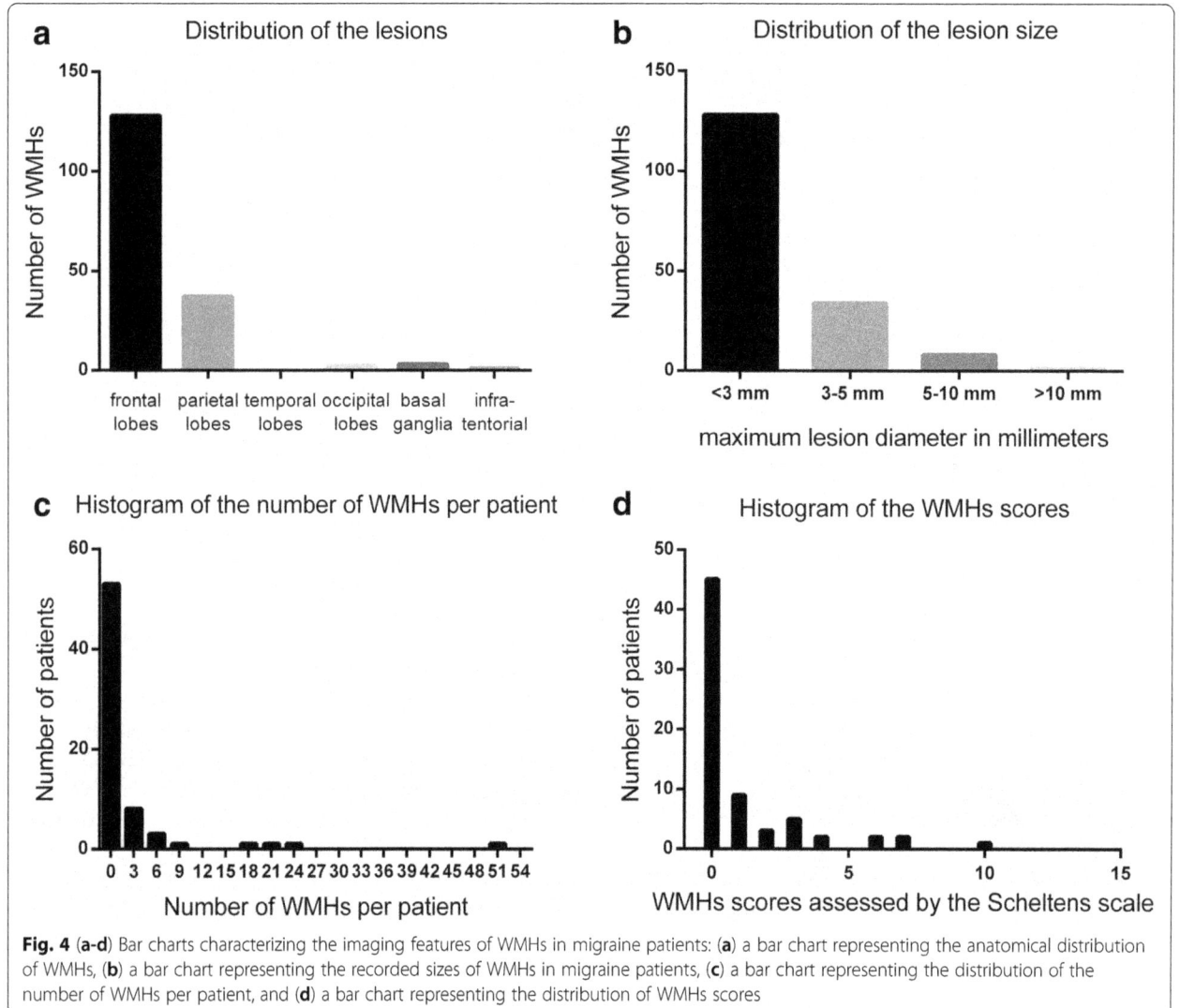

Fig. 4 (**a-d**) Bar charts characterizing the imaging features of WMHs in migraine patients: (**a**) a bar chart representing the anatomical distribution of WMHs, (**b**) a bar chart representing the recorded sizes of WMHs in migraine patients, (**c**) a bar chart representing the distribution of the number of WMHs per patient, and (**d**) a bar chart representing the distribution of WMHs scores

Multivariate logistic regression analysis was conducted to analyze the independent risk factor associated with the non-improved outcome. The impact of age, aura, disease duration, VAS and the presence of WMHs were examined. Our results showed that WMHs (OR = 12.6, 95% CI (1.093~ 145.848) and aura (OR = 0.04, 95% CI (0.002 ~ 0.683) were the independent risk factors associated with the non-improved outcome.

In the follow up group, patients without aura were significantly older than those with aura (36.6 ± 9.1 vs. 23.8 ± 8.3, $P < 0.001$) and had a significantly longer disease duration (median: 162 months vs. 36 months, $P = 0.003$) and attack duration (median: 2 h vs. 11 h, P < 0.001). Patients without aura also had a higher incidence of WMHs than those with aura (45.4% vs. 18.2%, $P = 0.249$). The difference was obvious although it did not achieve the statistical significance.

Discussion

Migraine is a well-documented risk factor for WMHs [3, 5, 17, 18]. However, to date, the clinical significance of WMHs in migraine prognosis remains unclear. Therefore, in the present study, we explored the association between WMHs and migraine prognosis. Results demonstrated that the presence and degree of WMHs can be associated with unfavorable migraine prognosis. In addition, in the present study, we described the features of WMHs in migraine patients, and observed that WMHs were positively correlated with old age.

WMHs are commonly associated with physiological conditions such as aging and pathological conditions associated with vascular risks such as hypertension [19]. Pathologically, WMHs can result from local brain ischemia at the microvascular level [14, 19]. Several reports have demonstrated a higher incidence of WMHs in patients with migraine, compared to healthy control subjects

Table 2 Comparison of demographics and WMHs between the improved and non-improved groups

	Improved group ($n = 15$)	Non-improved group ($n = 18$)	P-value
Age (year, mean ± SD)	29.5 ± 9.8	34.7 ± 11.0	0.166
Gender			1.000
Female, n (%)	13 (86.7%)	16 (88.9%)	
Male, n (%)	2 (13.3%)	2 (11.1%)	
BMI (kg/m², mean ± SD)	19.9 ± 2.3	21.1 ± 2.9	0.203
Headache characteristics			
Aura, n (%)	9 (60.0%)	2 (11.1%)	0.008*
Disease duration (month, quartile)	72 (24, 144)	150 (48, 279)	0.096
Attack frequency (day/month, quartile)	4.0 (2.0, 7.0)	2.0 (2.0, 5.5)	0.555
Attack duration (hour, quartile)	4.5 (2.0, 10.0)	11.0 (3.4, 24.0)	0.204
Visual analogue scale, mean ± SD	7.0 (6.0, 7.9)	8.0 (7.0, 9.3)	0.051
Medications			
Prophylactic medications#, n (%)	5 (33.3%)	4 (22.2%)	0.697
Medication overuse#, n (%)	1 (6.7%)	2 (11.1%)	1.000

*A significance level, $P < 0.05$; #The number of patients who took regular prophylactic medications for more than 3 months or had medication overuse during the follow-up period; *SD* standard deviation, *BMI* body mass index

[3, 5]. In the same context, Schurks et al. demonstrated that migraine is a definite risk of stroke, especially in young women [20]. This suggests the role of ischemia in the mechanism of WMHs in association with migraine. To date, the exact pathophysiology of WMHs is not well-understood. Accumulating evidence revealed that migraine patients may have abnormal platelet activation, impaired endothelial function and hypercoagulability [21–23], which can be potential causes for the development of WMHs. These abnormal vascular conditions might favor the persistence or even the progression of migraine. Consequently, it is reasonable to speculate that WMHs can be correlated with unfavorable migraine prognosis. Indeed, results obtained from the present study demonstrate that both the degree and frequency of WMHs were positively correlated with unfavorable migraine prognosis. To the best of our knowledge, this is the first report that demonstrated the prognostic value of WMHs in migraine patients.

Aging is another important risk factor of the development of WMHs [4, 19]. Among the examined clinical variables, only age and disease duration were correlated to WMHs in our patient cohort. However, a moderate positive correlation was observed between age and disease

Table 3 Fisher's exact test representing the correlation between WMHs and patient prognosis

	Improved	Non-improved	Total
WMHs group	2	10	12
Non-WMHs group	13	8	21
Total	15	18	33

Fisher's exact test: two-tailed P-value = 0.027

duration. The disease duration of patients with WMHs was not higher than that of patients without WMHs within the same age brackets. These results imply that the association between disease duration and WMHs could result from the confounding effect of age. Furthermore, we investigated whether age had a confounding effect on the association of WMHs and migraine prognosis. There was no significant difference in age between the improved and non-improved groups. Regression analysis showed WMHs was the independent risk factor for the non-improved outcome with the control of the cofounding effect of age. Finally, the rate of prophylactic treatment was also comparable between these two groups. Collectively, these results indicate that the association between WMHs and migraine prognosis were not affected by age or medications in our patient cohort. However, it is recognized that the prevalence of migraine increases with age from childhood to adulthood, and it peaks at 35 to 39 years of age, after which it gradually decreases, particularly among women after menopause [3]. Meanwhile, WMHs are not static, and in most cases WMHs progress with aging [24, 25]. Therefore, for older migraine patients, WMHs will not serve as a reliable marker for prognosis. It is worth mentioning that a 3-year longitudinal follow-up study revealed a non-significant increase in the number of WMHs in 19.5% of the patient cohort [26]. These results suggest that WMHs would not significantly progress within a relatively short period (3 years). In the present study, patients were re-evaluated after 2–4 years (mean: 3 years). Therefore, this might indicate that the validity of WMHs in migraine prognosis is at least applicable over a relatively short interval (3-year window). Future research should examine its validity through long-term follow ups.

In this study, our results demonstrated that migraineurs with favorable outcome had a higher incidence of aura. Studies analyzing the relationship between the presence of aura and migraine prognosis are scarce. Dahlof et al. observed that aura was associated with poor migraine prognosis in females, but a similar relationship was not observed in male patients [27]. A 5-year follow-up study that investigated the outcome of migraine in children and adolescents failed to find a significant difference between migraine with and without aura, although the percentage of subjects who were free from migraine at follow-up was 30.6% in the case of migraine with aura and 20.3% in the case of migraine without aura [28]. In our study cohort, patients with aura were significantly younger than those without aura. Disease duration and attack duration were significantly lower in patients with aura than those without aura. Patients with aura had a lower incidence of WMHs than those without aura although the difference was not significant. On the other hand, Gozke et al. previously suggested a higher incidence of WMHs in migraine with aura [29]. Moreover, it is well recognized that migraine with aura is a risk associated with ischemic stroke [20]. Therefore, it is plausible to speculate that the better baseline headache condition in patients with aura could contribute to better prognosis compared to patients without aura. However, the exact reason remains to be clarified in future studies.

There was no significant difference of SDS scores between WMHs group and Non-WMHs group. The relationship between depression and WMHs remains unclear [30, 31]. A meta-analysis showed a significant weak association between WMHs and depression (OR: 1.02~1.22) [32]. The burden of migraine can be assessed by disease duration, attack frequency, attack duration and headache intensity (VAS) [18]. In the present study, we investigated the impact of WMHs on disease burden. It was observed that WMHs were significantly associated with longer disease duration, while a significant correlation with attack frequency or its duration was not observed. To date, the association between WMHs and migraine features remain controversial [6, 18, 33, 34]. Earlier reports have consistently revealed that WMHs were not associated with migraine features, including disease duration or attack duration [35–37]. On the other hand, Gozke et al. demonstrated that WMHs were associated with a higher frequency of longer disease duration and higher attack frequencies [29]. Similarly, the CAMERA study supported the same conclusions [3]. However, the population of the CAMERA study had high proportions of vascular risk factors (32–42%

prevalence of hypertension, 60–66% prevalence of smoking, and 19–29% prevalence of oral contraceptive use), which may lead to confounding bias. This discrepancy might be attributed to the accuracy of the MRI techniques, especially the blurring artifact. Other factors include the demographic characteristics of the study population or discrepancies in the study design [3, 6, 29, 34, 35]. In addition, the measurements of disease burden are usually not stable; that is, disease duration was always affected by age, and attack frequency and attack duration often show changeable patterns over time; while the VAS had strong subjectivity. Therefore, future research should focus on more stable parameters to assess the disease burden of migraine.

Taken together, the results obtained from the study suggest that WMHs may predict unfavorable migraine prognosis. Therefore, our results could lead to the alteration of the treatment protocol for migraineurs with WMHs. That is, physicians could apply more positive treatment strategies to achieve a more favorable prognosis in patients with high WMHs scores. Furthermore, our results also indicate that WMHs have a closer association with age than the clinical features of migraine.

Nevertheless, the present study had a few limitations. The relatively small number of enrolled patients is considered to be the main limitation. Furthermore, the absence of a control group precluded definitive conclusions about the nature of the observed alterations in WMHs or whether their degree is beyond normal aging. Age should be controlled in the design of the study. Thus, future work should focus on investigating the implication of WMHs among relatively young migraine patients. Similarly, the heterogeneity of the patient cohort such as migraine with and without aura, episodic migraine and chronic migraine, should be improved. Different migraine types possibly have different effects on the prognosis. The relatively low migraine frequency at baseline in our study is also a major limitation as prognostic information may be of greater value in high frequency migraine states. However, the small sample size limited the stratified analysis of frequency in the case of controlling the effect of age. The method for migraine prognosis categorization was one-sided. It reflected the change of frequency but it did not investigate the current frequency level, headache intensity or even response to acute therapy. However, there is no standard prognostic categorization for migraine yet. Future prospective multicenter studies with more controlled conditions (migraine type and age) and long-term follow up should be conducted to confirm these results. Future studies should also employ more stable parameters that assess disease burden, in order to further confirm the clinical significance of WMHs. It is worth mentioning that in the present study, we could not definitively investigate other

WMH-associated risk factors, including hypertension, diabetes, hyperlipidemia, hyperhomocysteinemia, hyperuricemia, hypercoagulability, heart diseases, kidney diseases, inflammation and autoimmune diseases. These conditions may impact the strength of our conclusions regarding the nature of WMHs and their effect on migraine. Future studies should be controlled for the confounding effects of the above mentioned conditions.

Conclusion

This study suggests that WMHs can predict short-term unfavorable migraine prognosis, thereby providing a new insight into the clinical significance of WMHs in migraine. Meanwhile, it demonstrates that WMHs in migraine patients are generally mild, mostly located in the frontal and parietal lobes, and may have a closer association with age than headache characteristics.

Abbreviations

FLAIR: Fluid-attenuated inversion recovery; VAS: Visual analogue scale; WMHs: White matter hyperintensities

Funding

This work was supported by the National Key Technology R&D Program of China (No. 2014BAI04B05) and the National Natural Science Foundation of China (No. 81271127).

Authors' contributions

GGL, HX, KH and JY designed the study. HX, QZ, RL, ZJJ, YTB, DZ and LHZ collected and analyzed the data. HX, QZ and KH drafted and wrote the manuscript. HX, GGL, RL, ZJJ, DZ, LHZ, GLL and JY revised the manuscript critically for intellectual content. All authors provided intellectual input to the study and approved the final version of the manuscript.

Competing interests

The authors declare that they have no competing interests.

Author details

[1]Department of Neurology, The First Affiliated Hospital of Xi'an Jiaotong University, No. 277 Yanta West Road, Xi'an 710061, Shaanxi, China. [2]Department of Neurology, Shaanxi Provincial People's Hospital, Xi'an 710068, China. [3]Department of Radiology, The First Affiliated Hospital of Xi'an Jiaotong University, Xi'an 710061, China. [4]Arrhythmia Unit, Department of Cardiovascular Medicine, The First Affiliated Hospital of Xi'an Jiaotong University, Xi'an 710061, China.

References

1. Headache Classification Committee of the International Headache S. The international classification of headache disorders, 3rd edition (beta version). Cephalalgia. 2013;33:629–808.
2. Steiner TJ, Stovner LJ, Birbeck GL. Migraine: the seventh disabler. J Headache Pain. 2013;14:1.
3. Kruit MC, van Buchem MA, Hofman PA, Bakkers JT, Terwindt GM, Ferrari MD, et al. Migraine as a risk factor for subclinical brain lesions. JAMA. 2004;291: 427–34.
4. Lin J, Wang D, Lan L, Fan Y. Multiple factors involved in the pathogenesis of white matter lesions. Biomed Res Int. 2017;2017:9372050.
5. Swartz RH, Kern RZ. Migraine is associated with magnetic resonance imaging white matter abnormalities: a meta-analysis. Arch Neurol. 2004;61:1366–8.
6. Trauninger A, Leel-Ossy E, Kamson DO, Poto L, Aradi M, Kover F, et al. Risk factors of migraine-related brain white matter hyperintensities: an investigation of 186 patients. J Headache Pain. 2011;12:97–103.
7. Toghae M, Rahimian E, Abdollahi M, Shoar S, Naderan M. The prevalence of magnetic resonance imaging Hyperintensity in migraine patients and its association with migraine headache characteristics and cardiovascular risk factors. Oman Med J. 2015;30:203–7.
8. Zhang Q, Datta R, Detre JA, Cucchiara B. White matter lesion burden in migraine with aura may be associated with reduced cerebral blood flow. Cephalalgia. 2016;
9. Uggetti C, Squarza S, Longaretti F, Galli A, Di Fiore P, Reganati PF, et al. Migraine with aura and white matter lesions: an MRI study. Neurol Sci. 2017; 38:11–3.
10. Friedman DI, Dodick DW. White matter hyperintensities in migraine: reason for optimism. JAMA. 2012;308:1920–1.
11. Dufouil C, Godin O, Chalmers J, Coskun O, MacMahon S, Tzourio-Mazoyer N, et al. Severe cerebral white matter hyperintensities predict severe cognitive decline in patients with cerebrovascular disease history. Stroke. 2009;40: 2219–21.
12. Kurth T, Mohamed S, Maillard P, Zhu YC, Chabriat H, Mazoyer B, et al. Headache, migraine, and structural brain lesions and function: population based epidemiology of vascular ageing-MRI study. BMJ. 2011;342:c7357.
13. Bigal ME, Lipton RB. The prognosis of migraine. Curr Opin Neurol. 2008;21: 301–8.
14. Eggers AE. Migraine white matter hyperintensities and cerebral microinfarcts are silent cryptogenic strokes and relate to dementia. Med Hypotheses. 2017;102:1–3.
15. Scheltens P, Barkhof F, Leys D, Pruvo JP, Nauta JJP, Vermersch P, et al. A semiquantitative rating scale for the assessment of signal hyperintensities on magnetic resonance imaging. J Neurol Sci. 1993;114:7–12.
16. Adami A, Rossato G, Cerini R, Thijs VN, Pozzi-Mucelli R, Anzola GP, et al. Right-to-left shunt does not increase white matter lesion load in migraine with aura patients. Neurology. 2008;71:101–7.
17. Kruit MC, van Buchem MA, Launer LJ, Terwindt GM, Ferrari MD. Migraine is associated with an increased risk of deep white matter lesions, subclinical posterior circulation infarcts and brain iron accumulation: the population-based MRI CAMERA study. Cephalalgia. 2010;30:129–36.
18. Yilmaz Avci A, Lakadamyali H, Arikan S, Benli US, Kilinc M. High sensitivity C-reactive protein and cerebral white matter hyperintensities on magnetic resonance imaging in migraine patients. J Headache Pain. 2015;16:9.
19. Pantoni L. Cerebral small vessel disease: from pathogenesis and clinical characteristics to therapeutic challenges. Lancet Neurol. 2010;9:689–701.
20. Schurks M, Rist PM, Bigal ME, Buring JE, Lipton RB, Kurth T. Migraine and cardiovascular disease: systematic review and meta-analysis. Br Med J. 2009;339
21. Tietjen GE, Collins SA. Hypercoagulability and migraine. Headache. 2018;58: 173–83.
22. Danese E, Montagnana M, Lippi G. Platelets and migraine. Thromb Res. 2014;134:17–22.
23. Tietjen GE, Khubchandani J. Vascular biomarkers in migraine. Cephalalgia. 2015;35:95–117.
24. Palm-Meinders IH, Koppen H, Terwindt GM, Launer LJ, Konishi J, Moonen JM, et al. Structural brain changes in migraine. JAMA. 2012;308:1889–97.
25. Rozen TD. Images from headache: white matter lesions of migraine are not static. Headache. 2010;50:305–6.
26. Dinia L, Bonzano L, Albano B, Finocchi C, Del Sette M, Saitta L, et al. White matter lesions progression in migraine with aura: a clinical and MRI longitudinal study. J Neuroimaging. 2013;23:47–52.
27. Dahlof CG, Johansson M, Casserstedt S, Motallebzadeh T. The course of frequent episodic migraine in a large headache clinic population: a 12-year retrospective follow-up study. Headache. 2009;49:1144–52.
28. Cuvellier JC, Tourte M, Lucas C, Vallee L. Stability of pediatric migraine subtype after a 5-year follow-up. J Child Neurol. 2016;31:1138–42.
29. Gozke E, Ore O, Dortcan N, Unal Z, Cetinkaya M. Cranial magnetic resonance imaging findings in patients with migraine. Headache. 2004; 44:166–9.
30. Versluis CE, van der Mast RC, van Buchem MA, Bollen EL, Blauw GJ, Eekhof JA, et al. Progression of cerebral white matter lesions is not associated with development of depressive symptoms in elderly subjects at risk of cardiovascular disease: the PROSPER study. Int J Geriatr Psychiatry. 2006;21:375–81.
31. Firbank MJ, O'Brien JT, Pakrasi S, Pantoni L, Simoni M, Erkinjuntti T, et al. White matter hyperintensities and depression–preliminary results from the LADIS study. Int J Geriatr Psychiatry. 2005;20:674–9.
32. Wang L, Leonards CO, Sterzer P, Ebinger M. White matter lesions and depression: a systematic review and meta-analysis. J Psychiatr Res. 2014; 56:56–64.

33. Gaist D, Garde E, Blaabjerg M, Nielsen HH, Kroigard T, Ostergaard K, et al.
     Migraine with aura and risk of silent brain infarcts and white matter
     hyperintensities: an MRI study. Brain. 2016;139:2015–23.
34. Galli A, Di Fiore P, D'Arrigo G, Uggetti C, Squarza S, Leone M, et al. Migraine
     with aura white matter lesions: preliminary data on clinical aspects. Neurol
     Sci. 2017;38:7–10.
35. Pavese N, Canapicchi R, Nuti A, Bibbiani F, Lucetti C, Collavoli P, et al. White
     matter MRI hyperintensities in a hundred and twenty-nine consecutive
     migraine patients. Cephalalgia. 1994;14:342–5.
36. De Benedittis G, Lorenzetti A, Sina C, Bernasconi V. Magnetic resonance
     imaging in migraine and tension-type headache. Headache. 1995;35:264–8.
37. Cooney BS, Grossman RI, Farber RE, Goin JE, Galetta SL. Frequency of
     magnetic resonance imaging abnormalities in patients with migraine.
     Headache. 1996;36:616–21.

2

The subtleties of cognitive decline in multiple sclerosis: an exploratory study using hierarchichal cluster analysis of CANTAB results

Hideraldo Luis Souza Cabeça[1†], Luciano Chaves Rocha[2†], Amanda Ferreira Sabbá[2], Alessandra Mendonça Tomás[2], Natali Valim Oliver Bento-Torres[2,3], Daniel Clive Anthony[4] and Cristovam Wanderley Picanço Diniz[2*] (iD)

Abstract

Background: It is essential to investigate cognitive deficits in multiple sclerosis (MS) to develop evidence-based cognitive rehabilitation strategies. Here we refined cognitive decline assessment using the automated tests of the Cambridge Neuropsychological Test Automated Battery (CANTAB) and hierarchical cluster analysis.

Methods: We searched for groups of distinct cognitive profiles in 35 relapsing-remitting MS outpatients and 32 healthy controls. All individuals participated in an automated assessment (CANTAB) and in a pencil and paper general neuropsychological evaluation.

Results: Hierarchical cluster analysis of the CANTAB results revealed two distinct groups of patients based mainly on the Simple Reaction Time (RTI) and on the Mean Latency of Rapid Visual Processing (RVP). The general neuropsychological assessment did not show any statistically significant differences between the cluster groups. Compared to the healthy control group, all MS outpatients had lower scores for RTI, RVP, paired associate learning, and delayed matching to sample. We also analyzed the associations between CANTAB results and age, education, sex, pharmacological treatment, physical activity, employment status, and the Expanded Disability Status Scale (EDSS). Although limited by the small number of observations, our findings suggest a weak correlation between performance on the CANTAB and age, education, and EDSS scores.

Conclusions: We suggest that the use of selected large-scale automated visuospatial tests from the CANTAB in combination with multivariate statistical analyses may reveal subtle and earlier changes in information processing speed and cognition. This may expand our ability to define the limits between normal and impaired cognition in patients with Multiple Sclerosis.

Keywords: Multiple sclerosis, Cognitive dysfunction, Reaction time, Rapid visual processing, Information processing speed, Working memory

* Correspondence: cwpdiniz@gmail.com
†Hideraldo Luis Souza Cabeça and Luciano Chaves Rocha contributed equally to this work.
2Laboratório de Investigações em Neurodegeneração e Infecção, Hospital Universitário João de Barros Barreto, Universidade Federal do Pará, Instituto de Ciências Biológicas, Belém, PA, Brazil
Full list of author information is available at the end of the article

Background

Multiple sclerosis (MS) is a chronic inflammatory disease of the central nervous system that is associated with motor, cognitive, and neuropsychiatric symptoms that appear independently as the disease progresses [1]. Despite the high prevalence rates of cognitive dysfunction in MS, for many decades physicians and patients focused on the overt motor dysfunctions that affect the activities of daily life. It was not until 1991 that cognitive dysfunction began to be assessed in terms of its frequency, patterns, and prediction [2]. Until this time, cognitive function was not routinely assessed in patients [3–5], and the implications of cognitive deficits on the quality of life of MS patients remained unknown [6]. The prevalence of cognitive decline showed that information processing, episodic memory, and, to a lesser extent, attention and executive functions, were about 43% to 70% lower than age, sex and years of schooling matched controls [7], suggesting that several brain regions are impaired in MS. Neuroimaging continues to confirm this, and is helping define the extent and localization of areas in the central nervous system that are impaired in MS. [8, 9]

It is essential to determine the limits between normal and subtle cognitive decline in order to develop and implement clinical interventions that target cognitive rehabilitation [4] in chronic neurodegenerative diseases, including MS. In a previous report, we compared the use of the Cambridge Neuropsychological Test Automated Battery (CANTAB) and language tests to detect subtle differences in cognitive performance in two age groups. To distinguish the limits between normal and abnormal cognitive decline as age progresses we suggested, as an alternative to language tests, large-scale application of automated visuospatial cognitive tests [10].

The CANTAB is a nonverbal visuospatial stimulus battery that uses touchscreen technology to obtain nonverbal responses from participants. This is in line with recent recommendations to use more precise automated neuropsychological tests in MS. [11] Both longitudinal and cross-sectional studies have shown that the CANTAB is particularly well suited for cognitive assessments of patients from various cultures as it involves minimal interference from the researcher or clinician during data acquisition [12].

In this study, we aimed to utilize the CANTAB with multivariate analysis to assess cognitive function in MS patients to investigate the performance limits in cognitively impaired and unimpaired subjects as compared to control groups. A few studies have used the CANTAB to measure cognitive decline in MS patients [13–18], but none have searched for subgroups of patients with different patterns of cognitive impairment using multivariate statistical procedures. We hypothesized that there may be distinct subgroups of MS patients based on cognitive decline and that hierarchical cluster analysis of CANTAB results may be able to detect such groups. We expect that an improved understanding of cognitive deficits in MS could help guide evidence-based cognitive rehabilitation programs, and the selection of therapy, based on the cognitive profiles of MS patients [19, 20].

Methods

This observational exploratory study investigated whether the CANTAB in combination with hierarchical cluster analysis could detect subtle cognitive declines in MS to classify MS patients according to their performance on selected CANTAB tests. All subjects provided informed written consent prior to their participation, in accordance with the Declaration of Helsinki, which was voluntary. Patient data were coded to preserve confidentiality. This study was approved by the local ethics committee (Comitê de Ética em Pesquisa do Hospital Universitário João de Barros Barreto, protocol number 2.160.639), and it followed the International Ethical Guidelines for Health-related Research involving Humans (CIOMS/WHO).

Subjects

Thirty-five outpatients diagnosed with relapsing-remitting MS subtype (revised McDonald criteria, 2010) [21] were invited to participate. MS patients from a demyelinating clinic of a tertiary hospital were invited to participate. The inclusion criteria limited the studied group to MS relapsing-remitting subtype patients (revised McDonald criteria, 2010), less than 60 years old age, visual acuity (20/20 in Snellen's test) and at least eight years of formal education. Patients with previous cranioencephalic trauma, stroke, dementia, or other neurological diseases including past or actual criteria for primary depression (DSM IV) were excluded.

Study design

All of the MS participants, who were in remission at the time of testing, and all of the control subjects met the inclusion criteria, participated in a standardized pencil and paper neuropsychological assessment as well as the CANTAB on a single day. The neuropsychological assessment results were subjected to an initial cluster analysis limited to multimodal variables, resulting in the formation of a selected multiple sclerosis group (MS group, with only MS patients), healthy control group (HC group, with only healthy control subjects) and Group 1 and Group 2 (where MS and HC appeared together in the same cluster). To investigate the influence of exercise and employee as significant variables that may change cognitive assessment results we defined as exercised individuals, those practicing exercise for at least six months, three times a week, and as employed subjects, those citizens that work in any job for, at least, six months.

Standard neuropsychological assessment

The standard pencil and paper neuropsychological assessment was adjusted for use in a Brazilian population, including the Mini-Mental State Examination, the Verbal Fluency test and the Word List Memory, Recall, and Recognition tests [22]. Trained investigators administered these tests in about 30–45 min in an environment that had adequate lighting and reduced noise conditions.

Automated neuropsychological assessment (the CANTAB)

The three cognitive domains explored by the CANTAB are working memory and planning; attention; and visuospatial memory. All the tests in the battery utilize touchscreen responses, which minimizes potential interference through verbal instruction. All participants were assessed individually. The assessment started with a motor screening task to introduce the CANTAB touchscreen basic procedure. This task gives a general idea of potential sensorimotor or other difficulties that could limit valid data collection. After they become familiar with the touchscreen procedure, each participant was assessed on the following tasks: Rapid Visual Information Processing (RVP), which measures sustained attention; Reaction Time (RTI), which reflects motor and mental response speeds as well as movement time, reaction time, response accuracy, and impulsivity; Paired Associate Learning (PAL), which assesses visual memory and new learning; Spatial Working Memory (SWM), which measures the retention and manipulation of visuospatial information; and Delayed Matching to Sample (DMS), which, through forced choice, assesses recognition memory of visual patterns and tests both simultaneous matching and short-term visual memory. All battery generally lasts between 30 and 60 min, depending on the subject's performance. Additional file 1: Table S1 describes the cognitive tests based on the CANTAB user manual. For further details of the neuropsychological test, please see: http://www.cambridgecognition.com/cantab/cognitive-tests/.

Data analysis

We analyzed all data using Biostat 5.3®, Statistica 7®, and Graphpad Prism® software. Continuous variables are represented as means and standard deviations, and p values lower than 0.05 were considered significant. The statistical tests for intergroup comparisons included Student's t test for normally distributed data or the Mann-Whitney test for non-parametric analysis. A correlation matrix was used to assess potential associations between variables inside or between groups. All quantitative variables were submitted to an initial cluster analysis (Ward's method, Euclidean distance). We applied this multivariate

statistical procedure to our sample of behavioral data to search for possible group of patients sharing similar performances. The classes suggested by cluster analysis were assessed by a forward stepwise discriminant function analysis. Discriminant function analysis classifies and predicts the probability of unknown individuals to be classified into a certain group indicating the variables that best contributed to group formation. It assumes that the sample is normally distributed and as such, uses these variables to determine whether groups differ about the mean of a variable. The purpose of the analysis is to learn how one can discriminate between potential groups of distinct cognitive performances, based on the scores of each individual test results. Hierarchical cluster analysis (Ward's method and Euclidian distances) used multimodal or at least bimodal distributions. We measured the relative contribution of each variable for cluster formation using discriminant analysis.

We also expressed the results as Z-scores which is the number of standard deviations from the mean a data point is, which allows to compare the results with a normal distribution.

Table 1 Descriptive demographic data for the Multiple Sclerosis (MS) and Healthy Control groups

	Multiple Sclerosis	Healthy Control
N	35	32
Age (years)	34.2 ± 10 (18–55)	32.03 ± 8.40
Education (years)	13.8 ± 3.5 (8–23)	14.70 ± 3.42
Expanded Disability Status Scale (EDSS) score	1.44 ± 1.4 (0–6)	–
Average duration of disease (years)	4.66 ± 4 (0.25–13.6)	–
Average acute exacerbations (n)	1.82 ± 0.5 (1–3)	–
SEX		
Men (n)	6 (17%)	9 (28%)
Women (n)	29 (83%)	23 (72%)
Pharmacologic treatment		
Interferon-β 1a (n)	16 (45.7%)	–
Interferon-β 1b (n)	8 (22.85%)	–
Glatiramer acetate (n)	3 (8.6%)	–
Natalizumabe (n)	2 (5.7%)	–
None (n)	6 (17.15%)	32 (100%)
Physical activity		
Exercised (n)	9 (25.7%)	12 (37.5%)
Sedentary (n)	26 (74.3%)	20 (62.5%)
Employment status		
Yes (n)	28 (80%)	32 (100%)
No (n)	7 (20%)	0 (0%)

Results

Multiple sclerosis patients profile

The mean age of MS patients was 34.2 ± 10 years (range: 18–55) with mean education years of 13.8 ± 3.5 years (range: 8–23), mean Expanded Disability Status Scale (EDSS) score of 1.44 ± 1.4 (median: 1; range: 0–6), average duration of disease of 4.66 ± 4 years (range: 0.25–13.6) and average acute exacerbations of 1.82 ± 0.5 times (range: 1–3). Thus, this MS group consists of mostly patients in the early years of their disease and disability.

In this study cohort, which comprised an MS group (n = 35) and a healthy control (HC) group (n = 32), most of the participants were female. In the MS group, subcutaneous (44 μg) or intramuscular interferon β-1a was the main disease-modifying drug therapy. Others included subcutaneous interferon β-1b, subcutaneous

glatiramer acetate (20 mg), intravenous Natalizumab and none. There were no significant intergroup differences in age and education ($p > 0.05$, Student's t test).

Table 1 shows the descriptive demographic data as absolute values and percentages, and Table 2 shows the descriptive performance data as means and standard deviations and effect sizes (Cohen's d, Hedges' g and Glass' delta for variables with high variance).

Cognitive performance in the MS and HC groups

The MS and HC groups had significantly different mean scores on CANTAB tests, with the Spatial Working Memory (SWM) being the exception. Table 2 and Fig. 1 show that the MS group had lower average scores than the HC group. Table 2 also shows the Effects' sizes (Cohen's d, Hegdes' g and Glass' Δ) of intergroup

Table 2 Performances of Multiple Sclerosis (MS) and Healthy Control groups and intergroup effects' sizes (Cohen's d, Hedge's G and Glass' Δ for high variances values). Values are shown as mean and standard deviation. Effects' sizes with significant T Student's Test or Mann-Whitney Test ($p < 0.05$) are identified with *

	Multiple Sclerosis	Healthy Control	Cohen's D	Hedge's G	Glass' Δ
Spatial Working Memory (SWM)					
Strategy (STG)	38.28 ± 3.63	35.71 ± 6.95	0.487*	0.494*	0.388*
Total Errors (TE)	49.11 ± 20.22	41.56 ± 23.55	0.325	0.327	0.296
Rapid Visual Processing (RVP)					
A'	0.84 ± 0.06	0.88 ± 0.04	0.766*	0.759*	1.012*
Probability of Hit (PH)	0.49 ± 0.16	0.57 ± 0.16	0.401	0.409	0.433
Mean Latency (ML)	567.67 ± 167.17	446.19 ± 72.97	1.115*	1.099*	1.790*
Paired Associate Learning (PAL)					
First Trial Memory Score (FTMS)	11.8 ± 4.43	13.18 ± 3.02	4.623	0.396	0.517
Mean Trials to Success (MTS)	3.17 ± 1.68	2.07 ± 0.76	0.870*	0.857*	1.486*
Total Errors Adjusted (TEA)	37.71 ± 35.62	17.84 ± 14.28	0.776*	0.763*	1.597*
Reaction Time (RTI)					
5-Choice Accuracy Score (5CAS)	14.71 ± 0.62	14.93 ± 0.24	0.483	0.475	0.932
5-Choice Movement Time (5CMT)	675.92 ± 182.6 ms	598.55 ± 131.31 ms	0.655	0.649	0.862
5-Choice Reaction Time (5CRT)	446.31 ± 94.19 ms	403.93 ± 76.61 ms	0.424	0.422	0.474
Simple Accuracy Score (SAS)	14.54 ± 0.95	14.81 ± 0.47	0.223*	0.223*	0.221*
Simple Movement Time (SMT)	688.01 ± 198.74 ms	663.33 ± 220.78 ms	0.267	0.267	0.258
Simple Reaction Time (SRT)	425.19 ± 87.09 ms	377.23 ± 76.04 ms	0.657*	0.654*	0.699*
Delayed Matched to Sample (DMS)					
Total Correct (TC)	16.31 ± 2.98	17.96 ± 1.46	0.660*	0.650*	1.141*
Mini-Mental State Examination (MMSE)	28.17 ± 2.35	29.25 ± 0.85	0.611	0.600	1.270
Verbal fluency 1 (ANIMALS)	15.65 ± 5.72	18.61 ± 3.68	0.615*	0.610*	0.804*
Verbal fluency 2 (FRUITS)	14.54 ± 4.06	16.74 ± 3.24	0.599*	0.596*	0.679*
Verbal fluency 3 (A)	10.94 ± 4.89	12.96 ± 4.33	0.437*	0.436*	0.466*
Verbal fluency 4 (F)	12.37 ± 4.9	16.09 ± 3.76	0.852*	0.847*	0.989*
Word list Memory task	20.2 ± 3.27	20.51 ± 3.43	0.092	0.093	0.090
Word list recall	6.85 ± 1.73	7.16 ± 1.63	0.184	0.184	0.190
Word list recognition	9.12 ± 1.07	9.51 ± 0.99	0.378	0.378	0.394

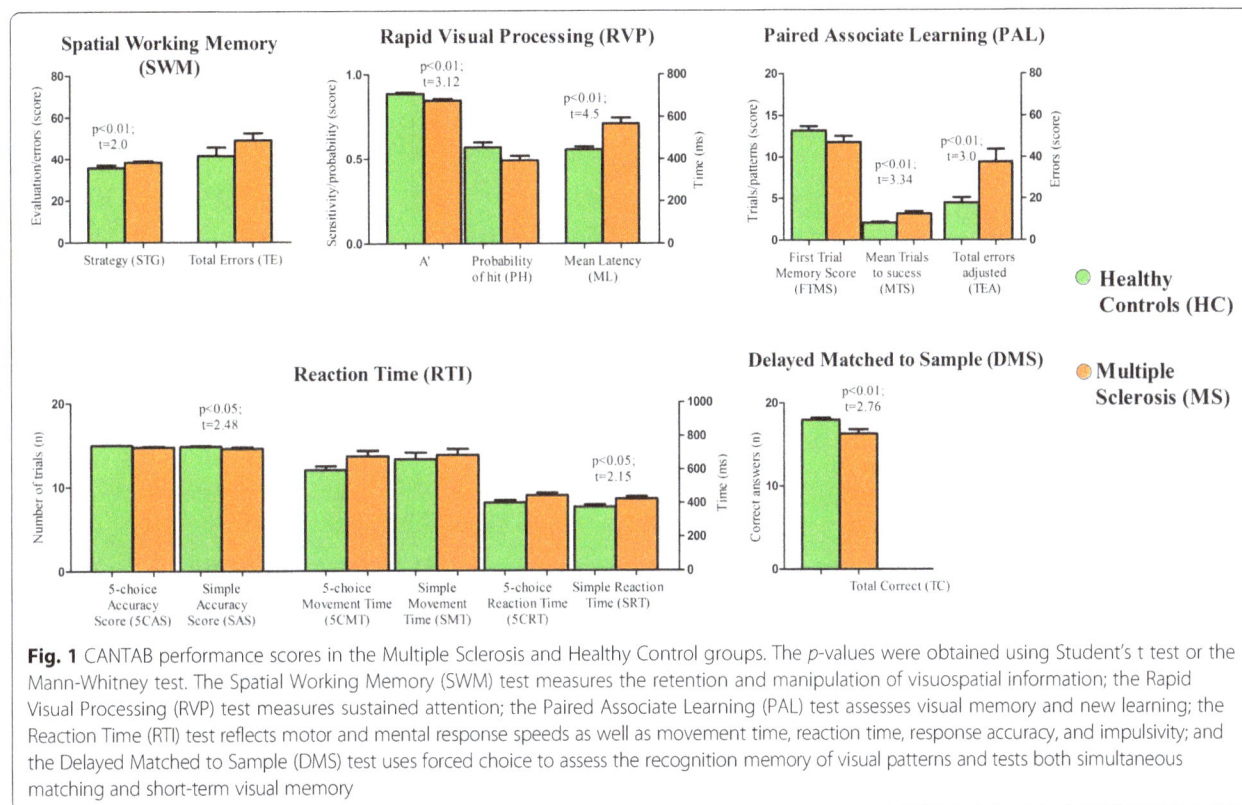

Fig. 1 CANTAB performance scores in the Multiple Sclerosis and Healthy Control groups. The *p*-values were obtained using Student's t test or the Mann-Whitney test. The Spatial Working Memory (SWM) test measures the retention and manipulation of visuospatial information; the Rapid Visual Processing (RVP) test measures sustained attention; the Paired Associate Learning (PAL) test assesses visual memory and new learning; the Reaction Time (RTI) test reflects motor and mental response speeds as well as movement time, reaction time, response accuracy, and impulsivity; and the Delayed Matched to Sample (DMS) test uses forced choice to assess the recognition memory of visual patterns and tests both simultaneous matching and short-term visual memory

disparities by Student's t test and Mann-Whitney test to quantify these performance differences. These findings reflect the impairment of a variety of cognitive domains.

Age, education, pharmacological treatment, physical activity, sex, and employment status all influenced the results of intergroup analysis

Table 3 shows descriptive data (score means and correspondent standard deviations) of all neuropsychological tests scores of Groups 1 and 2. There were, respectively, significant positive and negative correlations between age, education, and EDSS and the CANTAB tests, with r values ranging from -0.478 to 0.532. Age and education correlated significantly with Reaction Time (RTI), Paired Associate Learning (PAL), and Delayed Matched to Sample tests. Yet, education alone correlated with all CANTAB tests, including Rapid Visual Processing (RVP) and EDSS score correlated with SWM and DMS tests scores. Table 4 summarizes all the correlations results reported with *p*-values and correlation coefficients.

Notably, unemployed subjects had lower scores for SWM, A' (RVP), and PH (one-way ANOVA; *p* < 0.05, *p* < 0.01, and *p* < 0.01, respectively). Subjects who were being treated with interferon β-1a and β-1b based therapy (*n* = 24) did not impact on outcome compared to subjects who were being treated with other therapy or who

were not being treated with any reported medication (*n* = 11; one-way ANOVA, *p* > 0.05).

Multivariate analysis: Multimodal index, hierarchical cluster analysis, and discriminant analysis

Cluster analyses were performed using either a combination of general neuropsychological assessment data and CANTAB test results or using CANTAB results alone. Only bimodal or multimodal variables (Multimodal index > 0.5) were selected for cluster analysis (see Schweitzer and Renehan [23] for details). Thus, the following variables were used for the general hierarchical cluster analysis: mean latency (ML), mean trials to success (MTS), total errors adjusted (TEA), 5-choice accuracy score (5CAS), 5-choice reaction time (5CRT), simple accuracy score (SAS), and simple reaction time (SRT) from the CANTAB; the Mini-Mental State Examination (MMSE); and the Word List Recognition (WLR). In addition, we performed a separate cluster analysis that was limited to CANTAB variables. The results of the cluster analyses were similar when we used the dataset of multimodal variables of the general neuropsychological assessment + CANTAB and when we used the dataset that was limited to CANTAB variables. However, almost only CANTAB variables contributed to cluster formation in the general assessment, so we decided to limit the subsequent

Table 3 Test performance descriptive data, represented as means and standard deviations for Group 1 and Group 2. Values are shown as mean and standard deviation

	GROUP 1 (MEAN ± SD, N = 44)	GROUP 2 (MEAN ± SD, N = 23)
Spatial Working Memory (SWM)		
Strategy (STG)	36.06 ± 5.9	38.95 ± 4.43
Total Errors (TE)	38.9 ± 21.37	58.13 ± 17.61
Rapid Visual Procesing (RVP)		
A'	0.88 ± 0.04	0.82 ± 0.06
Probability of Hit (PH)	0.56 ± 0.16	0.46 ± 0.15
Mean Latency (ML)	442.03 ± 71.71	639 ± 158.80
Paired Associate Learning (PAL)		
First Trial Memory Score (FTMS)	13.77 ± 3,14	9.95 ± 3.91
Mean Trials to Success (MTS)	2.06 ± 0.82	3.77 ± 1.68
Total Errors (TEA)	17.47 ± 15.08	48.78 ± 37.83
Reaction Time (RTI)		
5-choice Accuracy Score (5CAS)	584.12 ± 115.41	746.96 ± 197.67
5-choice Movement Time (5CMT)	584.13 ± 115.42 ms	750.6 ± 194 ms
5-choice Reaction Time (5CRT)	392.37 ± 54.5 ms	490.54 ± 104.51 ms
Simple Accuracy Score (SAS)	14.8 ± 0.51	14.43 ± 1.08
Simple Movement Time (SMT)	599.33 ± 161.57 ms	823.33 ± 211.45 ms
Simple Reaction Time (SRT)	359.91 ± 43.02 ms	483.32 ± 86.85 ms
Delayed Matched to Sample (DMS)		
Total Correct (TC)	18.25 ± 1.33	14.91 ± 2.79
Mini-Mental State Examination (MMSE)	28.04 ± 4.01	27.65 ± 2.7
Verbal fluency 1 (ANIMALS)	18.81 ± 4.15	13.73 ± 5.02
Verbal fluency 2 (FRUITS)	16.67 ± 3.46	13.52 ± 3.71
Verbal fluency 3 (A)	13.04 ± 4.59	9.74 ± 4.23
Verbal fluency 4 (F)	15.67 ± 4.03	11.21 ± 4.7
Word list memory task	20.65 ± 3.75	19.78 ± 2.31
Word list recall	7.07 ± 1.65	6.87 ± 1.76
Word list recognition	9.39 ± 0.95	9.15 ± 1.21

analysis to the CANTAB dataset. This analysis distinguished two groups based on test results: Group 1, which included control subjects and a subset of MS patients, and Group 2, which comprised mostly of MS patients and a few control subjects (Figs. 2 and 3). Figure 3 exhibits X-Y plot of the discriminant analysis results related to the data set of Fig. 2.

Discriminant analysis of the dataset in Fig. 2 revealed that the RTI test was the variable that contributed most to cluster formation, showing that RTI could easily differentiate the cognitive status of MS patients. In addition, the ML of the RVP test, which is a reaction time measurement based on the median latency response after recognition of a sequence of visual stimuli, could also discriminate between Groups 1 and 2. This confirmed that the most significant change in these MS patients was a reduction in information processing speed

(IPS). Although it had a more limited influence, Total Errors (adjusted) from PAL test also discriminated between Groups 1 and 2 (please see the table under the dendrogram in Fig. 2, as well as Fig. 3 for details). Pharmacological treatment, physical activity, employment status, and sex did not map to the Group 1 and Group 2 distribution patterns in.

Yet, we also utilized cluster analysis without RVP and RTI tests (Fig. 4) and with only MMSE and language tests (Fig. 5), resulting in group formation with lower Euclidean distances.

Table 5 shows quantitative summary of z-score cognitive deficits based on means of Healthy Control (HC) group. Fig. 6 shows graphs that illustrate the differences and similarities between Group 1 and Group 2. Group 2, but not Group 1 showed significantly lower performance than the HC Group. The SWM scores of the MS Group

Table 4 Correlation Matrix (Spearman Rank Order Correlations) with Age, Education, EDSS score and CANTAB tests' measures. Correlations in bold are statistically significant ($p < 0.05$) with r values shown ranging from −0.884 to 0.959. Note that Age, Education and EDSS score had only mild to moderate correlations with CANTAB tests' measures (r values ranging from -0.478 to 0.532). Abbreviations utilized from the List of Abbreviations in this paper

	AGE	ED	EDSS	STG	TE	A'	PH	ML	FTMS	MTS	TEA	FCAS	5CMT	5CRT	SAS	SMT	SRT	TC
AGE	1.000	−0.034	0.271	0.333	0.429	−0.137	−0.074	−0.144	−0.478	0.502	0.502	−0.079	0.207	0.066	−0.084	0.383	0.169	−0.389
ED	−0.034	1.000	−0.166	−0.189	−0.392	0.532	0.456	0.225	0.304	−0.267	−0.267	0.276	−0.197	−0.192	0.194	−0.297	−0.353	0.367
EDSS	0.271	−0.166	1.000	0.428	0.384	−0.189	−0.254	−0.254	−0.191	0.301	0.241	0.133	0.302	0.080	−0.123	0.151	0.166	−0.396
STG	0.333	−0.189	0.428	1.000	0.750	−0.191	−0.098	−0.192	−0.280	0.266	0.307	−0.014	0.321	0.105	−0.157	0.447	0.263	−0.311
TE	0.429	−0.392	0.384	0.750	1.000	−0.278	−0.135	−0.238	−0.422	0.392	0.401	−0.219	0.237	0.097	−0.184	0.401	0.260	−0.308
A'	−0.137	0.532	−0.189	−0.191	−0.278	1.000	0.891	0.407	0.393	−0.427	−0.439	0.324	−0.168	−0.135	0.397	−0.302	−0.299	0.550
PH	−0.074	0.456	−0.254	−0.098	−0.135	0.891	1.000	0.385	0.243	−0.259	−0.275	0.276	−0.111	−0.126	0.281	−0.212	−0.233	0.406
ML	−0.144	0.225	−0.254	−0.192	−0.238	0.407	0.385	1.000	0.165	−0.281	−0.246	0.292	−0.200	−0.259	0.251	−0.093	−0.380	0.314
FTMS	−0.478	0.304	−0.191	−0.280	−0.422	0.393	0.243	0.165	1.000	−0.850	−0.884	0.305	−0.205	−0.005	0.187	−0.378	−0.182	0.489
MTS	0.502	−0.267	0.301	0.266	0.392	−0.427	−0.259	−0.281	−0.850	1.000	0.959	−0.242	0.216	−0.005	−0.261	0.348	0.152	−0.546
TEA	0.502	−0.267	0.241	0.307	0.401	−0.439	−0.275	−0.246	−0.884	0.959	1.000	−0.241	0.276	−0.020	−0.243	0.407	0.136	−0.540
FCAS	−0.079	0.276	0.133	−0.014	−0.219	0.324	0.276	0.292	0.305	−0.242	−0.241	1.000	−0.149	−0.308	0.307	−0.124	−0.289	0.222
5CMT	0.207	−0.197	0.302	0.321	0.237	−0.168	−0.111	−0.200	−0.205	0.216	0.276	−0.149	1.000	0.270	−0.221	0.776	0.294	−0.303
5CRT	0.066	−0.192	0.080	0.105	0.097	−0.135	−0.126	−0.259	−0.005	−0.005	−0.020	−0.308	0.270	1.000	−0.257	0.235	0.795	−0.414
SAS	−0.084	0.194	−0.123	−0.157	−0.184	0.397	0.281	0.251	0.187	−0.261	−0.243	0.307	−0.221	−0.257	1.000	−0.098	−0.116	0.297
SMT	0.383	−0.297	0.151	0.447	0.401	−0.302	−0.212	−0.093	−0.378	0.348	0.407	−0.124	0.776	0.235	−0.098	1.000	0.421	−0.400
SRT	0.169	−0.353	0.166	0.263	0.260	−0.299	−0.233	−0.380	−0.182	0.152	0.136	−0.289	0.294	0.795	−0.116	0.421	1.000	−0.506
TC	−0.389	0.367	−0.396	−0.311	−0.308	0.550	0.406	0.314	0.489	−0.546	−0.540	0.222	−0.303	−0.414	0.297	−0.400	−0.506	1.000

Tree Diagram for 67 Cases (All subjects - CANTAB battery)

Ward's method

Euclidean distances

	Wilks' Lambda	Partial Lambda	F-remove (1,62)	p-level	Toler.	1-Toler. (R-Sqr.)
Simple Reaction Time (RTI)	0.5501652	0.3570826	111.6293	0.000000	0.6285781	0.3714219
Mean Latency (RVP)	0.3184666	0.6168761	38.50642	0.000000	0.6307721	0.3692279
Total Errors Adjusted (PAL)	0.2107944	0.9319717	4.525628	0.037376	0.7225643	0.2774357
5-choice Accuracy Score (RTI)	0.205059	0.9580385	2.715563	0.104433	0.8662129	0.1337871

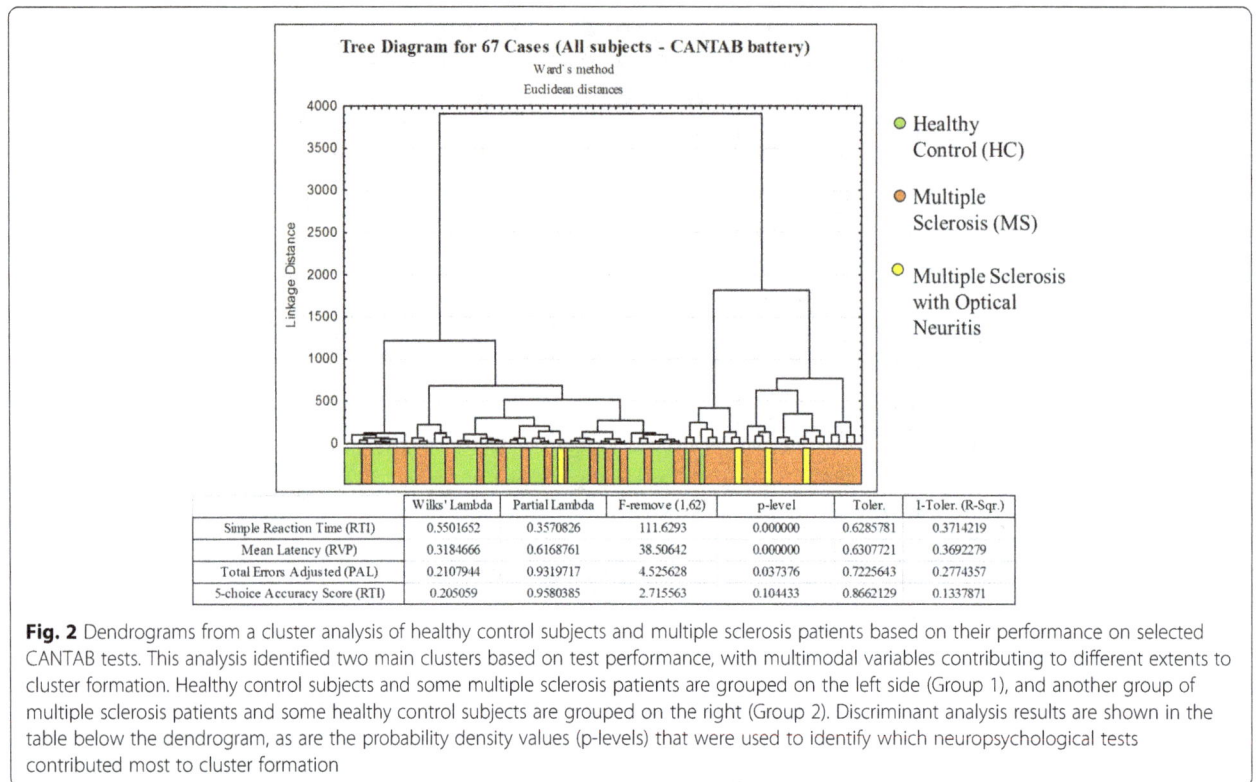

Fig. 2 Dendrograms from a cluster analysis of healthy control subjects and multiple sclerosis patients based on their performance on selected CANTAB tests. This analysis identified two main clusters based on test performance, with multimodal variables contributing to different extents to cluster formation. Healthy control subjects and some multiple sclerosis patients are grouped on the left side (Group 1), and another group of multiple sclerosis patients and some healthy control subjects are grouped on the right (Group 2). Discriminant analysis results are shown in the table below the dendrogram, as are the probability density values (p-levels) that were used to identify which neuropsychological tests contributed most to cluster formation

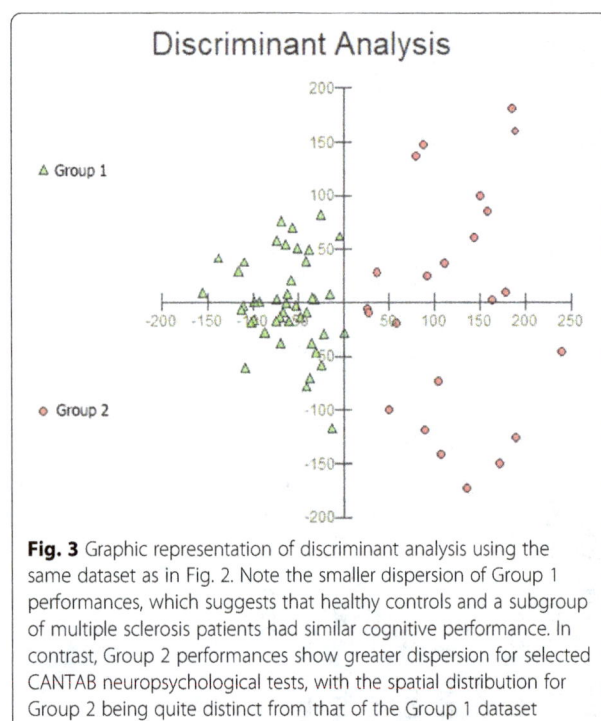

Fig. 3 Graphic representation of discriminant analysis using the same dataset as in Fig. 2. Note the smaller dispersion of Group 1 performances, which suggests that healthy controls and a subgroup of multiple sclerosis patients had similar cognitive performance. In contrast, Group 2 performances show greater dispersion for selected CANTAB neuropsychological tests, with the spatial distribution for Group 2 being quite distinct from that of the Group 1 dataset

were not significantly different than those of the HC Group; however, Group 2 showed lower scores than Group 1, which suggests that cluster analysis of the Groups that is based on CANTAB results of multimodal variables could detect subtle cognitive deficits that were previously undetectable using pencil and paper general neuropsychological assessment.

Although only total errors (TE; SWM), 5-choice reaction time (5CRT; RTI), simple movement time (SMT; RTI), simple reaction time (SRT; RTI), and total correct (TC; DMS) were significantly different with each other (Student's t test; $p < 0.05$), Group 2 and MS groups had lower performance than Group 1 on the majority of CANTAB tests, as shown by the z-scores (Fig. 7). In addition, almost all MS subjects (97.1%) had, at least, z-score subtle cognitive deficits based on Healthy Control (HC) means (standard deviation ≥ 0.5, Table 5).

Supplementary clinical data is shown in Additional file 2: Table S2. As observed, only 4 patients showed optical neuritis one of which in Group 1 and 3 in Group 2 suggesting that optical neuritis cannot explain lower scores in CANTAB cognitive tests of MS group.

Discussion

This study investigated the extent to which general neuropsychological pencil and paper tests and CANTAB tests, either alone or in combination, can detect subtle

Tree Diagram for 67 Cases (All subjects - CANTAB battery without RVP and RTI tests)

Ward's method
Euclidean distances

	Wilks' Lambda	Partial Lambda	F-remove (1,62)	p-level	Toler.	1-Toler. (R-Sqr.)
Mean Trials to Success (MTS)	1	0.435213	84.35233	0	1	0

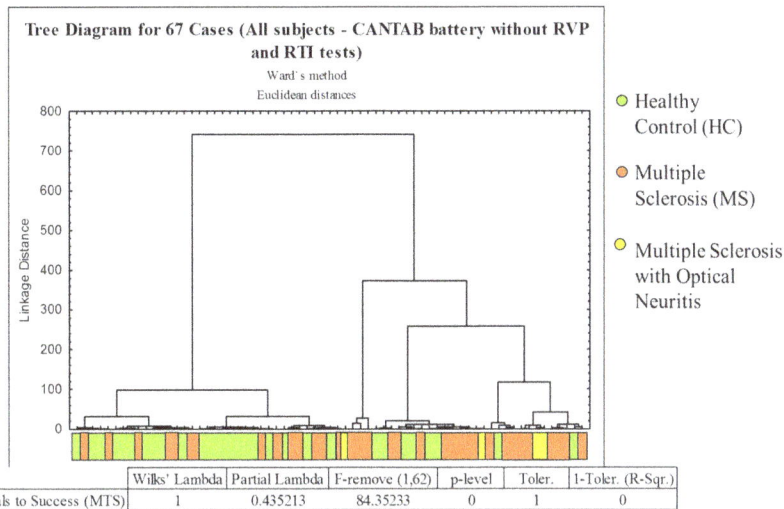

Coment: Eventhough similar patterns were present when comparing to the cluster analysis with all CANTAB battery, the euclidean distance in this figure (near 750) contrasts with the one previously found (near 4000). Optical neuritis were in concordance with previous analysis, as it can be perceived in yellow collors. Also, two MS subjects moved from group 2 to group 1 and 7 HC subjects moved from group 1 to group 2. In this image, we did not utilize memory tests and verbal fluency scores due to the lack of eligibility criterea (multimodal index). Finally, Mean Trials to Success (MTS) and Total Errors Adjusted (TEA) were the only eligible variables in this analysis and MTS is the isolated discriminant one.

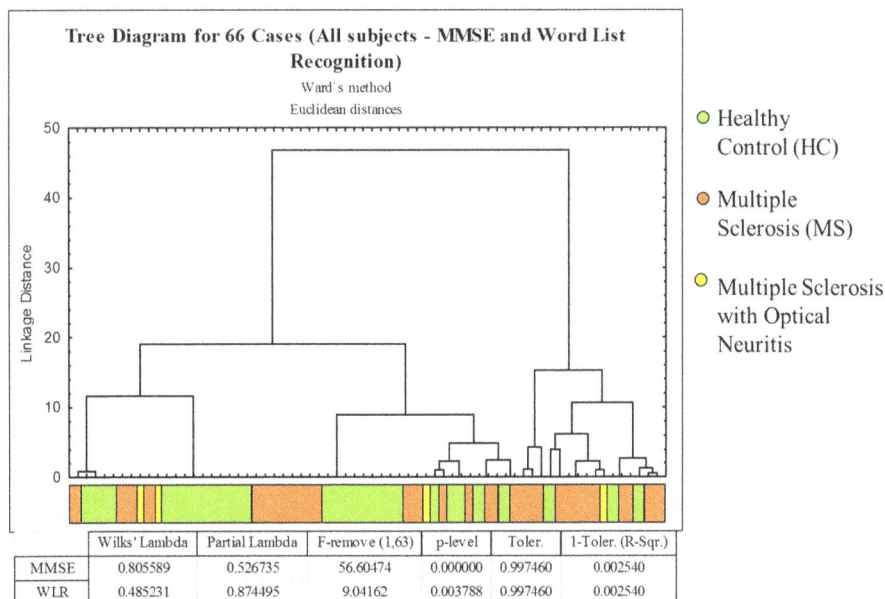

Fig. 4 Dendrograms from a cluster analysis of healthy control subjects and multiple sclerosis patients based on their performance on selected CANTAB tests without Rapid Visual Processing (RVP) and Reaction Time (RTI) scores. Even though similar patterns were present when comparing to the cluster analysis with all CANTAB battery, the Euclidean distance in this figure (near 750) contrasts with the one previously found (near 4000). Optical neuritis were in concordance with previous analysis, as it can be perceived in yellow colors. Also, two MS subjects moved from group 2 to group 1 and 7 HC subjects moved from group 1 to group 2. In this image, we did not utilize memory tests and verbal fluency scores due to the lack of eligibility criteria (multimodal index). Finally, Mean Trials to Success (MTS) and Total Errors Adjusted (TEA) were the only eligible variables in this analysis and MTS is the isolated discriminant one

Tree Diagram for 66 Cases (All subjects - MMSE and Word List Recognition)

Ward's method
Euclidean distances

	Wilks' Lambda	Partial Lambda	F-remove (1,63)	p-level	Toler.	1-Toler. (R-Sqr.)
MMSE	0.805589	0.526735	56.60474	0.000000	0.997460	0.002540
WLR	0.485231	0.874495	9.04162	0.003788	0.997460	0.002540

Fig. 5 Dendrograms from a cluster analysis of healthy control subjects and multiple sclerosis patients based on their performance on Mini-Mental State Examination (MMSE) and Word List Recognition (WLR). The Euclidean distance in this figure (near 50) highly contrasts with the analysis with only CANTAB battery (near 4000). Three subjects with optical neuritis move from group 2 to group 1. Some MS patients in group 2 of the previous analysis (CANTAB) migrated to group 1 in this analysis, diminishing the size of group 2. Finally, Mini-Mental State Examination (MMSE) and Word List Recognition (WRL) were the only analyzed variables and MMSE is the one that contributes most to group differentiation

Table 5 Quantitative summary of Multiple Sclerosis patients z-score cognitive deficits based on means of Healthy Control (HC) group performance. All variables showed statistical intergroup difference (T test or Mann Whitney test) between Multiple Sclerosis (MS) and Healthy Control (HC) groups. Variables with significant outcomes in discriminant analysis are identified with (*). In addition, tests' measures of Information Processing Speed (IPS) are marked with blue color and memory tests' scores, in general, are marked with orange color. Note that almost all subjects showed, at least, subtle cognitive deficits (91.4%) in information processing speed, and most of them showed, at least, subtle cognitive deficit (71.4%) in memory. Only one subject did not present any cognitive deficit based on z-scores. Abbreviations utilized from the List of Abbreviations in this paper

Analyzed Measures	Z-score Deficits	N (%)
All Measures	≥0.5	34 (97.1%)
	≥1.0	30 (85.7%)
	≥1.5	23 (65.7%)
Simple Reaction Time (SRT, RTI test)*	≥0.5	19 (54.3%)
	≥1.0	8 (22.8%)
	≥1.5	7 (20%)
Mean Latency (ML, RVP test)*	≥0.5	22 (62.9%)
	≥1.0	20 (57.1%)
	≥1.5	14 (40%)
Total Errors Adjusted (TEA, PAL test)*	≥0.5	21 (60%)
	≥1.0	14 (40%)
	≥1.5	11 (31.4%)
A' (RVP)	≥0.5	22 (62.8%)
	≥1.0	15 (42.8%)
	≥1.5	11 (31.4%)
Mean Trials to Success (MTS, PAL test)	≥0.5	18 (51.4%)
	≥1.0	16 (45.7%)
	≥1.5	13 (37.1%)
Simple Accuracy Score (SAS, RTI test)	≥0.5	11 (31.4%)
	≥1.0	11 (31.4%)
	≥1.5	11 (31.4%)
Total Correct (TC, DMS test)	≥0.5	19 (54.3%
	≥1.0	15 (42.9%)
	≥1.5	12 (34.3%)
Information Processing Speed (IPS)	≥0.5	32 (91.4%)
	≥1.0	28 (80%)
	≥1.5	22 (62.8%)
Memory (General)	≥0.5	25 (71.4%)
	≥1.0	20 (57.1%)
	≥1.5	16 (42.8%)

cognitive deficits in MS patients early in the course of their disease. Hierarchical cluster and discriminant analyses revealed that CANTAB tests could better distinguish between the cognitive performance of MS Groups than the general neuropsychological assessment. Although the present study sample is small, and the results may not be generalizable, this exploratory study strongly suggests that CANTAB test results may improve the signal-to-noise ratio and thereby distinguish the performance of subgroups of MS patients better than general paper and pencil neuropsychological tests. Thus, we suggest that the use of large-scale automated visuospatial tests to assess the information processing speed, learning, and memory on CANTAB tests may help discriminate between normal and impaired cognitive performance in MS patients.

Impairment in information processing speed (IPS) is the most common cognitive dysfunction in MS patients [7]. This impairment is associated with unemployment [24, 25], which can cause additional suffering and worse quality of life, as it affects self-esteem and overall mental and physical health and can lead to depression and somatization [26]. Neuropsychological tests, with cluster analysis, have previously been used to demonstrate in a large group of subjects that IPS and memory deficits can be used to differentiate between MS patients with versus without cognitive impairments, highlighting the central role of IPS in cognitive impairment [27]. However, the study employed individuals with a higher mean EDSS and the age range included many older patients. Furthermore, cluster analysis of event-related potentials from EEG signals and behavioral responses [28, 29] found that IPS is an early and important marker of cognitive dysfunction in MS. In this context, the Brief International Cognitive Assessment for Multiple Sclerosis (BICAMS) [30] brought together cognitive tests with distinct domains with the Symbol Digit Modalities Test (SDMT) for assessing IPS impairment, as it is sensitive to cognitive changes, correlates with brain MRI parameters, and is associated with employment status.

The Minimal Assessment of Cognitive Function in MS (MACFIMS), a 90-min overall cognitive assessment, covers more cognitive domains that are affected in MS than does the BICAMS assessment [31], but it has limited scale measurements compared to the CANTAB tests, which measure reaction times in milliseconds. However, different from BICAMS, MACFIMS or other cognitive assessments, CANTAB battery lacks validation in MS and, also, as a limitation of this study, were not compared to such validated assessments in MS to identify similar or more accurate outcomes.

Thus, in the present report, we suggest that the use of additional automated cognitive assessment tools from the CANTAB may detect subtle early cognitive dysfunction. This will help researchers develop earlier evidence-based interventions programs for cognitive rehabilitation.

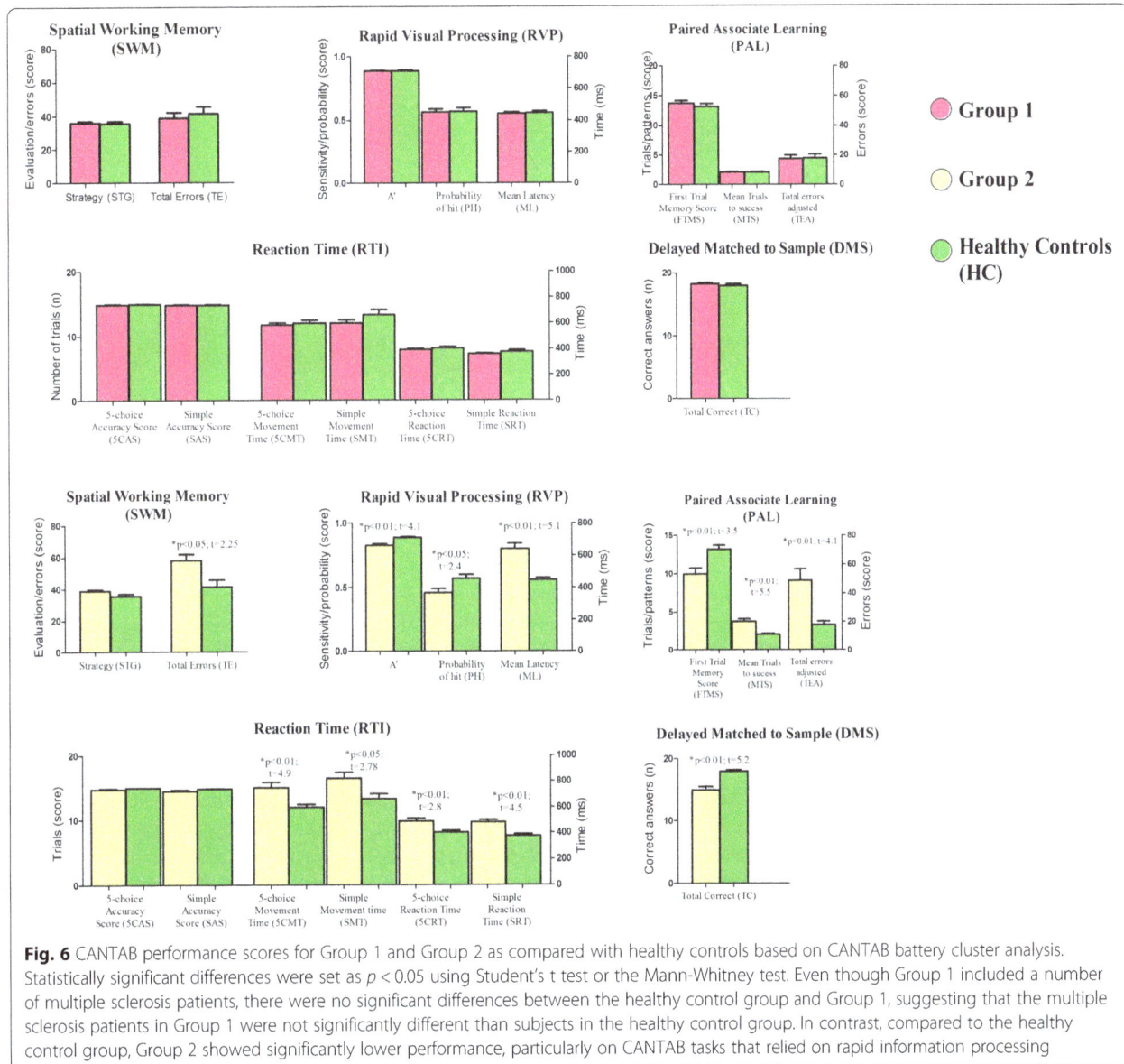

Fig. 6 CANTAB performance scores for Group 1 and Group 2 as compared with healthy controls based on CANTAB battery cluster analysis. Statistically significant differences were set as *p* < 0.05 using Student's t test or the Mann-Whitney test. Even though Group 1 included a number of multiple sclerosis patients, there were no significant differences between the healthy control group and Group 1, suggesting that the multiple sclerosis patients in Group 1 were not significantly different than subjects in the healthy control group. In contrast, compared to the healthy control group, Group 2 showed significantly lower performance, particularly on CANTAB tasks that relied on rapid information processing

To our knowledge, this is the first study to use hierarchical cluster analysis of multimodal CANTAB variables in a clinical study of cognitive dysfunction in MS patients. Consistent with previous studies, RTI measures, which reflect IPS, were the main variables in discriminant analysis, demonstrating the ability of this test to classify cognitive decline using hierarchical cluster analysis. In accordance with previous reports [32–35], learning and memory were less affected than IPS in MS patients. Thus, we suggest that PAL, DMS, and SWM test scores contribute less to cluster formation because the impact of reduced IPS is greater than the impact of impairments in learning and memory per se. Indeed, RTI and RVP contributed the most to cluster formation. We found significant differences in SWM scores in Group 1 versus Group 2, but not in the MS Group

versus the HC Group. This is consistent with a previous report [35] and suggests that the CANTAB is a good choice for assessing executive function in MS.

Executive function impairment has been associated with higher EDSS score. Since the mean EDSS of the MS group utilized in this study was quite low (mean EDSS: 1.44 ± 45), we might have expected a less pronounced cognitive domain in the MS cognitive dysfunction of this sample comparing to other MS populations [36]. However, the significant impairment in RVP and RTI measures scores in low EDSS scores subjects, as presented in this study, shows not only that there is early cognitive impairment in the least disabled MS patients, but our study also reveals the power of the CANTAB assessment to detect this early impairment. In a recent report [36], CANTAB utilization without RTI or RVP tests

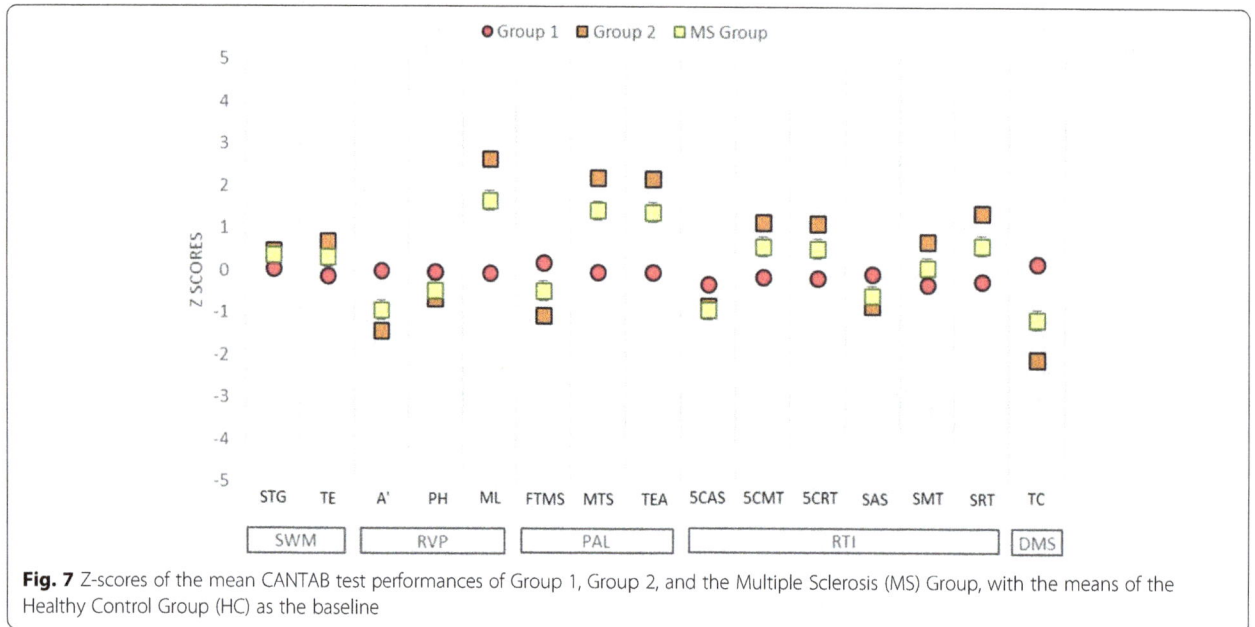

Fig. 7 Z-scores of the mean CANTAB test performances of Group 1, Group 2, and the Multiple Sclerosis (MS) Group, with the means of the Healthy Control Group (HC) as the baseline

in MS subjects displayed IPS and attention as the least prevalent cognitive domain impaired in MS, which contrasts with our findings regarding the centrality of IPS impairment in MS cognitive dysfunction, but also suggests that the utilization of IPS-sensitive CANTAB tests are, indeed, necessary.

The first studies that utilized the CANTAB in MS used the SWM and Spatial Span tests to investigate the executive function of patients with frontal lobe lesions [15]; to study deficits after acute relapse [14]; to correlate scores with magnetic resonance spectroscopy imaging [16]; and to compare cognitive dysfunction in MS subtypes [37]. Other studies investigated different aspects of MS cognition, such as memory [17] and decision making [18].

The first report of the use of the CANTAB in MS in a Brazilian population was published in 2011 [38]. That report described MS patients and patients with Duchenne muscular dystrophy as well as children and adult controls moving towards CANTAB norms in Brazil. The present study assessed cognitive dysfunction in MS patients living in the North Region of Brazil and used cluster analysis to differentiate patterns. Interestingly, patients with a benign MS subtype often perform worse on cognitive assessment tests and display a more heterogeneous pattern of cognitive dysfunction, suggesting silent deterioration of cognitive function [28, 29]. Our analysis grouped some healthy subjects with some MS patients because the MS group included both cognitively impaired and unimpaired patients, which is consistent with a previous study [28].

It is important to note that disease-modifying therapies such as interferon β-1a [39], interferon β-1b [40],

and natalizumab [41] can help preserve cognitive function in MS patients. These therapies play important roles in stabilizing or delaying cognitive dysfunction in relapsing-remitting MS. Thus, patients who do not receive these therapies could experience more severe cognitive deterioration, as observed in patients with non-cognitive impaired MS patients [29]. Compared to patients taking other disease-modifying drugs or taking no drugs, patients treated with interferon-based therapy showed no statistically significant differences in cognitive performance in this study.

Finally, despite the limited associations between education and test performance in our sample, formal education was associated previously with cognitive reserve in MS patients [42], with highly educated subjects showing better performance. Thus, it is important to include multisensory and cognitive stimulation in MS clinical intervention programs.

Conclusions

Our results suggest that the use of large-scale automated visuospatial tests, such as the CANTAB could improve the signal-to-noise ratio and reveal subtle and earlier changes in information processing speed (RTI and RVP) and learning and memory (PAL and DMS) in MS patients. This could help distinguish between normal and pathological decline in MS and contribute to the development of evidence-based individualized rehabilitation programs. Notably, most studies of CANTAB tests of MS patients have been conducted in the United Kingdom, while other countries lack normative data for CANTAB tests in MS patients. Thus, we further suggest that large-scale studies are needed in Brazil to determine whether the CANTAB can, in fact, be used as a diagnostic tool to detect cognitive impairment in MS.

Abbreviations

5CAS: 5-choice accuracy score; 5CRT: 5-choice reaction time; CANTAB: Cambridge neuropsychological test automated battery; DMS: Delayed matching to sample; EDSS: Expanded disability status scale; HC: Healthy control; IPS: Information processing speed; ML: Mean latency; MS: Multiple sclerosis; MSRT: Mean simple reaction time; MTS: Mean trials to success; PAL: Paired associate learning; PH: Probability of hit; RTI: Reaction time; RVP: Rapid visual processing; SAS: Simple accuracy score; SMT: Simple movement time; SRT: Simple reaction time; STG: Strategy; SWM: Spatial working memory; TC: Total correct; TEA: Total errors adjusted; WLR: Word list recognition

Acknowledgements
We are in debt with Dr. Paul Kretchmer for proofreading and edition.

Funding
Fundação de Amparo à Pesquisa do Pará – FADESP/ Pró-Reitoria de Pesquisa e Pós-Graduação da Universidade Federal do Pará – PROPESP Edital 02–2018-PIAPA; Coordenação de Aperfeiçoamento de Pessoal de Nível Superior – CAPES – Pró-Amazônia, Grant No. 3311/2013; Brazilian Research Council – CNPq Grant No: 307749/2004–5 and 471077/2007–0 for CWPD, Fundação Amazônia de Amparo a Estudos e Pesquisas do Pará – FAPESPA, ICAAF No 039/2017.

Author's contributions
LR, NVBT, CWPD and HC contributed to conception and design of the study. HC, LR, AS and AT were responsible for patient recruitment, assessment and data collection. NVBT, CWPD and AT selected appropriate cognitive tests. LR, AS and AT organized the database. LR and CWPD performed the statistical analysis. LR, NVBT, CWPD, DA and HC interpreted the data. LR wrote the first draft of the manuscript. LR, CWPD and DA wrote sections of the manuscript. All authors contributed to the manuscript revision, read and approved the submitted version.

Competing interests
The authors declare that they have no competing interests.

Author details
[1]Departamento de Neurologia, Hospital Ophir Loyola, Belém, PA, Brazil.
[2]Laboratório de Investigações em Neurodegeneração e Infecção, Hospital Universitário João de Barros Barreto, Universidade Federal do Pará, Instituto de Ciências Biológicas, Belém, PA, Brazil. [3]Faculdade de Fisioterapia e Terapia Ocupacional, Instituto de Ciências da Saúde, Universidade Federal do Pará, Belém, PA, Brazil. [4]Laboratory of Experimental Neuropathology, Department of Pharmacology, University of Oxford, Oxford, UK.

References
1. Baecher-Allan C, Kaskow BJ, Weiner HL. Multiple sclerosis: mechanisms and immunotherapy. Neuron. 2018;97(4):742–68. https://doi.org/10.1016/j.neuron.2018.01.021.
2. Rao SM, Leo GJ, Bernardin L, Unverzagt F. Cognitive dysfunction in multiple sclerosis. I. Frequency, patterns, and prediction. Neurology. 1991;41(5):685–91.
3. Messinis L, Kosmidis MH, Lyros E, Papathanasopoulos P. Assessment and rehabilitation of cognitive impairment in multiple sclerosis. Int Rev Psychiatry. 2010;22(1):22–34. https://doi.org/10.3109/09540261003589372.
4. Goverover Y, Chiaravalloti ND, O'Brien AR, DeLuca J. Evidenced-based cognitive rehabilitation for persons with multiple sclerosis: an updated review of the literature from 2007 to 2016. Arch Phys Med Rehabil. 2018; 99(2):390–407. https://doi.org/10.1016/j.apmr.2017.07.021.
5. Højsgaard Chow H, Schreiber K, Magyari M, Ammitzbøll C, Börnsen L, Romme Christensen J, et al. Progressive multiple sclerosis, cognitive function, and quality of life. Brain Behav. 2018;8(2):e00875. https://doi.org/10.1002/brb3.875.
6. Benito-León J, Morales JM, Rivera-Navarro J. Health-related quality of life and its relationship to cognitive and emotional functioning in multiple sclerosis patients. Eur J Neurol. 2002;9(5):497–502.
7. Chiaravalloti ND, DeLuca J. Cognitive impairment in multiple sclerosis. Lancet Neurol. 2008;7(12):1139–51. https://doi.org/10.1016/S1474-4422(08)70259-X.
8. Turner MP, Hubbard NA, Sivakolundu DK, Himes LM, Hutchison JL, Hart J, et al. Preserved canonicality of the BOLD hemodynamic response reflects healthy cognition: insights into the healthy brain through the window of multiple sclerosis. NeuroImage. 2018; https://doi.org/10.1016/j.neuroimage.2017.12.081.
9. Peterson DS, Fling BW. How changes in brain activity and connectivity are associated with motor performance in people with MS. Neuroimage Clin. 2018;17:153–62. https://doi.org/10.1016/j.nicl.2017.09.019.
10. Soares FC, de Oliveira TC, de Macedo LD, Tomás AM, Picanço-Diniz DL, Bento-Torres J, et al. CANTAB object recognition and language tests to detect aging cognitive decline: an exploratory comparative study. Clin Interv Aging. 2015;10:37–48. https://doi.org/10.2147/CIA.S68186.
11. Benedict RHB, DeLuca J, Enzinger C, Geurts JJG, Krupp LB, Rao SM. Neuropsychology of multiple sclerosis: looking back and moving forward. J Int Neuropsychol Soc. 2017;23(9–10):832–42. https://doi.org/10.1017/S1355617717000959.
12. Sahakian BJ, Owen AM. Computerized assessment in neuropsychiatry using CANTAB: discussion paper. J R Soc Med. 1992;85(7):399–402.
13. Barry A, Cronin O, Ryan AM, Sweeney B, O'Toole O, Allen AP, et al. Impact of short-term cycle ergometer training on quality of life, cognition and depressive symptomatology in multiple sclerosis patients: a pilot study. Neurol Sci. 2017; https://doi.org/10.1007/s10072-017-3230-0.
14. Foong J, Rozewicz L, Quaghebeur G, Thompson AJ, Miller DH, Ron MA. Neuropsychological deficits in multiple sclerosis after acute relapse. J Neurol Neurosurg Psychiatry. 1998;64(4):529–32.
15. Foong J, Rozewicz L, Quaghebeur G, Davie CA, Kartsounis LD, Thompson AJ, et al. Executive function in multiple sclerosis. The role of frontal lobe pathology. Brain. 1997;120(Pt 1):15–26.
16. Foong J, Rozewicz L, Davie CA, Thompson AJ, Miller DH, Ron MA. Correlates of executive function in multiple sclerosis. the use of magnetic resonance spectroscopy as an index of focal pathology J Neuropsychiatry Clin Neurosci. 1999;11(1):45–50. https://doi.org/10.1176/jnp.11.1.45.
17. Muhlert N, Atzori M, De Vita E, Thomas DL, Samson RS, Wheeler-Kingshott CA, et al. Memory in multiple sclerosis is linked to glutamate concentration in grey matter regions. J Neurol Neurosurg Psychiatry. 2014;85(8):833–9. https://doi.org/10.1136/jnnp-2013-306662.
18. Simioni S, Schluep M, Bault N, Coricelli G, Kleeberg J, Du Pasquier RA, et al. Multiple sclerosis decreases explicit counterfactual processing and risk taking in decision making. PLoS One. 2012;7(12):e50718. https://doi.org/10.1371/journal.pone.0050718.
19. Sumowski JF, Benedict R, Enzinger C, Filippi M, Geurts JJ, Hamalainen P, et al. Cognition in multiple sclerosis: State of the field and priorities for the future. Neurology. 2018;90(6):278–88. https://doi.org/10.1212/WNL.0000000000004977.
20. Rocca MA, Amato MP, De Stefano N, Enzinger C, Geurts JJ, Penner IK, et al. Clinical and imaging assessment of cognitive dysfunction in multiple sclerosis. Lancet Neurol. 2015;14(3):302–17. https://doi.org/10.1016/S1474-4422(14)70250-9.
21. Polman CH, Reingold SC, Banwell B, Clanet M, Cohen JA, Filippi M, et al. Diagnostic criteria for multiple sclerosis: 2010 revisions to the McDonald criteria. Ann Neurol. 2011;69(2):292–302. https://doi.org/10.1002/ana.22366.
22. Bertolucci PH, Okamoto IH, Brucki SM, Siviero MO, Toniolo Neto J, Ramos LR. Applicability of the CERAD neuropsychological battery to Brazilian elderly. Arq Neuropsiquiatr 2001;59 3-A:532–536.
23. Schweitzer L, Renehan WE. The use of cluster analysis for cell typing. Brain Res Brain Res Protoc. 1997;1(1):100–8.
24. Strober LB, Christodoulou C, Benedict RH, Westervelt HJ, Melville P, Scherl WF, et al. Unemployment in multiple sclerosis: the contribution of personality and disease. Mult Scler. 2012;18(5):647–53. https://doi.org/10.1177/1352458511426735
25. Strober L, Chiaravalloti N, Moore N, DeLuca J. Unemployment in multiple sclerosis (MS): utility of the MS functional composite and cognitive testing. Mult Scler. 2014;20(1):112–5. https://doi.org/10.1177/1352458513488235.
26. Linn MW, Sandifer R, Stein S. Effects of unemployment on mental and physical health. Am J Public Health. 1985;75(5):502–6.
27. Nocentini U, Pasqualetti P, Bonavita S, Buccafusca M, De Caro MF, Farina D, et al. Cognitive dysfunction in patients with relapsing-remitting multiple sclerosis. Mult Scler. 2006;12(1):77–87. https://doi.org/10.1191/135248506ms1227oa.

28. Gonzalez-Rosa JJ, Vazquez-Marrufo M, Vaquero E, Duque P, Borges M, Gomez-Gonzalez CM, et al. Cluster analysis of behavioural and event-related potentials during a contingent negative variation paradigm in remitting-relapsing and benign forms of multiple sclerosis. BMC Neurol. 2011;11:64. https://doi.org/10.1186/1471-2377-11-64.

29. Gonzalez-Rosa JJ, Vazquez-Marrufo M, Vaquero E, Duque P, Borges M, Gamero MA, et al. Differential cognitive impairment for diverse forms of multiple sclerosis. BMC Neurosci. 2006;7:39. https://doi.org/10.1186/1471-2202-7-39.

30. Langdon DW, Amato MP, Boringa J, Brochet B, Foley F, Fredrikson S, et al. Recommendations for a brief international cognitive assessment for multiple sclerosis (BICAMS). Mult Scler 2012;18 6:891–8; doi: https://doi.org/10.1177/1352458511431076.

31. Benedict RH, Fischer JS, Archibald CJ, Arnett PA, Beatty WW, Bobholz J, et al. Minimal neuropsychological assessment of MS patients: a consensus approach. Clin Neuropsychol 2002;16 3:381–97; doi: https://doi.org/10.1076/clin.16.3.381.13859.

32. Costa SL, Genova HM, DeLuca J, Chiaravalloti ND. Information processing speed in multiple sclerosis: past, present, and future. Mult Scler. 2017;23(6): 772–89. https://doi.org/10.1177/1352458516645869.

33. Leavitt VM, Lengenfelder J, Moore NB, Chiaravalloti ND, DeLuca J. The relative contributions of processing speed and cognitive load to working memory accuracy in multiple sclerosis. J Clin Exp Neuropsychol. 2011;33(5): 580–6. https://doi.org/10.1080/13803395.2010.541427.

34. Lengenfelder J, Bryant D, Diamond BJ, Kalmar JH, Moore NB, DeLuca J. Processing speed interacts with working memory efficiency in multiple sclerosis. Arch Clin Neuropsychol. 2006;21(3):229–38. https://doi.org/10.1016/j.acn.2005.12.001.

35. DeLuca J, Chelune GJ, Tulsky DS, Lengenfelder J, Chiaravalloti ND. Is speed of processing or working memory the primary information processing deficit in multiple sclerosis? J Clin Exp Neuropsychol. 2004;26(4):550–62. https://doi.org/10.1080/13803390490496641.

36. Cotter J, Vithanage N, Colville S, Lyle D, Cranley D, Cormack F, et al. Investigating domain-specific cognitive impairment among patients with multiple sclerosis using touchscreen cognitive testing in routine clinical care. Front Neurol. 2018;9:331. https://doi.org/10.3389/fneur.2018.00331.

37. Foong J, Rozewicz L, Chong WK, Thompson AJ, Miller DH, Ron MA. A comparison of neuropsychological deficits in primary and secondary progressive multiple sclerosis. J Neurol. 2000;247(2):97–101.

38. Roque DT, Teixeira RAA, Zachi EC, DF V. The use of the Cambridge neuropsychological test automated battery (CANTAB) in neuropsychological assessment: application in Brazilian research with control children and adults with neurological disorders. Psychol Neurosci. 2011;4(2):255–65.

39. Patti F, Morra VB, Amato MP, Trojano M, Bastianello S, Tola MR, et al. Subcutaneous interferon β-1a may protect against cognitive impairment in patients with relapsing-remitting multiple sclerosis: 5-year follow-up of the COGIMUS study. PLoS One. 2013;8(8):e74111. https://doi.org/10.1371/journal.pone.0074111.

40. Lacy M, Hauser M, Pliskin N, Assuras S, Valentine MO, Reder A. The effects of long-term interferon-beta-1b treatment on cognitive functioning in multiple sclerosis: a 16-year longitudinal study. Mult Scler. 2013;19(13):1765–72. https://doi.org/10.1177/1352458513485981.

41. Portaccio E, Stromillo ML, Goretti B, Hakiki B, Giorgio A, Rossi F, et al. Natalizumab may reduce cognitive changes and brain atrophy rate in relapsing-remitting multiple sclerosis--a prospective, non-randomized pilot study. Eur J Neurol. 2013; 20(6):986–90. https://doi.org/10.1111/j.1468-1331.2012.03882.x.

42. Luerding R, Gebel S, Gebel EM, Schwab-Malek S, Weissert R. Influence of formal education on cognitive Reserve in Patients with multiple sclerosis. Front Neurol. 2016;7:46. https://doi.org/10.3389/fneur.2016.00046.

3

Interactive effect of acute and chronic glycemic indexes for severity in acute ischemic stroke patients

Keon-Joo Lee[1], Ji Sung Lee[2] and Keun-Hwa Jung[3*]

Abstract

Background: Diabetes mellitus is a well-established risk factor for ischemic stroke and is known to increase stroke risk by 2–6 fold. Numerous studies have reported the relationship between parameters for glycemic status and stroke-related outcomes; however, studies focusing on the interaction between acute and chronic glycemic status indexes with stroke phenotype are lacking.

Methods: Acute ischemic stroke patients who were admitted to a tertiary hospital stroke center from 2002 to 2015 were consecutively enrolled in this study. Fasting blood sugar (FBS) and serum glycated hemoglobin (HbA1c) levels were recorded as acute and chronic glycemic indexes, respectively. The associations between initial stroke severity and both glycemic indexes were evaluated with consideration of the interaction between the glycemic indexes. Moreover, the distinct effects of stroke subtypes were evaluated.

Results: A total of 2595 patients were included in the final analysis. After adjustment for covariates, FBS was associated with initial stroke severity ($P < 0.001$), while HbA1c was not ($P = 0.16$). However, an interaction between FBS and HbA1c in association with initial stroke severity was observed ($P < 0.001$). The association between FBS and initial stroke severity was stronger, with a relatively normal HbA1c level. Among stroke subtypes, the interactions were significant for the large artery disease and cardioembolism subtypes (all, $P < 0.001$), but for the small vessel occlusion subtype ($P = 0.63$).

Conclusions: This study shows that HbA1c is an effect modifier for the association between FBS and initial stroke severity, and the interactive effect differs among stroke subtypes.

Keywords: Glucose, Ischemic stroke, Etiology, Hemoglobin A1c, Hyperglycemia

Background

Diabetes mellitus is an established modifiable risk factor for ischemic stroke, which accounts for approximately 3–20% of stroke risk [1, 2]. The risk of stroke is 2–6 times higher in diabetes patients than in non-diabetic individuals [3]. In the acute stroke stage, glycemic parameters, such as fasting blood sugar (FBS) or serum glycated hemoglobin (HbA1c), are known to be related to post-stroke outcomes, and the current guideline recommends strict glycemic control (normoglycemia) for the management of acute ischemic stroke [4].

However, results that focus on the simultaneous or interactive effects for the two glycemic indexes, representing immediate changes in the glycemic status at the acute stage of ischemic stroke and previously cumulative changes in the glycemic status (HbA1c), are limited. The impact of glucose level in the acute stage of ischemic stroke might vary between different HbA1c statuses. Moreover, as ischemic stroke is a heterogenous disease entity, the effect of glycemic status might differ among stroke subtypes with distinct pathophysiological mechanisms [3, 5]. Estimating the effect of acute glycemic status based on different underlying conditions would be useful for optimizing care in acute stroke patients.

* Correspondence: jungkh@gmail.com
[3]Department of Neurology, Seoul National University Hospital, 101, Daehangno, Jongno-gu, Seoul 03080, South Korea
Full list of author information is available at the end of the article

This study investigated the interaction between the indexes for acute and chronic glycemic status and examined whether the effects differed among stroke subtypes.

Methods

Study subjects

Acute ischemic stroke patients who were admitted to a tertiary hospital between January 2002 and May 2015 were included according to the following eligibility criteria (Additional file 1: Figure S1): 1) age older than 18 years, 2) relevant ischemic lesion confirmed with brain imaging (computed tomography or magnetic resonance imaging), 3) admission within 7 days of symptom onset, and 4) clearly determined stroke subtype of large artery disease (LAD), small vessel occlusion (SVO), or cardioembolism (CE). Stroke subtypes were classified according to the TOAST classification [5] and were determined at the time of the patient's discharge via consensus between at least two trained neurologists. Medical history and results of work-ups during hospitalization (e.g., cerebral angiography, transcranial Doppler sonography, transthoracic and transesophageal echocardiography, electrocardiogram, and 24-h Holter monitoring) were reviewed for subtype determination. The patients with 1) missing glycemic status indicators, 2) an unclear previous diagnosis of diabetes mellitus, and 3) missing outcome data were excluded.

Data collection

Demographic data and clinical parameters, namely age, sex, body mass index, time from symptom onset to hospital arrival, hyperacute reperfusion therapy administration, antithrombotic use at the acute stage, risk factor profiles including previous history, initial blood pressure, and lipid panel results at admission, were collected.

Glycemic indexes, which use the FBS level as an indicator for the acute glycemic status and glycated hemoglobin index (HbA1c) as an indicator for the chronic status, were measured in each subject after at least 8 h of fasting on the first or second day of admission according to an institutional protocol of blood sampling [6]. FBS was selected instead of the initial glucose level to minimize the effect of meals [7].

The outcome parameters included the National Institute of Health Stroke scale (NIHSS) score measured at hospital arrival, which represented initial stroke severity, and the modified Rankin scale (mRS) scores, which represented functional status at discharge [8]. These stroke scales were measured and recorded by the attending neurologist at both the times of hospital arrival and discharge.

The study design and subject data collection were approved by the Institutional Review Board.

Statistical analysis

The characteristics of study subjects are described as numbers and percentages for categorical variables and as mean ± standard deviation for interval variables. Stroke scale scores and interval between stroke onset and hospital arrival are presented as medians and interquartile ranges.

A bivariate correlation analysis between the two glycemic indexes (FBS and HbA1c) was performed using Spearman's rank correlation coefficient. FBS and HbA1c were centered for the arithmetic mean of each parameter, and the interaction terms of the centered FBS and HbA1c (FBS*HbA1c) were introduced into a multivariable linear regression model along with predetermined covariates (age, sex, interval between stroke onset and hospital arrival, body-mass index, hypertension, diabetes, hyperlipidemia, heart disease, previous stroke history, smoking, stroke subtype, systolic and diastolic blood pressure, LDL cholesterol, HDL cholesterol, and triglyceride level) and the centered glycemic indexes to examine their associations with the admission NIHSS scores.

To evaluate the association between the discharge mRS score and the glycemic indexes, a shift analysis using a multivariable ordinal regression model and an analysis for mRS scores dichotomized into good (mRS scores: 0–1) and poor (mRS scores: 2–6) using a multivariable binary logistic regression model were performed. In these analyses, the NIHSS score at admission along with additional covariates, including the variables indicating acute treatment status (acute antithrombotics administration and hyperacute reperfusion therapy), were included in the model in order to evaluate whether the glycemic indexes had a secondary effect on patient outcome independently of their effect on initial stroke severity (Additional file 2: Table S1).

Linear fit line from scatter plots showing the estimated correlation between FBS and outcome measurements according to HbA1c levels in the normal (HbA1c < 5.7%), pre-diabetes (5.8% ≤ HbA1c < 6.5%), and diabetes (6.5% ≤ HbA1c) range was presented in figures (Figs. 1, 2 and 3) [6].

In order to evaluate the interaction between glycemic indexes and stroke subtypes, the interactions between the original variables and every combination of terms for each variable (FBS*HbA1c, FBS*stroke subtypes, HbA1c*stroke subtypes, and FBS*HbA1c*stroke subtypes) were introduced into the model (Additional file 2: Table S2).

As an interaction between glycemic indexes and stroke subtypes was demonstrated to exist, a subgroup analysis among the three subtypes was performed and an additional subgroup analysis of the relationship between patients who had a previous history of diabetes and those who had not was conducted at the post-hoc level.

Two-tailed P values < 0.05 were considered statistically significant. All statistical analyses were performed with the use of R software, version 3.4 (R Foundation for Statistical Computing, Vienna, Austria).

Results

A total of 2595 patients were included in the final analysis (Additional file 1: Figure S1). The basic characteristics of the study subjects are presented in Table 1. There were 1047 (40.3%) patients classified as LAD, 832 (32.1%) as SVO, and the remaining 716 (27.6%) as CE. The mean age of the subjects was 66.9 ± 11.9 years, and most patients (61.4%) were male. Thirty-five percent of the patients were previously diagnosed with diabetes. The median time to hospital arrival was approximately 17 h. The median NIHSS score at arrival was 3, and 7.3% of patients received hyperacute reperfusion therapy.

Table 1 Baseline characteristics of all study subjects ($N = 2595$)

	Values
Age	66.9 ± 11.9
Male	1593 (61.4)
Time to hospital arrival (hours)	17 (4–49)
Body-mass index (kg/m^2)	23.86 ± 3.30
Hypertension	1821 (70.2)
Diabetes	918 (35.4)
Hyperlipidemia	688 (26.5)
Smoking	881 (33.9)
Heart disease	632 (24.4)
Previous stroke	550 (21.2)
Reperfusion therapy	189 (7.3)
Acute medication	
Antiplatelet	2081 (80.2)
Anticoagulation	511 (19.7)
Stroke subtype	
Large artery disease	1047 (40.3)
Small vessel occlusion	832 (32.1)
Cardioembolism	716 (27.6)
Initial NIHSS	3 (1–6)
Discharge mRS	2 (2–4)
SBP (mmHg)	153.3 ± 27.3
DBP (mmHg)	85.6 ± 15.6
Total cholesterol level (mg/dL)	177.3 ± 40.0
LDL cholesterol level (mg/dL)	107.6 ± 35.2
HDL cholesterol level (mg/dL)	45.1 ± 12.8
Triglyceride (mg/dL)	123.8 ± 72.3
Fasting blood sugar (mg/dL)	112.8 ± 40.5
HbA1c (%)	6.4 ± 1.3

NIHSS National Institute of Health Stroke Scale score, mRS modified Rankin's scale, SBP systolic blood pressure, DBP diastolic blood pressure, LDL low-density lipoprotein, HDL high density-lipoprotein

FBS and HbA1c were moderately positively correlated ($\rho = 0.52$, $P < 0.001$; Additional file 3: Figure S2). Thus, it was necessary to introduce an interaction term in further analysis models. When FB and HbA1c and their interaction term (FBS*HbA1c) were inputted to a multivariable linear regression model, FBS ($P < 0.001$), but not HbA1c ($P = 0.16$), was shown to have an association with the initial NIHSS score (Table 2). Moreover, these two glycemic indexes had an interaction ($P < 0.001$) regarding their effect on initial stroke severity. The interaction plot displayed in Fig. 1 shows the estimated correlation between FBS and initial NIHSS scores in different HbA1c ranges. The correlations appeared stronger when HbA1c was within a relatively normal range than when it was higher for both unadjusted (A) and adjusted (B) models.

There was an interaction between the glycemic indexes for the mRS score at discharge in the shift analysis ($P = 0.04$). However, neither an association nor an interaction between the glycemic indexes and the functional outcome at discharge was shown when the initial NIHSS scores were included in the models (Additional file 2: Table S1).

There was an interaction between the stroke subtypes and the glycemic indexes and their interaction term (Additional file 2: Table S2); thus, a subgroup analysis for stroke subtypes was performed (Table 3 and Fig. 2). FBS and the interaction term, FBS*HbA1c, were shown to be associated with the initial NIHSS score in the LAD and CE subtypes (all $P < 0.001$), while the association was absent in the SVO subtype (Table 3). The linear fit lines from the scatter plots showed a stronger correlation in patients with an HbA1c range lower than 6.5% in the LAD and CE subtypes (Fig. 2).

In the post-hoc analysis, in which the patients were categorized based on the diagnosis of diabetes before admission, the interaction between the glycemic indexes was significant regardless of diabetes history (Table 4 and Fig. 3). However, the HbA1c level was not negatively correlated with initial stroke severity in patients previously diagnosed with diabetes ($B = -0.26$, $P = 0.03$).

Discussion

In this study, we demonstrated that FBS and HbA1c interact with initial stroke severity in acute ischemic stroke patients. The chronic glycemic status, represented by the HbA1c level, seemed to modify the effect of acute glycemic status on stroke severity. Moreover, this effect differed among stroke subtypes in that the interaction was significant in patients with the LAD and CE subtypes, while insignificant in those with the SVO subtype.

Numerous prior studies have shown the association between glucose levels in the acute stage and outcomes in ischemic stroke patients. Higher blood glucose level on admission is known to be correlated with stroke progression [9, 10], poor functional outcomes [9, 11], and

Table 2 Association between glycemic parameters and initial stroke severity, considering interactions

Variables	Coefficient (B)	Standard error (ε)	t-value	P-value
FBS (mg/dL)	0.03	0.004	9.81	< 0.001
HbA1c (%)	−0.18	0.12	− 1.42	0.16
FBS * HbA1c	−0.007	0.001	−4.81	< 0.001
Age (y)	0.040	0.009	4.28	< 0.001
Sex	0.33	0.24	1.41	0.16
Stroke subtype				
LAD (reference)	–	–	–	–
SVO	−1.64	0.24	−6.93	< 0.001
CE	1.90	0.34	5.60	< 0.001
Time to hospital arrival (hour)	−0.01	0.003	−5.38	< 0.001
Body-mass index	−0.16	0.032	−5.12	< 0.001
Hypertension	−0.30	0.23	−1.28	0.20
Diabetes	−0.78	0.30	−2.60	0.009
Hyperlipidemia	−0.21	0.24	−0.90	0.37
Heart disease	0.24	0.33	0.73	0.47
Previous stroke history	0.74	0.25	3.01	0.003
Smoking	−0.03	0.24	−0.11	0.92
SBP (mmHg)	−0.007	0.005	−1.42	0.16
DBP (mmHg)	0.02	0.009	2.51	0.01
LDL cholesterol (mg/dL)	0.007	0.0	2.27	0.02
HDL cholesterol (mg/dL)	−0.03	0.008	−3.78	< 0.001
Triglyceride (mg/dL)	−0.002	0.002	−1.26	0.21

FBS fasting blood sugar, *LAD* large artery disease, *SVO* small vessel occlusion, *CE* cardioembolism, *SBP* systolic blood pressure, *DBP* diastolic blood pressure, *LDL* low-density lipoprotein, *HDL* high-density lipoprotein

mortality [12, 13]. In addition, high blood glucose levels have been associated with poor outcomes after reperfusion therapy [14–16] or hemorrhagic transformation following initial ischemic stroke occurrence [17]. Another glycemic index, HbA1c, is known to represent glycemic control status within the past 2–3 months [18], but relatively few studies have addressed the effect of HbA1c on stroke outcomes. For example, one study involving patients from the Fukuoka stroke registry showed that

HbA1c predicts neurological deterioration and functional outcome at discharge [19], while another observational study did not find an association between HbA1c and functional outcomes [20].

To date, no study has considered the interactive effect of these two glycemic indexes. A recent study by Chinese investigators showed that newly diagnosed diabetes with isolated elevation of HbA1c that was not accompanied by elevated blood glucose level was not associated with poor

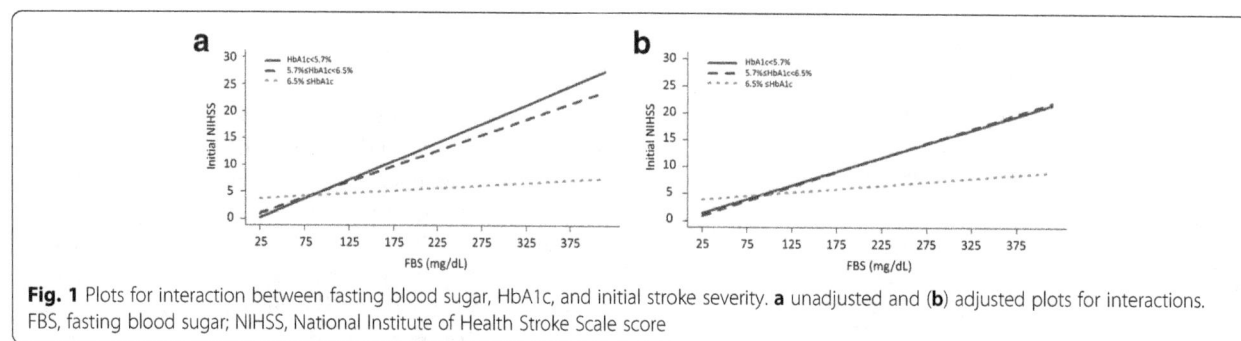

Fig. 1 Plots for interaction between fasting blood sugar, HbA1c, and initial stroke severity. **a** unadjusted and (**b**) adjusted plots for interactions. FBS, fasting blood sugar; NIHSS, National Institute of Health Stroke Scale score

Table 3 Interaction between glycemic parameters and initial stroke severity among stroke subtypes

	Coefficient (B)	Standard error (ε)	t-value	P-value
Large artery disease (N = 1047)				
FBS (mg/dL)	0.05	0.006	8.47	< 0.001
HbA1c (%)	−0.25	0.18	−1.34	0.18
FBS * HbA1c	−0.01	0.002	−4.89	< 0.001
Small vessel occlusion (N = 832)				
FBS (mg/dL)	0.02	0.003	0.65	0.52
HbA1c (%)	0.04	0.12	0.34	0.74
FBS * HbA1c	0.0006	0.001	0.48	0.63
Cardioembolism (N = 716)				
FBS (mg/dL)	0.06	0.009	6.91	< 0.001
HbA1c (%)	−0.66	0.33	−1.96	0.05
FBS * HbA1c	−0.02	0.005	−3.36	< 0.001

FBS fasting blood sugar

Adjusted for age, sex, time before hospital arrival, body-mass index, hypertension, diabetes, hyperlipidemia, heart disease, previous stroke history, smoking, systolic and diastolic blood pressure, LDL cholesterol, HDL cholesterol and triglyceride level

Table 4 Interaction between glycemic parameters for initial stroke severity based on history of diabetes

	Coefficient (B)	Standard error (ε)	t-value	P-value
Diabetes (N = 918)				
FBS (mg/dL)	0.02	0.003	6.18	< 0.001
HbA1c (%)	−0.26	0.12	−2.19	0.03
FBS * HbA1c	−0.006	0.002	−3.43	< 0.001
Non-diabetes (N = 1677)				
FBS (mg/dL)	0.06	0.007	8.56	< 0.001
HbA1c (%)	−0.53	0.31	−1.71	0.09
FBS * HbA1c	−0.23	0.0009	−2.45	0.02

FBS fasting blood sugar

Adjusted for age, sex, time to hospital arrival, body-mass index, stroke subtype, hypertension, hyperlipidemia, heart disease, previous stroke history, smoking, systolic and diastolic blood pressure, LDL cholesterol, HDL cholesterol and triglyceride level

outcome after ischemic stroke [21]. This result implies that the glycemic status before a stroke might have a different effect than the acute glycemic status.

Several pathophysiological mechanisms have been proposed regarding how a high glucose level may result in poor outcomes after ischemic stroke. Notably, reperfusion injury is suggested to be a mainstay of the harmful effect in which hyperglycemia would augment oxidative stress [22]. According to this background, the current clinical guideline recommends avoiding hyperglycemia and instead maintaining normoglycemia within the range of 140 to 180 mg/dL during the acute stage of ischemic stroke [4]. In addition, a high glucose level is known to compromise the recruitment of collateral circulation in ischemic stroke animal models or clinical studies [23, 24]. The lack of association in the SVO subtype might be explained by a relatively small infarct size and lesser influence of the collateral circulation due to the different pathophysiology

of this subtype [25]. However, considering that the hyperglycemic status supplies sufficient glucose and energy to the brain, the effect of hyperglycemia seems to be complicated in the ischemic brain [22]. Our result, which showed a weaker association of acute hyperglycemia with stroke severity in patients with higher HbA1c levels, may be an implication of this beneficial effect of hyperglycemia.

Because the glycemic indicators in our study were measured after stroke onset, the bi-directional effect of glycemic change and stroke should be considered. The increase in glucose level during the acute stroke period is sometimes noted with the term "stress hyperglycemia," which results partly from an elevated sympathetic tone [22, 26]. Stress hyperglycemia might be a marker of impaired glucose regulation in patients with insulin resistance and is known to be associated with poor outcome after stroke [26, 27]. The association between FBS level and stroke severity in the patients of our study with a relatively normal HbA1c might indicate the effect of stress hyperglycemia; however, stress hyperglycemia might be understood as a protective response that may help survival [28]. The pathophysiological or

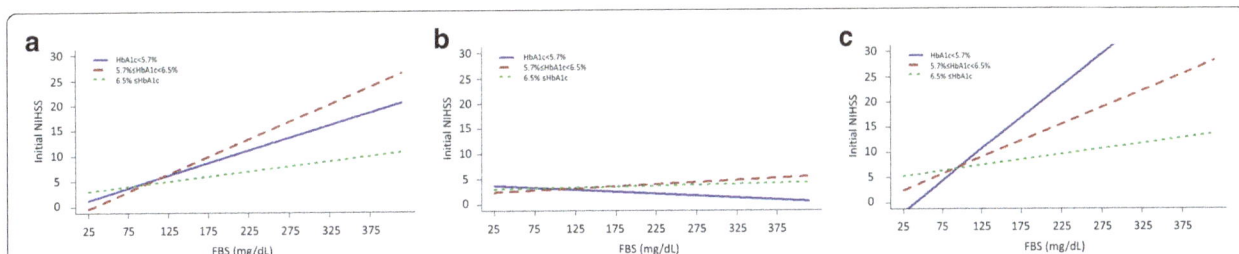

Fig. 2 Adjusted plots for interaction among stroke subtypes. **a** large artery disease, **b** small vessel occlusion, and (**c**) cardioembolism. FBS, fasting blood sugar; NIHSS, National Institute of Health Stroke Scale score

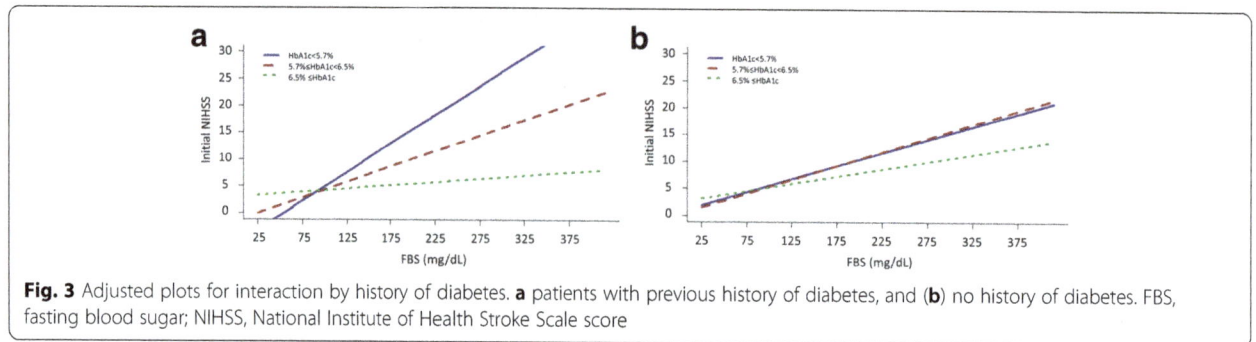

Fig. 3 Adjusted plots for interaction by history of diabetes. **a** patients with previous history of diabetes, and (**b**) no history of diabetes. FBS, fasting blood sugar; NIHSS, National Institute of Health Stroke Scale score

clinical implications of stress hyperglycemia should be revealed by future studies.

The association between FBS and stroke severity was weaker when the HbA1c level was higher. The patients with higher HbA1c level had several other cardiovascular risk factors and were using medication including antidiabetic agents, statins, and antithrombotics. Considering that such agents are potentially beneficial for protecting the brain against ischemic insult [29–33], the effect of FBS on stroke severity in those patients might be attenuated. However, when we conducted a post-hoc subgroup analysis comparing the patients who were previously diagnosed with diabetes with those who were not, the noted interaction between the glycemic indexes remained valid in both groups (Table 4 and Fig. 3).

There are several limitations to our study. First, as discussed above, a reversed temporal relationship between the measurements of the glycemic indexes and the stroke severity scale should be considered, and a causal relationship could not be determined from this study. Second, the outcome measurements in our study consisted of stroke scales, which might not directly implicate the pathological status of the study subjects [8]. Parameters derived from brain images, such as infarct volume, might be more useful in this respect. Third, information on medications prior to stroke was not collected, although prior antithrombotics, statins, and some oral hypoglycemic agents may influence the stroke phenotype. Fourth, the period of patient enrollment spanned more than a decade, and changes in clinical practice during this period would be considerable.

Conclusion

Our study results showed that HbA1c was an effect modifier for the association between FBS and stroke severity and that stroke subtypes affected the intensity of the association. Further studies are warranted for evaluating the pathophysiological aspects of these findings and their implications for acute stroke management.

Abbreviations
CE: Cardioembolism; FBS: Fasting blood sugar; HbA1c: Serum glycated hemoglobin; HDL: High density lipoprotein; LAD: Large artery disease; LDL: Low density lipoprotein; mRS: Modified Rankin scale; NIHSS: National Institute of Health Stroke scale; SVO: Small vessel occlusion; TOAST: Trial of Org 10,172 in Acute Stroke Treatment

Funding
This research was supported by the Brain Research Program through the National Research Foundation of Korea (NRF) funded by the Ministry of Science, ICT & Future Planning (2016M3C7A1914002). Jung KH was supported by a research grant from CJ HealthCare Corp. (Republic of Korea, 0620160450).

Authors' contributions
KJL designed the study, analyzed and interpreted the patient data, and was a major contributor in writing the manuscript. JSL made substantial contributions to statistical conception and design and analyzed the patient data. KHJ contributed to design, revised the manuscript, and supervised the study. All authors read and approved the final manuscript.

Competing interests
The authors declare that they have no competing interests.

Author details
[1]Department of Neurology, Seoul National University Bundang Hospital, Seoul, South Korea. [2]Clinical Research Center, Asan Medical Center, Seoul, South Korea. [3]Department of Neurology, Seoul National University Hospital, 101, Daehangno, Jongno-gu, Seoul 03080, South Korea.

References
1. Donnell MJO, Chin SL, Rangarajan S, Xavier D, Liu L, Zhang H, et al. Global and regional eff ects of potentially modifiable risk factors associated with acute stroke in 32 countries (INTERSTROKE): a case-control study. Lancet. 2016;388:761–5. https://doi.org/10.1016/S0140-6736(16)30506-2.
2. Willey JZ, Moon YP, Kahn E, Rodriguez CJ, Rundek T, Cheung K, et al. Population attributable risks of hypertension and diabetes for cardiovascular disease and stroke in the northern Manhattan study. J Am Heart Assoc. 2014;3:e001106. https://doi.org/10.1161/JAHA.114.001106.
3. Sander D, Kearney MT. Reducing the risk of stroke in type 2 diabetes: pathophysiological and therapeutic perspectives. J Neurol. 2009;256:1603–19. https://doi.org/10.1007/s00415-009-5143-1.
4. Jauch EC, Saver JL, Adams HP, Bruno A, Connors JJ, Demaerschalk BM, et al. Guidelines for the early management of patients with acute ischemic stroke: a guideline for healthcare professionals from the American Heart Association/American Stroke Association. Stroke. 2013;44:870–947. https://doi.org/10.1161/STR.0b013e318284056a.
5. Adams HP, Bendixen BH, Kappelle LJ, Biller J, Love BB, Gordon DL, et al. Classification of subtype of acute ischemic stroke. Definitions for use in a multicenter clinical trial. TOAST. Trial of org 10172 in acute stroke treatment. Stroke. 1993;24:35–41. https://doi.org/10.1161/01.STR.24.1.35.

6. American Diabetes Association. 2. Classification and Diagnosis of Diabetes: Standards of Medical Care in Diabetes—2018. Diabetes Care. 2018;41:S13–27. https://doi.org/10.2337/dc18-S002.

7. Moebus S, Göres L, Lösch C, Jöckel KH. Impact of time since last caloric intake on blood glucose levels. Eur J Epidemiol. 2011;26:719–28. https://doi.org/10.1007/s10654-011-9608-z.

8. Kasner SE. Clinical interpretation and use of stroke scales. Lancet Neurol. 2006;5:603–12. https://doi.org/10.1016/S1474-4422(06)70495-1.

9. Baird TA, Parsons MW, Phanh T, Butcher KS, Desmond PM, Tress BM, et al. Persistent poststroke hyperglycemia is independently associated with infarct expansion and worse clinical outcome. Stroke. 2003;34:2208–14. https://doi.org/10.1161/01.STR.0000085087.41330.FF.

10. Shimoyama T, Kimura K, Uemura J, Saji N, Shibazaki K. Elevated glucose level adversely affects infarct volume growth and neurological deterioration in non-diabetic stroke patients, but not diabetic stroke patients. Eur J Neurol. 2014;21:402–10. https://doi.org/10.1111/ene.12280.

11. Ntaios G, Egli M, Faouzi M, Michel P. J-shaped association between serum glucose and functional outcome in acute ischemic stroke. Stroke. 2010;41:2366–70. https://doi.org/10.1161/STROKEAHA.110.592170.

12. Hyvärinen M, Qiao Q, Tuomilehto J, Laatikainen T, Heine RJ, Stehouwer CD, et al. Hyperglycemia and stroke mortality: comparison between fasting and 2-h glucose criteria. Diabetes Care. 2009;32:348–54. https://doi.org/10.2337/dc08-1411.

13. Williams LS, Rotich J, Qi R, Fineberg N, Espay A, Bruno A, et al. Effects of admission hyperglycemia on mortality and costs in acute ischemic stroke. Neurology. 2002;59:67–71. http://www.ncbi.nlm.nih.gov/pubmed/12105309

14. Alvarez-Sabín J, Molina CA, Montaner J, Arenillas JF, Huertas R, Ribo M, et al. Effects of admission hyperglycemia on stroke outcome in reperfused tissue plasminogen activator-treated patients. Stroke. 2003;34:1235–40. https://doi.org/10.1161/01.STR.0000068406.30514.31.

15. Poppe AY, Majumdar SR, Jeerakathil T, Ghali W, Buchan AM, Hill MD. Admission hyperglycemia predicts a worse outcome in stroke patients treated with intravenous thrombolysis. Diabetes Care. 2009;32:617–22. https://doi.org/10.2337/dc08-1754.None.

16. Kim JT, Jahan R, Saver JL. Impact of glucose on outcomes in patients treated with mechanical thrombectomy: a post hoc analysis of the solitaire flow restoration with the intention for thrombectomy study. Stroke. 2016;47:120–7. https://doi.org/10.1161/STROKEAHA.115.010753.

17. Paciaroni M, Agnelli G, Corea F, Ageno W, Alberti A, Lanari A, et al. Early hemorrhagic transformation of brain infarction: rate, predictive factors, and influence on clinical outcome: results of a prospective multicenter study. Stroke. 2008;39:2249–56. https://doi.org/10.1161/STROKEAHA.107.510321.

18. Sacks DB. Hemoglobin A1c in diabetes: panacea or pointless? Diabetes. 2013;62(1):41–3. https://doi.org/10.2337/db12-1485.

19. Kamouchi M, Matsuki T, Hata J, Kuwashiro T, Ago T, Sambongi Y, et al. Prestroke glycemic control is associated with the functional outcome in acute ischemic stroke: the Fukuoka stroke registry. Stroke. 2011;42:2788–94. https://doi.org/10.1161/STROKEAHA.111.617415.

20. Murros K, Fogelholm R, Kettunen S, Vuorela AL, Valve J. Blood glucose, glycosylated haemoglobin, and outcome of ischemic brain infarction. J Neurol Sci. 1992;111:59–64. http://www.ncbi.nlm.nih.gov/pubmed/1402998

21. Jing J, Pan Y, Zhao X, Zheng H, Jia Q, Li H, et al. Prognosis of ischemic stroke with newly diagnosed diabetes mellitus according to hemoglobin A1c criteria in Chinese population. Stroke. 2016;47:2038–44. https://doi.org/10.1161/STROKEAHA.116.013606.

22. Robbins NM, Swanson RA. Opposing effects of glucose on stroke and reperfusion injury: acidosis, oxidative stress, and energy metabolism. Stroke. 2014;45:1881–6. https://doi.org/10.1161/STROKEAHA.114.004889.

23. van Seeters T, Biessels GJ, Kappelle LJ, van der Graaf Y, Velthuis BK. Dutch acute stroke study (DUST) investigators. Determinants of leptomeningeal collateral flow in stroke patients with a middle cerebral artery occlusion. Neuroradiology. 2016;58:969–77. https://doi.org/10.1007/s00234-016-1727-5.

24. Reeson P, Jeffery A, Brown CE. Illuminating the effects of stroke on the diabetic brain: insights from imaging neural and vascular networks in experimental animal models. Diabetes. 2016;65:1779–88. https://doi.org/10.2337/db16-0064.

25. Caplan LR. Lacunar infarction and small vessel disease: pathology and pathophysiology. J Stroke. 2015;17:2–6. https://doi.org/10.5853/jos.2015.17.1.2.

26. Lindsberg PJ, Roine RO. Hyperglycemia in acute stroke. Stroke. 2004;35:363–4. https://doi.org/10.1161/01.STR.0000115297.92132.84.

27. Capes SE, Hunt D, Malmberg K, Pathak P, Gerstein HC. Stress hyperglycemia and prognosis of stroke in nondiabetic and diabetic patients: a systematic overview. Stroke. 2001;32:2426–32. https://doi.org/10.1161/hs1001.096194.

28. Marik PE, Bellomo R. Stress hyperglycemia: an essential survival response! Crit Care. 2013;17:305. https://doi.org/10.1186/cc12514.

29. Marso SP, Daniels GH, Brown-Frandsen K, Kristensen P, Mann JF, Nauck MA, et al. Liraglutide and cardiovascular outcomes in type 2 diabetes. N Engl J Med. 2016;375:311–22. https://doi.org/10.1056/NEJMoa1603827.

30. Marso SP, Bain SC, Consoli A, Eliaschewitz FG, Jódar E, Leiter LA, et al. Semaglutide and cardiovascular outcomes in patients with type 2 diabetes. N Engl J Med. 2016;375:1834–44. https://doi.org/10.1056/NEJMoa1607141.

31. Hong J, Zhang Y, Lai S, Lv A, Su Q, Dong Y. Effects of metformin versus glipizide on cardiovascular outcomes in patients with type 2 diabetes and coronary artery disease. Diabetes Care. 2012;36:1304–11. https://doi.org/10.2337/dc12-0719.

32. Park JM, Kang K, Cho YJ, Hong KS, Lee KB, Park TH, et al. Comparative effectiveness of Prestroke aspirin on stroke severity and outcome. Ann Neurol. 2016;79:560–8. https://doi.org/10.1002/ana.24602.

33. Ishikawa H, Wakisaka Y, Matsuo R, Makihara N, Hata J, Kuroda J, et al. Influence of statin pretreatment on initial neurological severity and short-term functional outcome in acute ischemic stroke patients: the Fukuoka stroke registry. Cerebrovasc Dis. 2016;42:395–403. https://doi.org/10.1159/000447788.

4

Cardiac autonomic neuropathy in type 1 and type 2 diabetes patients

Anca Moţăţăianu[1*], Smaranda Maier[1], Zoltan Bajko[1], Septimiu Voidazan[2], Rodica Bălaşa[1] and Adina Stoian[3]

Abstract

Background: Cardiac autonomic neuropathy (CAN) in diabetes is among the strongest risk markers for future global and cardiovascular mortality. The aim of this study was to analyse CAN prevalence and to compare the associations between CAN, the glycaemic control, cardiovascular risk factors, peripheral neuropathy, retinopathy and macroangiopathy in patients with type 1 (T1DM) and type 2 diabetes mellitus (T2DM).

Methods: One hundred ninety-five diabetic patients were included in this study. All patients were evaluated for detection of CAN (with standardised cardiovascular reflex tests), diabetes-related microvascular complications (polyneuropathy, retinopathy), common carotid artery intima-media thickness (IMT) and ankle-brachial index (ABI).

Results: The prevalence of CAN was 39.1% in T2DM and 61.8% in T1DM patients. Multivariate logistic regression analysis demonstrated that in T2DM, the odds [OR (95% confidence intervals)] of CAN increased with diabetes duration [1.67(1.42–1.92)], HbA1c [1.74(1.34–2.27)], cholesterol [1.01(1.00–1.01)], triglycerides [1.01(0.99–1.00)], smoking [2.35(1.23–4.49)], systolic blood pressure [1.01(1.00–1.03)], BMI [1.16(1.08–1.24)], glomerular filtration rate [0.91(0.88–0.93)], peripheral neuropathy [25.94(11.04–44.25)], retinopathy [13.13(3.03–84.73)] and IMT [10.12 (7.21–15.32)]. In T1DM, the odds of CAN increased with diabetes duration [1.62(1.13–2.31)], HbA1c [4.49(1.27–15.9)], age of patients [1.14(1.03–1.27)], glomerular filtration rate [0.94(0.89–0.99)], peripheral neuropathy [31.6(4.5–45.8)] and IMT [5.5(2.3–8.3)].

Conclusion: This study indicated that CAN is a more frequent complication in T1DM. Apart from glycaemic control, the existence of CAN is associated with potentially modifiable cardiovascular risk only in T2DM patients. The presence of other micro- and macrovascular complications increases the probability of having CAN in both types of DM (but more pronounced in T2DM).

Keywords: Cardiac autonomic neuropathy, Type 1 diabetes, Type 2 diabetes, Microvascular complication, Macrovascular complication, Cardiovascular risk factors, Glycaemic control

Background

Diabetes is a problem of major concern and has been characterised as the primary health care challenge of the twenty-first century. The prevalence of diabetes, along with its complications, has risen rapidly. Currently, type 2 diabetes mellitus (DM) is an epidemic development throughout the world. Data from the International Diabetes Federation (IDF) show that in 2015 almost 5 million patients across the world died due to diabetes and its complications. The prevalence of type 1 diabetes mellitus (T1DM) shows a rapid increase as well as the rise of type 2 diabetes mellitus (T2DM) in younger patients [1].

Cardiac autonomic neuropathy (CAN) is one of the most overlooked of all serious complications of diabetes. Although silent in the earlier stages, it is a powerful predictor of mortality risk in diabetic patients and is a major challenge for all physicians dealing with people suffering from diabetes. Patients with CAN have a five-fold increased risk of mortality due to a high-risk of cardiac arrhythmias, silent myocardial ischaemia and sudden death. The burden of DM is reflected not only in the increasing number of patients but also in the growing number of premature deaths due to diabetes [2–4].

The purpose of this study was to evaluate the CAN characteristics in T1DM versus T2DM patients and to identify the relationship between CAN, cardiovascular risk factors (CVRF) and other microvascular and

* Correspondence: motataianuanca@gmail.com
[1]Department of Neurology, University of Medicine and Pharmacy Târgu Mureş, Gh Marinescu 50, 540136 Târgu Mureş, Romania
Full list of author information is available at the end of the article

macrovascular complications. Currently, more studies are required when considering the global increase of DM in order to improve the strategies for fresh CAN prevention.

Methods

This was a cross-sectional study in which 212 consecutive inpatients with T1DM and T2DM were selected among diabetic subjects who presented to the Diabetes Department of the TirguMures University Hospital (Romania). Exclusion criteria were as follows: presence of cardiac arrhythmia, heart blockage, clinical coronary artery disease, presence of thyroid disease, presence of hypo- or hyperglycaemia in the previous 24 h, presence of acute illness, severe systemic disease, medication that affects the autonomic nervous system (anti-arrhythmic medication, antidepressants, antihistamine and sympathomimetic cough preparations), alcohol abuse, use of neurotoxic medication or malignant disease, history of diabetic ketoacidosis and other secondary causes of diabetes [3]. Based upon these exclusion criteria, 17 patients were excluded from the study group. The majority of our patients were hospitalised for periodical control, not for acute comorbidities. This study protocol was approved by the University of Medicine and Pharmacy Tirgu Mures Review Board, and all subjects gave their written informed consent.

Clinical examination was performed and stress on heart rate, systolic and diastolic blood pressure (SBP/DBP), body weight, waist circumference and body mass index (BMI) were recorded. Complete blood count and chemistry tests (including complete renal, hepatic and other metabolic testing panels) were collected in the morning after an overnight fast. Glycated haemoglobin (HbA1c) was determined by high-performance liquid chromatography with a non-diabetic reference range of 4.1–6.0. Renal function was assessed by estimated glomerular filtration rate (eGFR), which was calculated using the Modification of Diet in Renal Disease study (MDRD) formula [5].

Diabetic retinopathy was evaluated by an experienced independent ophthalmologist. Direct funduscopy was performed on dilated pupils, and the findings were classified as normal, pre-proliferative retinopathy (including maculopathy) or proliferative retinopathy. For statistical analysis, we considered those patients without retinopathy with normal funduscopy and pre-proliferative retinopathy, and patients with retinopathy with proliferative retinopathy.

Neuropathic symptoms were assessed based upon neuropathy symptom scores as previously described [6].

Peripheral nerve function was assessed using nerve conduction studies (NCS), by an electrodiagnostic protocol as recommended by the American Diabetes Association [7]. For each patient, NCS were performed bilaterally on the median, ulnar, peroneal, tibial and sural nerves according to standard techniques [8]. NCSs were performed with a four-channel electromyography (EMG) apparatus (Neuro-MEP-4, Russia) with surface electrodes. Reduced amplitudes in the motor or sensory responses less than the normal limit (mean−2 standard deviations, SD) and slowness in the motor or sensory conduction velocity less than the normal limit (mean−2 SD) were identified as abnormal values [8]. When two or more nerves were abnormal, NCS were considered abnormal according to the Mayo Clinic staging criteria [9]. The patients were classified as having subclinical peripheral neuropathy in the absence of signs or symptoms of neuropathy if they had abnormal NCS. They were classified as having confirmed peripheral neuropathy in the presence of abnormal NCS and signs or symptoms of polyneuropathy (PNP), and they were considered to have no PNP if NCS were normal with no symptoms or signs of neuropathy on clinical examination [10].

Patients were requested to avoid strenuous physical exercise in the 24 h preceding the cardiovascular testing and to avoid smoking, eating or coffee consumption for at least 2 h prior to autonomic testing. All antidiabetic and other medications were administered at the end of the examination.

Cardiovascular autonomic reflex tests were performed by one examiner early in the morning according to Ewing's method, which includes a battery of five noninvasive autonomic tests [11]. Testing of autonomic parasympathetic dysfunctions was assessed by the heart rate variability (HRV) to slow deep breathing with a rate of six breaths per minute Valsalva manoeuvring and a postural change from lying to standing. HRV was assessed from electrocardiographic recordings of R-R intervals automatically using an ELI 350 electrocardiograph system (Mortara Instrument Inc., Milwaukee, USA). For HRV to the Valsalva manoeuvring, the ratio between the longest R-R interval to the shortest R-R interval was assessed during forced exhalation into a mouthpiece of a manometer to 40 mmHg for 15 s. The HRV to postural changes was evaluated by the ratio of the longest R-R interval during beats 20–40 after standing to the shortest R-R interval during beats 5–25 after standing and HRV to deep breathing was asseseed by recording the difference between the maximum and minimum heart rates (beats/minute). These tests were performed using technique-specific normative data as previously described [12]. The test results of the deep-breathing test were interpreted according to normal age-related values [13]. Sympathetic dysfunction was assessed by measuring blood pressure response to postural change from lying to standing and to sustained handgrip. Orthostatic hypotension was defined as a reduction of systolic blood pressure of at least 20 mmHg, or diastolic blood pressure of at least 10 mmHg, within 3 min of standing. The blood pressure measurement point while standing-was at heart level. Details of these assessments of cardio-vascular autonomic function have been previously described [3]. CAN was defined as the presence of at least two abnormal standard tests [10]. The patients were divided into two groups according to the presence or absence of CAN.

The common carotid artery intima-media thickness (IMT) was assessed using ultrasonography (Siemens Accuson Antares Ultrasound System) on both bilateral common carotid arteries with a linear array 5-mHz transducer as reported previously [14]. Scanning was performed at three different longitudinal projection sites (anterior-oblique, lateral and posterior-oblique). The IMT was measured at the thickest portion of the scanning area, and at two other points: 1 cm upstream and 1 cm downstream from the site of greatest thickness. The mean of these three IMT measurements was used as the individual's IMT. We also evaluated the ankle-brachial index (ABI) with a handheld 5-mHz Doppler device (HI Dop Vascular Doppler set) in all patients.

Statistical analyses

Statistical analyses were performed using MedCalc Software (Version 12.3.0 bvba, Mariakerke, Belgium). Data were considered as nominal or quantitative variables. Nominal variables were characterized using frequencies. Quantitative variables were tested for normality of distribution using Kolmogorov-Smirnov test and were characterized by median and range or by mean and standard deviation (SD), when appropriate. A chi-square test was used in order to compare the frequencies of nominal variables. Quantitative variables were compared using t test, Mann-Whitney test, when appropriate. Multivariate analysis was carried out using linear regressions. We used as dependent variable the CAN: CAN+ code 1 vs CAN- code 0. We used the Bonferroni correction in order to account for multiple comparisons. The level of statistical significance was set at $p < 0.05$.

Results

General characteristics of study patients

Baseline characteristics of the studied patients are shown in Table 1. At the time of the study, the patients with T2DM were older than those with T1DM and had a shorter duration of diabetes, but had better glycaemic control than the T1DM patients group as reflected by HbA1c levels. Despite the better glycaemic control in T2DM, the prevalence of hypertension, BMI, triglyceride levels and abdominal obesity reflected by waist-to-hip ratios were significantly higher in T2DM patients. The incipient macrovascular complications reflected by IMT were more evident in T2DM patients than in those with

T1DM, but the prevalence of the advanced microvascular complications, clinical polyneuropathy and proliferative retinopathy were significantly higher in T1DM patients.

Comparing the study patients with and without CAN

Table 2 compares the diabetic patients with and without CAN between the T1DM and T2DM.

Of 34 patients with T1 DM, 21 (61.8%) were diagnosed with CAN. T1DM patients with CAN had a higher duration of diabetes, poorer glycaemic control as indexed by HbA1c levels, a lowere GFR, a higher prevalence of clinical polyneuropathy and proliferative retinopathy and an increased IMT than patients without CAN.

Of 161 patients with T2DM, 63 (39.1%) were diagnosed with CAN. Compared with T2DM patients without CAN, the T2DM patients with CAN were younger at the time of diabetes diagnosis and had a longer duration of diabetes, poorer glycaemic control reflected by HbA1c levels, a significantly higher BMI, a significantly higher systolic blood pressure level, higher cholesterol levels and were more frequently smokers. The prevalence of pre-proliferative retinopathy, proliferative retinopathy and clinical polyneuropathy were significantly higher in the group of T2DM patients with CAN than in those without CAN.

Logistic regression analysis

Univariate logistic regression analysis (Table 3) was performed to identify determinants of CAN in both types of DM. In T2DM patients, the odds [OR (95% confidence intervals)] of CAN increased with age at diabetes diagnosis, diabetes duration, BMI, smoking, systolic blood pressure, cholesterol level, triglyceride level, HbA1c level, increased IMT, existence of PNP and retinopathy.

For T1DM patients, the significant predictors for the existence of CAN were age of patients, diabetes duration, HbA1c, peripheral neuropathy and IMT. The traditional CVRF (hypertension, obesity, smoking, dyslipidemia) had no effect on the risk of developing CAN in T1DM patients.

Discussion

The differences between T1DM and T2DM in terms of prevalence, disease mechanism (deficiency of insulin versus insulin resistance), age of onset, typical conformation of the patient and the treatment are well known. Five percent of patients with DM have T1DM, a disease mostly seen in children and young adults, which is characterised by autoimmune destruction of beta cells with loss of insulin production. The remaining 95% patients have T2DM, a metabolic disease with high pancreatic insulin production in the setting of insulin resistance. In a recent meta-analysis, the authors concluded that the neuropathy in T1DM and T2DM are substantially

Table 1 Baseline characteristics of studied patients

Variable	DM type 1	DM type 2	p value
Patients number	34	161	
Male/Female, nr (%)	12 (35.3)/22 (64.7)	76 (47.2)/85 (52.8)	0.20[#]
Age (years)	36.7 ± 9.5	58.1 ± 8.2	0.0001**
Age at diabetes diagnosis (years)	22.2 ± 7.5	49.8 ± 9.2	0.0001**
Diabetes duration (years)	14.5 (1–27)	6 (1–37)	0.0001*
Diabetes duration			
< 5 years, nr (%)	4 (11.8)	61 (37.9)	0.01[#]
5–10 years, nr (%)	6 (17.6)	28 (17.4)	0.78[#]
11–15 years, nr (%)	10 (29.43)	54 (33.5)	0.54[#]
> 15 yers, nr (%)	14 (41.2)	18 (11.2)	0.001[#]
Body mass index (kg/m2)	22.6 ± 3.9	30.8 ± 5.3	0.001**
Systolic BP(mmHg)	123.6 ± 13.8	143.4 ± 19.6	0.001**
Diastolic BP (mmHg)	72.6 ± 10.4	81.4 ± 9.9	0.001**
Pulse pressure	51.8 ± 10.4	61.5 ± 16.1	0.001**
Hypertension (yes), nr (%)	9 (26.5)	106 (65.8)	0.001[#]
Ex-smokers, nr (%)	21 (61.8)	92 (57.1)	0.32[#]
Smokers (yes), nr (%)	13 (38.2)	69 (42.9)	0.42[#]
< 20 cigarettes/day, nr (%)	10 (71.4)	33(47.8)	0.38[#]
> 20 cigarettes/day, nr (%)	4 (28.6)	36 (52.2)	0.38[#]
Triglycerides (mg%)	142.0 (76–478)	178 (60–1100)	0.003*
HgbA1c	9.2 ± 1.3	8.3 ± 1.4	0.004**
FPG (mg%)	231.8 ± 63.5	183.9 ± 64.0	0.001**
eGFR (ml/min per 1.73 m2)	71.1 ± 24.7	75.6 ± 20.5	0.26**
PNP			
Clinical, nr (%)	22 (64.7)	68 (42.2)	0.02[#]
Subclinical, nr (%)	0 (0.0)	46 (28.6)	0.005[#]
No PNP, nr (%)	12 (35.3)	44 (29.2)	0.78[#]
Retinopathy			
Proliferative, nr (%)	8 (23.5)	10 (6.2)	0.002[#]
Preproliferative, nr (%)	12 (35.3)	49 (30.4)	0.82[#]
No retinopathy, nr (%)	14 (41.2)	102 (63.4)	0.001[#]
ABI*	1 (0.75–1.3)	0.95 (0.75–1.35)	0.32[#]
QTc	431.5 ± 37.2	426.4 ± 31.6	0.41**
IMT	0.76 ± 0.19	0.91 ± 0.19	0.001**
Waist to hip ratio	0.81 ± 0.02	0.90 ± 0.08	0.001**
Abdominal circumference	83.8 ± 9.9	104.6 ± 12.3	0.001**

Data were expressed as mean ± SD, – student t test**; median (range) - Mann Whitney test* and no (%) - chi square test[#]
CAN- cardiac autonomic neuropathy, *BP*- blood pressure, *FPG* - fasting plasma glucose, HgbA1c-glycosylated hemoglobine, *eGFR* - estimated glomerular filtration rate, *PNP*-peripheral neuropathy, *ABI*- ankle-brachial index, *IMT* - intima-media thickness, *QTc*- corrected QT interval

different complications with disparate mechanisms. Glucose control in T1DM has a large effect on prevention of neuropathy, but in T2DM, glucose control has a small effect on the prevention of neuropathy [15].

In a recent study that evaluated long-term clinical outcomes and survival in young-onset T1DM compared with T2DM at the same age at onset, the results established that the young-onset T2DM was the most lethal phenotype of diabetes because is associated with a greater mortality, more diabetic complications and unfavourable cardiovascular disease risk factors when compared to T1DM [16].

Table 2 Characteristics of the study patients according to the presence (CAN+) or absence of CAN (CAN−)

Variable	DM type 1			DM type 2		
	CAN −	CAN +	p value	CAN −	CAN +	p value
Nr (%)	13 (38.2)	21(61.8)		98 (60.9)	63 (39.1)	
Male/Female, nr (%)	5(38.5)/8 (61.5)	7 (33.3)/14 (66.7)	0.76#	47 (48.0)/51 (52.0)	29 (46.0)/34 (54.0)	0.81#
Age (years)	30.8 ± 8.2	40.3 ± 8.5	0.003**	57.4 ± 8.5	59.1 ± 7.7	0.22**
Age at diabetes diagnosis (years)	24.4 ± 7.3	20.7 ± 7.4	0.16**	53.1 ± 8.6	45.0 ± 7.9	0.0001**
DM duration (years)	7 (1–11)	22 (6–27)	0.0001*	4 (1–15)	12 (5–37)	0.0001*
DM duration						
< 5 years, nr (%)	4 (30.8)	0 (0.0)	0.02#	61 (62.2)	0 (0.0)	0.0001#
5–10 years nr (%)	8 (61.5)	2 (9.5)	0.04#	8 (8.2)	20 (31.7)	0.002#
11–15 years, nr (%)	1 (7.7)	5 (23.8)	0.52#	29 (29.6)	25 (39.7)	0.24#
> 15 years, nr (%)	0 (0.0)	14 (66.7)	0.001#	0 (0.0)	18 (28.6)	0.0001#
BMI (kg/m2)	21.1 ± 4.1	23.5 ± 3.5	0.08**	29.3 ± 4.9	33.2 ± 5.1	0.0001**
SBP (mmHg)	119.4 ± 11.3	126.3 ± 14.8	0.16**	140.6 ± 18.4	149.9 ± 20.7	0.01**
DBP (mmHg)	70.7 ± 7.2	73.9 ± 11.9	0.38**	80.9 ± 9.4	82.1 ± 10.7	0.44**
Pulse pressure	48.7 ± 8.2	53.8 ± 11.3	0.16**	59.5 ± 15.4	64.6 ± 16.5	0.04**
Hypertension (yes)	1 (7.7)	8 (38.1)	0.051#	62 (63.3)	44 (69.8)	0.39#
Nonsmokers	7 (53.8)	14 66.7)	0.45#	64 (65.3)	28 (44.4)	0.03#
Smokers	6 (46.2)	7 (33.3)	0.45#	34 (34.7)	35 (55.6)	0.02#
< 20cigarettes/day	5 (38.5)	5 (23.8)	0.5#	17 (17.3)	16 (25.4)	0.78#
> 20cigarettes/day	2 (15.4)	2 (9.5)	0.5#	17 (17.3)	19 (30.2)	0.54#
Triglycerides (mg%)	142 (76–188)	143 (78–478)	0.22*	154.5 (60–996.0)	204 (95–1100)	0.001*
Cholesterol (mg%)	170.5 ± 26.3	200.6 ± 68.3	0.14**	204.5 ± 29.1	228.7 ± 49.1	0.002**
HgbA1c	8.4 ± 0.72	9.6 ± 1.37	0.01**	7.9 ± 1.4	9.1 ± 1.2	0.001**
FPG (mg%)	229.2 ± 55.8	233.4 ± 69.2	0.85**	173.6 ± 68.2	199.7 ± 53.7	0.01**
eRFG	86.9 ± 17.4	60.7 ± 23.6	0.001**	85.6 ± 17.2	60.4 ± 14.6	0.0001**
PNP						
Clinical	3 (23.1)	19 (90.5)	0.0001#	16 (17.5)	52 (82.5)	0.0001#
Subclinical	0 (0.0)	0 (0.0)	–	40 (40.8)	6 (9.5)	0.0001#
No PNP	10 (76.9)	2 (9.5)	0.0001#	42 (42.9)	5 (7.9)	0.0001#
Retinopathy						
Proliferative	0 (0.0)	8 (38.1)	0.003#	2 (2.0)	8 (12.7)	0.002#
Preproliferative	0 (0.0)	12 (57.2)	0.001#	12 (12.2)	37 (58.7)	0.0001#
No rethinopathy	13 (100.0)	1 (4.8)	0.001#	84 (85.7)	18 (28.6)	0.0001#
ABI	1.02 (0.91–1.1)	0.92 (0.75–1.3)	0.30*	1.01 (0.78–0.14)	0.86(0.75–1.35)	0.0001*
QTc	402.8 ± 33.4	449.2 ± 27.4	0.001**	412.7 ± 27.6	447.8 ± 25.1	0.0001**
IMT	0.60 ± 0.13	0.86 ± 0.16	0.001**	0.82 ± 0.17	1.03 ± 0.15	0.0001**

Data were expressed as mean ± SD, – student t test**; median (range) - Mann Whitney test* and no (%) - chi square test#

CAN - cardiac autonomic neuropathy, BP- blood pressure, FPG - fasting plasma glucose, HgbA1c-glycosylated hemoglobine, eGFR - estimated glomerular filtration rate, PNP- peripheral neuropathy, ABI- ankle-brachial index, IMT - intima-media thickness, QTc- corrected QT interval

In T1DM, there is clear evidence for genetic predisposition but also strong evidence for an autoimmune mechanism for destruction of the beta cells leading to absolute dependence on insulin treatment. Neurons and pancreatic beta cells have a neuroectodermal origin and therefore share common antigens, especially in the early stage of evolution. Granberg et al. [17] provided epidemiological data that support the implication of autoimmunity in autonomic neuropathy in T1DM by demonstrating the existence of antibodies against the autonomic nervous system (sympathetic ganglion, vagus nerve,

Table 3 Univariate linear regression analysis: ORs and 95% CIs for CAN in T1 DM and T2 DM patients

CAN in T1DM patients			CAN in T2DM patients	
Variable	OR (CI 95%)	p-value	OR (CI 95%)	p-value
Male/Female, nr (%)	0.80 (0.18–3.37)	0.76	0.92 (0.49–1.75)	0.81
Age (years)	1.14 (1.03–1.27)	0.0009	1.02 (0.98–1.06)	0.22
Age at DM diagnosis (years)	0.93 (0.83–1.03)	0.17	0.89 (0.85–0.94)	< 0.0001
DM duration (years)*	1.62 (1.13–2.31)	0.0007	1.67 (1.42–1.92)	0.0001
BMI (kg/m2)	1.19 (0.96–1.48)	0.09	1.16 (1.08–1.24)	0.0003
SBP (mmHg)	1.04 (0.98–1.10)	0.16	1.01 (1.00–1.03)	0.02
DBP(mmHg)	1.01 (0.96–1.10)	0.38	1.004 (0.97–1.03)	0.44
Hypertension (yes)	7.38 (0.80–68.1)	0.07	1.34 (0.68–2.68)	0.39
Smoking (yes vs. no)	0.62 (0.15–2.61)	0.52	2.35 (1.23–4.49)	0.0009
Cholesterol (mg%)	1.01 (0.98–1.04)	0.14	1.01 (1.00–1.01)	0.004
Triglyceride (mg%)	1.01 (0.99–1.02)	0.16	1.00 (0.99–1.00)	0.03
HgbA1c	4.49 (1.27–15.9)	0.01	1.74 (1.34–2.27)	< 0.0001
FPG (mg%)	1.01 (0.99–1.01)	0.85	1.00 (1.00–1.01)	0.01
eRFG (ml/min/1.73 m2)	0.94 (0.89–0.99)	0.007	0.91 (0.88–0.93)	< 0.0001
ABI	1.13 (0.01–76.01)	0.95	0.01 (0.00–0.20)	0.001
QTc	1.05 (1.01–1.1)	0.007	1.20 (1.03–1.07)	< 0.0001
IMT	5.5 (2.3–8.3)	0.007	10.12 (7.21–15.32)	< 0.0001
RD (yes vs no)	1.25 (0.56–1.9)	0.88	13.13 (3.03–84.73)	0.002
PNP (yes vs no)	31.6 (4.5–45.8)	0.001	25.94 (11.04–44.25)	0.0001

BP- blood pressure, FPG - fasting plasma glucose, HgbA1c-glycosylated hemoglobine, eGFR - estimated glomerular filtration rate, PNP- peripheral neuropathy, ABI- ankle-brachial index, IMT - intima-media thickness, QTc- corrected QT interval, *- median range

adrenal medulla) in T1DM patients with autonomic neuropathy.

In our study, poor glycaemic control and the long duration of diabetes were the key risk factors for developing CAN in either T1DM or T2DM. We found that the patients with T1DM have a longer duration of diabetes compared with T2DM patients (22 vs 12.5 years). This difference can be explained by the fact that the patients with T2DM often have a history of many years without symptoms during which blood glucose peaks occur unnoticed, but diabetes is not yet diagnosed and treated. So, in T2DM, the diabetes complications may exist at the time of initial presentation, but in T1DM, there is likely to be a window between initial diagnosis and the onset of organ damage [18].

Poor glycaemic control is a major risk factor for the development and progression of CAN in both types of DM. In our study, poor glycaemic control was associated with the increased risk of having CAN. This result suggests that glycaemic control is a more important driver of cardiac autonomic dysfunction in T1DM than in T2DM. Brownlee [19] demonstrated that the high blood glucose level in the past determined the risk for later diabetic complication. Due to the asymptomatic period in T2DM with inadequate control of hyperglycaemia before the establishment of the diagnosis, further diabetic

complications will occur later despite the optimal glycaemic control. This phenomenon is called 'hyperglycaemic or metabolic memory', and it is responsible for the initial damage that occurs very early on, even before diabetes has been initially diagnosed. Because we evaluated glycaemic control by HbA1c levels, which reflects the average blood glucose level over the past 3 months, a possible explanation of the differences in OR between T1DM and T2DM patients could be not that our T2DM patients have better glycaemic control in the past 3 months, but a history of 'silent' and untreated hyperglycaemia, which plays a major role in hyperglycemia-induced late complications of T2DM.

The Action to Control Cardiovascular Risk in Diabetes (ACCORD) study on 10,251 participants demonstrated that in the patients with T2DM and high cardiovascular risk or preexisting cardiovascular and microvascular damage, the mortality rate was increased in the arm receiving intensive treatment with forced HbA1c reduction. Also, the ACCORD study demonstrated that neuropathies (somatic and autonomic) are significant risk factors for cardiovascular disease, and this particular group of patients represents a high-risk group in which intensive glucose control should be well-balanced against the mortality risk [20, 21]. The basic approach for living with DM and having as few complications as possible is to start treatment immediately after onset of the diabetes with the purpose of achieving metabolic control as much as possible. The actual trend throughout the world is to restrict the prognostic perspective of diabetes to the HbA1c value, but this is not justified by the complex mechanism implicated in vascular complications of DM.

In T1DM, two important epidemiological studies, Diabetes Control and Complications Trial (DCCT) and Epidemiology of Diabetes Interventions and Complications study (EDIC), demonstrated that early intensive glycaemic control can decrease the incidence of CAN, and this protective effect persisted for more than 14 years after the end of the study despite the disappearance of intensive glycaemic control [22, 23]. In a recent Cochrane meta-analysis, it was demonstrated that enhanced glucose control significantly prevents the development of clinical neuropathy only in T1DM [24].

In T2DM, the effect of glycaemic control was not so evident. The United Kingdom Prospective Diabetes Study (UKPDS) on 3867 recently diagnosed T2DM patients demonstrated that at 10 years from inclusion in the study, there were no differences on developing neuropathy between the group with intensive glycaemic control versusthe group with conventional glycaemic control, irrespective of other CVRF. In other studies that followed the UKPDS study (the VA Cooperative study, Duckworth study and Steno-2 study), intensive glycaemic control resulted in a small decrease in diabetic neuropathy incidence, suggesting that in T2DM, factors that are independent from glycaemic control are responsible for the damage of somatic and autonomic nervous system. In the Steno-2 study, there was clear evidence that intensive pharmacological treatment targeting hypertension, hyperlipidemia and microalbuminuria combined with lifestyle changes (diet, smoking cessation and physical exercise) reduced the risk of autonomic neuropathy over the course of almost 8 years of follow-up [25–28].

In the present study, we found that among T2DM patients, the odds of CAN increased with the existence of traditional CVRF (hypertension, smoking, obesity, higher cholesterol level), but CVRF had no effect on cardiac autonomic dysfunction in T1DM patients. Smoking was associated with increased odds of CAN among T2DM patients in our study, but there was no significant association between smoking and CAN in T1DM patients. Although there are no data to explain the effect of smoking on autonomic function in T2DM patients, the studies performed on the non-diabetic population demonstrated that smoking is associated with autonomic dysfunction related to increased oxidative stress and increased inflammatory activity [29].

Our results confirm that in T2DM when CVRF are associated with poor glycaemic control, the risk of developing CAN increased. In order prevent or to slow the progression of CAN, improving glycaemic control, lifestyle changes and cardiovascular risk factor management are the mainstays of treatment,but in T1DM patients, our results are not in accordance with previous studies that demonstrated the associations between CAN and CVRF [30, 31]. This observed difference between T1DM and T2DM patients can be explained by (a) implication of hyperglycaemia and autoimmune mechanisms in developing CAN in T1DM and of hyperglycaemia and CVRF in developing CAN in T2DM or (b) because of the small number of T1DM patients in our study, which can be accepted as a limitation.

In the group of T1DM and T2DM patients, the risk for developing CAN increased in the presence of peripheral neuropathy, retinopathy and accelerated atherosclerosis (reflected by increased IMT and decreased ABI). These associations between cardiac autonomic dysfunction and micro- and macrovascular complications were more evident in T2DM. Microvascular complications of DM share a common pathogenetic factor with atherosclerosis represented by functional disturbances in the vascular endothelium induced by hyperglycaemia and increased oxidative stress. Endothelial dysfunction is considered to be an early stage and precursor of atherosclerosis. Our results are consistent with previous data from Yokoyama and coworkers [32], who reported a positive relationship between diabetic neuropathy (including autonomic neuropathy), increased IMT and arterial stiffness assessed by brachial-ankle pulse wave velocity in T2DM patients. In previous DDCT and EDIC studies on T1DM patients, it was demonstrated that microvascular complication per se conferred an independent risk for macrovascular disease [33, 34].

Conclusions

As the incidence of diabetes rises, so too does the requirement for healthcare, and in order to prevent CAN in patients with T1DM, we must focus on glycaemic control, but in T2DM we should focus not only on glycaemic control but also on improving adherence to cardiovascular risk factor intervention. In T2DM patients, enhanced glycaemic control can delay development of CAN but increase the risk of severe hypoglycaemic episodes, which need to be taken into account when evaluating the risk/benefits ratio. There is a need for further studies to discover the optimal level of glycaemic control in order to reduce the development of CAN without increasing the risk of death.

Abbreviations
ABI: ankle-brachial index; ACCORD: The Action to Control Cardiovascular Risk in Diabetes; BMI: body mass index; CAN: cardiac autonomic neuropathy; CVRF: cardiovascular risk factors; DBP: diastolic blood pressure; DCCT: Diabetes Control and Complications Trial; EDIC: Epidemiology of Diabetes Interventions and Complications; eGFR: estimated glomerular filtration rate; EMG: electromyography; FPG: fasting plasma glucose;

HbA1c: glycated haemoglobin; HRV: heart rate variability; IMT: intima-media thickness; MDRD: Modification of Diet in Renal Disease study; NCS: nerve conduction studies; PNP: polyneuropathy; QTc: corrected QT interval; SBP: systolic blood pressure; SD: standard deviations; T1DM: type 1 diabetes mellitus; T2DM: type 2 diabetes mellitus; UKPDS: The United Kingdom Prospective Diabetes

Funding
This study was supported by the internal research grant of UMF Tîrgu-Mureş 18/23.12.2014.

Authors' contributions
AM, AS, RB designed the study. AM, SV, SM, ZB collected and analyzed the data. AM, ZB, SV, SM drafted and wrote the manuscript. RB, AS revised the manuscript critically for intellectual content. All authors read and approved the final version of the manuscript.

Competing interest
The authors declare that they have no competing interests.

Consent for publication
A written consent form was obtained from all participants for potentially publishing their clinical data while protecting their personal information.

Author details
[1]Department of Neurology, University of Medicine and Pharmacy Târgu Mureş, Gh Marinescu 50, 540136 Târgu Mureş, Romania. [2]Department of Epidemiology, University of Medicine and Pharmacy Târgu Mureş, Târgu Mureş, Romania. [3]Department of Pathophysiology, University of Medicine and Pharmacy Târgu Mureş, Târgu Mureş, Romania.

References

1. Ogurtsova K, da Rocha Fernandes JD, Huang Y, Linnenkamp U, Guariguata L, Cho NH, et al. IDF diabetes atlas: global estimates for the prevalence of diabetes for 2015 and 2040. Diabetes Res Clin Pract. 2017;128:40–50.
2. Vinik AI, Erbas T, Casellini CM. Diabetic cardiac autonomic neuropathy, inflammation and cardiovascular disease. J Diabetes Investig. 2013;4:4–18.
3. Vinik AI, Maser RE, Mitchell BD, et al. Diabetic autonomic neuropathy. Diabetes Care. 2003;26:1553–79.
4. What PBR. Do we know and what we do not know about cardiovascular autonomic neuropathy in diabetes. J of Cardiovasc Trans Res. 2012;5:463–78.
5. Levey AS, Eckardt KU, Tsukamoto Y, Levin A, Coresh J, Rossert J, De Zeeuw D, Hostetter TH, Lameire N, Eknoyan G. Definition and classification of chronic kidney disease: a position statement from kidney disease: improving global outcomes (KDIGO). Kidney Int. 2005;67:2089–100.
6. Meijer JW, Smit AJ, Sonderen EV, Groothoff JW, Eisma WH, Links TP. Symptom scoring systems to diagnose distal polyneuropathy in diabetes: the diabetic neuropathy symptom score. Diabet Med. 2002;19:962–5.
7. American Diabetes Association American Academy of Neurology. Consensus statement: report and recommendations of the San Antonio conference on diabetic neuropathy. Diabetes Care. 1988;11:592–7.
8. Kimura J. Anatomy and physiology of the peripheral nerve. In: Kimura J, editor. Electrodiagnosis in diseases of the nerve and muscle:principles and practice. New York: OxfordUniversity Press; 2013. p. 47–73.
9. Dyck PJ. Detection, characterization, and staging of polyneuropathy: assessed in diabetics. Muscle Nerve. 1988;11:21–32.
10. Tesfaye S, Boulton AJ, Dyck PJ, Freeman R, Horowitz M, Kempler P, Lauria G, Malik RA, Spallone V, Vinik A, Bernardi L, Valensi P, Toronto Diabetic Neuropathy Expert Group. Diabetic neuropathies: update on definitions, diagnostic criteria, estimation of severity, and treatments. Diabetes Care. 2010;33:2285–93.
11. Ewing DJ, Martyn CN, Young RJ, Clarke BF. The value of cardiovascular autonomic function tests: 10 years experience in diabetes. Diabetes Care. 1985;8:491–8.
12. Spallone V, Ziegler D, Freeman R, Bernardi L, Frontoni S, Pop-Busui R, Stevens M, Kempler P, Hilsted J, Tesfaye S, Low P, Valensi P. On behalf of the Toronto consensus panel of diabetic neuropathy. Cardiovascular

autonomic neuropathy in diabetes: clinical impact, assessment, diagnosis, and management. Diabetes Metab Res Rev. 2011;27:639–53.
13. Ziegler D, Laux G, Dannehl K, Spuler M, Muhlen H, Mayer P, Gries FA. Assessment of cardiovascular autonomic function: age-related normal ranges and reproducibility of spectral analysis, vector analysis, and standard tests of heart rate variation and blood pressure responses. Diabet Med. 1992;9:166–75.
14. Wendelhag I, Gustavsson T, Suurkula M, et al. Ultrasound measurement of wall thickness in the carotid artery: fundamental principles and description of computerized image analyzing system. Clin Physiol. 1991;11:565–77.
15. Callaghan BC, Hur J, Feldman EL. Diabetic neuropathy: one disease or two. Curr Opin Neurol. 2012;25:536–41.
16. Constantino MI, Molyneaux L, Limacher-Gisler F, et al. Long-term complications and mortality in young-onset diabetes- type 2 is more hazardous and lethal than type 1 diabetes. Diabetes Care. 2013;36:3863–9.
17. Granberg V, Ejskjaer N, Peakman M, et al. Autoantibodies to autonomic nerves associated with cardiac and peripheral autonomic neuropathy. Diabetes Care. 2005;28:1959–64.
18. Hammes HP. Diabetic nerve, vascular and organ damage from the pathogenetic key to new therapeutic approaches. In: Rett K, editor. Better chances for nerves and vessels. Stuttgart: Georg Thieme Verlag KG; 2011. p. 9–19.
19. Brownlee M. Diabetic complications: pathobiology of hyperglycemic damage and potential impact on treatment. In: Thornalley PJ, Kempler P, editors. Complications of diabetes mellitus: pathophysiology and pathogenetically-based treatment options. Stuttgart: Georg Thieme Verlag KG; 2009. p. 1–8.
20. Calles-Escandon J, Lovato LC, Simons-Morton DG, et al. Effect of intensive compared with standard glycemia treatment strategies on mortality by baseline subgroup characteristics: the action to control cardiovascular risk in diabetes (ACCORD) trial. Diabetes Care. 2010;33:721–7.
21. Pop-Busui R, Evans GW, Gerstein HC, et al. Effects of cardiac autonomic dysfunction on mortality risk in the action to control cardiovascular risk in diabetes (ACCORD) trial. Diabetes Care. 2010;33:1578–84.
22. DCCT Research Group. The effect of intensive diabetes therapy on measures of autonomic nervous system function in the diabetes control and complications trial (DCCT). Diabetologia. 1998;41:416–23.
23. Pop-Busui R, Low PA, Waberski BH, et al. Effects of prior intensive insulin therapy on cardiac autonomic nervous system function in type 1 diabetes mellitus: the diabetes control and complications trial/epidemiology of diabetes interventions and complications study (DCCT/EDIC). Circulation. 2009;119:2886–93.
24. Callaghan B, Littlle AA, Feldman EL, et al. Enhanced glucose control for preventing and treating diabetic neuropathy. Cochrane Database Syst Rev. 2012;6:CD007543.
25. UK Prospective Diabetes Study (UKPDS) Group. Intensive blood-glucose control with sulphonylureas or insulin compared with conventional treatment and risk of complication in patients with type 2 diabetes (UKPDS 33). Lancet. 1998;352:837–53.
26. Gaede P, Vedel P, Larsen GV, et al. Multifactorial intervention and cardiovascular disease in patients with type 2 diabetes. N Engl J Med. 2003; 348:383–93.
27. Azad N, Emanuele NV, Abraira C, et al. The effects of intensive glycemic control on neuropathy in the VA cooperative study on type II diabetes mellitus. J Diabetes Complicat. 1999;13:307–13.
28. Duckworth W, Abraira C, Moritz T, et al. Glucose control and vascular complications in veterans with type 2 diabetes. N Engl J Med. 2009;360: 129–39.
29. Shinozaki N, Yuasa T, Takata S. Cigarette smoking augments sympathetic nerve activity in patients with coronary heart disease. Int Heart J. 2008;49:261–72.
30. Tesfaye S, Chaturvedi N, Eaton SE, et al. Vascular risk factors and diabetic neuropathy. N Engl J Med. 2005;352:341–50.
31. Voulgari C, Psallas M, Kokkinos A. The association between cardiac autonomic neuropathy with metabolic and other factors in subjects with type 1 and type 2 diabetes. J Diabetes Complicat. 2011;25:159–67.
32. Yokoyama H, Yokota Y, Tada J, Kanno S. Diabetic neuropathy is closely associated with arterial stiffening and thickness in type 2 diabetes. Diabet Med. 2007;24:1329–35.
33. Anonymus. Effect of intensive diabetes management on macrovascular events and risk factors in the diabetes control and complications trial. Am J Cardiol. 1995;75:894–903.

5

Hyperuricemia and dementia – a case-control study

Bettina Engel[1,2], Willy Gomm[3], Karl Broich[4], Wolfgang Maier[3,5], Klaus Weckbecker[1] and Britta Haenisch[3,4,6*] (iD)

Abstract

Background: There is evidence that uric acid may have antioxidant and neuroprotective effects and might therefore alter the risk for neurodegenerative diseases such as dementia. So far, the relation between serum uric acid (SUA) levels or hyperuricemia and dementia remains elusive. Most studies focused on the disease or SUA levels. Effects of anti-hyperuricemic treatment have not been considered yet. This study investigated the association between hyperuricemia and dementia taking into account anti-hyperuricemic treatment.

Methods: We used longitudinal German public health insurance data and analyzed the association between hyperuricemia with and without different treatment options and dementia in a case-control design. Applying logistic regression the analysis was adjusted for several potential confounders including various comorbidities and polypharmacy.

Results: We identified 27,528 cases and 110,112 matched controls of which 22% had a diagnosis of hyperuricemia or gout and 17% received anti-hyperuricemic drugs. For patients with a diagnosis of hyperuricemia we found a slightly reduced risk for dementia (adjusted odds ratio [OR] 0.94, 95% confidence interval [CI] 0.89 to 0.98). The risk reduction was more pronounced for patients treated with anti-hyperuricemic drugs (adjusted OR 0.89, 95% CI 0.85 to 0.94, for regular treatment).

Conclusions: Our results showed a slight reduction for dementia risk in patients with hyperuricemia, both with and without anti-hyperuricemic treatment.

Keywords: Epidemiology, Gout, Hyperuricemia, Treatment, Dementia

Background

Hyperuricemia and dementia are both well-known and common diseases. Alzheimer's disease (AD) is the most common cause of dementia; vascular dementia is very common in older individuals with dementia, often occurring in mixed dementia pathologies together with AD [1]. Although the exact biological mechanisms by which neuronal damage in dementia takes place are still not fully understood, there are risk factors that have been shown to potentially alter dementia risk [1]. Stroke and metabolic syndrome have been detected as risk factors for vascular and all-cause dementia [2, 3]. Gout and hyperuricemia have previously been found to be associated with metabolic syndrome and cardiovascular diseases

[4, 5]. Therefore, patients with gout or hyperuricemia might have a modified- maybe higher- risk of dementia. On the contrary, uric acid has antioxidant properties and could therefore exert potentially neuroprotective effects [6, 7]. Evidence suggests that gout is associated with a lower risk for Parkinson's disease (PD) [8–10]. The exact underlying mechanism by which uric acid protects against PD is still unclear, but it has been hypothesized that uric acid may ameliorate oxidative stress, a pathogenic pathway in PD [11], as well as in other neurodegenerative diseases such as dementia [12]. Indeed, previous studies detected that serum uric acid (SUA) levels in patients with mild cognitive impairment or AD are lower compared to healthy controls [13, 14]. However, studies on the association of SUA levels with cognitive decline or dementia are conflicting [15]. A cohort study by Euser et al. revealed that higher SUA levels are associated with a better cognitive function in late life and a decreased risk of dementia

* Correspondence: britta.haenisch@bfarm.de
[3]German Center for Neurodegenerative Diseases (DZNE), Bonn, Germany
[4]Federal Institute for Drugs and Medical Devices (BfArM),
Kurt-Georg-Kiesinger-Allee 3, D-53175 Bonn, Germany
Full list of author information is available at the end of the article

[16]. A recent study by Latourte et al. detected a higher risk for AD and vascular or mixed dementia with high SUA levels [17]. However, Latourte et al. excluded patients receiving urate-lowering treatments so they calculated the association within normal SUA level ranges while Euser et al. did not exclude gout or hyperuricemia patients. Another limitation of both studies is that SUA level was assessed only at baseline and up to 12 years before dementia was diagnosed. Furthermore, the sample size of cohort data studies is generally small, limiting the generalizability of the results. Currently, only two studies examined the connection between gout or hyperuricemia and dementia on a population-based level: one study involved claims data from Taiwan, examining the effect on vascular and non-vascular dementia, the other one is based on computerized medical records from general practitioners in the UK and was restricted to Alzheimer's disease as the outcome parameter [18, 19]. None of the previous studies included the effects of different anti-hyperuricemic treatment. In the present study, we use a large longitudinal German claims dataset and apply a matched case-control design to evaluate the effect of hyperuricemia on the risk of incident any dementia. To increase generalizability and assess an unselected patient population we include patients who did or did not receive anti-hyperuricemic drugs. We further differentiate between occasional and intensive treatment with anti-hyperuricemic drugs.

Methods
Data source and study design
A longitudinal sample of the largest German statutory health insurance, Allgemeine Ortskrankenkasse (AOK), was used to conduct case-control analyses. The AOK covers about 50% of the German population at least 80 years old and one third of the total population at least 50 years old [20]. The AOK data set includes the ambulatory as well as the hospital sector of the health care system. The ambulatory sector is an important source of medical care as it consists of a network of ambulatory primary and specialist care professionals.

The data include information on basic demographics like age and gender, as well as inpatient and outpatient diagnoses (coded by the International Classification of Diseases-10, ICD-10) and filled drug prescriptions (categorized according to the Anatomical-Therapeutic-Chemical classification system, ATC code). Data are compiled on a quarterly basis for the years 2004–2013. As a baseline interval where initially no dementia was claimed we used the year 2004 in the data set. A lag time of two years before the first valid diagnosis of dementia was introduced. The index date is the first valid dementia diagnosis. The observation time is defined from study start until begin of the lag time before index date. The minimal

follow-up time is three years (one year minimal observation time plus two years lag time).

Dementia diagnosis and case-control matching
Patients aged 60 years or older were included. Cases were defined as patients who had a dementia diagnosis in at least 75% of all quarters after the first valid diagnosis within the study period and had no data inconsistencies (missing birthdate, date of death before start of study, different gender in different years). The following ICD-10 codes for dementia were used: G30 (Alzheimer's disease), F00 (Dementia in Alzheimer's disease), F01 (Vascular dementia), F02 (Dementia in other diseases), F03 (Unspecified dementia), F05.1 (Delirium superimposed on dementia), G31.1 (Senile degeneration of brain), G31.82 (Lewy bodies dementia), and G31.9 (Degenerative disease of nervous system, unspecified). We considered diagnoses as valid if they were hospital diagnoses or reported as verified by the physician for the outpatient sector. Patients were excluded if they had less than three years of follow-up in the study, if they had any dementia diagnosis in the baseline interval (year 2004), or if they had less than 75% of all quarters after the index quarter with a valid dementia diagnosis. Cases were matched to four controls without replacement on age (± one year) at study begin and gender. Matched cases and controls have the same study begin and index date; thus, all patients have the same follow-up time in each match group.

Hyperuricemia/gout diagnosis
Cases and controls were categorized into six groups according to hyperuricemia/ gout diagnoses (ICD-10: E79, M10, M11.8, M11.9) and use of anti-hyperuricemic drugs (ATC codes: M04AA01, M04AA02, M04AA03, M04AA51, M04AB01, M04AB02, M04AB03, M04AB04, M04AX01, M04AX02, V03AF07). As the aim of our study was to show the correlation between hyperuricemia and dementia, we did not differentiate gout and hyperuricemia. The diagnosis gout implicates hyperuricemia. Drug use was separated into two categories: occasional use defined as one to three quarters, and intensive use: four and more quarters with prescriptions in the observation time. Combining the status of hyperuricemia diagnosis and drug use led to the following six groups. The reference category was no diagnosis and no drug use. The exposed groups were: no diagnosis with occasional drug use, no diagnosis with intensive drug use, diagnosis but no drug use, diagnosis with occasional drug use, and diagnosis with intensive drug use.

Statistical analyses
We adjusted the analysis for the following potential confounders: age, gender, polypharmacy (defined as five or more drug prescriptions besides anti-hyperuricemic

drugs) and the comorbidities depression (ICD-10: F32-F34, F38, F39), stroke (ICD-10: I63, I64, I69.3, I69.4, G45), ischemic heart disease (ICD-10: I20-I25), other cerebrovascular diseases (ICD-10: I65-I67,I69.8), diabetes (ICD-10: E10-E14, E89.1), polyarthritis (ICD-10: M05-M09), atherosclerosis (ICD-10: I70), hypertension (ICD-10: I10-I13, I15), renal impairment (ICD-10: N18, N19) and hyperlipidemia (ICD-10: E78.0-E78.5, E78.8, E78.9). The covariates were selected based on existing evidence and previous publications on the topic of dementia risk and gout diagnoses [18, 20–22]. We considered comorbidity as present if it was reported in at least one quarter during the observation time, and in at least two quarters during the study time.

We examined the effect of hyperuricemia diagnosis and drug use status on incident any dementia using a multinomial variable including the following values 0: reference category with no diagnosis and no drug use, 1: no diagnosis with occasional drug use, 2: no diagnosis with intensive drug use, 3: diagnosis without any drug use, 4: diagnosis with occasional drug use, 5: diagnosis with intensive drug use. Conditional logistic regression was applied. The match groups were used as strata. The dependent variable was the occurrence of incident any dementia. The analysis was adjusted for potential confounding factors as described above. We applied backward selection to remove variables with non-significant effects on the outcome. All calculations were done using SAS 9.3 for Windows. We considered $p < 0.05$ (two tailed) to be statistically significant.

Results

Sample characteristics

We identified 33,331 persons aged 60 years or older at the beginning of the study period in 2004 with no dementia at baseline, a valid dementia diagnosis afterwards, and at least three years of follow-up. Of these, 5803 were excluded after filtering for quality control criteria (see Fig. 1). In total, we included 137,640 patients, 27,528 cases and 110,112 controls in our study (Table 1). The overall mean age of these patients in 2004 was 73.9 (±6.5) years; 63% were female, 37% were male patients (Table 1).The mean age at first dementia diagnosis was 80.9 (±6.3) years.

Anti-hyperuricemic drugs

In our sample, we detected 23,370 patients with a prescription of anti-hyperuricemic drugs. Allopurinol was by far the most frequently prescribed drug (98.4%), followed by Benzbromarone (1.8%), Allopurinol combinations (1.3%), Febuxostat (0.2%), Probenecid (0.06%), and Rasburicase (0.01%; including multiple different

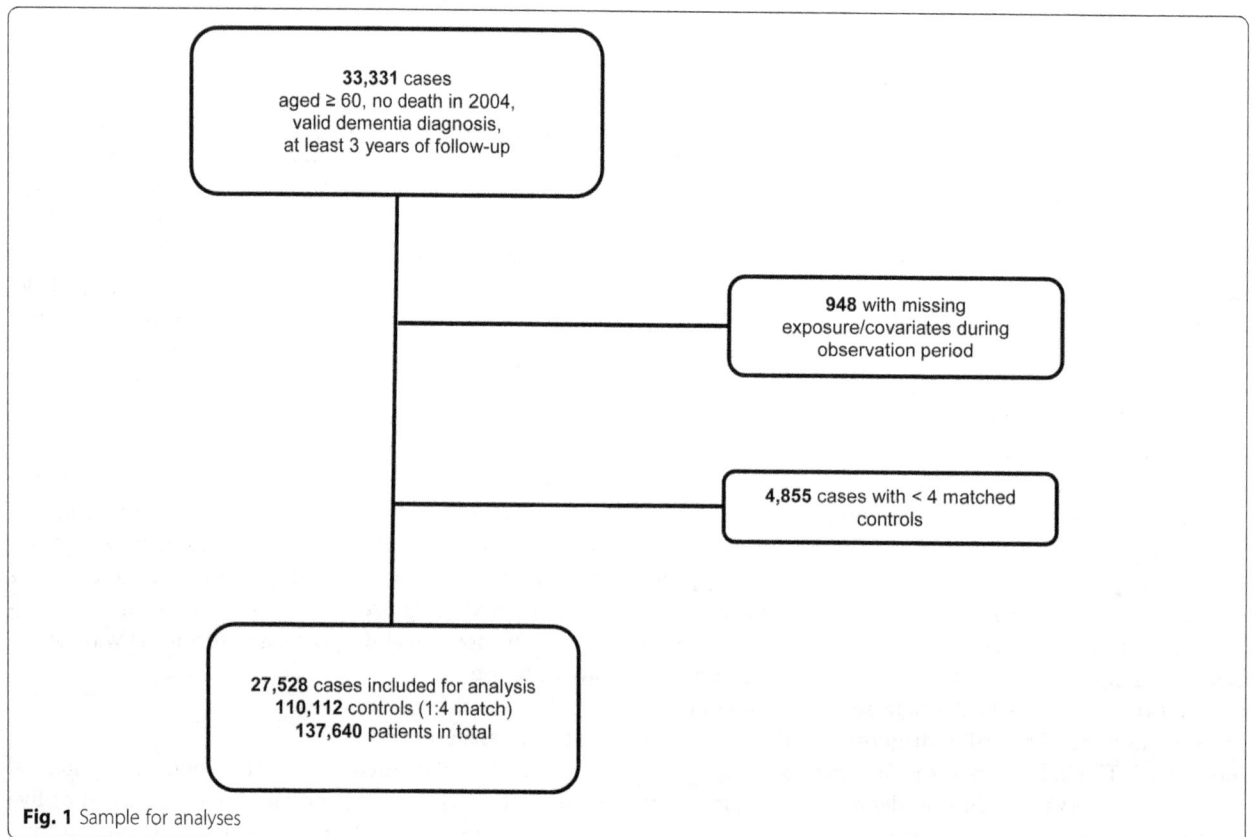

Fig. 1 Sample for analyses

Table 1 Descriptive results

	N (% from 137,640)	Cases (% from 27,528)	Controls (% from 110,112)
Female	86,910 (63.1)	17,382 (63.1)	69,528 (63.1)
Male	50,730 (36.9)	10,146 (36.9)	40,584 (36.9)
Mean age in 2004 (SD)	73.9 (6.5)	74.0 (6.5)	73.9 (6.5)

prescriptions at a time). We analyzed the daily prescribed dose of Allopurinol (DDD 0.4 g/d, 90d/quarter). 35.5% of patients received 300 mg/d, another 35.7% less than 200 mg/d, 12.1% 200–300 mg/d, and 16.8% received more than 300 mg/d allopurinol (see Table 2).

Association between hyperuricemia and dementia

After grouping the cases in six categories according to hyperuricemia/gout diagnosis and use of any anti-hyperuricemic drugs as described in material and methods we found 2379 patients (8.6% of all cases; Table 3) with the diagnosis of any type dementia and the diagnosis of hyperuricemia or gout as well as at least four quarters with a prescription of anti-hyperuricemic drugs (intensive drug use). 1168 patients (4.2% of all cases; Table 3) had the diagnosis of hyperuricemia or gout, but received anti-hyperuricemic drugs in less than four quarters (occasional drug use). 2590 patients (9.4% of all cases; Table 3) had the diagnosis of hyperuricemia or gout but received no anti-hyperuricemic drugs. Another group included patients without a diagnosis of hyperuricemia or gout and intensive ($n = 558$; Table 3) or occasional ($n = 629$; Table 3) anti-hyperuricemic drug use. The category of patients with neither diagnosis of hyperuricemia or gout nor anti-hyperuricemic therapy ($n = 20,204$, 73.4% of all cases; Table 3) represented the cases within our reference group.

Patients with a diagnosis of hyperuricemia or gout (D:1) without and with anti-hyperuricemic therapy have a slight, but significant reduced risk for incident any dementia. This finding is consistent for no drug use (OR 0.94 [CI 0.89–0.98]; Table 2), for occasional (T:1 < =qu < 4: OR 0.89 [CI 0.83–0.95]; Table 2) as well as intensive anti-hyperuricemic drug use (T:qu ≥ 4: OR 0.89 [0.85–0.94];

Table 2 Dose categories for allopurinol prescriptions

Daily Dose Allopurinol (mg) (DDD 0.4 g/d, 90d/quarter)	%
< 200	35.7
200–300	12.1
300	35.5
300–400	12.7
400–600	3.7
> 600	0.4

Table 2). Patients with no diagnosis of hyperuricemia or gout, but with anti-hyperuricemic drug prescription showed no significant risk reduction, neither for occasional (OR 0.93 [0.85–1.02]) nor for intensive anti-hyperuricemic drug use (OR 0.95 [0.86–1.04], Table 2).

Our analysis was adjusted for potential confounders as shown in Table 4. Of the included covariates, we detected the highest risk increase for incident any dementia with stroke, depression, cerebrovascular diseases, and diabetes (OR 1.53 [CI 1.47–1.59], OR 1.50 [CI 1.46–1.55], OR 1.32 [CI 1.27–1.37], and OR 1.29 [CI 1.25–1.33], respectively; Table 4). Polypharmacy (OR 1.15 [CI 1.11–1.19]) and renal impairment (OR 1.11 [CI 1.06–1.15]) also increased dementia risk (see Table 4). The use of anti-hyperuricemic drugs (OR 0.94 [CI 0.90–0.99]), hyperuricemia (OR 0.94 [CI 0.90–0.98]), hyperlipidemia (OR 0.87 [CI 0.84–0.89]), and hypertension (OR 0.92 [CI 0.89–0.96]) slightly decreased dementia risk (see Table 3). Two covariates (atherosclerosis and polyarthritis) were removed by backward selection with $p \geq 0.05$.

Discussion

Our results showed a slight reduction for dementia risk in patients with a diagnosis of hyperuricemia or gout and occasional or intensive anti-hyperuricemic treatment. This category of patients is supposed to have the highest uric acid levels because the disease requires treatment. Similarly, patients with a hyperuricemia or gout diagnosis, but without treatment also displayed a reduced risk for dementia. The groups of patients without a particular hyperuricemia or gout diagnosis, but with occasional or intensive anti-hyperuricemic drug prescription, showed no significantly reduced dementia risk.

In theory, the prescription of anti-hyperuricemic drugs should correlate with the diagnosis of gout or hyperuricemia. Giersiepen et al. used German statutory health insurance data and showed a correlation of anti-hyperuricemic drug prescription in 27.7% of patients with gout diagnosis and in a further 16.2% of patients with hyperuricemia after three years of prescription of anti-hyperuricemic drugs [23]. This displays a considerable amount of under-documentation of hyperuricemia or gout in Germany, similar to other countries [24, 25].

Uric acid is the pathogenic factor for the development of gout. Hyperuricemia can lead to gout that is characterized by deposition of urate crystals, mostly in joints, connective tissue and kidneys. The aim of gout treatment is to reduce the uric acid level (below the solubility product of 6.5 mg/dl) [26]. Different anti-hyperuricemic drugs are available. The most common drug used is Allopurinol [27]. Our study showed that Allopurinol accounts for 98% of all anti-hyperuricemic drug prescriptions. Further anti-hyperuricemic drug prescriptions are for Benzbromarone, Febuxostat, Rasburicase and Probenecid

Table 3 Association between gout or hyperuricemia and dementia, different treatment/diagnosis groups

Diagnosis (hyperuricemia or gout), Treatment regimen (antihyperuricemic drug use)[a]	Controls (n=110,112) (% from 137,640)	Cases (n=27,528) (% from 137,640)	OR (95% CI), adjusted	p-value, adjusted for covariates
D:0, T:0	81,091 (58.9)	20,204 (14.7)	Ref	
D:0, T:1 < =qu < 4	2445 (1.8)	629 (0.5)	0.93 (0.85,1.02)	0.11
D:0, T:qu > =4	2084 (1.5)	558 (0.4)	0.95 (0.86,1.04)	0.26
D:1, T:0	10,385 (7.6)	2590 (1.9)	0.94 (0.89,0.98)	0.0065
D:1, T:1 < =qu < 4	4718 (3.4)	1168 (0.9)	0.89 (0.83,0.95)	< 0.001
D:1, T:qu > =4	9389 (6.8)	2379 (1.7)	0.89 (0.85,0.94)	< 0.001

Global test: Wald X^2 = 2403.13, DF = 14, $p < 0.001$
[a]Treatment: T:0 means no anti-hyperuricemic treatment, qu > =x: means x or more quarters with treatment in the observation period, D:0 means no hyperuricamia diagnosis

as described in the results. In our study we calculated that 47.8% of patients received less than 300 mg/d Allopurinol, and 35.5% received 300 mg/d. As described in other studies, about 300 mg/d of the anti-hyperuricemic drug Allopurinol is needed to reach the SUA target level [28, 29]. However, some studies showed that patients requiring anti-hyperuricemic treatment often receive insufficient dosage of anti-hyperuricemic drugs (e.g. < 300 mg/d Allopurinol) [28, 29]. This suggests that a large proportion of patients requiring treatment in our study presumably displays SUA levels which are above the SUA target level. A main reason for insufficient therapy can be that regular SUA level control after treatment initiation is neglected [30]. Hence, no or insufficient dose adjustment takes place. Thus, the effect of a slightly reduced dementia risk in patients with anti-hyperuricemic drug treatment could be interpreted as a result from still elevated SUA levels in these patients. We did not find evidence that anti-hyperuricemic drug treatment itself has a significant modifying effect on dementia risk.

Exact biological mechanisms by which SUA levels might contribute to the observed inverse association with dementia risk are yet to be explored. The frequently discussed hypothesis includes that uric acid has antioxidative properties and might be able to reduce oxidative stress by being a scavenger of biological oxidants such as peroxynitrite radicals which have been shown to be involved in the pathology of neurodegenerative diseases [31]. In this way, uric acid exerts neuroprotective effects by ameliorating free-radical-induced protein and DNA damage [32]. Furthermore, uric acid has been shown to act as an electron donor that increases antioxidant enzyme activity (e.g. superoxide dismutase) [33]. The brain is especially susceptible to oxidative stress and a dysfunction of antioxidative properties has been reported to contribute to neurodegenerative diseases [34].

Our results are in line with other claims data studies. A Taiwanese study with national health insurance data also showed that patients with gout have a lower risk for incident dementia (HR 0.77 CI 0.72–0.82, for all gout

Table 4 Association between gout/hyperuricemia and dementia including covariates, all patients, no selection according to treatment

Covariate	N (% from 137,640)	Cases (% from 27,528)	Controls (% from 110,112)	OR (CI)	p-value
Anti-hyperuricemia drugs	23,370 (17.0)	4.734 (17.2)	18,636 (16.9)	0.94 (0.90,0.99)	0.01
Hyperuricemia	30,629 (22.3)	6137 (22.3)	24,492 (22.2)	0.94 (0.90,0.98)	0.0025
Polypharmacy[a]	90,418 (65.7)	19,495 (70.8)	70,923 (64.4)	1.15 (1.11,1.19)	< 0.001
Diabetes	48,553 (35.3)	11,247 (40.9)	37,306 (33.9)	1.29 (1.25,1.33)	< 0.001
Ischemic heart disease	55,307 (40.2)	11,862 (43.1)	43,445 (39.5)	1.04 (1.01,1.07)	0.005
Stroke	16,429 (11.9)	4716 (17.1)	11,713 (10.6)	1.53 (1.47,1.59)	< 0.001
Other cerebrovascular diseases	21,754 (15.8)	5670 (20.6)	16,084 (14.6)	1.32 (1.27,1.37)	< 0.001
Atherosclerosis	17,339 (12.6)	3898 (14.2)	13,441 (12.2)	Removed from model	0.078
Hypertension	113,640 (82.6)	22.978 (83.5)	90,662 (82.3)	0.92 (0.89,0.96)	< 0.001
Renal impairment	18,769 (13.6)	4285 (15.6)	14,484 (13.2)	1.11 (1.06,1.15)	< 0.001
Hyperlipidemia	70,373 (51.1)	13,877 (50.4)	56,496 (51.3)	0.87 (0.84,0.89)	< 0.001
Depression	27,567 (20.0)	7257 (26.4)	20,310 (18.4)	1.50 (1.46,1.55)	< 0.001
Polyarthritis	5692 (4.1)	1196 (4.3)	4496 (4.1)	Removed from model	0.73

Global test: Wald X^2 = 2402.99, DF = 11, $p < 0.001$
[a]Polypharmacy means prescription of 5 or more different drugs (ATC codes) besides anti-hyperuricemic drugs in a quarter

patients in the adjusted model) [18]. Lu et al. used medical record data from general practitioners in the UK and detected an inverse association between gout and the risk of developing AD, supporting the potential neuroprotective role of uric acid [19]. The authors observed an hazard ratio (HR) of 0.76 (CI 0.66–0.87) for AD risk with gout in the adjusted model [19]. However, our results are slightly less pronounced.

Our findings do not support the results by Latourte et al. who reported elevated risks for dementia with higher SUA levels [17]. This might be due to differences in study populations. Latourte et al. analyzed the effect of different SUA levels mostly within the normal, not elevated range and excluded patients receiving urate-lowering medication [17]. It is therefore difficult to judge if further confounding factors that were not addressed in their study might have contributed to the effect. Furthermore, the sample size was limited, including only 110 all-cause dementia cases, leading to non-significant effects for most SUA level categories [17]. In a sensitivity analysis with an usual hyperuricemia threshold the effect was not significant [17]. Time-varying effects were not taken into account as SUA levels were based on a single measurement, up to 12 years prior dementia diagnosis [17].

Our study has several strengths. For our study we included a large data set of treated and untreated hyperuricemia or gout patients and controls. The sample is population-based and covers longitudinal data from 2004 to 2013 extracted from the largest German statutory public health insurance. This allowed us to perform the analysis in an unselected patient population. Health claims data cover the total population, not only community-dwelling individuals. The sample also includes people who are excluded in most cohort studies, namely persons who live in institutions such as assisted living or nursing homes. Furthermore, with the use of routine database records selection bias or recall bias is avoided.

There are also limitations. Because we make use of claims data we cannot completely rule out residual confounding. However, we adjusted our analysis by including potential confounding factors such as polypharmacy and comorbidities. Because we analyzed claims data with a high number of diagnoses of unspecified and mixed dementia, we were not able to differentiate between different dementia etiologies, such as dementia in the course of AD or vascular dementia. This is why we do not perform subgroup analyses for different dementia types. In addition, claims data lack data on SUA levels. Thus, we rely on prescription data and are not able to confirm SUA level ranges of treated or untreated patients.

Conclusion

Using German claims data our study showed a slight reduction for dementia risk in patients with hyperuricemia or gout diagnosis and occasional as well as regular anti-hyperuricemic treatment. Patients without targeted treatment also displayed a decreased risk for dementia. Our finding confirms previous studies with medical record and claims data from the UK and Taiwan that hyperuricemia or gout is inversely associated with dementia risk. More research is needed to gain more evidence of a potential neuroprotective mechanism of high SUA levels.

Abbreviations
AD: Alzheimer's disease; AOK: Allgemeine Ortskrankenkasse; ATC: Anatomical-Therapeutic-Chemical; CI: Confidence interval; DDD: Defined daily dose; ICD-10: International Classification of Diseases, tenth revision; OR: Odds ratio; PD: Parkinson's disease; SUA: Serum uric acid

Acknowledgements
The authors are grateful to the Scientific Research Institute of the AOK (WIdO) for providing the data.

Funding
No funding was received to carry out the work described in this article.

Authors' contributions
All authors contributed to the study design and to the analysis and interpretation of data. BE, WG and BH drafted the manuscript. All authors critically revised the manuscript and approved the final version.

Competing interests
The authors declare that they have no competing interests.

Author details
[1]Institute of General Practice and Family Medicine, University of Bonn, Bonn, Germany. [2]Department of Health Services Research, Division of General Medicine, University of Oldenburg, Oldenburg, Germany. [3]German Center for Neurodegenerative Diseases (DZNE), Bonn, Germany. [4]Federal Institute for Drugs and Medical Devices (BfArM), Kurt-Georg-Kiesinger-Allee 3, D-53175 Bonn, Germany. [5]Department of Psychiatry, University of Bonn, Bonn, Germany. [6]Center for Translational Medicine, University of Bonn, Bonn, Germany.

References
1. Alzheimer's Association. 2016 Alzheimer's disease facts and figures. Alzheimers Dement. 2016;12:459–509.
2. Raffaitin C, Gin H, Empana J-P, Helmer C, Berr C, Tzourio C, et al. Metabolic syndrome and risk for incident Alzheimer's disease or vascular dementia: the Three-City study. Diabetes Care. 2009;32:169–74.
3. Mijajlovic MD, Pavlovic A, Brainin M, Heiss WD, Quinn TJ, Ihle-Hansen HB, et al. Post-stroke dementia - a comprehensive review. BMC Med. 2017;15:11.
4. Li C, Hsieh M-C, Chang S-J. Metabolic syndrome, diabetes, and hyperuricemia. Curr Opin Rheumatol. 2013;25:210–6.
5. Borghi C, Rosei EA, Bardin T, Dawson J, Dominiczak A, Kielstein JT, et al. Serum uric acid and the risk of cardiovascular and renal disease. J Hypertens. 2015;33:1729–41.
6. Bowman GL, Shannon J, Frei B, Kaye JA, Quinn JF. Uric acid as a CNS antioxidant. J Alzheimers Dis. 2010;19:1331–6.
7. Mendez-Hernandez E, Salas-Pacheco J, Ruano-Calderon L, Téllez-Valencia A, Cisneros-Martínez J, Barraza-Salas M, et al. Lower uric acid linked with cognitive dysfunction in the elderly. CNS Neurol Disord Drug Targets. 2015;14:564–6.
8. De Vera M, Rahman MM, Rankin J, Kopec J, Gao X, Choi H. Gout and the risk of Parkinson's disease: a cohort study. Arthritis Rheum. 2008;59:1549–54.

9. Alonso A, Rodríguez LA, Logroscino G, Hernán MA. Gout and risk of Parkinson disease: a prospective study. Neurology. 2007;69:1696–700.

10. Weisskopf MG, O'Reilly E, Chen H, Schwarzschild MA, Ascherio A. Plasma urate and risk of Parkinson's disease. Am J Epidemiol. 2007;166:561–7.

11. Parkinson Study Group SURE-PD Investigators, Schwarzschild MA, Ascherio A, Beal MF, Cudkowicz ME, Curhan GC, et al. Inosine to increase serum and cerebrospinal fluid urate in Parkinson disease: a randomized clinical trial. JAMA Neurol. 2014;71:141–50.

12. Devore EE, Grodstein F, van Rooij FJ, Hofman A, Stampfer MJ, Witteman JC, et al. Dietary antioxidants and long-term risk of dementia. Arch Neurol. 2010;67:819–25.

13. Schirinzi T, Di Lazzaro G, Colona VL, Imbriani P, Alwardat M, Sancesario GM, et al. Assessment of serum uric acid as risk factor for tauopathies. J Neural Transm. 2017;124:1105–8.

14. Tuven B, Soysal P, Unutmaz G, Kaya D, Isik AT. Uric acid may be protective against cognitive impairment in older adults, but only in those without cardiovascular risk factors. Exp Gerontol. 2017;89:15–9.

15. Khan AA, Quinn TJ, Hewitt J, Fan Y, Dawson J. Serum uric acid level and association with cognitive impairment and dementia: systematic review and meta-analysis. Age. 2016;38:16.

16. Euser SM, Hofman A, Westendorp RG, Breteler MM. Serum uric acid and cognitive function and dementia. Brain. 2009;132:377–82.

17. Latourte A, Soumaré A, Bardin T, Perez-Ruiz F, Debette S, Richette P. Uric acid and incident dementia over 12 years of follow-up: a population-based cohort study. Ann Rheum Dis. 2017;77:328–35.

18. Hong JY, Lan TY, Tang GJ, Tang CH, Chen TJ, Lin HY. Gout and the risk of dementia: a nationwide population-based cohort study. Arthritis Res Ther. 2015;17:139.

19. Lu N, Dubreuil M, Zhang Y, Neogi T, Rai SK, Ascherio A, et al. Gout and the risk of Alzheimer's disease: a population-based, BMI-matched cohort study. Ann Rheum Dis. 2016;75:547–51.

20. Gomm W, von Holt K, Thomé F, Broich K, Maier W, Weckbecker K, et al. Regular benzodiazepine and Z-substance use and risk of dementia: an analysis of German claims data. J Alzheimers Dis. 2016;54:801–8.

21. Chen PH, Cheng SJ, Lin HC, Lee CY, Chou CH. Risk factors for the progression of mild cognitive impairment in different types of neurodegenerative disorders. Behav Neurol. 2018;2018:6929732.

22. Fiolaki A, Tsamis KI, Milionis HJ, Kyritsis AP, Kosmidou M, Giannopoulos S. Atherosclerosis, biomarkers of atherosclerosis and Alzheimer's disease. Int J Neurosci. 2014;124:1–11.

23. Giersiepen K, Pohlabeln H, Egidi G, Pigeot I. Quality of diagnostic ICD coding for outpatients in Germany. Bundesgesundheitsblatt Gesundheitsforschung Gesundheitsschutz. 2007;50:1028–38.

24. Kuo CF, Grainge MJ, Mallen C, Zhang W, Doherty M. Rising burden of gout in the UK but continuing suboptimal management: a nationwide population study. Ann Rheum Dis. 2015;74:661–7.

25. Rashid N, Levy GD, Wu YL, Zheng C, Koblick R, Cheetham TC. Patient and clinical characteristics associated with gout flares in an integrated healthcare system. Rheumatol Int. 2015;35:1799–807.

26. Engel B, Prautzsch H. Management of gout- new guidelines published by the German College of General Practitioners and Family Physicians (DEGAM). Z Allg Med. 2014;90:7–12.

27. Engel B, Just J, Bleckwenn M, Weckbecker K. Treatment options for gout. Dtsch Arztebl Int. 2017;114:215–22.

28. Jennings CG, Mackenzie IS, Flynn R, et al. Up-titration of allopurinol in patients with gout. Semin Arthritis Rheum. 2014;44:25–30.

29. Perez-Ruiz F, Carmona L, Yébenes MJ, Pascual E, de Miguel E, Ureña I, et al. An audit of the variability of diagnosis and management of gout in the rheumatology setting: the gout evaluation and management study. J Clin Rheumatol. 2011;17:349–55.

30. Singh JA, Hodges JS, Asch SM. Opportunities for improving medication use and monitoring in gout. Ann Rheum Dis. 2009;68:1265–70.

31. Squadrito GL, Cueto R, Splenser AE, Valavanidis A, Zhang H, Uppu RM, et al. Reaction of uric acid with peroxynitrite and implications for the mechanism of neuroprotection by uric acid. Arch Biochem Biophys. 2000;376:333–7.

32. Muraoka S, Miura T. Inhibition by uric acid of free radicals that damage biological molecules. Pharmacol Toxicol. 2003;93:284–9.

33. Hink HU, Santanam N, Dikalov S, McCann L, Nguyen AD, Parthasarathy S, et al. Peroxidase properties of extracellular superoxide dismutase: role of uric acid in modulating in vivo activity. Arterioscler Thromb Vasc Biol. 2002;22:1402–8.

6

Shanghai cognitive intervention of mild cognitive impairment for delaying progress with longitudinal evaluation-a prospective, randomized controlled study (SIMPLE): rationale, design, and methodology

Yiqi Lin[†], Binyin Li[†], Huidong Tang, Qun Xu, Yuncheng Wu, Qi Cheng, Chunbo Li, Shifu Xiao, Lu Shen, Weiguo Tang, Hui Yu, Naying He, Huawei Lin, Fuhua Yan, Wenwei Cao, Shilin Yang, Ye Liu, Wei Zhao, Dong Lu, Bin Jiao, Xuewen Xiao, Lin Zhou and Shengdi Chen[*]

Abstract

Background: Mild cognitive impairment is an early stage of Alzheimer's disease. Increasing evidence has indicated that cognitive training could improve cognitive abilities of MCI patients in multiple cognitive domains, making it a promising therapeutic approach for MCI. However, the effect of long-time training has not been widely explored. It is also necessary to evaluate the extent how it could reduce the convertion rate from MCI to AD.

Methods/design: The SIMPLE study is a multicenter, randomized, single-blind prospective clinical trial assessing the effects of computerized cognitive training on different cognitive domains in MCI patients. It is carried out in 7 centers in China. The study population includes patients aged 50–85, and they are randomly allocated to the training or control group. The primary outcome is to compare the conversion rate of MCI within 36-month follow-up. Structural and functional MRI will be used to interpret the effect of cognitive training. The cognitive training comprises a variety of games related with cognitive domains such as attention, memory, visualspatial ability and executive function. We cautiously set 50% reduction in the rate of conversion as estimated effect. With 80–90% statistical power and 12% as the overall probability of conversion within the study period, 600–800 patients are finally required in the study. The first patent has been recruited in April 2017.

Discussion: Previous studies suggested the benefit of cognitive training for MCI, but neither long-time nor Chinese culture were investigated. The SIMPLE designs and utilizes an improved computerized cognitive training approach and assesses its effects on MCI progress. In addition, neural activities explaining the effects on cognition function changes will be revealed, which could in turn to imply more useful therapeutic approaches.

Trial registration: ClinicalTrials.gov Identifier: NCT03119051.

Keywords: Mild cognitive impairment, Cognitive training, China, Longitude evaluation, Randomized controlled trial

* Correspondence: chen_sd@medmail.com.cn
[†]Yiqi Lin and Binyin Li contributed equally to this work.
Department of Neurology & Institute of Neurology, Rui Jin Hospital affiliated to Shanghai Jiao Tong University School of Medicine, Shanghai 200025, China

Background

Alzheimer's disease (AD) is one of the most common neurodegenerative diseases. Its symptoms usually emerge gradually after the age of 65 and get worse over time. The disease seriously impaired cognitive functions and daily living abilities, posing heavy care and economic burden on patients' families and the society. The American Cognitive Function and Aging Study (ACFAS) indicates that the prevalence of AD among people over 65 is 6.5% [1]. In Shanghai, one of the most biggest cities in China, the prevalence of cognition impairment in people over 60 in rural regions and over 55 in urban areas are reported to be 7 and 8.38% respectively [2, 3]. The number of AD patients in China is estimated to reach 23.3 million in 2030 [4].

So far there have been a few effective treatment for AD, though cognitive decline may be slowed down by medications like cholinesterase inhibitors and N-methyl-D-aspartate receptor antagonists. Once dementia happens, no treatment could stop or reverse disease progression by now. The latest studies of AD medications, for example, phase II or III clinical trials using monoclonal antibodies for immunomodulatory therapy [5, 6], all failed in the end. In April of 2011, the National Institute on Aging Alzheimer's Association (NIA-AA) extended the definition of AD and described three stages of AD [7]. The updated diagnostic guidelines describe preclinical stage before dementia: asymptomatic stage with underlying amyloid deposit and neural injury. In the mildly symptomatic predementia stage, mild cognitive impairment due to AD (MCI) is marked by mild symptoms (no interference with independence) with at least one positive biomarker, including β-amyloid deposits or evidence of neuronal injury. Among the three stages in the NIA-AA guideline, MCI is of greatest significance for clinical interventions. First, approximately 10–12% of MCI patients progressed to AD every year and the 3-year MCI-AD conversion rate reached up to 25–30%. Overall, more than 60% of MCI patients developed AD [8]. So interventions for MCI patients are highly necessary. Secondly, presence of cognitive symptoms makes it possible for identification and diagnosis. Finally, since symptoms are relatively mild, patients could cooperate well with various therapeutic interventions.

Pharmacological and non-pharmacological treatments have been greatly concerned about their effects. Donepezil, rivastigmine, galantamine, and memantine are the drugs presently approved by the Food and Drug Administration (FDA) for treatment of AD. However, both cholinesterase inhibitors (ChEIs) and antiglutamatergic treatments are not indicated for MCI patients. A review and meta-analysis concluded that treatment with ChEIs merely affected MCI progression to dementia or improved cognitive test scores [9]. In one study of data from Alzheimer's Disease Neuroimaging Initiative, MCI patients who received ChEIs with or without memantine were more impaired, showed greater decline in scores, and progressed to dementia sooner than patients who did not receive ChEIs [10].

In addition, as cognitive symptoms of MCI patients are still mild, drug compliance could be another problem. Moreover, costs and side effects of drugs are important negative factors of early medical treatment.

In recent years, cognitive training has gradually become an important therapeutic approach due to its convenience and effectiveness. It describes a group of brain games exercising mental processing ability such as attention, memory, calculation and so on [11]. An increasing number of studies have proved that cognitive training has beneficial effects on delaying cognitive decline in the elderly. The Advanced Cognitive Training for Independent and Vital Elderly (ACTIVE) study which did a 5-year follow-up of 2802 healthy aging people found that there was a significantly smaller proportion of cognitive decline and higher score of living abilities in the intervention group receiving various cognitive training [12]. Similar effects of cognitive training are also found in MCI patients. Sylvie Belleville et al. [13] found that both MCI patients and healthy elders who received an 8-week intervention focusing on teaching episodic memory strategies had better performance in episodic memory assessment than the control group. An randomized clinical trial of 100 MCI patients found that 6-month cognitive training improved significantly cognitive functions of the intervention group in multiple domains and this improvement was well maintained during a 18-month follow-up [14].

However, there are some limitations in present cognitive training [15]. First, not all cognitive domains are involved in the training. For example, in the ACTIVE study [16], participants received training related with the ability of memory, attention and reasoning, while other cognitive domains like visuospatial and executive functions were not involved. Second, in the traditional pencil-and-paper training, difficulty levels hardly vary from person to person according to their different cognitive abilities. In addition, most clinical trials only performed neuropsychological assessment without objective biomarkers or imaging evaluation. Finally, most clinical trials lack a stable longer-term follow-up of a large number of MCI patients.

Computerized cognitive training has been considered as a convenient, flexible and scalable intervention, which might protect cognition from aging and AD [17]. A meta-analysis suggested its efficacy on global cognition, select cognitive domains, and psychosocial functioning in MCI patients [18]. Our preliminary data analysis suggested that computerized cognitive training improved the MCI participants' cognitive functions. We once performed a human-computer interaction-based comprehensive training for 66 MCI or dementia patients in Shanghai, and found that the training delayed cognitive decline in visualspatial ability [19]. Thus, based on the previous studies, a 3-year follow-up prospective multi-center trial will be conducted for MCI patients to investigate the role of the computerized-cognitive training in cognitive improvement and its possible mechanisms. Neuropsychological assessment and both structural and functional neuroimaging will be used for evaluation at baseline and follow-up.

Methods/design

Study aims

The primary aim of SIMPLE is to evaluate the effect of the computerized cognitive training on the conversion rate of MCI to AD in the 3-year follow-up.

The secondary aims of this study are to investigate how the cognitive training affects global cognitive function, daily living function and brain activities, and to determine whether patients should receive such intervention at MCI stage.

The main research topics are:

1. Are there significantly less MCI patients convert to AD if they receive computerized cognitive training in the 3 years period?
2. Could the scores of cognitive assessments and daily living activities be improved after training?
3. Does computerized cognitive training have effect on the brain structure or activities (both regional and neural connectivity) changes? If so, how are they linked with cognitive function?

Study design

SIMPLE is a 3-year multicenter prospective single-blind clinical cohort study with two parallel arms in 1:1 ratio. Patients are randomized into the training group the control group (absence of training). The total training dose will be around 200 h, with 3–4 sessions per week and 30 min per session. Though dose effect was not well studied, we will give the training dose that is acceptable by MCI patients according to previous studies and our preliminary data. Global cognitive function and daily living activity will be assessed at baseline and every 6 months afterwards (in month 6, 12, 18, 24, 30 and 36), while specific cognitive domains (memory, executive function, attention and language) will be evaluated at baseline and every 12 months afterwards (in month 12, 24 and 36). In addition, brain structure and function will be assessed by MRI at baseline and in month 12 and 36. During the follow-up period, medications for dementia (ChEIs or memantine) are not indicated. If a patients converts to AD during follow-up, pharmacological therapy starts. Cognitive assessments for all cognitive domains and MRI will be performed at that time. Meanwhile, telephone follow-ups will be conducted every two weeks in both groups. As an single-blind trial, neuropsychological assessor will be blinded to the group

allocation. The total duration of the study will be approximately 5 years, from June 2017 (first in) until June 2022 (last out).

Patients

In total, 600–800 MCI patients will be enrolled from memory clinic of four centers in Shanghai, one in Zhejiang Province, one center in Hu'nan Province and one in An'hui Province: Ruijin Hospital affiliated to Shanghai Jiaotong University School of Medicine, Renji Hospital affiliated to Shanghai Jiaotong University School of Medicine, Shanghai General Hospital affiliated to Shanghai Jiaotong University School of Medicine, Shanghai Mental Health Center, Suzhou municipal hospital in Anhui Province, Zhoushan Hospital in Zhejiang Province and Xiangya Hospital in Hu'nan Province. Among them, Ruijin Hospital is the leader of SIMPLE, in charge of patients enrollment, quality control and ethical problems. The inclusion and exclusion criteria are shown as follows.

Inclusion criteria are

  Male or female, aged 50–85;
- MCI diagnosed according to the National Institute on Aging-Alzheimer's Association (NIA-AA) workgroups [20];
- $24 \leq$ Mini-Mental State Examination (MMSE) ≤ 28;
- The Hamilton Depression Scale/17-item (HAMD) score ≤ 10;
- Not on medication for dementia (Table 1);
- MRI T2 weighted imaging (T2WI) scan: if aged ≤ 70, Fazeca scale for White Matter lesions rating level ≤ 1; if > 70 years, white matter damage rating scale ≤ 2. The number of lacunar infarcts larger than 2 cm in diameter ≤ 2. No infarcts in hypothalamus, entorhinal cortex, para-hypothalamus, cortical and subcortical cavity infarction near gray matter nuclei. The medial temporal lobe atrophy (MTA) score: Grade II or above.
- Accompanied by reliable caregivers (at least intensive contact of 4 days every week and 2 h every day) who are expected to participate in the follow-up visits and provide useful information for scores of scales;
- Education level: primary school (grade 6) or above.
- Expected good compliance with the therapy and follow-up. Each patient gives a written informed consent, and the study has been approved by Ruijin Hospital's ethical committees.

Exclusion criteria are

- Cognitive decline caused by other diseases (including but not limited to: cerebrovascular disease, central nervous system infections, Parkinson's disease,

Table 1 Forbidden and restricted medication in the trial

Forbidden medication	Cholinesterase inhibitors
	N-methyl-D-aspartate (NMDA) antagonists
	Synthetic adrenal corticosteroids
	Central nervous system stimulants
	Chinese and western cognitive improvement medication
Restricted medication[a]	Antipsychotics
	Antidepressants
	Sedative-hypnotics[b]

Restricted medication[a]: The dose of these medications should not be increased during the trial. Patients with these medications for a long time should keep the dose stable

Sedative-hypnotics[b]: If necessary, temporary use of zopiclone, alprazolam or estazolam is allowed. Last dose before psychological assessment should not be given later than 22:00 last night

metabolic encephalopathy, deficiency of folic acid/vitamin B12 and hypothyroidism);
▪ Medical history of other neurological disorders (including stroke, Parkinson's disease, epilepsy, etc.);
▪ Psychiatric disorders defined by Diagnostic and Statistical Manual of Mental Disorders (DSM)-IV criteria;
▪ Severe disease of heart, lung, liver, kidney or hematopoietic system;
▪ History of alcohol or drug abuse;
▪ Participation in other clinical trials within 30 days before the screening of this study;
▪ Other reasons that make one inability to complete the study.

Withdrawal criteria are
Patients should withdraw from the trial if they meet the following criteria:

▪ Poor compliance to the protocol;
▪ A serious complication or other severe disease happens in the trial.
▪ Patients refuse to be followed up or become lost at the point of follow-up.

Endpoint criteria
Patients finish their training when either of the criteria is met:

▪ Patients finish 3-year cognitive training;
▪ Patients meet the diagnostic criteria of dementia due to AD, according to the National Institute on Aging-Alzheimer's Association (NIA-AA) workgroups [7].

Recruitment, screening and run-in period
Patients will be recruited from the memory clinic of 7 centers above. During the first week, each patient will perform

MMSE and HAMD as screen. Then eligible patients will enter a run-in period of 2 weeks, during which they will receive blood tests, electrocardiogram, cranial MRI and a basic computer operation test. The blood tests contain complete blood count, liver and kidney function test, syphilis, folic acid level, vitamin B12 level, thyroid function and ApoE genotype. The purpose of the run-in period is to collect basic clinical data, rule out other causes of cognitive decline and evaluate participants' compliance. Then all the eligible patients will be registered before baseline assessment.

Baseline assessment and randomization
Baseline demographics include sex, age, education level, occupation, concomitant disease and medications. Physical exercise and diet style will also be recorded.

A neuropsychological battery for multiple cognitive domains will be performed by neuropsychological assessors who are blind to the following grouping. These tests included MMSE, the Chinese version of Alzheimer's Disease Assessment Scale-Cognitive subscale(ADAS-Cog) [21], Alzheimer's Disease Cooperative Study-Activities of Daily Living (ADCS-ADL) [21], the Auditory Verbal Learning Test (AVLT)-Huashan version [22], the Shape Trail Test (STT, including Part A and B) [23], the Rey-Osterrieth Complex Figure Test (CFT) [24], the Stroop Color-World Test (SCWT) and Boston Naming Test (see Additional file 1).

After the baseline assessment, patients will be randomly allocated into two groups, which will be managed by Ruijin Hospital with interactive web response system. The stratification factors will be balanced between two groups when allocation, including education level (university or not) and age (older than 65 years or not). Assessors will be specific in each center and blinded to the grouping.

Ethics and informed consent
Conformed to the ethical principles proclaimed in the Declaration of Helsinki in 1964, and revised in Tokyo in 2004, the study protocol has been reviewed and thus approved by independent ethics committees in the Ruijin Hospital, which is the leading center of the study. Before the inclusion, written informed consent forms will be signed by patients or their surrogate family member after a detailed explanation. The SIMPLE study is registered with Chinese Trial Registry.gov and ClinicalTrial.gov (Register number: ChiCTR-INR-16008959 and NCT03119051).

Intervention and follow-up
All the participants in the intervention group will login an online training website with their own passwords by either cell phone or tablet computer. A variety of cognitive domains will be involved in the training including memory, calculation, attention, visualspatial and executive skills. The

difficulty level of each game will be adjusted automatically according to patients' last training results so that patients' accuracy rate will be kept between 70 and 80%. Patients will be required to play 3–4 times of 30 min' training game every week. Training time and results will be uploaded immediately to a web server which could be monitored by investigators. In contrast, participants in the control group will be required to neither alter their daily lifestyle nor receive any additional cognitive training.

Investigators will conduct telephone follow-ups for both groups every two weeks to obtain their feedback and offer encouragement. On the other hand, follow-up assessment will be performed every six months (in month 6, 12, 18, 24, 30, 36 ± 2 weeks). In month 6, 18, 30, brief assessment including MMSE, ADAS-Cog and ADL would be done, while in month 12, 24 and 36, the neuropsychological battery at baseline for multiple cognitive domains will be performed. MRI is given in month 12 and 36 (Fig. 1).

Outcome measures

The primary outcome is the incidence of AD during the follow-up. The diagnosis of AD will be made according to NIA-AA criteria. The performance in each cognitive domain will be compared as secondary outcomes. ADAS-Cog will be used to assess the global cognitive

performance of MCI patients. Memory will be assessed using the AVLT-H. Attention and executive functions will be evaluated by TMT and the Stroop task. Language will be assessed by Boston naming test (30-item version). Visual spatial ability and visual memory will be evaluated by the Rey–Osterrieth complex figure test (CFT). Activities of daily living will be assessed by ADCS-ADL. Structural and functional MRI will help to uncover the potential neural activity changes during training. The schedule of all the outcome measures is shown in the Table 2.

Neuroimaging markers

Structural and functional brain MRI will be performed at baseline, one-year follow-up and endpoint (Table 2). The MRI protocol is described in the Table 3. In structural MRI analysis, medial temporal lobe atrophy visual rating scale is used to indicate the level of atrophy in the medial temporal lobes (ranging from 0 to 3) [25]. According to cognitive ability changes, we also use voxel based morphometry (VBM) to quantitatively compare the volume of specific areas in brain. With regard to functional MRI, we use blood oxygen level dependent (BOLD) signal to find out functional changes related with cognitive performance changes. Fractional amplitude of low frequency fluctuation (fALFF), regional homogeneity (Reho) will be used to

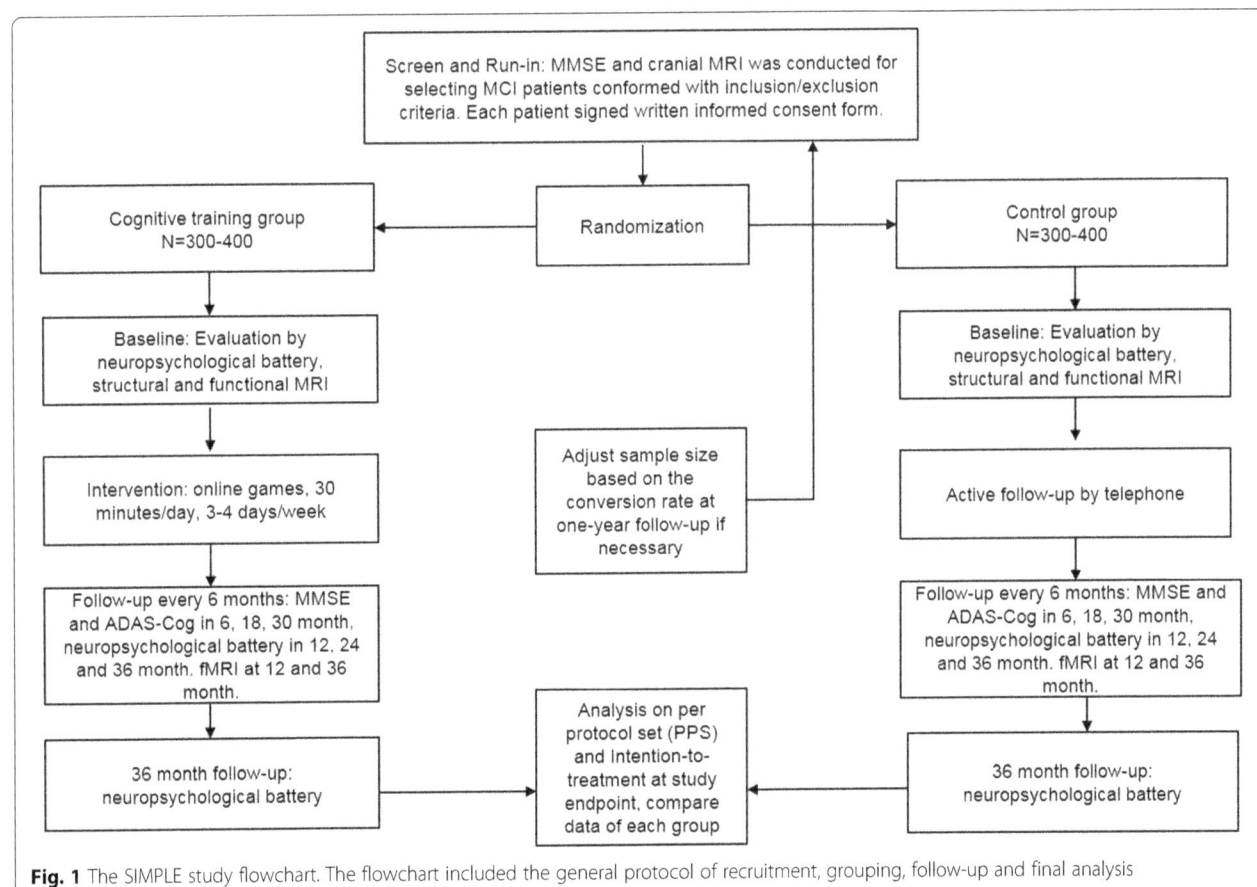

Fig. 1 The SIMPLE study flowchart. The flowchart included the general protocol of recruitment, grouping, follow-up and final analysis

Table 2 Outline and timelines of the trial

Time Points	Screening −3 weeks	Run-in −2 weeks	Baseline 0	1st Visits 6 months	2nd Visit 2 months	3rd Visit 18 months	4th Visit 24 months	5th Visit 30 months	Endpoint[a] 36 months
Written informed consent		×							
Inclusion/exclusion criteria	×	×	×						
Blood test		×							
Electrocardiogram		×							
Cranial MRI examination		×			×				×
MMSE	×		×	×	×	×	×	×	×
ADAS-Cog			×	×	×	×	×	×	×
ADCS-ADL			×	×	×	×	×	×	×
HAMD/GDS	×		×		×		×		×
AVLT			×		×		×		×
TMT			×		×		×		×
CFT			×		×		×		×
Stroop Test			×		×		×		×
Boston Naming Test			×		×		×		×

[a]Endpoint is either the ending of 36-month follow-up or the diagnosis of AD during follow-up

represent regional neural activities, while neural network changes are indicated by functional connectivity [26, 27].

Sample size and statistical analysis

Sample size was estimated based on conversion rate from MCI to AD in the SAS study [28]. In the SAS sample, it was 6.0 per 100 person-years. In the three-year follow-up, the overall probability of conversion event would be 17%. We use hazard ratio (HR) to represent the converting difference of the training group per unit time as the control group. HR represents instantaneous risk over the all period, and is clinically significant due to its indication risks that happen before the endpoint. A power calculation was performed with the online freeware program by "time-to-event" method [29] (http://powerandsamplesize.com).

Due to HR as an almost unprecedented outcome in such sort of trial, we cautiously set 50% reduction in the rate of conversion as estimated effect. With 80–90% statistical power and 12% as the overall probability of conversion within the study period, 544–728 patients in total are considered the minimal number necessary to estimate the hazard ratio. Considering 10% dropout, we plan to enroll approximately 600–800 patients, with 300–400 patients in each group.

As an exploring study, we used per-protocol set instead of intention-to-treat (ITT) analysis as primary endpoint analysis in order to strictly estimate the effect of training. If participants were indicated cholinesterase inhibitors or memantine, or they could not insist on training, they would be excluded from per-protocol sets. ITT approach will also be done to avoid the effects of crossover and dropout. The results of these two analysis will be carefully interpreted.

The randomization is stratified by age and education years according to the Ruijin center using SAS statistical software (SAS Institute Inc., Cary, NC, USA) by a statistician (Qi Cheng) with no access to information on the patients or physicians. Patients will be randomized in a ratio of 1:1 to receive the training or only follow-up. In the randomization process, the randomized code is generated and assigned to physicians in a sealed envelope by the statistician. Afterwards, the sealed randomization codes are sent out to each center. The odd number means the training group, while the even number means the control group. If the patient cannot be trained because of difficulty in operating computer or cellphone, the patient will be managed as off-trial.

Continuous variables (scores of each cognitive assessment) will undergo mixed model analysis in the two

Table 3 Brain MRI protocol

Sequence name/ Acquisition method	Field of View (mm)	Matrix	Slices	Inter-slice gap (mm)	Thickness (mm)	Voxel (mm³)	TR /TE (ms)
3D FSPGR	256 × 256	256 × 256	192	0	1	1 × 1 × 1	5.52/1.72
BOLD	240 × 240	64 × 64	33	0.7	3.5	3.5 × 3.5 × (3.5 + 0.7)	2000/30

Abbreviations: TR repetition time, *TE* echo time, *3D FSPGR* three-dimensional fast spoiled gadient-recalled

groups for the secondary outcomes. At the same time, the effect of ApoE genotype on primary outcome will be observed through analysis of subgroups divided by ApoE genotype in both groups. With regard to MRI, VBM measures and BOLD signal will be used to find out structural and functional changes related with cognitive performance changes.

Discussion

The SIMPLE trial is leaded by Ruijin Steering Committee (Binyin Li, Huidong Tang, Shengdi Chen), which is assisted by an independent data safety and monitoring board from Public Health College of Shanghai Jiaotong University School of Medicine (leaded by Qi Chen). The Board includes epidemiologists and statisticians, who are not otherwise participating in the trial. The Steering Committee members and principal investigators of each center (Qun Xu in Shanghai Renji Hospital, Yunchen Wu in Shanghai General Hospital, Chunbo Li and Shifu Xiao in Shanghai Mental Health Center, Hui Yu in Suzhou municipal hospital, Anhui Province, Weiguo Tang in Zhoushan Hospital, Zhejiang Province, Lu Shen in Xiangya Hospital, Hu'nan Province) are in charge of the ethics and patient safety. They will have a face-to-face or online meeting every month to monitor the status and progress of the trial. The diagnosis of AD will be reviewed by independent experts in each center and steering committee. The sponsor of the SIMPLE trial is the Clinical Research Center, Shanghai Jiao Tong University School of Medicine. The sponsor has no influence on the study design, data collection, data analysis, and final drafting of the manuscript.

The primary object of this multicenter randomized clinical trial is to explore the effect of multi-model online cognitive intervention for MCI patients. Seven centers are enrolled in the trial and the first patient will be recruited into the study in April 2017. The results are expected for publications in 2022.

Abbreviations

ACFAS: the American Cognitive Function and Aging Study; ACTIVE: The Advanced Cognitive Training for Independent and Vital Elderly; AD: Alzheimer's disease; ADAS-Cog: Alzheimer's Disease Assessment Scale-Cognitive subscale; ADCS-ADL: Alzheimer's Disease Cooperative Study-Activities of Daily Living; AVLT: Auditory Verbal Learning Test; BOLD: Blood oxygen level dependent; CFT: Complex Figure Test; ChEIs: cholinesterase inhibitors; DSM: Diagnostic and Statistical Manual of Mental Disorders; fALFF: Fractional amplitude of low frequency fluctuation; FDA: Food and Drug Administration; HAMD: Hamilton Depression Scale; HR: Hazard ratio; ITT: intention-to-treat; MCI: mild cognitive impairment due to AD; MMSE: Mini-Mental State Examination; NIA-AA: National Institute on Aging Alzheimer's Association; Reho: Regional homogeneity; SCWT: Stroop Color-

World Test; STT: Shape Trail Test; T2WI: T2 weighted imaging; VBM: Voxel based morphometry

Acknowledgements

The Department of Radiology in Shanghai Ruijin Hospital, Shanghai Renji Hospital, Shanghai General Hospital, Shanghai Mental Health Center, Suzhou municipal hospital in Anhui Province, Zhoushan Hospital in Zhejiang Province and Xiangya Hospital in Hu'nan Province are in charge of neuroimaging of participants in each medical center. We will appreciate their contribution to the study.

Funding

The SIMPLE trial is supported by the Clinical Research Center, Shanghai Jiao Tong University School of Medicine (DLY201603) and National Key R&D Program of China (2016YFC1305804), which has no influence on the study design, data collection, data analysis, and final drafting of this manuscript.

Authors' contributions

YQL and BYL drafted the manuscript. SDC is a principal investigator, and SDC and HDT are participated in the study design and helped to revise the manuscript. QX, YCW, CBL, SFX, HY, WGT, LS are the principal investigator of each center and participated in coordination. QC participated in statistics of the study data. NYH and FHY drafted and revised the MRI part of the manuscript. All authors read and approved the final manuscript.

Competing interests

The authors declare that they have no competing interests.

References

1. Matthews FE, et al. A two-decade comparison of prevalence of dementia in individuals aged 65 years and older from three geographical areas of England: results of the cognitive function and ageing study I and II. Lancet. 2013;382(9902):1405–12.
2. Zhang ZX, et al. Dementia subtypes in China: prevalence in Beijing, Xian, shanghai, and Chengdu. Arch Neurol. 2005;62(3):447–53.
3. Yao YH, Xu RF, Tang HD, Jiang GX, Wang Y, Wang G. Cognitive Impairment and Associated factors among the elderly in the shanghai suburb: findings from a low-education population. Neuroepidemiology. 2010;34:4.
4. Xu J, et al. The economic burden of dementia in China, 1990-2030: implications for health policy. Bull World Health Organ. 2017;95(1):18–26.
5. Salloway S, Sperling R, Brashear HR. Phase 3 trials of solanezumab and bapineuzumab for Alzheimer's disease. N Engl J Med. 2014;10(370):15.
6. Richard Dodel AR. Peter Bartenstein et al, Intravenous immunoglobulins for the treatment of mild to moderate Alzheimer's disease: a phase II, randomised, doubleblind, placebo-controlled dose-finding trial. Lancet Neurol. 2013;12(3):10.
7. McKhann GM, et al. The diagnosis of dementia due to Alzheimer's disease: recommendations from the National Institute on Aging-Alzheimer's Association workgroups on diagnostic guidelines for Alzheimer's disease. Alzheimers Dement. 2011;7(3):263–9.
8. Grundman M, et al. Mild cognitive impairment can be distinguished from Alzheimer disease and normal aging for clinical trials. Arch Neurol. 2004; 61(1):59–66.
9. Russ TC, Morling JR. Cholinesterase inhibitors for mild cognitive impairment. Cochrane Database Syst Rev. 2012;9:CD009132.
10. Schneider LS, et al. Treatment with cholinesterase inhibitors and memantine of patients in the Alzheimer's disease neuroimaging initiative. Arch Neurol. 2011;68(1):58–66.
11. Simons DJ, et al. Do "brain-training" programs work? Psychol Sci Public Interest. 2016;17(3):103–86.
12. Karlene Ball P, Berch DB, Helmers KF, Jobe JB, Mary, et al. Effects of cognitive training interventions with older adults: a randomized controlled trial. JAMA Neurol. 2002;288(18):2271–81.
13. Belleville S, et al. Improvement of episodic memory in persons with mild cognitive impairment and healthy older adults: evidence from a cognitive intervention program. Dement Geriatr Cogn Disord. 2006;22(5–6):486–99.

14. Suzuki H, et al. Cognitive intervention through a training program for picture book reading in community-dwelling older adults: a randomized controlled trial. BMC Geriatr. 2014;14:122.

15. Bin-Yin Li H-DT, Qiao Y, Chen S-D. Mental training for cognitive improvement in elderly people: what have we learned from clinical and neurophysiologic studies? Curr Alzheimer Res. 2015;12(6):543–52.

16. Jobe JB, et al. ACTIVE: a cognitive intervention trial to promote independence in older adults. Control Clin Trials. 2001;22(4):453–79.

17. Barban F, et al. Protecting cognition from aging and Alzheimer's disease: a computerized cognitive training combined with reminiscence therapy. Int J Geriatr Psychiatry. 2016;31(4):340–8.

18. Hill NT, et al. Computerized cognitive training in older adults with mild cognitive impairment or dementia: a systematic review and meta-analysis. Am J Psychiatry. 2017;174(4):329–40.

19. Zhuang JP, et al. The impact of human-computer interaction-based comprehensive training on the cognitive functions of cognitive impairment elderly individuals in a nursing home. J Alzheimers Dis. 2013;36(2):245–51.

20. Alberta MS, Steven T, DeKosky, Dickson D. *The diagnosis of mild cognitive impairment due to Alzheimer's disease: Recommendations from the National Institute on Aging-Alzheimer's Association workgroups on diagnostic guidelines for Alzheimer's disease*. Alzheimers Dement. 2011;7:9.

21. Zhang ZX, et al. Rivastigmine patch in Chinese patients with probable Alzheimer's disease: a 24-week, randomized, double-blind parallel-group study comparing Rivastigmine patch (9.5 mg/24 h) with capsule (6 mg twice daily). CNS Neurosci Ther. 2016;22(6):488–96.

22. Zhao Q, et al. Short-term delayed recall of auditory verbal learning test is equivalent to long-term delayed recall for identifying amnestic mild cognitive impairment. PLoS One. 2012;7(12):e51157.

23. Zhao Q, et al. The Shape Trail test: application of a new variant of the trail making test. PLoS One. 2013;8(2):e57333.

24. Zhao Q, et al. Auditory verbal learning test is superior to Rey-Osterrieth complex figure memory for predicting mild cognitive impairment to Alzheimer's disease. Curr Alzheimer Res. 2015;12(6):520–6.

25. Scheltens P, et al. Atrophy of medial temporal lobes on MRI in "probable" Alzheimer's disease and normal ageing: diagnostic value and neuropsychological correlates. J Neurol Neurosurg Psychiatry. 1992;55(10):967–72.

26. Zou QH, et al. An improved approach to detection of amplitude of low-frequency fluctuation (ALFF) for resting-state fMRI: fractional ALFF. J Neurosci Methods. 2008;172(1):137–41.

27. Liu Y, et al. Regional homogeneity, functional connectivity and imaging markers of Alzheimer's disease: a review of resting-state fMRI studies. Neuropsychologia. 2008;46(6):1648–56.

28. Ding D, et al. Progression and predictors of mild cognitive impairment in Chinese elderly: a prospective follow-up in the shanghai aging study. Alzheimers Dement (Amst). 2016;4:28–36.

29. Scheltens P, van de Pol L. Impact commentaries. Atrophy of medial temporal lobes on MRI in "probable" Alzheimer's disease and normal ageing: diagnostic value and neuropsychological correlates. J Neurol Neurosurg Psychiatry. 2012;83(11):1038–40.

7

A gaze-independent audiovisual brain-computer Interface for detecting awareness of patients with disorders of consciousness

Qiuyou Xie[1†], Jiahui Pan[2,3†], Yan Chen[1], Yanbin He[1], Xiaoxiao Ni[1], Jiechun Zhang[1], Fei Wang[3], Yuanqing Li[3*] and Ronghao Yu[1*] (iD)

Abstract

Background: Currently, it is challenging to detect the awareness of patients who suffer disorders of consciousness (DOC). Brain-computer interfaces (BCIs), which do not depend on the behavioral response of patients, may serve for detecting the awareness in patients with DOC. However, we must develop effective BCIs for these patients because their ability to use BCIs does not as good as healthy users.

Methods: Because patients with DOC generally do not exhibit eye movements, a gaze-independent audiovisual BCI is put forward in the study where semantically congruent and incongruent audiovisual number stimuli were sequentially presented to evoke event-related potentials (ERPs). Subjects were required to pay attention to congruent audiovisual stimuli (target) and ignore the incongruent audiovisual stimuli (non-target). The BCI system was evaluated by analyzing online and offline data from 10 healthy subjects followed by being applied to online awareness detection in 8 patients with DOC.

Results: According to the results on healthy subjects, the audiovisual BCI system outperformed the corresponding auditory-only and visual-only systems. Multiple ERP components, including the P300, N400 and late positive complex (LPC), were observed using the audiovisual system, strengthening different brain responses to target stimuli and non-target stimuli. The results revealed the abilities of three of eight patients to follow commands and recognize numbers.

Conclusions: This gaze-independent audiovisual BCI system represents a useful auxiliary bedside tool to detect the awareness of patients with DOC.

Keywords: Audiovisual brain-computer interface (BCI), Event-related potential (ERP), Semantic congruency, Disorders of consciousness (DOC), Awareness detection

Background

Brain-computer interfaces (BCIs) decode brain activities into computer control signals with the aim at providing a non-muscular communication pathway with external devices [1]. Among these brain activities, event-related potentials (ERPs) have been widely used in electroencephalography (EEG)-based BCI systems [2]. ERP BCIs use visual/auditory/tactile stimuli that correspond to control operations [3, 4]. The user selects an operation by focusing on the corresponding stimulus (target) while ignoring other stimuli (non-targets). For instance, the P300 speller described by Farwell and Donchin presented a selection of characters in a 6×6 matrix from a computer display [5]. The user was required to focus attention on the row and the column that contained the target character, while each row and column of the matrix flashed at random. In this case, the target character flashed with a probability of 0.167 (2/12). The visual P300 ERP

* Correspondence: auyqli@scut.edu.cn; gesund@139.com
†Qiuyou Xie and Jiahui Pan contributed equally to this work.
³Center for Brain Computer Interfaces and Brain Information Processing, South China University of Technology, Guangzhou 510640, China
¹Coma Research Group, Centre for Hyperbaric Oxygen and Neurorehabilitation, Guangzhou General Hospital of Guangzhou Military Command, Guangzhou 510010, China
Full list of author information is available at the end of the article

elicited by the oddball was identified and translated into a character.

BCIs can potentially detect the awareness of patients with disorders of consciousness (DOC), such as unresponsive wakefulness syndrome (UWS, formerly known as the vegetative state [6]) and minimally conscious state (MCS). The UWS is defined by the preservation of spontaneous or stimulus-induced arousal without self or environmental awareness, whereas the MCS is characterized by the presence of inconsistent but discernible behaviors. Keystones in diagnosis lies in recovering the voluntary response, such as the ability to follow commands and functional use two different objects, which indicates emergence from the UWS and the MCS, respectively [7]. At present, the clinical diagnosis of patients with DOC is conducted on the basis of behavioral scales in general, such as the Coma Recovery Scale-Revised (CRS-R), which takes use of overt motor actions to external stimuli during observation [8]. However, in recent years, electroencephalography (EEG), functional magnetic resonance imaging (fMRI) and other neuroimaging methods have shown that misdiagnosis of patients with DOC who display a severe lack of motor function is possible [9]. For instance, Cruse et al. tested a motor imagery-related BCI with a group of 16 patients with UWS. Three of these patients achieved offline accuracies ranging from 61 to 78% during the motor imagery tasks [10]. Monti et al. instructed 54 patients (23 with UWS and 31 with MCS) to "imagine playing tennis" and "walk through houses" during an fMRI experiment and found that five (4 with UWS and 1 with MCS) were able to modulate their sensorimotor rhythms [11]. Recently, many BCI paradigms have been proposed for patients with DOC [12–16]. Lule et al. [13] proposed an auditory oddball EEG-based BCI paradigm based on data from 16 healthy subjects, 3 patients with UWS, 13 patients with MCS, and 2 patients with locked-in syndrome (LIS). One patient with MCS and one patient with LIS achieved significant offline accuracies over the chance level. In our previous study [17], we detected command following in eight patients with DOC (4 with UWS, 3 with MCS and 1 with LIS) using a visual hybrid P300 and SSVEP BCI, and successfully revealed that one UWS patient, one MCS patient and one LIS patient possessed residual awareness. However, the use of BCI for detecting awareness of patients with DOC remains in primary stage. These patients exhibit a generally weak BCI performance as they have a much lower cognitive ability than healthy individuals. Furthermore, substantial differences in EEG signals have been observed between patients with DOC and healthy individuals because of severe brain injuries in the patients. Therefore, many efforts should be taken for developing novel BCIs to enhance the performance of awareness detection.

For BCI-based awareness detection, an important issue lies in the type of stimulus modality. Up to now, most BCI studies have focused on unimodal (e.g., auditory-only or visual-only) stimuli. Compared to unimodal stimuli, congruent multisensory stimuli may activate additional neurons and result in faster behavioral responses and more accurate perception/recognition [18, 19]. However, multisensory stimulus paradigms have rarely received attentions in the field of BCIs [20]. In this study, we concentrated on the potential benefits of employing audiovisual stimuli to improve BCI performance. To the best of our knowledge, only three BCI studies focused on investigating audiovisual stimuli [21–23]. Belitski and colleagues compared different types of auditory-only, visual-only and audiovisual speller BCIs to assess their relative performance. Their experimental results involved 11 subjects reported that the positive effects of an audiovisual ERP-BCI paradigm compared with the corresponding visual-only and auditory-only variants [21]. Sellers and Donchin tested a P300-based BCI in the visual, auditory, and audiovisual modes, and reported that auditory mode exhibited a significantly worse classification accuracy compared with visual or audiovisual mode [22]. In our recent study [23], we designed an audiovisual BCI for detecting awareness of DOC patients, in which the audiovisual stimuli were semantically congruent visual and spoken numbers. The patients were required to give respond to target stimuli through following the instructions. According to the results regarding 8 healthy subjects, the use of the audiovisual BCI resulted in a better performance than the corresponding auditory-only or visual-only BCI, and multiple ERP components were strengthened by the audiovisual congruent target stimuli, which were useful for improving target detection. In the above audiovisual BCIs, two or more than two buttons were used in the GUIs. Thus, the GUIs were not completely gaze-independent.

Since most of the patients with DOC lack the ability to control eye movements, this study proposed a gaze-independent audiovisual BCI (Fig. 1) for detecting their awareness. Specifically, the stimuli included semantically congruent and incongruent audiovisual numbers. Furthermore, all audiovisual stimuli were presented individually, and thus the paradigm was completely gaze-independent. Ten healthy subjects and eight patients with DOC participated in our experiments. With this study, we aimed to (1) develop and validate a novel gaze-independent audiovisual BCI using semantically congruent and incongruent audiovisual stimuli; and (2) test whether this audiovisual BCI system assessed the covert conscious awareness of patients with DOC.

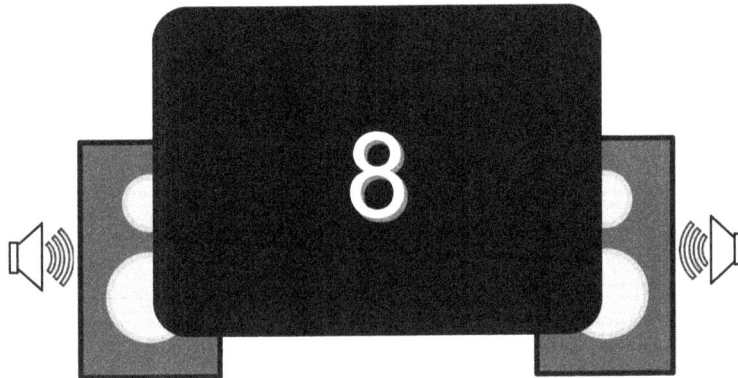

Fig. 1 GUI of the audiovisual BCI. A pair of audiovisual stimuli were presented, which were semantically congruent (e.g., a visual number "8" and a spoken number "8") or incongruent (e.g., a visual number "5" and a spoken number "6")

Methods

Subjects

The experiment included ten healthy subjects (nine males; average age ± SD: 29 ± 2 years) and eight patients with severe brain injuries (seven males; five with UWS and three with MCS; mean age ± SD: 42 ± 12 years; Table 1) in a local hospital. The recruitment was conducted based on pre-arranged inclusion/exclusion criteria. There were five inclusion criteria: 1) the patient had not taken centrally acting drugs; 2) the patient had not accepted sedation in the past 48 h; 3) the patient should keep eye opening for a period; 4) the patient had not suffered impaired visual or auditory acuity; 5) the patient had been diagnosed with VS or MCS after anoxic brain damage, traumatic brain injury (TBI), or cerebrovascular disease. There are three exclusion criteria: 1) the patient had a documented history of brain injury; 2) the patient once suffered an acute illness; 3) the patient had accepted hospitalization for less than 2 consecutive months. This study was approved by the Ethical Committee of the General Hospital of Guangzhou Military Command of PLA.

UWS and MCS are diagnosed clinically on the basis of CRS-R. which contains 23 items organized in subscales that involve auditory, visual, motor, oromotor, communication, and arousal functions [24]. Each subscale is scored based on whether there is behavioral response to certain sensory stimuli defined in operation. For example, once the visual fixation of mirror occurs for more than 2 seconds at least twice in four directions, the score of visual subscale is 2 points, which means the patient exhibits MCS. Each patient participated in two CRS-R evaluations, one in the week before the experiment and another at 1 month after the experiment. Each evaluation contains five CRS-R assessments conducted in different days. The CRS-R scores for each patient presented in Table 1 were based on his/her best responses to the repeated CRS-R assessments.

GUI and audiovisual paradigm

Figure 1 shows GUI employed in the study. A visual button was positioned in the central of a LED monitor (22 in.) (the area ration of button to monitor is 0:1).

Table 1 Summary of patients' clinical statuses. The clinical diagnosis listed in the brackets were obtained 1 month after the experiment

Patient	Age	Gender	Clinical Diagnosis	Etiology	Time Since Injury (months)	CRS-R Score (subscores)	
						Before the experiment	After 1 month
UWS1	34	M	UWS (UWS)	ABI	2	5 (1–1–1-1-0-1)	5 (1–1–1-1-0-1)
UWS2	55	M	UWS (MCS)	TBI	5	7 (1–1–2-2-0-1)	9 (1–1–4-2-0-1)
UWS3	41	M	UWS (UWS)	CVA	1	6 (1–1–1-1-0-2)	7 (1–1–2-1-0-2)
UWS4	48	M	UWS (MCS)	ABI	3	6 (1–1–2-1-0-1)	12 (1–3–5-1-0-1)
UWS5	22	M	UWS (UWS)	TBI	18	5 (1–1–1-1-0-1)	5 (1–1–1-1-0-1)
MCS1	53	F	MCS (MCS)	ABI	3	9 (1–3–2-1-0-2)	9 (1–3–2-1-0-2)
MCS2	37	M	MCS (EMCS)	TBI	4	8 (1–3–1-1-0-2)	19 (3–5–6-2-1-2)
MCS3	38	M	MCS (EMCS)	TBI	2	9 (1–3–2-1-0-2)	18 (3–5–6-1-1-2)

ABI anoxic brain injury, *CRS-R* Coma Recovery Scale-Revised, *CVA* cerebrovascular accident, and *TBI* traumatic brain injury, *CRS-R subscales* auditory, visual, motor, oromotor, communication, and arousal functions

Two loudspeakers were located in the back of monitor which is used to show auditory stimuli. The visual stimuli consisted of 10 visual numbers (0, 1, ..., 9), whereas the auditory stimuli included 10 spoken numbers (0, 1, ..., 9; 22 kHz, 16 bit). The root mean square of power of all sound files was equalized to adjust sound intensities. Each stimulus presentation (300 ms) included a pair of the visual and spoken numbers that were semantically congruent (such as a visual number 8 and a spoken number 8) or incongruent (such as a visual number 5 and a spoken number 6). Furthermore, a 700-ms interval was employed between two consecutive stimulus appearances. Notably, all audiovisual stimuli are presented individually, with the visual stimuli appearing in the same location of the screen (the foveal visual field). Thus, the paradigm was gaze-independent.

Here, we used semantically congruent and incongruent audiovisual stimuli for two reasons. First, we constructed an oddball paradigm for evoking P300. Second, semantically congruent and incongruent audiovisual stimuli may produce more ERP components, such as the N400 and the late positive complex (LPC, also described as P600) [25–27], which might be useful for improving BCI performance.

Experimental procedures

In the experiment, subjects seated comfortably in wheelchair and were required to avoid blinking eyes or moving bodies. The healthy subjects attended Experiment I, and the patients with DOC participated in Experiment II.

Experiment I

The experiment comprises three sessions which were performed randomly. The three sessions correspond to visual (V), auditory (A) as well as audiovisual (AV) stimulus, respectively. In each session, a calibration run of 10 trials was first employed to train the support vector machine (SVM) model, followed by an evaluation run of 40 trials. Notably, a small training dataset was

collected specific to each subject, because this BCI system was designed mainly for patients with DOC who are easily fatigued during the experiment.

Figure 2 illustrates the experimenting process of one trail of audiovisual session. We firstly constructed four pairs of audiovisual stimuli where one pair was semantically congruent (such as a visual number 8 and a spoken number 8) and the other three pairs were semantically incongruent (such as a visual number 5 and a spoken number 6). Under the condition of semantic congruency/incongruency, these visual stimuli and auditory stimuli were pseudo-randomly chosen from the visual and spoken numbers (0, 1, ..., 9). Each trial started as task instruction was presented visually and auditorily and lasted for 8 s. The instruction was "Count the number of times that the spoken number is the same as the visual number." Following the presentation of the instruction, the four audiovisual stimulus pairs constructed as described above were individually presented 8 times in a random order. Specifically, four number buttons flashed from appearance to disappearance in a random order, with each appearance lasting 300 ms and with a 700-ms interval between two consecutive appearances. The appearance of a number button was accompanied by a spoken number for 300 ms. The subject was instructed to count the appearances of the congruent audiovisual stimuli (target) while ignoring the incongruent audiovisual stimuli (non-target). In this manner, the "oddball" effect was produced [28]. After 32 s, the BCI system performed online P300 detection for determining the audiovisual stimulus pair patients focused on. A feedback result determined by the BCI algorithm appeared in the center of the monitor. With correct result, positive audio feedback (applause) lasted for 4 s to encourage the subject. Otherwise, no feedback was presented and the screen was blank for 4 s. A short 6-s interval between two consecutive trials was utilized. Since four pairs of audiovisual stimuli were presented, one of which was the target, the chance level of accurate detection was 25%.

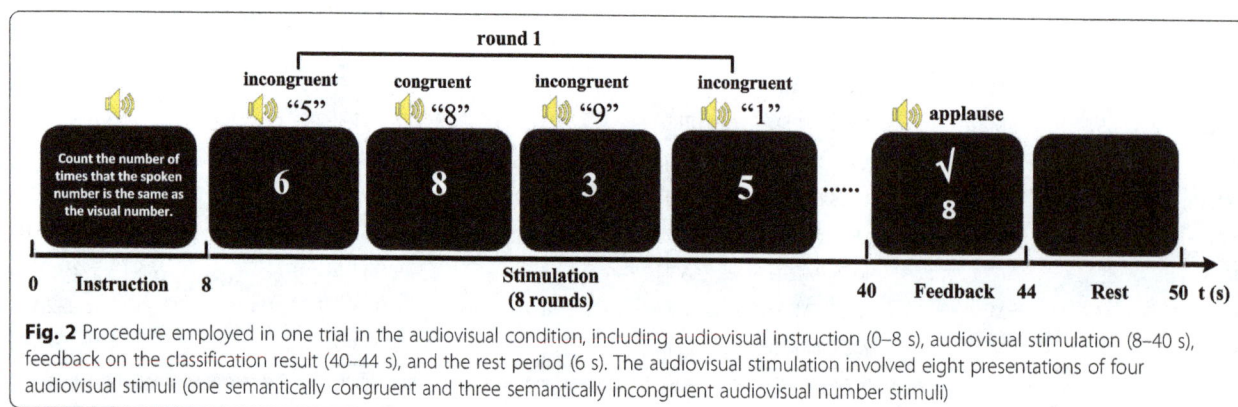

Fig. 2 Procedure employed in one trial in the audiovisual condition, including audiovisual instruction (0–8 s), audiovisual stimulation (8–40 s), feedback on the classification result (40–44 s), and the rest period (6 s). The audiovisual stimulation involved eight presentations of four audiovisual stimuli (one semantically congruent and three semantically incongruent audiovisual number stimuli)

The experimental process of visual session and auditory session exhibited a similarity to audiovisual session, and there were two obvious exceptions. First, the instruction was "Focus on the target number (e.g., 8), and count the presenting times of target number". Second, visual session used visual-only stimuli and auditory session adopted auditory-only stimuli.

Experiment II

Experiment II consisted of an audiovisual session in which each trial was conducted in the same procedure as the audiovisual session described in Experiment I. Eight patients with DOC participated in this experiment, in which 10 trials were calibrated and an online evaluation run of 40 trials were performed. Because patients were subject to fatigue, the calibration and evaluation runs were divided into five blocks, and each block contained 10 trials performed in different days. For these patients, the experiment lasted for 1–2 weeks. Based on the EEG data obtained in the calibration run, the SVM classifier on the first evaluation block was trained. For each of the later blocks, the classification model was updated using the data obtained from the previous block [12, 29]. For instance, data from Block 3 was used to update the SVM model for online classification of Block 4. During the experiment, the experimenters and families kept explaining these instructions to ensure that the patient concentrate themselves on audiovisual target stimuli. An experienced doctor carefully observed the patient to make sure the task engagement. Once the arousal degree was decreased (i.e., the patient closed eyes) or the patient kept moving body (e.g., severe eye blinking/moving) for over 4 s, the trail would be excluded. Additionally, according to the fatigue level of patients, the interval between two continuous trails was extended to at least 10 s.

Data acquisition

A NuAmps device (Neuroscan, Compumedics Ltd., Victoria, Australia) was used to collect scalp EEG signals. Each patient was required to wear an EEG cap (LT 37) equipped with Ag-AgC1 electrodes. The EEG signals were referenced to the right mastoid. The EEG signals used for analysis were obtained from 32 electrodes which were positioned standardly in the 10–20 international system [30]. EEG signals over multiple trails were averaged, followed by the time lock, so as to identify ERPs. "HEOR" and "HEOL", and "VEOU" and "VEOL" were used to record an electrooculogram (EOG). Then, a time-domain regression method which can record EOG was applied to reduce ocular artifacts. The impedances of all electrodes were maintained at less than 5μk. The EEG signals were amplified, sampled at 250 Hz and band-pass filtered between 0.1 Hz and 30 Hz.

Data processing

Online detection algorithm

The same online analysis was performed for each session in Experiments I as well as II. We illustrated the online detection in an audiovisual session as an example. In term of each trial in the calibration and evaluation runs, EEG signals were first filtered at 0.1–20 Hz. The EEG signal epoch (0–900 ms after the stimulus onset) was extracted for each channel and stimulus appearance. This EEG epoch was down-sampled at a rate of 5 for obtaining a data vector which is composed of 45 data points to reduce computation of online processing. The vectors from all 30 channels were concatenated to obtain a new data vector of 1350 data points (45 × 30), which corresponded to a stimulus appearance. Second, we constructed a feature vector containing 1350 data points for each audiovisual stimulus pair by averaging the data vectors across the 8 appearances in a trial to improve the signal-to-noise ratio (SNR). Notably, these features contained several ERP components within 900 ms after stimulus onset. Third, we trained an SVM classifier by virtue of these feature vectors from calibration data. The SVM classifier was based on the popular LibSVM toolbox with the linear kernel. The parameters for the SVM were identified by five-fold cross-validation. Finally, for each online trial, we applied the SVM classifier for the four feature vectors (4×1350 data points) which corresponded to four pairs of audiovisual stimuli, thereby obtaining four SVM scores. The detection result obtained from this trial was determined as the audiovisual stimulus pair corresponding to the maximum of the SVM scores.

Offline data analysis for experiment I

We used the data from the evaluation run in each session of Experiment I to analyze the ERP. Specifically, after the band-pass filtering at 0.1–20 Hz, the EEG epochs of each channel were extracted from 100 ms pre-stimulus to 900 ms post-stimulus, and corrected baseline relying on the data from the 100-ms interval before stimulus. For artifact rejection, once the potential was larger than 60 μV in any channel, the epochs were excluded from averaging. The missing data for the ERP amplitudes were replaced with the mean value for the subject, as recommended for psychophysiological research [31]. During the evaluation run of each stimulus condition, we conducted time-lock averaging on EEG signals of 40 trials to extract the ERP responses.

The ERPs for target stimuli and non-target stimuli were compared to illustrate the effectiveness of the proposed audiovisual BCI paradigm. Specifically, a statistical analysis of the ERP components were conducted as described below [32–34]. First, based on the averaged ERP waveforms extracted above, the ERP components and their corresponding time windows were selected for all conditions. The width of the time window for each ERP component was 200 ms, as described in previous studies [26]. Then, the peak latency of each component was computed separately for each subject/condition. The latencies of maximum peaks were individually computed to ensure that the peak of each individual component was enclosed in its corresponding time window. Next, the mean amplitudes of these components were computed using a small window (50 ms in this study) surrounding the peak maximum. Finally, differences in the amplitudes of the signals between targets and non-targets were tested with two-way repeated measures analyses of variance (ANOVA) using the stimulus condition (the A, V, and AV conditions) and electrode site ("Pz", "Cz", and "Fz") as within-subject factors for each of the ERP components. The missing data for ERP amplitudes were replaced with the mean value of the subject, as recommended for psychophysiological research [31]. Post hoc t-tests (Tukey's test to correct for multiple comparisons) were further performed, when necessary. Results were considered significant when p values were less than 0.05.

Performance measures for experiment II

For each session, the accuracy represented the ratio of the number of all correct responses (hits) among the total number of presented trials. This study used two classes (hit and miss). A hit referred to the situation that output class of a trial was congruent stimulus (i.e. a true positive); otherwise, it was regarded as a miss (i.e. a false positive). Our paradigm employed four choices, namely, one congruent stimulus and three incongruent stimuli. The congruent stimulus (hit) exhibited a chance level of 25%, whereas the incongruent stimuli (miss) exhibited a chance level of 75%. A Jeffreys' Beta distribution-based binomial test was used to compute the significance level of the four-class paradigm, which was expressed as follows [35]:

$$\lambda = \left\{ a + \frac{2(N-2m)z\sqrt{0.5}}{2N(N+3)} \right\} + z\sqrt{\frac{a(1-a)}{N+2.5}} \quad (1)$$

In the equation, N represents the number of trial, m represents the expected number of successful trial, a represents the expected accuracy (here it is 0.25), λ denotes the accuracy rate, and z denotes the z-score according to the standardized normal distribution. As one-sided test exhibited a significance level of 0.05, z is set as 1.65. Based on Eq. (1), the accuracy rate λ

corresponding to the significance level (37.3% for 40 trials) was obtained.

Results
Results for healthy subjects

Ten healthy subjects participated in Experiment I. Table 2 summarizes the online classification accuracies for all healthy subjects. Among the visual-only, auditory-only, and audiovisual conditions, the online accuracy of auditory-only condition was the lowest for each healthy subject. For nine of the ten healthy subjects, the online audiovisual accuracy was larger than or equivalent to the visual-only online accuracy. The average online accuracies for all subjects were 92% for audiovisual condition, 84.75% for visual-only condition, and 74.75% for the audiovisual conditions (Table 2). A one-way repeated measures ANOVA was conducted to test the effect of the stimulus condition on the online accuracy. The stimulus condition exerted a significant effect ($F_{(2, 27)} = 7.849$, $p = 0.005$). Furthermore, according to the post hoc Tukey-corrected t-tests, online average accuracy for audiovisual condition was significantly higher compared with visual-only ($p = 0.031$ corrected) or auditory-only condition ($p = 0.002$ corrected).

We compared the brain responses evoked by target stimuli and non-target stimuli in the three conditions in our ERP analysis. The group mean ERP waveforms from 0 to 900 ms post-stimulus at the "Fz", "Cz", and "Pz" electrodes are shown in Fig. 3(a). Three ERP components, P300, N400, and LPC, were observed. We further determined the time windows for these ERP components (P300 window: 300–500 ms; N400 window: 500–700 ms; and LPC window: 700–900 ms). A two-way ANOVA did not reveal a significant interaction between the stimulus condition and electrode site for each of the ERP components. The electrode site did not exert a significant effect

Table 2 Online classification accuracies of the auditory-only (A), visual-only (V) and audiovisual (AV) sessions for healthy subjects

Subject	Accuracy (%)		
	A	V	AV
H1	75	80	90
H2	70	85	85
H3	55	85	85
H4	87.5	87.5	92.5
H5	70	80	90
H6	82.5	90	100
H7	67.5	80	100
H8	80	90	85
H9	82.5	87.5	97.5
H10	77.5	82.5	95
Average	74.75 ± 0.09	84.75 ± 0.04	92 ± 0.06

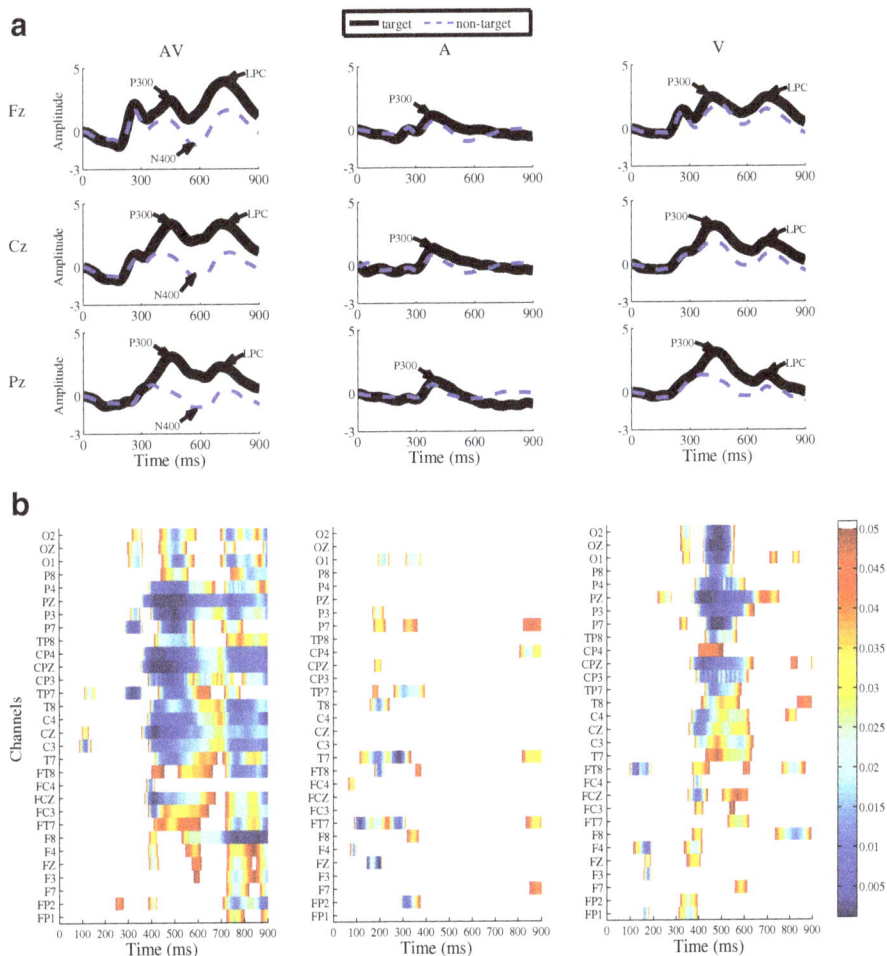

Fig. 3 ERP waveforms and comparison of the results obtained from the audiovisual (AV, left panel), auditory-only (A, middle panel) and visual-only (V, right panel) conditions. **a** Average ERP waveforms of all healthy subjects recorded from the "Fz", "Cz", "Pz" electrodes. The solid and dashed curves correspond to the target and nontarget stimuli, respectively. **b** Point-wise running t-tests compared target with nontarget responses among all healthy subjects for 30 electrodes. Significant differences were plotted when data points met an alpha criterion of 0.05 with a cluster size greater than seven

on each of the ERP components. However, according to the analysis, the stimulus condition can greatly affect each of the ERP components (P300: $F_{(2,63)} = 7.928$, $p = 0.005$; N400: $F_{(2,63)} = 8.708$, $p = 0.004$; LPC: $F_{(2,63)} = 12.557$, $p = 0.003$). Furthermore, post hoc Tukey-corrected t-tests revealed the following: (i) for the P300 component, the target and non-target stimuli in audiovisual condition delivered greater differences in amplitude from that in auditory-only condition ($p = 0.003$, corrected). (ii) For the N400 component, the greater differences in amplitude were observed between the target and non-target stimuli in audiovisual condition compared with visual-only ($p = 0.031$, corrected) or auditory-only condition ($p = 0.006$, corrected). (iii) For the LPC component, greater differences in amplitude were observed between the target and non-target stimuli in the audiovisual condition than in the visual-only ($p = 0.004$, corrected) or auditory-only condition ($p = 0.002$, corrected).

Point-wise running two-tailed t-tests were performed to evaluate the discriminative characteristics of target response and non-target response in the three conditions. From Fig. 3(b), certain time windows, such as 300–500 ms, 500–700 ms, and 700–900 ms, could show more discriminative characteristics in audiovisual condition compared with the other two conditions.

Patients' results

Eight patients attended Experiment II, with online results presented in Table 3. Three patients (UWS4, MCS2, and MCS3) exhibited an obviously higher accuracy (40–45%) than the chance level 25% (accuracy ≥37.3% or $p < 0.05$, binomial test). For patients UWS1, UWS2, UWS3, UWS5, and MCS1, the accuracies

Table 3 Online accuracy of each patient

Subject	Trials	Hits	Accuracy	p-value
UWS1	40	11	27.5%	$p = 0.7150$
UWS2	40	9	22.5%	$p = 0.7150$
UWS3	40	12	30%	$p = 0.4652$
UWS4	40	16	**42.5%**	$p = 0.0106$
UWS5	40	13	32.5%	$p = 0.2733$
MCS1	40	14	35%	$p = 0.1441$
MCS2	40	16	**40%**	$p = 0.0285$
MCS3	40	18	**45%**	$p = 0.0035$

The accuracies that were significantly greater than the chance level 25% (accuracy ≥37.3% or $p < 0.05$) are highlighted in bold

were not significant (i.e., ≤37.3%; ranging from 22.5 to 35%).

The ERP waveforms were calculated for the eight patients with DOC. Specifically, the ERP waveforms in 0–900 ms post-stimulus were obtained by averaging the EEG channel signals across all 40 trials. Note that three trial epochs from patient UWS2 and two trial epochs from patients UWS5 and MCS2 were excluded from further data processing due to noise artifacts (the amplitude exceeded 60 μV). Fig. 4 presents the mean EEG signal amplitudes of eight patients recorded at "Fz", "Cz" and "Pz" electrodes, with solid red curves representing target stimuli and dashed blue curves representing non-target stimuli. Furthermore, the meaningful ERP components were then determined for each patient. Since the ERP latencies were delayed in patients with acquired brain damage [36, 37], a wider time window of 300 ms (P300 window: 300–600 ms; N400 window: 500–800 ms; and LPC window: 700–1000 ms) was used for compensating the delayed latency of each ERP component in patients with DOC. If obvious positive/negative deflection emerged in the three time windows, the corresponding ERP component was elicited in this patient. For the three patients (UWS4, MCS2, and MCS3) who exhibited an obviously higher accuracy than the chance level, a P300-like component was apparent in each target curve, whereas the N400 and LPC responses were not evoked to the same extent as in the healthy controls. For the other five patients (UWS1, UWS2, UWS3, UWS5, and MCS1), none of the P300, N400, and LPC components were observed.

In the five entirely vegetative patients diagnosed by CRS-R assessments, patients UWS2 and UWS4 progressed to MCS 1 month after the experiment. Besides, patient UWS4 subsequently emerged from MCS in the follow-up (4 months after the experiment). Patients MCS2 and MCS3 subsequently emerged from their conditions and exhibited motor-dependent behavior 1 month after experiment. Other patients (UWS1, UWS3, UWS5, and MCS1) remained clinically unchanged at

follow-up. More interestingly, according to the CRS-R, three patients (patients UWS4, MCS2 and MCS3) who obtained accuracy rates that were significantly higher than the chance level 25% (accuracy ≥37.3% or $p < 0.05$, binomial test), which greatly enhanced improved their consciousness levels to a large degree. Specifically, their CRS-R score of these patients improved from 6, 8, and 9 (before experiment) to 12, 19, and 18 (1 month after experiment), respectively.

Discussion

In the present study, we developed a novel audiovisual BCI system using semantically congruent and incongruent audiovisual numerical stimuli. All audiovisual stimuli were presented sequentially, and thus the BCI system was gaze-independent. The experimental results obtained from ten healthy subjects indicted that the audiovisual BCI system achieved higher classification accuracy than the corresponding auditory-only and visual-only BCI systems. Furthermore, the audiovisual BCI was applied to detecting the awareness of DOC patients. Among the eight DOC patients (5 with UWS and 3 with MCS) who participated in the experiment, three (1 with UWS and 2 with MCS) achieved an obviously higher accuracy compared with the chance level (Table 3). According to our results, these three patients exhibited the abilities to follow commands and residual number recognition.

Here, our paradigm was unlike the standard oddball paradigms. The stimuli in our paradigm included semantically congruent and incongruent audiovisual numbers (25% congruent and 75% incongruent audiovisual stimuli), which were presented individually. This paradigm was applied in our experiment for healthy subjects, which indicated two main ERP correlates between the semantic processing (N400 and LPC) and the P300 component in the audiovisual condition. As shown in Fig. 3(a), the ERP responses to semantic processing first included a negative shift (N400) exhibiting a latency of 500–700 ms at electrodes "Fz", "Cz" and "Pz" for semantically incongruent stimuli (nontarget). Then, a subsequent positive peak (LPC) was observed from 700 to 900 ms for semantically congruent stimuli (target) at electrodes "Fz", "Cz" and "Pz". These experimental results well fit previous reports focusing on semantic processing [38–40]. The time windows of P300, N400 and LPC are generally 200–400 ms, 400–600 ms, and 600–800 ms, respectively [26]. In the present study, the delayed latencies of ERP components might be due to the increased difficulty of the experimental task (i.e., distinguishing the semantically congruent audiovisual stimuli from the semantically incongruent stimuli). This finding was consistent with previous studies showing that an increase in the difficulty of the task results in prolonged

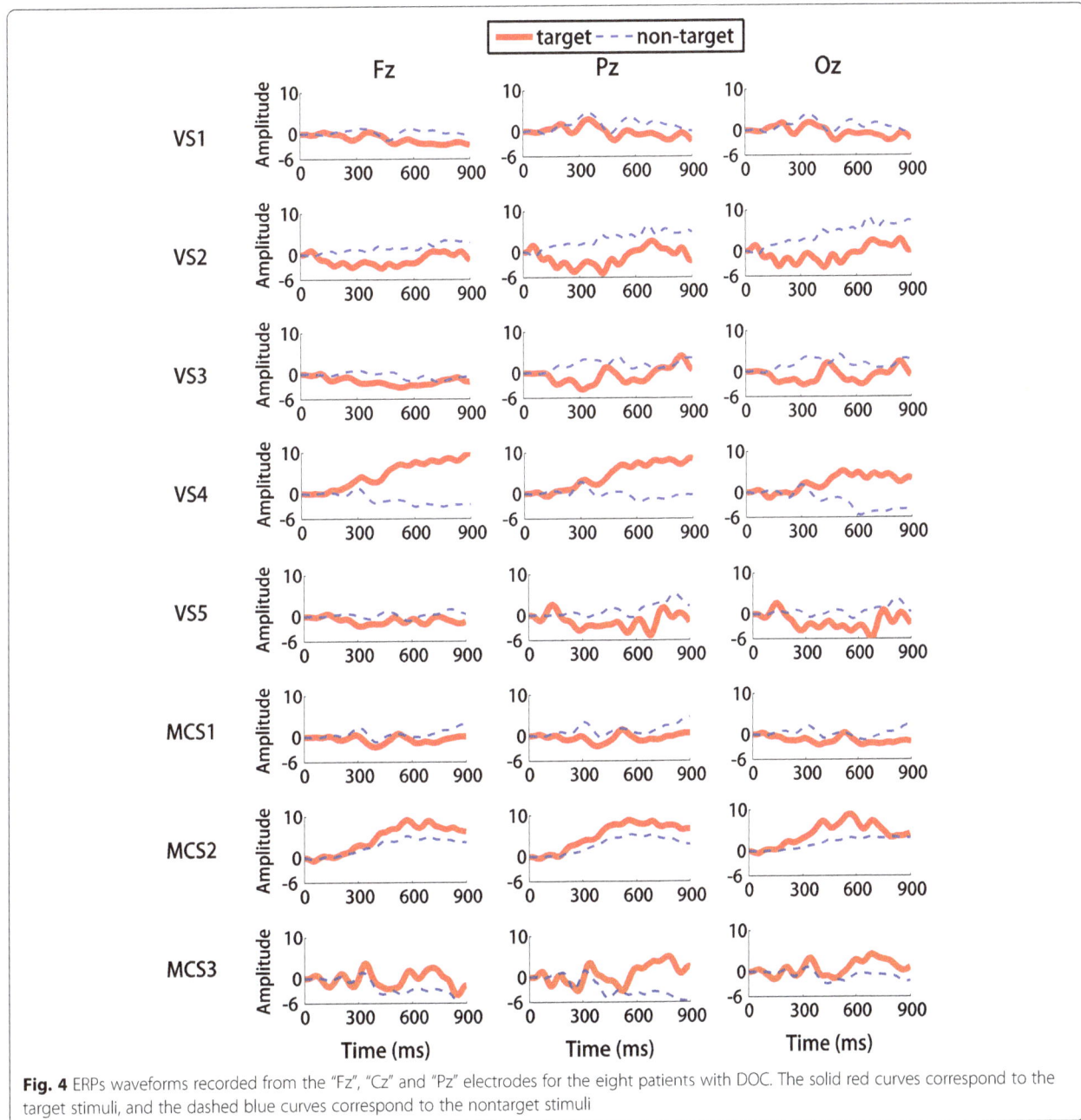

Fig. 4 ERPs waveforms recorded from the "Fz", "Cz" and "Pz" electrodes for the eight patients with DOC. The solid red curves correspond to the target stimuli, and the dashed blue curves correspond to the nontarget stimuli

latencies of ERP components [41, 42]. In our ERP analysis of healthy subjects, a stronger P300 response appeared in AV condition compared with A condition, and stronger responses for both N400 and LPC were detected in AV condition compared with A and V conditions. Furthermore, as shown in Fig. 3(b), in several time windows corresponding to the P300, N400 and LPC components, there was a greater difference between the target response and non-target responses for audiovisual condition compared with visual-only condition and auditory-only condition, which was helpful to improve the BCI performance (Table 2). Taken together, the

potential benefits of our paradigm are described below. First, all the audiovisual stimuli were presented randomly in a serial manner to generate oddball effect. This gaze-independent oddball paradigm was partially supported by results from previous studies [43, 44]. Second, several ERP components, like the N400 and the LPC (Fig. 3), were enhanced using semantically congruent and incongruent audiovisual stimuli. The N400 component is a specific ERP component elicited by violations of a meaningful context [45]. Several studies used sentences or word-pair paradigms to record N400 components of semantic processing in patients with DOC [46, 47]. The LPC component was evoked in the semantic task, like memorizing congruous or incongruous auditory sentences [40, 48], memorizing words list [49, 50], as well as making decisions on congruency [51, 52]. In our audiovisual BCI system, we used all these enhanced ERP components and P300 for classification, which achieved performance improvement on proposed BCI in comparison by corresponding visual-only BCI and auditory-only BCI.

As reported earlier, behavioral observation scales such as CRS-R can yield a relatively high misdiagnosis rate in patients with DOC. BCIs represent an auxiliary bedside tool for detecting residual awareness of patients. Specifically, if the ability to follow commands and the experimental task-related cognitive functions appear in a UWS patient in virtue of a BCI system, we may conclude that the patient possesses awareness and a misdiagnosis might occur. In the present study, one UWS patient (UWS4) could implement the BCI experimental task accurately, which well fit previous fMRI [11] and EEG [53] data showing that some patients who are diagnosed with UWS based on the behavioral scales possessed residual cognitive functions and even exhibited consciousness to some extents. In fact, according to the behavioral CRS-R assessments, this patient with UWS progressed to MCS 1 month after the experiment and further emerged from MCS 3 months later. This behavioral observation supports the results of the conducted BCI assessment for the UWS patient.

Importantly, many cognitive functions, including the ability to understand instructions, selectively focusing on the target stimuli, and maintaining attentional focus on the target, are needed to perform the experimental tasks. One any abovementioned cognitive functions was missed, the experimental tasks may not be performed. Therefore, positive results in BCI experiments may indicate the existence of all these cognitive functions as well as residual awareness in these patients. However, negative results in BCI experiments should not be provided as final evidence for an absence of awareness, because even approximately 13% of healthy subjects exhibited BCI illiteracy, thus fail in effectively controlling a simple BCI [28].

In the study, DOC patients and healthy subjects exhibited a significant difference in ERP components (P300, N400 and LPC). For instance, the N400 or LPC responses were not evoked to the same extent in patients as in the healthy subjects (Fig. 4(a)). The main reason might be that the impairments of the brain networks might deteriorate the ability to evoke ERP components, such as N400 and LPC. Some patients might not simultaneously focus on the audiovisual stimuli, as observed for healthy subjects and patients UWS4, MCS2, and MCS3, and thus a neglect of the auditory or visual stimuli might also have allowed the deterioration of the

evoked ERP components. Another reason lies in the consciousness fluctuation in DOC patients with time. ERP correlates in relation to semantic process cannot be effectively evoked due to low consciousness level. Besides, it is impossible to collect enough training data before each block as patients were fatigued, which may impact classifier performance. Actually, data of previous blocks collected in different days were used for updating the classifier of current block. The separation of calibration and evaluation sessions over several days might be affected by unreliable brain responses on different days. For instance, in a previous study [37], the authors proposed an auditory oddball paradigm for differentiating UWS patients and MCS patients. The study was performed at two different time points (labelled as T1 and T2), with the interval of at least 1 week. The presence of the P300 component at T1 did not well prove that it presented at T2. Based on these findings, DOC patients suffered a much lower BCI performance compared with healthy subjects, although many patients exhibited an obviously higher accuracy (about 45%) compared with the chance level.

It is necessary to conduct further studies for confirming the way to enhance the BCI performance for DOC patients. One potential solution is to update the SVM classifier using the online data with labels. During online awareness detection experiment, DOC patients with DOC were required to pay attention to a target, according to the instructions. Therefore, the labels for online data were available. Furthermore, the online data must be selected to ensure that patients were engaged in the task.

Our study, however, has several limitations. The first CRS-R evaluation was carried out before the experiment, and the experiment lasted from one to 2 weeks. Some patients were more responsive before than during the experiment. Moreover, our study lacks sensitivity because it requires a relatively high level of cognitive ability to understand task instructions.

Conclusions

In summary, a gaze-independent audiovisual BCI was developed for detecting the awareness of patients with DOC in this study. Multiple ERP components, including the P300, N400 and LPC, were enhanced by the semantically congruent and incongruent audiovisual stimuli, which might be useful for improving audiovisual BCI performance. The audiovisual BCI system was first validated in ten healthy subjects and then applied for online detection of awareness of eight DOC patients. Our experimental results demonstrated both the abilities to follow commands and recognize residual number in three of the eight patients with DOC. The BCI system seems to be applicable for DOC patients with display both auditory and visual function. This audiovisual BCI paradigm should be extended to enable an application as simple "YES/NO" communication (e.g., patients focusing on the congruent audiovisual stimuli to communicate yes, and focusing on the incongruent audiovisual stimuli to communicate no) in this patient group.

Abbreviations
ANOVA: Analysis of variance; BCI: Brain-computer interface; CRS-R: Coma recovery scale-revised; DOC: Disorders of consciousness; EEG: Electroencephalography; ERP: Event-related potential; fMRI: Functional magnetic resonance imaging; GCS: Glasgow coma scale; LIS: Locked-in syndrome; LPC: Late positive complex; MCS: Minimally conscious state; SVM: Support vector machine; UWS: Unresponsive wakefulness syndrome; VS: Vegetative state

Acknowledgements
The authors greatly appreciate all subjects who volunteered to participate in the experiments described in this paper.

Funding
This work was supported by the National Key Basic Research Program of China (973 Program) under Grant 2015CB351703, the National Natural Science Foundation of China under Grants 61633010 and 61876067, the Guangdong Natural Science Foundation under Grant 2014A030312005, the Pearl River S&T Nova Program of Guangzhou under Grant 201710010038, and the Nansha District Science and Technology Project under Grant 2016CX014.

Authors' contributions
YL, QX, and RY designed this study. YL designed the BCI systems, experiments and paradigms. JP and FW implemented the BCI systems. RY, QX, YC, YH, JZ and XN conducted the clinical assessments of participants. JP, FW, and YH collected the BCI data. JP analyzed the data, and JP and YL wrote the manuscript. All authors read and approved the final manuscript.

Competing interests
The authors declare that they have no competing interests.

Author details
Coma Research Group, Centre for Hyperbaric Oxygen and Neurorehabilitation, Guangzhou General Hospital of Guangzhou Military Command, Guangzhou 510010, China. ²School of Software, South China Normal University, Guangzhou 510641, China. ³Center for Brain Computer Interfaces and Brain Information Processing, South China University of Technology, Guangzhou 510640, China.

References
1. Wolpaw JR, Birbaumer N, McFarland DJ, Pfurtscheller G, Vaughan TM. Brain-computer interfaces for communication and control. Clin Neurophysiol. 2002;113(6):767–91.
2. Allison BZ, Wolpaw EW, Wolpaw JR. Brain-computer interface systems: progress and prospects. Expert Rev Med Devices. 2007;4(4):463–74.
3. Kübler A, Furdea A, Halder S, Hammer EM, Nijboer F, Kotchoubey B. A brain-computer interface controlled auditory event-related potential (P300) spelling system for locked-in patients. Ann N Y Acad Sci. 2009;1157(1):90–100.
4. Thurlings ME, Brouwer A-M, Van Erp JB, Blankertz B, Werkhoven PJ. Does bimodal stimulus presentation increase ERP components usable in BCIs? J Neural Eng. 2012;9(4):045005.

5. Farwell LA, Donchin E. Talking off the top of your head: toward a mental prosthesis utilizing event-related brain potentials ☆. Electroencephalogr Clin Neurophysiol. 1988;70(6):510.
6. Laureys S, Celesia GG, Cohadon F, Lavrijsen J, Leóncarrión J, Sannita WG, et al. Unresponsive wakefulness syndrome: a new name for the vegetative state or apallic syndrome. Bmc Med. 2010;8:1–68.
7. Noirhomme Q, Lesenfants D, Lehembre R, Lugo Z, Chatelle C, Vanhaudenhuyse A, et al. Detecting consciousness with a brain-computer Interface. In: Converging Clinical and Engineering Research on Neurorehabilitation edn Springer Berlin Heidelberg; 2013. p. 1261–4.
8. Seel RT, Sherer M, Whyte J, Katz DI, Giacino JT, Rosenbaum AM, et al. Assessment scales for disorders of consciousness: evidence-based recommendations for clinical practice and research. Arch Phys Med Rehabil. 2010;91(12):1795–813.
9. Demertzi A, Vanhaudenhuyse A, Bruno M-A, Schnakers C, Boly M, Boveroux P, et al. Is there anybody in there? Detecting awareness in disorders of consciousness. Expert Rev Neurother. 2008;8(11):1719–30.
10. Cruse D, Chennu S, Chatelle C, Bekinschtein TA, Fernández-Espejo D, Pickard JD, et al. Bedside detection of awareness in the vegetative state: a cohort study. Lancet. 2011;378(9809):2088–94. https://doi.org/10.1016/S0140-6736(11)61224-5.
11. Monti MM, Vanhaudenhuyse A, Coleman MR, Boly M, Pickard JD, Tshibanda L, et al. Willful modulation of brain activity in disorders of consciousness. N Engl J Med. 2010;362(7):579–89. https://doi.org/10.1056/Nejmoa0905370.
12. Pan J, Xie Q, Huang H, He Y, Sun Y, Yu R, et al. Emotion-Related Consciousness Detection in Patients With Disorders of Consciousness Through an EEG-Based BCI System. Frontiers in Human Neuroscience. 2018;12.
13. Lulé D, Noirhomme Q, Kleih SC, Chatelle C, Halder S, Demertzi A, et al. Probing command following in patients with disorders of consciousness using a brain–computer interface. Clin Neurophysiol. 2013;124(1):101–6.
14. Müller-Putz G, Klobassa D, Pokorny C, Pichler G, Erlbeck H, Real R, et al.: The auditory p300-based SSBCI: A door to minimally conscious patients? In: Engineering in Medicine and Biology Society (EMBC), 2012 Annual international conference of the IEEE. IEEE; 2012: 4672–4675. http://ieeexplore.ieee.org/stamp/stamp.jsp?tp=&arnumber=6347009&isnumber=6345844.
15. Coyle D, Stow J, McCreadie K, McElligott J, Carroll Á. Sensorimotor modulation assessment and brain-computer interface training in disorders of consciousness. Arch Phys Med Rehabil. 2015;96(3):S62–70.
16. Müller-Putz GR, Pokorny C, Klobassa DS, Horki P. A single-switch BCI based on passive and imagined movements: toward restoring communication in minimally conscious patients. Int J Neural Syst. 2013;23(02):1250037.
17. Pan J, Xie Q, He Y, Wang F, Di H, Laureys S, et al. Detecting awareness in patients with disorders of consciousness using a hybrid brain–computer interface. J Neural Eng. 2014;11(5):056007.
18. Gondan M, Niederhaus B, Rösler F, Röder B. Multisensory processing in the redundant-target effect: a behavioral and event-related potential study. Atten Percept Psychophys. 2005;67(4):713–26.
19. Talsma D, Woldorff MG. Selective attention and multisensory integration: multiple phases of effects on the evoked brain activity. J Cogn Neurosci. 2005;17(7):1098–114.
20. Thurlings ME, Brouwer AM, Van Erp JB, Werkhoven P. Gaze-independent ERP-BCIs: augmenting performance through location-congruent bimodal stimuli. Front Syst Neurosci. 2014;8(143):143.
21. Belitski A, Farquhar J, Desain P. P300 audio-visual speller. J Neural Eng. 2011;8(2):025022.
22. Sellers EW, Donchin E. A P300-based brain–computer interface: initial tests by ALS patients. Clin Neurophysiol. 2006;117(3):538–48.
23. Wang F, He Y, Pan J, Xie Q, Yu R, Zhang R, et al. A novel audiovisual brain-computer interface and its application in awareness detection. Sci Rep. 2015;5:9962.
24. Giacino JT, Kalmar K, Whyte J. The JFK coma recovery scale-revised: measurement characteristics and diagnostic utility. Arch Phys Med Rehabil. 2004;85(12):2020–9.
25. Juottonen K, Revonsuo A, Lang H. Dissimilar age influences on two ERP waveforms (LPC and N400) reflecting semantic context effect. Cogn Brain Res. 1996;4(2):99–107.
26. Duncan CC, Barry RJ, Connolly JF, Fischer C, Michie PT, Näätänen R, et al. Event-related potentials in clinical research: guidelines for eliciting, recording, and quantifying mismatch negativity, P300, and N400. Clin Neurophysiol. 2009;120(11):1883–908.

27. Daltrozzo J, Wioland N, Kotchoubey B. The N400 and late positive complex (LPC) effects reflect controlled rather than automatic mechanisms of sentence processing. Brain Sci. 2012;2(3):267–97.

28. Guger C, Daban S, Sellers E, Holzner C, Krausz G, Carabalona R, et al. How many people are able to control a P300-based brain–computer interface (BCI)? Neurosci Lett. 2009;462(1):94–8.

29. Li Y, Pan J, He Y, Fei W, Laureys S, Xie Q, et al. Detecting number processing and mental calculation in patients with disorders of consciousness using a hybrid brain-computer interface system. Bmc Neurol. 2015;15(1):259.

30. Jasper HH. The 10–20 electrode system of the international federation. Electroencephalogr Clin Neurophysiol. 1958;10:370–5.

31. Blumenthal TD, Cuthbert BN, Filion DL, Hackley S, Lipp OV, Van Boxtel A. Committee report: guidelines for human startle eyeblink electromyographic studies. Psychophysiology. 2005;42(1):1–15.

32. Perrin F, Schnakers C, Schabus M, Degueldre C, Goldman S, Brédart S, et al. Brain response to one's own name in vegetative state, minimally conscious state, and locked-in syndrome. Arch Neurol. 2006;63(4):562–9.

33. Talsma D, Doty TJ, Woldorff MG. Selective attention and audiovisual integration: is attending to both modalities a prerequisite for early integration? Cereb Cortex. 2006;17(3):679–90.

34. Schnakers C, Perrin F, Schabus M, Majerus S, Ledoux D, Damas P, et al. Voluntary brain processing in disorders of consciousness. Neurology. 2008; 71(20):1614–20.

35. Noirhomme Q, Lesenfants D, Gomez F, Soddu A, Schrouff J, Garraux G, et al. Biased binomial assessment of cross-validated estimation of classification accuracies illustrated in diagnosis predictions. NeuroImage. 2014;4:687–94.

36. Guérit J-M, Verougstraete D, de Tourtchaninoff M, Debatisse D, Witdoeckt C. ERPs obtained with the auditory oddball paradigm in coma and altered states of consciousness: clinical relationships, prognostic value, and origin of components. Clin Neurophysiol. 1999;110(7):1260–9.

37. Real RG, Veser S, Erlbeck H, Risetti M, Vogel D, Müller F, et al. Information processing in patients in vegetative and minimally conscious states. Clin Neurophysiol. 2016;127(2):1395–402.

38. Anderson JE, Holcomb PJ. Auditory and visual semantic priming using different stimulus onset asynchronies: an event-related brain potential study. Psychophysiology. 1995;32(2):177–90.

39. Liotti M, Woldorff MG, Perez R, Mayberg HS. An ERP study of the temporal course of the Stroop color-word interference effect. Neuropsychologia. 2000;38(5):701–11.

40. Perrin F, García-Larrea L. Modulation of the N400 potential during auditory phonological/semantic interaction. Cogn Brain Res. 2003;17(1):36–47.

41. Dien J, Spencer KM, Donchin E. Parsing the late positive complex: mental chronometry and the ERP components that inhabit the neighborhood of the P300. Psychophysiology. 2004;41(5):665–78.

42. Hagen GF, Gatherwright JR, Lopez BA, Polich J. P3a from visual stimuli: task difficulty effects. Int J Psychophysiol. 2006;59(1):8–14.

43. Acqualagna L, Treder MS, Schreuder M, Blankertz B: A novel brain-computer interface based on the rapid serial visual presentation paradigm. In: Engineering in Medicine and Biology Society (EMBC), 2010 Annual international conference of the IEEE. IEEE; 2010: 2686–9. http://ieeexplore.ieee.org/stamp/stamp.jsp?tp=&arnumber=5626548&isnumber=5625939.

44. Acqualagna L, Blankertz B. Gaze-independent BCI-spelling using rapid serial visual presentation (RSVP). Clin Neurophysiol. 2013;124(5):901–8.

45. Marí-Beffa P, Valdés B, Cullen DJ, Catena A, Houghton G. ERP analyses of task effects on semantic processing from words. Cogn Brain Res. 2005;23(2):293–305.

46. Kotchoubey B, Lang S, Mezger G, Schmalohr D, Schneck M, Semmler A, et al. Information processing in severe disorders of consciousness: vegetative state and minimally conscious state. Clin Neurophysiol. 2005; 116(10):2441–53.

47. Balconi M, Arangio R, Guarnerio C. Disorders of consciousness and N400 ERP measures in response to a semantic task. J Neuropsychiatry Clin Neurosci. 2013;25(3):237–43.

48. McCallum W, Farmer S, Pocock P. The effects of physical and semantic incongruites on auditory event-related potentials. Electroencephalogr Clin Neurophysiol. 1984;59(6):477–88.

49. Martin A, Chao LL. Semantic memory and the brain: structure and processes. Curr Opin Neurobiol. 2001;11(2):194–201.

50. Kounios J, Green DL, Payne L, Fleck JI, Grondin R, McRae K. Semantic richness and the activation of concepts in semantic memory: evidence from event-related potentials. Brain Res. 2009;1282:95–102.

51. Kounios J, Holcomb PJ. Structure and process in semantic memory: Evidence from event-related brain potentials and reaction times. J Exp Psychol. 1992;121(4):459.

52. Salmon N, Pratt H. A comparison of sentence-and discourse-level semantic processing: an ERP study. Brain Lang. 2002;83(3):367–83.

53. Cruse D, Chennu S, Fernández-Espejo D, Payne WL, Young GB, Owen AM. Detecting awareness in the vegetative state: electroencephalographic evidence for attempted movements to command. PLoS One. 2012;7(11):e49933.

8

Hyponatremia is a potential predictor of progression in radiation-induced brain necrosis: a retrospective study

Huan Liao[1†], Zhuoting Zhu[2†], Xiaoming Rong[1], Hongxuan Wang[1] and Ying Peng[1,3*] (iD)

Abstract

Background: To investigate the prognostic value of hyponatremia, defined as serum sodium level < 135 mEq/L, in radiation-induced brain necrosis (RN) patients.

Methods: We performed a retrospective analysis of the RN patients (The patients included in our study had a history of primary cancers including nasopharyngeal carcinoma/glioma/oral cancer and received radiotherapy previously and then were diagnosed with RN) treated in Sun yat-sen Memorial Hospital from January 2013 to August 2015. Patients without cranial magnetic resonance imaging (MRI) scan and serum sodium data were excluded. Progression was identified when the increase of edema area ≥ 25% on the MRI taken in six months comparing with those taken at the baseline. Factors that might associate with prognosis of RN were collected. Multivariable logistic regression analyses were used to identify potential predictors.

Results: We total included 135 patients, 32 (23.7%) of them with hyponatremia and 36 (26.7%) with RN progression. Percentage of progression was roughly three fold in hyponatremia patients compared with nonhyponatremia patients (53.1% versus 18.4%), translating into a 5-fold increased odds ratio ($P < 0.001$). Multivariable analyses identified hyponatremia as a potential predictor of progression (OR, 4.82; 95% CI [1.94–11.94]; $P = 0.001$).

Conclusions: Hyponatremia was identified as a potential predictor for the progression of patients with RN. Hyponatremia management in patients with RN should be paid much more concern in clinical practice.

Keywords: Hyponatremia, Radiation-induced brain necrosis

Background

Radiotherapy is the standard treatment for nasopharyngeal carcinoma (NPC) and various brain tumors. NPC is the third most common malignant tumor in men in certain regions of East Asia, with an incidence of 15/100,000 to 50/100000 [1]. Moreover, since radiotherapy is invariably associated with radiation exposure of surrounding healthy tissues [2], nearly 100,000 primary and metastatic brain neoplasm patients/year survive long enough (> half a year) to suffer radiation-induced brain necrosis

(RN) in the US [3]. RN is a progressive disease, rendering impairments in attention, memory and executive function, which results in decreased patient quality of life [3].

There is consistent evidence demonstrating that hyponatremia not only acts as risk factors in various diseases such as cancer [4] and heart failure [5], but also has close relationship with central nervous system (CNS) diseases, such as stroke [6], subarachnoid hemorrhage [7, 8] and meningitis [9, 10], through inducing longer hospital stay, increased mortality, and raised complications [11–14]. In neurointensive care, it is usually the development of delayed cerebral infarctions, seizures, and cerebral edema that connects hyponatremia to prognosis [6]. Documentaries also suggest that hyponatremia probably serves as an onlooker reflecting the severity of diseases since it might be preexisting [6, 15, 16], which might be induced by cerebral salt wasting syndrome(CWS) and the syndrome

---

* Correspondence: docpengy123@163.com
†Huan Liao and Zhuoting Zhu contributed equally to this work.
[1]Department of Neurology, Sun Yat-sen Memorial Hospital, Sun Yat-Sen University, No. 107 West Yanjiang Road, Guangzhou 510120, China
[3]Guangdong Provincial Key Laboratory of Malignant Tumor Epigenetics and Gene Regulation, Sun Yat-sen Memorial Hospital, Sun Yat-sen University, Guangzhou, China
Full list of author information is available at the end of the article

of inappropriate antidiuretic hormone secretion(SIADH) [13, 17, 18].

Whereas, for RN, whether hyponatremia is related to the prognosis of RN has not been addressed. In this study, by facilitating a comprehensive coverage of patient characteristics, we aimed to clarify factors associated with prognosis of RN.

Methods

Patient selection

The study was approved by the Institutional Review Board of Sun yat-sen Memorial Hospital. We retrospectively collected the data of patients diagnosed with RN (The patients included in our study had a history of primary cancers including nasopharyngeal carcinoma/glioma/oral cancer and received radiotherapy previously and then were diagnosed with RN) and treated at Department of Neurology, Sun Yat-Sen Memorial Hospital from January, 2013 to August, 2015. The eligible criteria were listed as following: (1) Patients diagnosed with RN between January, 2013 and August, 2015 in the Department of Neurology, Sun Yat-Sen Memorial Hospital; (2) Patients with cranial MRI scan at baseline (the date of the first MRI performed for the diagnosis of RN for the patients in Sun Yat-Sen Memorial Hospital between January, 2013 and August, 2015) and six-month follow-up; (3) Available data of serum sodium during the period between the time of baseline and six-month follow-up.

Clinical details

Patients' characteristics including age, sex, in-hospital days, history of hypertension, epilepsy, dyslipidemia, cerebral infarction, pulmonary infection, paralysis of cranial nerves, nasopharyngeal carcinoma, glioma, oral cancer and baseline result of cranial MRI were retrieved from our institutional prospective electronic medical records. Serum sodium values were measured by use of Ion Selective Electrodes with automated specimen dilution (Cobas Integra 800, Roche) and the lowest values within the time period mentioned above were selected for analysis. Hyponatremia was defined as serum sodium values less than 135 mmol/L according to Hyponatremia Guidelines in Europe in 2014 [19] and was corrected by using hypertonic saline infusions (NaCl, 3%) or 0.9% sodium infusions aiming at an increase of ≤8 mg/dL per 24 h. In addition, all patients were treated with a conventional corticosteroid regimen as described in our prior study [20].

MRI acquisition and analysis

Diagnosis of RN was made by clinical history and MRI performance (Sonata; 1.5 T; Siemens), which included T1-weighted gadolinium contrast-enhanced and T2-weighted image. The MRI recognition of RN was referred to a prior study [21]. Typically, the most common feature of MRI in patients with RN is that the appearance of focal necrosis and finger like edema displays low signal intensity on T1WI while high signal on T2WI. We draw the edge of the maximum area of each edema manually which was then calculated automatically by software Volume Viewer 2(GE, AW Suite 2.0, 6.5.1.z). Two neuroradiologists who were blinded to clinical data reviewed the scans independently. Particularly, edema area was counted as the mean value of two measurements. Moreover, in cases of discrepancies, a second consensus analysis was made by the third author. Follow-up MRIs at six months were used to evaluate the end-point. The end-point is the edema progression occurrence, based on our prior methods [20]. Briefly, the edema progression occurrence was identified when the increase of edema area > 25%.

Statistical analysis

Student's t test (presented as mean ± SD) or Mann-Whitney test (median, range) was used to compare continuous variables, while Pearson Chi-square or Fisher's exact test was used for the comparison of categorical data where appropriate. Multivariable logistic analyses were calculated to investigate independent risk factors for progression. Parameters reaching a statistical trend in univariable analysis ($P < 0.30$) were included into the multivariable models. Collinearity was examined using variance inflation factors (VIF) procedure. Statistical significance was defined as a P value < 0.05 at 2-sided. All statistical analyses were performed with SPSS version 22.0 (SPSS Inc).

Results

A total of 135 patients were included in our study (Fig. 1), with a mean age of 50.9 ± 10.0 years old. 103 patients (76.3%) were male and 32 (23.7%) were female. Among the patients, 126 (93.3%) had a history of nasopharyngeal carcinoma, 8 (6.0%) had glioma and 1 (0.7%) had oral cancer. The median timing of the lowest concentration was one month after the first MRI performed. The mean of the lowest serum sodium values within the six-month period of each patients were 136.7 ± 5.1 mmol/L. Out of 135 patients enrolled for our analysis, 32 patients (23.7%) had hyponatremia and 36 (26.7%) occurred edema progression (increase of edema area > 25%) within a six-month follow-up.

Table 1 shows the comparison of clinical characteristics between patients with and without hyponatremia. Hyponatremia patients were showing statistical trends to have more male gender (87.5% versus 72.8%, $P = 0.088$) and more frequent existing of pulmonary infection (12.5% versus 3.0%, $P = 0.093$). In other aspects of clinical characteristics, there were no significant differences between these two groups.

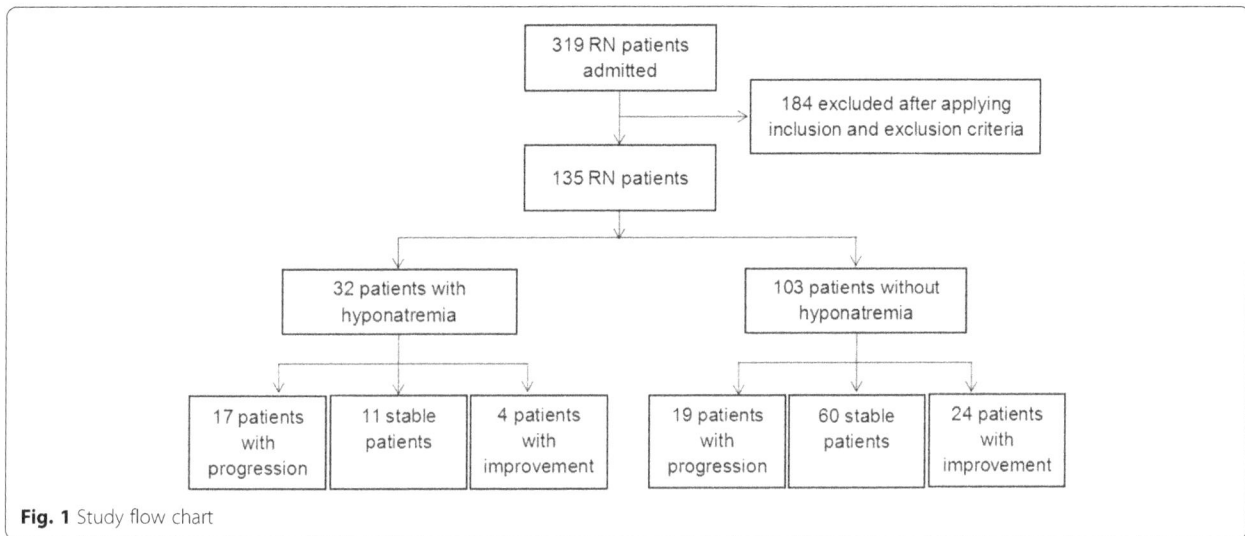

Fig. 1 Study flow chart

Table 2 displays the clinical characteristics of the patients divided into 2 groups according to the presence of edema progression. Patients whose cranial MRI indicating progression were more likely to have lower serum sodium concentration (132.9 ± 6.2 mmol/L versus 138.1 ± 3.8 mmol/L, $P < 0.001$) and higher incidence of medical history on hypertension (27.8% versus 13.1%, $P = 0.045$).

Percentage of progression was roughly three fold in hyponatremia compared with nonhyponatremia patients (53.1%; $n = 17$ versus 18.4%; $n = 19$), translating into a 5-fold increased odds ratio (95% CI, [2.13, 11.77]; $P < 0.001$). Multivariable analyses identified hyponatremia as an independent risk factor of progression (OR, 4.82; 95% CI, [1.94, 11.94]; $P = 0.001$), after adjustment with

covariables including age, in-hospital days, history of hypertension, cerebral infarction, pulmonary infection and edema area in baseline MRI scan, which were found no collinearity existing (Table 3).

Discussion

To the best of our knowledge, this is the first retrospective study to document the association between hyponatremia and outcome of cranial MRI in RN patients. Our findings show that hyponatremia is a potential predictor of progression of RN.

It's very common to have hyponatremia among inpatients and outpatients, with prevalence ranging from 11 to 28.2% [22]. In our study, we found 23.7% of the enrolled

Table 1 Comparison of characteristics between patients with or without hyponatremia

Characteristics	Hyponatremia $n = 32$	Nonhyponatremia $n = 103$	P-Value
Serum sodium, mmol/L (mean ± SD)	129.3 ± 4.3	139.0 ± 2.4	< 0.001
Age, yrs. (mean ± SD)	52.0 ± 9.8	50.5 ± 10.0	0.465
Male	28 (87.5%)	75 (72.8%)	0.088
In-hospital days (M)	8.3 (4–20)	7.5 (1.8–23)	0.546
Hypertension	7 (21.9%)	16 (15.5%)	0.405
Epilepsy	3 (9.4%)	15 (14.6%)	0.648
Dyslipidemia	4 (12.5%)	11 (9.7%)	1.000
Cerebral infarction	5 (15.6%)	8 (7.8%)	0.330
Pulmonary infection	4 (12.5%)	3 (3.0%)	0.093
Paralysis of cranial nerves	7 (21.9%)	16 (15.5%)	0.405
Nasopharyngeal carcinoma	31 (96.9%)	95 (92.2%)	0.607
Glioma	1 (3.1%)	7 (6.8%)	0.734
Oral cancer	0 (0%)	1 (1.0%)	1.000
Baseline T1-weight gadolinium-contrast area (cm2)(mean ± SD)	5.1 ± 2.3	5.3 ± 3.8	0.810
BaselineT2-weighted area (cm2) (mean ± SD)	10.6 ± 5.5	10.4 ± 6.6	0.843

M median, *SD* standard deviation

Table 2 Comparison of characteristics between patients with or without progression

Characteristics	With progression n = 36	Without progression n = 99	P-Value
Serum sodium, mmol/L (mean ± SD)	132.9 ± 6.2	138.1 ± 3.8	< 0.001
Age, yrs. (mean ± SD)	52.7 ± 11.0	50.2 ± 9.5	0.207
Male	27 (75%)	76 (76.8%)	0.831
In-hospital days (M)	8.3 (4.5–23)	7.3 (1.8–22)	0.119
Hypertension	10 (27.8%)	13 (13.1%)	0.045
Epilepsy	4 (11.1%)	14 (14.1%)	0.864
Dyslipidemia	3 (8.3%)	12 (12.1%)	0.757
Cerebral infarction	6 (16.7%)	7 (7.1%)	0.180
Pulmonary infection	4 (11.1%)	3 (3.0%)	0.152
Paralysis of cranial nerves	7 (19.4%)	16 (16.2%)	0.654
Nasopharyngeal carcinoma	33 (91.7%)	93 (94.0%)	0.938
Glioma	3 (8.3%)	5 (5.0%)	0.762
Oral cancer	0 (0%)	1 (1.0%)	1.000
Baseline T1-weight gadolinium-contrast area (cm2)(mean ± SD)	4.5 ± 2.4	5.5 ± 3.8	0.153
BaselineT2-weighted area (cm2) (mean ± SD)	9.3 ± 5.9	10.8 ± 6.4	0.200

M median, *SD* standard deviation

RN patients with hyponatremia. Hyponatremia has acquired broad recognition as a predictor being associated with poor outcome in various diseases [23, 24]. Two main hypothetical mechanisms of hyponatremia impacting on prognosis in disorders of CNS were SIADH and CSW [25]. Excessive antidiuretic hormone (ADH) release causing renal water reabsorption and expansion of the extracellular fluid volume (ECF) was the primary pathogenic mechanism underlying SIADH. When hypothalamus and pituitarium were under pressure or got injured, ADH would be secreted abnormally, causing hyponatremia. Meantime, the mechanism by which RN leads to renal salt wasting is also poorly understood. The most probable process involved central elaboration of a circulating natriuretic factor and/or disruption of neural input into the kidney. Atrial natriuretic peptide (ANP), brain natriuretic peptide (BNP), c-type natriuretic peptide (CNP)

and ouabainlike compound (OLC) had been demonstrated to play a vital role in CSW [26–30], whose releasing also was related to the disruption of hypothalamus and pituitarium. Of note, it is important to make an accurate diagnosis because the treatment of each condition is quite different. Fluid restriction is the treatment of choice in patients with SIADH while vigorous salt replacement is required in patients with CSW. Existing data suggested that fluid restriction was very likely to worsen the underlying neurological condition in the setting of CSW, even cause cerebral infarction [31], acute symptomatic seizures [32] or death. Moreover, the clinical symptoms of vomiting and headache, were often regarded as the results of intracranial hypertension caused by brain edema in RN patients, thus mannitol was usually applied to alleviate the symptom. Nevertheless, in fact, the symptoms could not get remission sometimes, which implied that

Table 3 The logistic regression for the relationship between progression of RN and factors

	Progression	Unadjusted		Adjusted	
		OR (95% CI)	P-Value	OR (95% CI)	P-Value
Hyponatremia (n = 32)	17 (53.1%)	5.01(2.13; 11.77)	< 0.001	4.82(1.94; 11.94)	0.001
Age	–	–		1.01(0.97; 1.06)	0.657
In-hospital days	–	–		1.05(0.95; 1.16)	0.350
Hypertension (n = 23)	10 (43.5%)	–		2.17(0.71; 6.60)	0.172
Cerebral infarction (n = 13)	6 (46.2%)	–		2.04(0.47; 8.82)	0.342
Pulmonary infection (n = 7)	4 (57.1%)	–		3.46(0.53; 22.43)	0.194
T1-weight gadolinium-contrast area	–	–		1.10(0.70; 1.73)	0.672
T2-weighted area	–	–		0.88(0.69; 1.12)	0.299

OR odds ratio, *CI* confidence interval

the symptoms were not caused by brain edema, but very likely by hyponatremia [33]. The information above concludes that, on one hand, when doing irradiation therapy for the primary tumors, avoiding radiation exposure of hypothalamus and pituitarium if possible may effectively reduce the occurrence of hyponatremia from the source [34, 35]. On the other hand, more proper dehydrants instead of those dehydrants which can cause hyponatremia should be chosen when dealing with brain edema of RN. Better management of hyponatremia in RN patients needs more attention.

There were several studies indicating that inflammatory cytokines such as Interleukin 6 (IL-6) [36] and Interleukin 1 beta (IL-1β) [37] play vital roles in the nonosmotic release of ADH. Under inflammatory conditions, this mechanism may be responsible for the occurrence of hyponatremia [38]. Interestingly, the mechanism of RN involves damage to the immune system [39]. In addition, previous studies found that after radiation, microglia in mouse brain tissue could secrete several inflammatory cytokines including IL-6, IL-1β, tumor necrosis factor alpha (TNF-α) and cyclooxygenase-2 (COX-2) [40]. Therefore, we speculate disorder of immune system could render the development of hyponatremia in patients with RN, which should be demonstrated by further studies.

However, despite these postulated pathophysiological considerations of hyponatremia-induced impacts on prognosis, it remains unsolved if hyponatremia merely stands for an onlooker of diseases, that is, preexisting polymedication or comorbidity mirroring worse overall status, which itself maybe responsible for poor prognosis. For instance, hyponatremia was independently associated with anemia on hospital admission, mentioning that hyponatremia was probably preexisting condition rather than developing acutely [6]. Accordingly, in our study, hypertension was also found to be associated with progression of RN. This need to be paid more attention because all hyponatremia patients present with hyponatremia on admission rather than developed it during the course of clinical management [6]. In addition, no existing evidence across a variety of disciplines and diseases demonstrated that correcting hyponatremia could result in better clinical end points so far [41].

Our study firstly demonstrated the association between hyponatremia and prognosis of RN, broadening the area of factors impacting on RN outcome and thus offered a new target on improving the prognosis in clinical practice. Nevertheless, this study still had some limitations. First, retrospective design left the unanswered question why hyponatremia patients presented increased progression of RN. Second, we did not collect the unavailable information regarding the irradiation strategy (radiation fields together with radiation dosages and schedule), though irradiation strategy has been demonstrated to be associated

with occurrence rate of RN [42], which may also have impacts on the outcome of the patients. Third, we could not exclude other causes besides radiation necrosis that might also lead to hyponatremia in RN patients. For example, Table 1 shows a 2× higher frequency of cerebral infarction and a 4× higher frequency of pulmonary infarction associated with hyponatremia. Probably, the limited number of patients studied explains that these observations are not significant. In addition, results may have been biased by excluded patients with uncompleted data. Moreover, the data in the paper failed to answer that when and how often to use hyponatremia detection, and once hyponatremia is detected when the next MRI should be done. Additionally, our data showed that the median timing of the lowest serum sodium concentration was one month after the first MRI performed. The potential explanation maybe that one month after the first MRI performed, patients suffered from bad symptoms (which might be a sign of RN progression) and had to go to hospital to have medical check including blood examination which showed low concentration of sodium including hyponatremia, furtherly surpporting that hyponatremia is a potential predictor for the progression of patients with RN. However, more studies are warranted to confirm and explain this. Lastly, MR spectroscopy is a potential better choice to distinguish recurrent tumor and radiation injury in patients previously radiated for brain neoplasm [43]. However, since the MR spectroscopy data of the enrolled patients wasn't available, we had to choose conventional MR imaging.

Conclusions

In summary, hyponatremia is a common phenomenon in the hospitalized RN patients and acts as a potential predictor of progression, which has clinical significance that doctors need to pay more attention to the management of hyponatremia in RN patients. Large and prospective studies are needed to verify these findings and provide further evidence.

Abbreviations
ADH: Antidiuretic hormone; CI: Confidence interval; CWS: Cerebral salt wasting syndrome; M: Median; MRI: Magnetic resonance imaging; OR: Odds ratio; RN: Radiation-induced brain necrosis; SD: Standard deviation; SIADH: The syndrome of inappropriate antidiuretic hormone secretion; VIF: Variance inflation factors

Funding
This study is supported by National Natural Science Foundation of China (No. 81572481, 81272197) to Ying Peng, International Collaboration Program of Universities in Guangdong Province (No.2012gjhz001) and the Key Project of Product, Study and Research of Guangzhou city (No. 201508020058) to Ying Peng, Grant KLB09001 from the Key Laboratory of Malignant Tumor Gene Regulation and Target Therapy of Guangdong Higher Education Institutes, Sun Yat-Sen University and Grant [2013]163 from Key Laboratory of Malignant Tumor Molecular Mechanism and Translational Medicine of Guangzhou Bureau of Science and Information Technology, National Natural Science Foundation of China (No. 81502167) and Natural Science Foundation of Guangdong Province (No. 2015A030313030) to Xiaoming Rong.

Authors' contributions

HL designed the study and wrote the manuscript. ZZ performed the analysis and interpretation of data as well as manuscript writing. XR and HW was responsible for the acquisition and interpretation of data and the manuscript revision. YP designed the study with HL and made a critical revision for the manuscript. All authors read and approved the final manuscript.

Consent for publication

Not applicable.

Competing interests

The authors declare that they have no competing interests.

Author details

[1]Department of Neurology, Sun Yat-sen Memorial Hospital, Sun Yat-Sen University, No. 107 West Yanjiang Road, Guangzhou 510120, China. [2]State Key Laboratory of Ophthalmology, Zhongshan Ophthalmic Center, Sun Yat-sen University, Guangzhou, China. [3]Guangdong Provincial Key Laboratory of Malignant Tumor Epigenetics and Gene Regulation, Sun Yat-sen Memorial Hospital, Sun Yat-sen University, Guangzhou, China.

References

1. Ho JH. An epidemiologic and clinical study of nasopharyngeal carcinoma. Int J Radiat Oncol Biol Phys. 1978;4(3–4):182–98.
2. Cole AM, Scherwath A, Ernst G, Lanfermann H, Bremer M, Steinmann D. Self-reported cognitive outcomes in patients with brain metastases before and after radiation therapy. Int J Radiat Oncol Biol Phys. 2013;87(4):705–12.
3. Greene-Schloesser D, Robbins ME, Peiffer AM, Shaw EG, Wheeler KT, Chan MD. Radiation-induced brain injury: a review. Front Oncol. 2012;2:73.
4. Castillo JJ, Glezerman IG, Boklage SH, et al. The occurrence of hyponatremia and its importance as a prognostic factor in a cross-section of cancer patients. BMC Cancer. 2016;16:564.
5. Hamaguchi S, Kinugawa S, Tsuchihashi-Makaya M, et al. Hyponatremia is an independent predictor of adverse clinical outcomes in hospitalized patients due to worsening heart failure. J Cardiol. 2014;63(3):182–8.
6. Kuramatsu JB, Bobinger T, Volbers B, et al. Hyponatremia is an independent predictor of in-hospital mortality in spontaneous intracerebral hemorrhage. Stroke. 2014;45(5):1285–91.
7. Bales J, Cho S, Tran TK, et al. The effect of hyponatremia and sodium variability on outcomes in adults with aneurysmal subarachnoid hemorrhage. World Neurosurg. 2016;96:340–9.
8. Mapa B, Taylor BE, Appelboom G, Bruce EM, Claassen J, Connolly ES. Impact of hyponatremia on morbidity, mortality, and complications after aneurysmal subarachnoid hemorrhage: a systematic review. World Neurosurg. 2016;85: 305–14.
9. Brouwer MC, van de Beek D, Heckenberg SG, Spanjaard L, de Gans J. Hyponatraemia in adults with community-acquired bacterial meningitis. QJM. 2007;100(1):37–40.
10. Misra UK, Kalita J, Bhoi SK, Singh RK. A study of hyponatremia in tuberculous meningitis. J Neurol Sci. 2016;367:152–7.
11. Astaf'eva LI, Kutin MA, Mazerkina NA, et al. The rate of hyponatremia in neurosurgical patients (comparison between the data from the Burdenko Neurosurgical Instutite and the literature) and recommendations for the diagnosis and treatment. Zh Vopr Neirokhir Im N N Burdenko. 2016;80(1): 57–70.
12. Moro N, Katayama Y, Igarashi T, Mori T, Kawamata T, Kojima J. Hyponatremia in patients with traumatic brain injury: incidence, mechanism, and response to sodium supplementation or retention therapy with hydrocortisone. Surg Neurol. 2007;68(4):387–93.
13. Hasan D, Wijdicks EF, Vermeulen M. Hyponatremia is associated with cerebral ischemia in patients with aneurysmal subarachnoid hemorrhage. Ann Neurol. 1990;27(1):106–8.
14. Lehmann L, Bendel S, Uehlinger DE, et al. Randomized, double-blind trial of the effect of fluid composition on electrolyte, acid-base, and fluid homeostasis in patients early after subarachnoid hemorrhage. Neurocrit Care. 2013;18(1):5–12.
15. Schrier RW, Sharma S, Shchekochikhin D. Hyponatraemia: more than just a marker of disease severity. Nat Rev Nephrol. 2013;9(1):37–50.
16. Hoorn EJ, Zietse R. Hyponatremia and mortality: moving beyond associations. Am J Kidney Dis. 2013;62(1):139–49.
17. Rahman M, Friedman WA. Hyponatremia in neurosurgical patients: clinical guidelines development. Neurosurgery. 2009;65(5):925–35. discussion 935–6
18. Diringer M, Ladenson PW, Borel C, Hart GK, Kirsch JR, Hanley DF. Sodium and water regulation in a patient with cerebral salt wasting. Arch Neurol. 1989;46(8):928–30.
19. Spasovski G, Vanholder R, Allolio B, et al. Clinical practice guideline on diagnosis and treatment of hyponatraemia. Eur J Endocrinol. 2014;170(3): G1–47.
20. Tang Y, Rong X, Hu W, et al. Effect of edaravone on radiation-induced brain necrosis in patients with nasopharyngeal carcinoma after radiotherapy: a randomized controlled trial. J Neuro-Oncol. 2014;120(2):441–7.
21. Shah R, Vattoth S, Jacob R, et al. Radiation necrosis in the brain: imaging features and differentiation from tumor recurrence. Radiographics. 2012;32(5):1343–59.
22. Upadhyay A, Jaber BL, Madias NE. Incidence and prevalence of hyponatremia. Am J Med. 2006;119(7 Suppl 1):S30–5.
23. Kovesdy CP, Lott EH, Lu JL, et al. Hyponatremia, hypernatremia, and mortality in patients with chronic kidney disease with and without congestive heart failure. Circulation. 2012;125(5):677–84.
24. Cárdenas A, Solà E, Rodríguez E, et al. Hyponatremia influences the outcome of patients with acute-on-chronic liver failure: an analysis of the CANONIC study. Crit Care. 2014;18(6):700.
25. Palmer BF. Hyponatremia in patients with central nervous system disease: SIADH versus CSW. Trends Endocrinol Metab. 2003;14(4):182–7.
26. Isotani E, Suzuki R, Tomita K, et al. Alterations in plasma concentrations of natriuretic peptides and antidiuretic hormone after subarachnoid hemorrhage. Stroke. 1994;25(11):2198–203.
27. Tomida M, Muraki M, Uemura K, Yamasaki K. Plasma concentrations of brain natriuretic peptide in patients with subarachnoid hemorrhage. Stroke. 1998;29(8):1584–7.
28. von BP, Ankermann T, Eggert P, Claviez A, Fritsch MJ, Krause MF. Diagnosis and management of cerebral salt wasting (CSW) in children: the role of atrial natriuretic peptide (ANP) and brain natriuretic peptide (BNP). Childs Nerv Syst. 2006;22(10):1275–81.
29. Fukui K, Inamura T, Nakamizo A, et al. Relationship between cardiac natriuretic peptide (ANP/BNP) and fluid intake in patients with subarachnoid hemorrhage. No To Shinkei. 2000;52(11):1019–23.
30. Yamada K, Goto A, Nagoshi H, Hui C, Omata M. Role of brain ouabainlike compound in central nervous system-mediated natriuresis in rats. Hypertension. 1994;23(6 Pt 2):1027–31.
31. Wijdicks EF, Vermeulen M, Hijdra A, van Gijn J. Hyponatremia and cerebral infarction in patients with ruptured intracranial aneurysms: is fluid restriction harmful. Ann Neurol. 1985;17(2):137–40.
32. Nardone R, Brigo F, Trinka E. Acute symptomatic seizures caused by electrolyte disturbances. J Clin Neurol. 2016;12(1):21–33.
33. Inamdar P, Masavkar S, Shanbag P. Hyponatremia in children with tuberculous meningitis: a hospital-based cohort study. J Pediatr Neurosci. 2016;11(3):182–7.
34. Lin YT, Huang CC, Chyau CC, Chen KC, Peng RY. Sixteen years post radiotherapy of nasopharyngeal carcinoma elicited multi-dysfunction along PTX and chronic kidney disease with microcytic anemia. BMC Urol. 2014;14:19.
35. Appelman-Dijkstra NM, Kokshoorn NE, Dekkers OM, et al. Pituitary dysfunction in adult patients after cranial radiotherapy: systematic review and meta-analysis. J Clin Endocrinol Metab. 2011;96(8):2330–40.
36. Swart RM, Hoorn EJ, Betjes MG, Zietse R. Hyponatremia and inflammation: the emerging role of interleukin-6 in osmoregulation. Nephron Physiol. 2011;118(2):45–51.
37. Landgraf R, Neumann I, Holsboer F, Pittman QJ. Interleukin-1 beta stimulates both central and peripheral release of vasopressin and oxytocin in the rat. Eur J Neurosci. 1995;7(4):592–8.
38. Ohta M, Ito S. Hyponatremia and inflammation. Rinsho Byori. 1999;47(5):408–16.
39. Schnegg CI, Kooshki M, Hsu FC, Sui G, Robbins ME. PPARδ prevents radiation-induced proinflammatory responses in microglia via transpression of NF-κB and inhibition of the PKCα/MEK1/2/ERK1/2/AP-1 pathway. Free Radic Biol Med. 2012;52(9):1734–43.

40. Xue J, Dong JH, Huang GD, Qu XF, Wu G, Dong XR. NF-κB signaling modulates radiation-induced microglial activation. Oncol Rep. 2014;31(6):2555–60.
41. Konstam MA, Gheorghiade M, Burnett JC, et al. Effects of oral tolvaptan in patients hospitalized for worsening heart failure: the EVEREST outcome trial. JAMA. 2007;297(12):1319–31.
42. Jen YM, Hsu WL, Chen CY, et al. Different risks of symptomatic brain necrosis in NPC patients treated with different altered fractionated radiotherapy techniques. Int J Radiat Oncol Biol Phys. 2001;51(2):344–8.
43. Sundgren PC. MR spectroscopy in radiation injury. AJNR Am J Neuroradiol. 2009;30(8):1469–76.

9

Effect of interferon beta-1a subcutaneously three times weekly on clinical and radiological measures and no evidence of disease activity status in patients with relapsing–remitting multiple sclerosis at year 1

Anthony Traboulsee[1]* ⓘ, David K. B. Li[1], Mark Cascione[2], Juanzhi Fang[3], Fernando Dangond[4] and Aaron Miller[5]

Abstract

Background: In the PRISMS study, interferon beta-1a subcutaneously (IFN β-1a SC) reduced clinical and radiological disease burden at 2 years in patients with relapsing–remitting multiple sclerosis. The study aimed to characterize efficacy of IFN β-1a SC 44 μg and 22 μg three times weekly (tiw) at Year 1.

Methods: Exploratory endpoints included annualized relapse rate (ARR), 3-month confirmed disability progression (1-point Expanded Disability Status Scale increase if baseline was < 6.0 [0.5-point if baseline was ≥6.0]), active T2 lesions, and no evidence of disease activity (NEDA; defined as no relapses [subanalyzed by relapse severity], 3-month confirmed progression, or active T2 lesions). Effect of IFN β-1a SC in prespecified patient subgroups was also assessed.

Results: Patients were randomized to IFN β-1a 22 μg ($n = 189$), 44 μg ($n = 184$), or placebo ($n = 187$). At 1 year, IFN β-1a SC tiw reduced ARR ($p < 0.001$), risk of disability progression ($p ≤ 0.029$), and mean number of active T2 lesions per patients per scan ($p < 0.001$) versus placebo. Clinical and radiological benefits were seen as early as Month 2 and 3. Outcomes in subgroups were consistent with those in the overall population. More patients treated with IFN β-1a SC tiw achieved NEDA status, versus placebo, regardless of relapse severity ($p ≤ 0.006$).

Conclusion: Clinical, radiological, and NEDA outcomes at Year 1 were consistent with Year 2 results. Treatment efficacy was consistent in pre-specified patient subgroups.

Keywords: Relapsing–remitting multiple sclerosis, Clinical trials, Interferon-beta subcutaneously, Disability progression, MRI, No evidence of disease activity

* Correspondence: t.traboulsee@ubc.ca
[1]University of British Columbia, S113-2211 Wesbrook Mall, Vancouver, BC V6T 1Z7, Canada
Full list of author information is available at the end of the article

Background

PRISMS (Prevention of Relapses and disability by Interferon beta-1a Subcutaneously in Multiple Sclerosis) was a 2-year, double-blind, placebo-controlled study in patients with relapsing–remitting multiple sclerosis (RRMS), which demonstrated that interferon beta-1a (IFN β-1a) subcutaneously (SC) three times weekly (tiw) significantly reduced the number of relapses, risk of 3-month confirmed disability progression, and number of active T2 lesions, compared with placebo [1]. In the 2-year extension phase of PRISMS, these clinical and radiological benefits were sustained following continuous IFN β-1a SC tiw therapy [2].

While clinical trials evaluating disease-modifying drugs for the treatment of RRMS typically last 2 years or more, some recent trials have been designed to evaluate outcomes over 1 year; additionally, a recent cohort study has found that no evidence of disease activity (NEDA) status at 1 year predicts a lack of disability progression at 7 years [3–5]. The current post hoc analyses were conducted to characterize the efficacy of IFN β-1a SC tiw compared with placebo on clinical and radiological endpoints, and NEDA, during the first year of the PRISMS study. Additional subgroup analyses were conducted to assess the relationship between baseline and clinical characteristics and the treatment effect of IFN β-1a SC tiw on NEDA endpoints, and the impact of relapse severity on NEDA.

Methods

Study design and treatment

The full details of the PRISMS-2 study have been published previously [1]. Eligible patients (18–50 years of age) had clinically definite or laboratory-supported definite RRMS based on the Poser criteria [6], a history of two or more relapses in the previous 2 years, and an Expanded Disability Status Scale (EDSS) score of 0–5.0. Patients were assigned randomly (1:1:1) to IFN β-1a 44 or 22 µg SC tiw or placebo for 2 years. The amount of study drug administered was gradually increased (titrated) to the full dose at the beginning of treatment: patients received 20% of their assigned dose for 2–4 weeks, followed by 50% of this dose for another 2–4 weeks, before finally receiving the full dose.

Patients underwent neurological assessments every 3 months, and as needed for relapse assessment. All patients had magnetic resonance imaging (MRI) scans biannually (cohort 1), and a subset of patients had monthly proton density (PD)/T2 and T1 gadolinium-enhancing (Gd+) scans prior to treatment initiation and during the first 9 months of treatment (cohort 2).

Relapses were defined as a new or worsening symptom attributable to MS, accompanied by an appropriate new neurological abnormality or focal neurological

dysfunction lasting at least 24 h in the absence of fever, and preceded by stability or improvement for at least 30 days [1]. A visit to the study center within 7 days of relapse for confirmation and assessment of severity by the assessing neurologist was requested. Relapse severity was categorized according to quantitative changes in the Scripps Neurological Rating Scale (NRS) score, whereby the worst score during the relapse was compared with the patient's score prior to the start of the relapse: a decrease of 0–7 points was defined as mild, 8–14 as moderate, and ≥ 15 as severe. If it was not possible to evaluate a relapse using the Scripps NRS at the time of worst severity, the relapse was scored according to its effect on activities of daily living. All relapses, as defined by the study protocol, were reported.

Post hoc analyses examined between-treatment differences (IFN β-1a SC tiw compared with placebo) in the following clinical endpoints up to Year 1: annualized relapse rate (ARR); risk of 3-month confirmed disability progression (1-point increase in EDSS score if the baseline EDSS score was < 6.0, or 0.5-point increase if the baseline EDSS score was ≥6.0, with the increase being confirmed at a visit 3 months later); time to first relapse; and proportion of patients relapse-free over 3, 6, 9, and 12 months. The radiological endpoints assessed up to Year 1 included: mean number of active T2 lesions (defined as a new or newly enlarging lesion, or a recurrent lesion ['recurrent' lesions were those that appeared on one scan, were not present on the next scan, then appeared again on a third scan]) per patient per scan (total study cohort) [7]; monthly percentages of patients free of Gd + lesions; and cumulative mean numbers of active T2, Gd+, and combined unique active lesions (defined as an active lesion on T1 post-Gd, T2 sequences, or both, avoiding double counting) per patient per scan in the frequent-MRI cohort.

Further analyses assessed clinical and radiological efficacy results at Year 1 in patient subgroups stratified by prespecified baseline characteristics, including age (< 40 vs. ≥40 years), sex (male vs. female), baseline EDSS score (≤median vs. >median; median baseline EDSS score: 2.5), baseline number of relapses (< 3 vs. ≥3), baseline burden of disease (BOD; ≤median vs. >median; median baseline burden of disease: 1992.5 mm²), and time since MS onset (< 4 vs. ≥4 years).

Treatment differences at Year 1 were examined across a range of composite endpoints. These endpoints included the proportion of patients who had no evidence of clinical disease activity (defined as no protocol-defined relapses and no 3-month confirmed disability progression); were free of active T2 lesions; and achieved NEDA, defined as clinical activity free and no active T2 lesions. NEDA results were also analyzed using Scripps NRS score–assessed relapse definitions based on moderate and/or severe relapse and severe relapse criteria.

Statistical analyses

Comparison of ARR between treatment groups was based on a negative binomial model adjusting for baseline EDSS score (≤3.5 vs. > 3.5), age (< 40 vs. ≥40 years), number of relapses in 2 years prior to screening, and baseline T2 BOD (total area [mm^2] of all T2 lesions, outlined on the PD/T2 scan) with log time on study up to 1 year as an offset variable.

Treatment differences in the proportions of patients free from relapse (cumulative assessment up to 3, 6, 9, and 12 months) were examined using a logistic model adjusting for treatment center.

Comparison of mean number of active T2 lesions per patient per scan (Month 6 and Year 1) was based on a negative binomial model adjusting for baseline BOD, and treatment center with log number of MRI scans up to Year 1 as an offset variable.

Between-treatment comparisons of no evidence of clinical disease activity and NEDA endpoints were based on adjusted logistic models.

Results

Patients

The intent-to-treat population in PRISMS comprised 560 patients who had been randomly assigned to receive IFN β-1a 22 μg (n = 189) or 44 μg (n = 184) SC tiw, or placebo (n = 187). The monthly MRI cohort (cohort 2) comprised 205 patients who had been treated with IFN β-1a 22 μg or 44 μg SC tiw; or placebo (67, 68, and 70

randomized patients, respectively). Baseline demographic and clinical characteristics were similar across treatment groups (see Additional file 1: Table S1) [1].

Efficacy up to year 1

Relapses

Treatment with both IFN β-1a 44 and 22 μg SC tiw reduced clinical and MRI disease activity compared with placebo at Year 1. At Year 1, adjusted mean (95% confidence interval [CI]) ARRs were lower in patients treated with IFN β-1a 44 μg (0.92 [0.78–1.09]) and 22 μg (1.01 [0.86–1.19]) SC tiw compared with placebo (1.49 [1.29–1.72]), representing reductions of 38% and 32%, respectively (both $p < 0.001$). Compared with placebo, time to first relapse over 1 year was significantly delayed by IFN β-1a 44 and 22 μg SC tiw treatment ($p < 0.001$, Fig. 1). Increases in the proportion of IFN β-1a SC patients relapse free (compared with placebo) were significant beginning at Month 3 (71.7% vs. 60.8%; $p = 0.0230$) through Month 12 with IFN β-1a 44 μg SC tiw, and from Month 6 (56.5% vs. 40.3%; $p = 0.0019$) through Month 12 with IFN β-1a 22 μg SC tiw (Fig. 1). IFN β-1a 44 μg SC tiw also significantly reduced the mean cumulative number of relapses compared with placebo during each incremental 3-month period in Year 1, including at 0–3 months (0.30 vs. 0.43; $p = 0.0421$) and at > 3–6, > 6–9, and > 9–12 months ($p < 0.001$), while IFN β-1a 22 μg SC tiw significantly reduced mean cumulative relapse number compared with placebo over 6, 9, and 12 months ($p < 0.01$). Incremental relapse counts over each 3-month period up

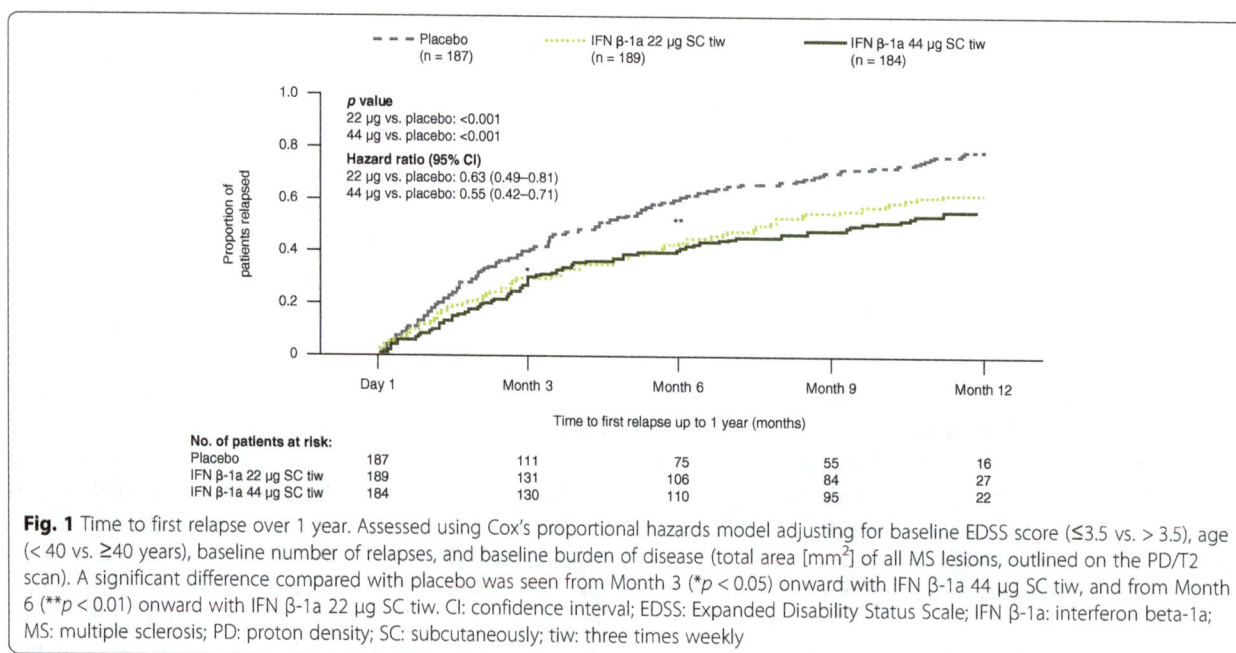

Fig. 1 Time to first relapse over 1 year. Assessed using Cox's proportional hazards model adjusting for baseline EDSS score (≤3.5 vs. > 3.5), age (< 40 vs. ≥40 years), baseline number of relapses, and baseline burden of disease (total area [mm^2] of all MS lesions, outlined on the PD/T2 scan). A significant difference compared with placebo was seen from Month 3 (*$p < 0.05$) onward with IFN β-1a 44 μg SC tiw, and from Month 6 (**$p < 0.01$) onward with IFN β-1a 22 μg SC tiw. CI: confidence interval; EDSS: Expanded Disability Status Scale; IFN β-1a: interferon beta-1a; MS: multiple sclerosis; PD: proton density; SC: subcutaneously; tiw: three times weekly

to Year 1 were lower in both IFN β-1a SC tiw groups compared with placebo (Additional file 2: Figure S1).

Disability progression

The risk of 3-month confirmed disability progression was significantly reduced with IFN β-1a 44 μg and 22 μg SC tiw over 1 year compared with placebo, showing reductions of 38% and 45%, respectively (Fig. 2).

MRI activity

For the entire cohort, IFN β-1a 44 μg and 22 μg SC tiw significantly reduced the mean (standard deviation) number of active T2 lesions per patient per scan compared with placebo over 1 year (1.16 [1.94] and 1.95 [3.41] vs. 3.83 [4.57], respectively; $p < 0.001$ for both comparisons). The proportion of patients free of T2 lesions over 1 year was significantly higher with IFN β-1a 22 μg and 44 μg SC tiw treatment, compared with placebo ($p < 0.001$; Fig. 3). Overall, 26.3%, 49.4%, and 63.9% of patients in the placebo, IFN β-1a 22 μg SC tiw, and IFN β-1a 44 μg SC tiw groups, respectively, were free of active T2 lesions on the scan at 1 year (that is, not considering the scan at 6 months; $p < 0.001$ for both IFN groups compared with placebo). Analyses of data from the frequent, monthly MRI cohort (cohort 2) showed that IFN β-1a SC tiw treatment significantly reduced MRI disease activity compared with placebo from as early as Month 2, as evidenced by a decrease in the mean number of Gd + lesions per patient per scan and an increase in the proportion of patients who were free of Gd + lesions (Additional file 3: Figure S2).

Subgroup analysis

Treatment effects on clinical and MRI outcomes in the prespecified patient subgroups were consistent with the overall population at Year 1. In all subgroups, point estimates and 95% CIs indicated treatment benefits in favor of IFN β-1a 44 μg SC tiw compared with placebo on the proportion of patients free from relapses (with the exception of patients aged ≥40 years; Fig. 4a) and number of active T2 lesions (Fig. 4b). A significant benefit of IFN β-1a 44 μg SC tiw treatment compared with placebo with regard to the proportion of patients free from 3-month confirmed disability progression was observed in females ($p = 0.013$) and in patients with BOD above the median level (1992.5 mm^2; $p = 0.007$). Although there was a consistent trend for estimates of relative treatment effects in favor of IFN β-1a 44 μg SC tiw compared with placebo across all other patient subgroups, it did not reach statistical significance. Significant treatment benefits on the proportion of patients free from relapses over 1 year were also seen in favor of IFN β-1a 22 μg SC tiw compared with placebo in all age and sex subgroups, and in the subgroups of patients with greater disease activity or duration at baseline; significant treatment benefits on the number of active T2 lesions up to 1 year were seen in favor of IFN β-1a 22 μg SC tiw compared with placebo in all prespecified patient subgroups (data not shown).

No evidence of clinical disease activity and NEDA outcomes

Compared with placebo, significantly more patients treated with IFN β-1a SC tiw were free from relapses, 3-month confirmed disability progression, and active T2 lesions (free at both 6-month and 1-year MRI scans)

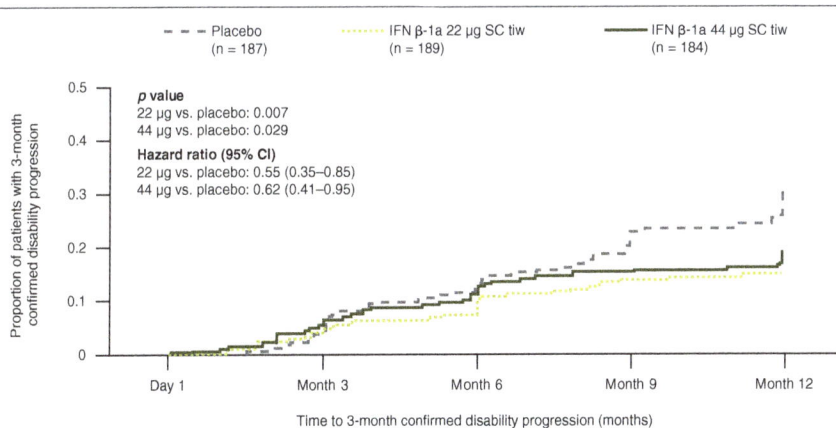

Fig. 2 Time to 3-month confirmed disability progression[a] over 1 year. Assessed using Cox's proportional hazards model adjusting for baseline EDSS score (≤3.5 vs. > 3.5) and age (< 40 vs. ≥40 years). [a]EDSS progression was defined as 1-point increase in EDSS score if the baseline EDSS score was < 6.0 or a 0.5-point increase if the baseline EDSS score was ≥6.0. (EDSS scores could be > 5 if scores increased between screening and baseline). CI: confidence interval; EDSS: Expanded Disability Status Scale; IFN β-1a: interferon beta-1a; SC: subcutaneously; tiw: three times weekly

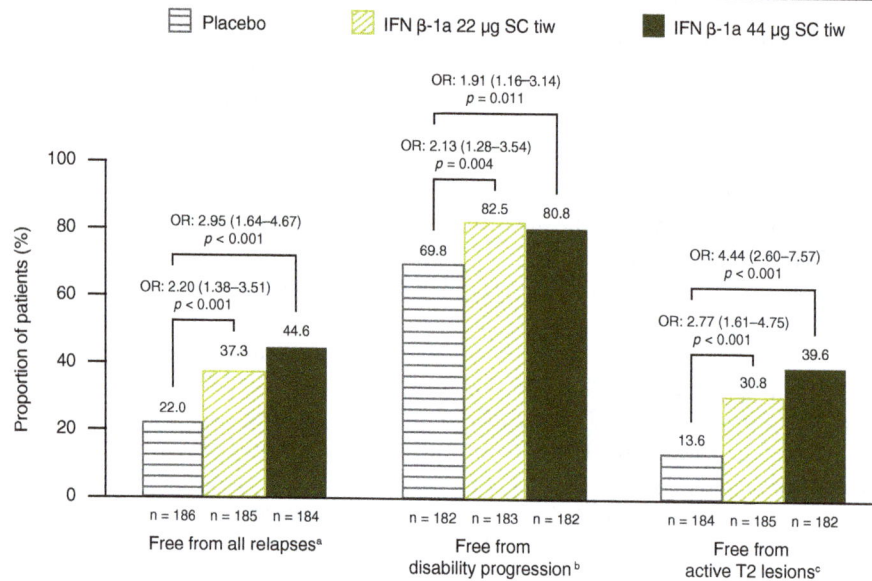

Fig. 3 Proportions free from relapses, disability progression, and active T2 lesions up to 1 year. Based on a logistic regression adjusting for age (< 40 vs. ≥40 years), sex, baseline EDSS score (≤3.5 vs. > 3.5), number of relapses prior to the study within 24 months, and time since MS onset; p values indicate effect of IFN β-1a SC tiw compared with placebo. Values within parentheses are 95% CI values. Active T2 lesions obtained at 6-month and 1-year scans were included. [a]Endpoint is missing if the patient withdrew before the first year and did not have any relapses. [b]Endpoint is missing if the patient withdrew before the first year and did not have 3-month confirmed EDSS progression before withdrawal; EDSS progression was defined as 1-point increase in EDSS score if the baseline EDSS score was < 6.0 or 0.5-point increase if the baseline EDSS score was ≥6.0 (EDSS scores could be > 5 if scores increased between screening and baseline). [c]Endpoint is missing if the patient withdrew before the first year and did not have any active T2 lesions. CI: confidence interval; EDSS: Expanded Disability Status Scale; IFN β-1a: interferon beta-1a; OR: odds ratio; SC: subcutaneously; tiw: three times weekly

over Year 1 (Fig. 3). These treatment effects were reflected in composite outcomes, with significantly more patients treated with IFN β-1a 22 and 44 μg SC tiw achieving no evidence of clinical disease activity (Fig. 5) and NEDA status (Fig. 6) over Year 1, compared with patients receiving placebo.

Across treatment groups, greater proportions of patients achieved NEDA as defined by no Scripps-assessed moderate and/or severe relapse (NEDA-2) and NEDA as defined by no Scripps-assessed severe relapse (NEDA-3) than achieved NEDA as defined by absence of any protocol-defined relapses (Fig. 6). Significant treatment benefits were seen in favor of IFN β-1a 22 and 44 μg SC tiw, regardless of the relapse criteria used. Odds ratios (ORs) for IFN β-1a 44 μg SC tiw versus placebo were larger when the definition of NEDA included absence of Scripps-assessed moderate and/or severe relapses (NEDA-2; OR: 3.55; $p < 0.001$) or the absence of Scripps-assessed severe relapses (NEDA-3; OR: 3.59; $p < 0.001$) rather than absence of all protocol-defined relapses (OR: 2.88; $p = 0.006$) (Fig. 6).

Discussion

The findings from these post hoc analyses over Year 1 from the PRISMS study demonstrated that both doses of IFN β-1a SC tiw therapy had significant, early benefits

on clinical, radiological, and NEDA endpoints compared with placebo. These results are consistent with the findings at 2 years in PRISMS [1].

In the analyses presented here, IFN β-1a SC tiw had sustained benefits on both clinical and radiological endpoints, with a statistically significant difference in time to first relapse between IFN β-1a SC tiw treatment groups and placebo, seen as early as Month 3 and continuing up to Year 1. Both doses of IFN β-1a SC tiw significantly reduced the risk of 3-month confirmed disability progression up to 1 year compared with placebo. In addition, improvements were seen as early as Month 2 for radiological endpoints and were maintained at Months 6, 9, and 12. Moreover, the results of prespecified subgroup analyses indicate that the effect of IFN β-1a SC tiw is consistent across a broad range of patient populations, regardless of baseline disease characteristics.

The finding of a treatment benefit for interferon therapy as early as Month 2 for radiological endpoints is noteworthy, as the modified Rio score in current use predicts response or nonresponse to interferon therapy based on MRI results after a full year [8]. It should be considered that the current analysis did not attempt to predict subsequent clinical responses based on MRI at 2 months, and that it is relatively uncommon to conduct MRI as often as every month and thus datasets used to

a)

	Number of patients				Percentage		
	IFN β-1a 44 µg SC tiw	Placebo			IFN β-1a 44 µg SC tiw	Placebo	OR (95% CI)
Total study population	184	186			44.6	22.0	2.92 (1.84–4.62)
Age							
<40 years	129	135			45.7	20.7	3.52 (2.02–6.12)
≥40 years	55	51			41.8	25.5	2.34 (0.98–5.58)
Sex							
Male	62	46			41.9	21.7	3.01 (1.23–7.36)
Female	122	140			45.9	22.1	2.99 (1.73–5.16)
Baseline EDSS[a]							
≤ median	106	114			46.2	29.8	2.01 (1.15–3.52)
> median	78	72			42.3	9.7	6.92 (2.80–17.20)
Baseline number of relapses							
<3	74	75			50.0	32.0	2.29 (1.16–4.50)
≥3	110	111			40.9	15.3	3.69 (1.92–7.06)
Baseline BOD (mm²)[b]							
≤ median	96	88			46.9	29.5	2.29 (1.22–4.29)
> median	88	98			42.0	15.2	4.01 (1.99–8.08)
Time since MS onset							
<4 years	65	83			56.9	22.9	4.40 (2.12–9.16)
≥4 years	119	103			37.8	21.4	2.35 (1.28–4.31)

0.5   1.0   2.0   10.0   20.0

Odds ratio of IFN β-1a 44 µg SC tiw vs placebo (95% CI)

← Favors placebo   Favors IFN β-1a 44 µg SC tiw

b)

	Number of patients				Rate ratio (95% CI)
	IFN β-1a 44 µg SC tiw	Placebo			
Total study population	182	184			3.33 (2.56–4.35)
Age					
<40 years	128	134			3.13 (2.33–4.35)
≥40 years	54	50			3.45 (2.13–5.56)
Sex					
Male	61	46			4.00 (2.50–6.67)
Female	121	138			3.03 (2.22–4.17)
Baseline EDSS[a]					
≤ median	104	114			3.70 (2.63–5.26)
> median	78	70			2.86 (1.89–4.17)
Baseline number of relapses					
<3	74	74			2.86 (1.85–4.55)
≥3	108	110			3.57 (2.56–5.00)
Baseline BOD (mm²)[b]					
≤ median	95	88			3.45 (2.17–5.26)
> median	87	96			3.13 (2.27–4.35)
Time since MS onset					
<4 years	64	83			4.55 (3.03–7.14)
≥4 years	118	101			2.63 (1.89–3.70)

0.5   1.0   2.0   10.0

Rate ratio of placebo vs IFN β-1a 44 µg SC tiw (95% CI)

← Favors placebo   Favors IFN β-1a 44 µg SC tiw →

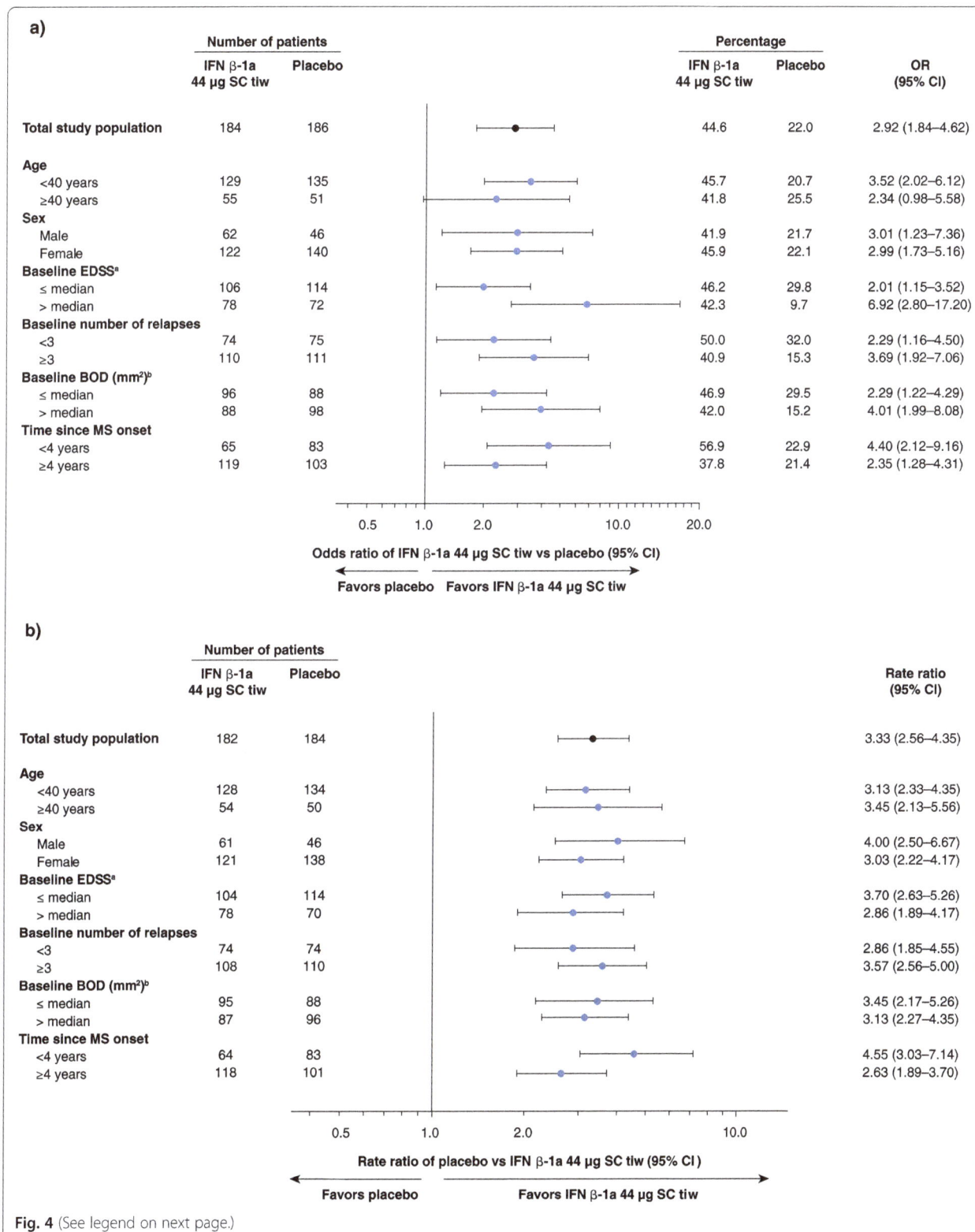

Fig. 4 (See legend on next page.)

(See figure on previous page.)

Fig. 4 Year 1 effect of IFN β-1a 44 μg SC tiw in prespecified subgroups of patients. **a** ORs of IFN β-1a 44 μg SC tiw compared with placebo for the proportion of patients free from relapse at Year 1. Based on logistic model adjusting for age, number of pre-study relapses, baseline EDSS score, and baseline BOD as covariates. (Age, number of pre-study relapses, baseline EDSS score, and baseline BOD were not covariates used in analysis of the subgroups determined by each of these respective characteristics.) **b** Rate ratios for placebo compared with IFN β-1a 44 μg SC tiw for the number of active T2 lesions up to Year 1. Based on a negative binomial model adjusting for baseline BOD as covariate, and log number of scans up to Year 1 as an offset variable. Baseline BOD was not a covariate used in the analysis of the baseline BOD subgroups. Active T2 lesions up to 1 year included those lesions detected at the 6-month or 1-year MRI assessments. [a]Median baseline EDSS score: 2.5. [b]Median baseline BOD: 1992.5 mm². BOD: burden of disease; CI: confidence interval; EDSS: Expanded Disability Status Scale; IFN β-1a: interferon beta-1a; MRI: magnetic resonance imaging; MS: multiple sclerosis; OR: odds ratio; SC: subcutaneously; tiw: three times weekly

predict clinical response based on later MRI results can be larger than our sample [9]. It has been recommended to "re-baseline" patients taking interferon therapy at 3–6 months for purposes of estimating future NEDA status [10]; although benefit was shown in this study as early as Month 2 we are not able to say that this would be a more efficient way of estimating future disease status in clinical practice.

Disease activity in the placebo arms of modern MS clinical trial populations has fallen due to changing diagnostic criteria, trial enrollment criteria, and endpoint definitions [11, 12]. For example, compared with PRISMS, more stringent definitions of relapse (e.g. a requirement for EDSS score changes in order for relapses to be confirmed) have been increasingly used in

subsequent clinical trials [11, 13]. Therefore, we also assessed the impact of relapse severity on the proportion of patients achieving the composite efficacy endpoints. More patients taking IFN β-1a SC tiw were able to achieve no evidence of clinical disease activity and NEDA status compared with placebo, regardless of relapse severity.

Finally, the early effect of IFN β-1a SC tiw treatment is consistent and maintained in the long-term follow-up. The early benefit of IFN β-1a SC tiw treatment was maintained through 4 years and in the long-term follow- up in this patient population with highly active disease at baseline [2, 14]. Through 15 years in PRISMS, patients with higher cumulative dose exposure and longer duration on treatment experienced better clinical outcomes [14].

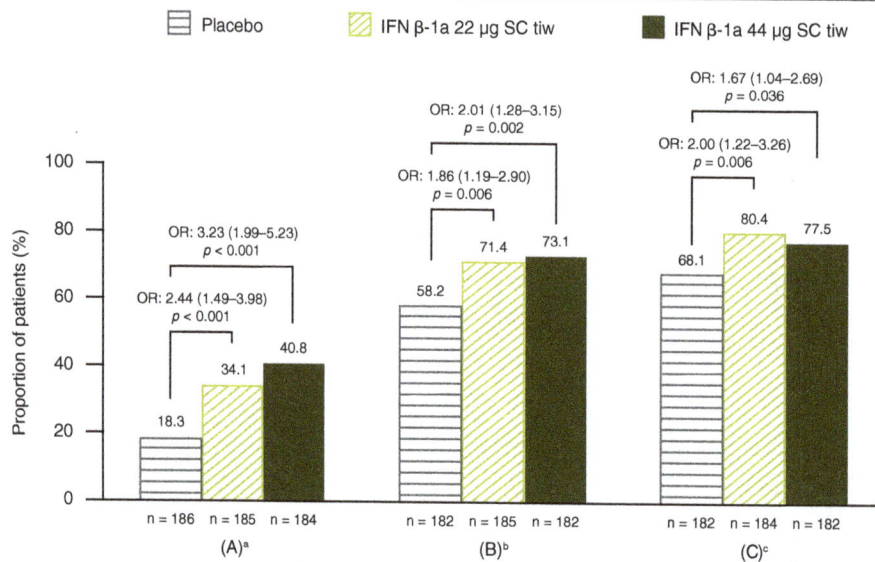

Fig. 5 Proportion of patients with no evidence of clinical disease activity. Based on (**a**) absence of all protocol-defined relapses, (**b**) absence of Scripps-assessed moderate and/or severe relapses, or (**c**) absence of severe relapses, at 1 year. Based on a logistic model adjusting for age (< 40 vs. ≥40 years), sex, baseline EDSS (≤3.5 vs. > 3.5), number of relapses in 2 years prior to screening, and time since MS onset. Values within parentheses are 95% CI values. [a]Defined as no relapses and no 3-month confirmed disability progression (1-point increase in EDSS score if the baseline EDSS score was < 6.0 or 0.5-point increase if the baseline EDSS score was ≥6.0). (EDSS score could be > 5 if scores increase between screening and baseline.) [b]Defined as no relapses and no 3-month confirmed disability progression (1-point increase in EDSS score if the baseline EDSS score was < 6.0 or 0.5-point increase if the baseline EDSS score was ≥6.0). (EDSS score could be > 5 if scores increase between screening and baseline.) Relapses are defined as Scripps-assessed moderate and/or severe. [c]Defined as no relapses and no 3-month confirmed disability progression (1-point increase in EDSS score if the baseline EDSS score was < 6.0 or 0.5-point increase if the baseline EDSS score was ≥6.0). (EDSS score could be > 5 if scores increase between screening and baseline.) Relapses are defined as Scripps-assessed severe. EDSS: Expanded Disability Status Scale; IFN β-1a: interferon beta-1a; OR: odds ratio; SC: subcutaneously; tiw: three times weekly

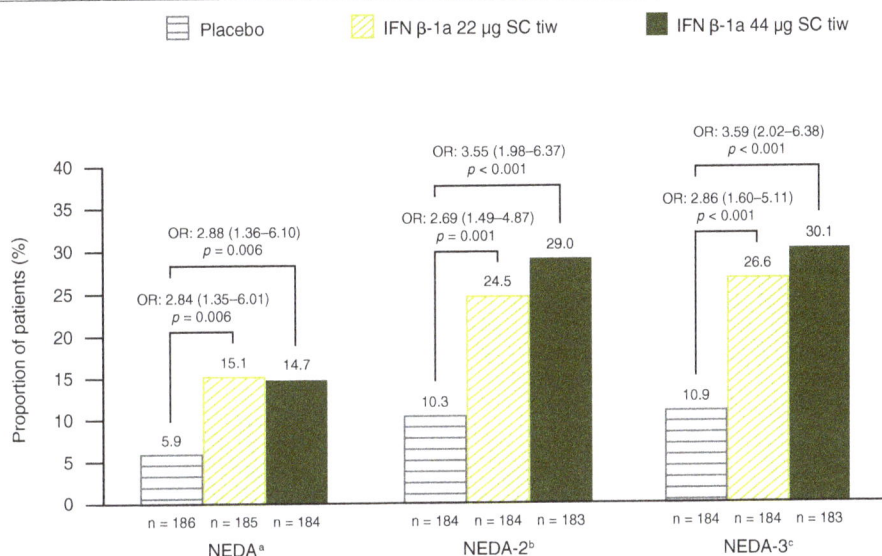

Fig. 6 Proportion of patients with NEDA status up to 1 year. Based on a logistic model adjusting for age (< 40 vs. ≥40 years), sex, baseline EDSS (≤3.5 vs. > 3.5), number of relapses in 2 years prior to screening, and time since MS onset. Active T2 lesions obtained at 6-month and 1-year scans were used. [a]NEDA defined as no relapses, no 3-month confirmed disability progression, and no active T2 lesions over 1 year; disability progression was defined as a 1-point increase in EDSS score if the baseline EDSS score was < 6.0 or 0.5-point increase if the baseline EDSS score was ≥6.0. (EDSS score could be > 5 if scores increase between screening and baseline.). [b]NEDA-2, defined as NEDA with relapses defined as Scripps-assessed moderate and/or severe. [c]NEDA-3, defined as NEDA with relapses defined as Scripps-assessed severe. EDSS: Expanded Disability Status Scale; IFN β-1a: interferon beta-1a; NEDA: no evidence of disease activity; OR: odds ratio; SC: subcutaneously; tiw: three times weekly

Conclusions

IFN β-1a SC tiw treatment had significant early benefits on clinical and radiological endpoints; efficacy was also confirmed using varying definitions of NEDA. Finally, the efficacy of IFN β-1a SC tiw across patient subgroups was consistent with effects seen in the overall treatment population.

Abbreviations

ARR: Annualized relapse rate; BOD: Burden of disease; CI: Confidence interval; EDSS: Expanded Disability Status Scale; Gd+: Gadolinium-enhancing; IFN: Interferon; MRI: Magnetic resonance imaging; MS: Multiple sclerosis; NEDA: No evidence of disease activity; NRS: Neurological Rating Scale; OR: Odds ratio; PD: Proton density; RRMS: Relapsing–remitting multiple sclerosis; SC: Subcutaneously; tiw: Three times weekly

Acknowledgements

The authors thank Stephen Craig, PhD, and Matthew Thomas, PhD, of Caudex, Oxford, UK (supported by EMD Serono, Inc., Rockland, MA, USA [a business of Merck KGaA, Darmstadt, Germany] and Pfizer Inc., New York, NY, USA) for editorial assistance in drafting the manuscript, collating the comments of authors, and assembling tables and figures.

Funding

This study and analyses were supported by EMD Serono, Inc., Rockland, MA, USA (a business of Merck KGaA, Darmstadt, Germany) and Pfizer Inc., New York, NY, USA. The sponsor planned the post hoc analyses reported here in cooperation with the authors. Analysis and interpretation was performed by the authors. The authors were involved in all stages of development and finalization of the manuscript and received editorial assistance from an independent medical-writing-services agency paid by EMD Serono, Inc., Rockland, MA, USA (a business of Merck KGaA, Darmstadt, Germany) and Pfizer Inc., New York, NY, USA.

Authors' contributions

AT, DKBL, MC, JF, FD and AM all made substantial contributions to the study conception and design; analysis and interpretation of data; and drafting and/or critically reviewing the manuscript. JF was involved in acquisition of data. AT, DKBL, MC, JF, FD and AM all reviewed and approved the final draft of the manuscript.

Ethics approval and consent to participate

Ethics approval was obtained from appropriate Institutional Ethics Committees/Institutional Review Boards: Royal Melbourne Hospital, Melbourne, Victoria, Australia; Central Sydney Area Health Service, Camperdown, Australia; University of Western Ontario, London, Ontario, Canada; Ottawa General Hospital, Ottawa, Ontario, Canada; University of British Columbia, Vancouver, British Columbia, Canada; Lund University Hospital, Lund, Sweden; Independent Review Board, Amsterdam, Netherlands; Newcastle & North Tyneside Health Authorities, Newcastle upon Tyne, UK; University Hospital, Nottingham, UK; St. Thomas's Hospital, London, UK; Central Oxford Research Ethics Committee, Headington, Oxford, UK; UZ Leuven, Leuven, Belgium; Limburgs Universitair Centrum, Diepenbeek, Belgium; Université catholique de Louvain, Louvain-la-Neuve, Belgium; Helsinki University Hospitals, Helsinki, Finland; Turku University Central Hospital, Turku, Finland; Würzburg University, Würzburg, Germany; Kantonsspital Basel, Basel, Switzerland; Academisch Ziekenhuis Rotterdam, Rotterdam, Netherlands; St George's Hospital, London, UK; and Hôpitaux Universitaires de Genève, Geneva, Switzerland.. All patients gave written informed consent.

Competing interests

A Traboulsee has acted as a consultant for Biogen, Genzyme, Roche, and Teva, and is Principal Investigator on clinical trials for Biogen, Chugai, Genzyme, and Roche.
D Li is the Director of the UBC MS/MRI Research Group, which has been contracted to perform central analysis of MRI scans for therapeutic trials with Genzyme, Hoffmann-La Roche, Merck Serono, Nuron, Perspectives, and Sanofi-Aventis. He has acted as a consultant to Vertex Pharmaceuticals; has served on scientific advisory boards for Novartis, Nuron, and Roche; has served

on a data and safety advisory board for Opexa; and has received research funding from the Canadian Institute of Health Research and Multiple Sclerosis Society of Canada.

M Cascione has received funding/honoraria for research, consultation, and speakers bureau participation from Acorda, Bayer HealthCare, Biogen, EMD Serono, Genentech, Genzyme/Sanofi, Novartis, Pfizer, Roche, and Teva Pharmaceuticals.

J Fang was an employee of EMD Serono, Inc., Rockland, MA, USA (a business of Merck KGaA, Darmstadt, Germany) at the time of writing.

F Dangond is an employee of EMD Serono, Inc., Billerica, MA, USA (a business of Merck KGaA, Darmstadt, Germany).

A Miller has received research support from Biogen, Genzyme/Sanofi, Mallinckrodt (Questcor), Novartis, and Roche/Genentech. He has acted as a consultant for Accordant Health Services (Caremark), Acorda Therapeutics, Alkermes, Biogen, EMD Serono, Sanofi Genzyme, GlaxoSmithKline, Mallinckrodt (Questcor), Novartis, and Roche/Genentech. He has served on the speakers bureau for Biogen, Genentech, and Sanofi Genzyme for unbranded disease awareness programs only.

Author details

[1]University of British Columbia, S113-2211 Wesbrook Mall, Vancouver, BC V6T 1Z7, Canada. [2]Tampa Neurology Associates, South Tampa Multiple Sclerosis Center, 2919 W. Swann Avenue, Suite 401, South Tampa, FL 33609, USA. [3]EMD Serono, Inc., One Technology Place, Rockland, MA 02370, USA. [4]EMD Serono, Inc, 45A Middlesex Tpke, Billerica, MA 01821, USA. [5]Mount Sinai Hospital, 5 East 98th Street, 1st Floor, New York, NY 10029, USA.

References

1. PRISMS Study Group. Randomised double-blind placebo-controlled study of interferon beta-1a in relapsing/remitting multiple sclerosis. Lancet. 1998;352: 1498–504.

2. PRISMS Study Group, University of British Columbia MS/MRI Analysis Group. PRISMS-4: long-term efficacy of interferon-beta-1a in relapsing MS. Neurology. 2001;56:1628–36.

3. Calabresi PA, Kieseier BC, Arnold DL, Balcer LJ, Boyko A, Pelletier J, et al. Pegylated interferon beta-1a for relapsing-remitting multiple sclerosis (ADVANCE): a randomised, phase 3, double-blind study. Lancet Neurol. 2014;13:657–65.

4. Gold R, Giovannoni G, Selmaj K, Havrdova E, Montalban X, Radue EW, et al. Daclizumab high-yield process in relapsing-remitting multiple sclerosis (SELECT): a randomised, double-blind, placebo-controlled trial. Lancet. 2013; 381:2167–75.

5. Rotstein DL, Healy BC, Malik MT, Chitnis T, Weiner HL. Evaluation of no evidence of disease activity in a 7-year longitudinal multiple sclerosis cohort. JAMA Neurology. 2015;72:152–8.

6. Poser CM, Paty DW, Scheinberg L, McDonald WI, Davis FA, Ebers GC, et al. New diagnostic criteria for multiple sclerosis: guidelines for research protocols. Ann Neurol. 1983;13:227–31.

7. Li DK, Paty DW, UBC MS/MRI Analysis Research Group, PRISMS Study Group. Magnetic resonance imaging results of the PRISMS trial: a randomized, double-blind, placebo-controlled study of interferon-beta1a in relapsing-remitting multiple sclerosis. Ann Neurol. 1999;46:197–206.

8. Sormani MP, Rio J, Tintore M, Signori A, Li D, Cornelisse P, et al. Scoring treatment response in patients with relapsing multiple sclerosis. Mult Scler. 2013;19:605–12.

9. Sormani MP, Gasperini C, Romeo M, Rio J, Calabrese M, Cocco E, et al. Assessing response to interferon-beta in a multicenter dataset of patients with MS. Neurology. 2016;87:134–40.

10. Giovannoni G, Turner B, Gnanapavan S, Offiah C, Schmierer K, Marta M. Is it time to target no evident disease activity (NEDA) in multiple sclerosis? Mult Scler Relat Disord. 2015;4:329–33.

11. Uitdehaag BM, Barkhof F, Coyle PK, Gardner JD, Jeffery DR, Mikol DD. The changing face of multiple sclerosis clinical trial populations. Curr Med Res Opin. 2011;27:1529–37.

12. Sormani MP, Tintore M, Rovaris M, Rovira A, Vidal X, Bruzzi P, et al. Will Rogers phenomenon in multiple sclerosis. Ann Neurol. 2008;64:428

13. Giovannoni G, Comi G, Cook S, Rammohan K, Rieckmann P, Soelberg SP, et al. A placebo-controlled trial of oral cladribine for relapsing multiple sclerosis. N Engl J Med. 2010;362:416–26.

14. Kappos L, Kuhle J, Multanen J, Kremenchutzky M, Verdun di Cantogno E, Cornelisse P, et al. Factors influencing long-term outcomes in relapsing remitting multiple sclerosis: PRISMS-15. J Neurol Neurosurg Psychiatry. 2015; 86:1202–7.

10

Sleep quality, daytime sleepiness, fatigue, and quality of life in patients with multiple sclerosis treated with interferon beta-1b: results from a prospective observational cohort study

Sylvia Kotterba[1], Thomas Neusser[2], Christiane Norenberg[3], Patrick Bussfeld[4], Thomas Glaser[2], Martin Dörner[2] and Markus Schürks[2]* (iD)

Abstract

Background: Sleep disorders and fatigue are common in multiple sclerosis (MS). The underlying causes are not fully understood, and prospective studies are lacking. Therefore, we conducted a prospective, observational cohort study investigating sleep quality, fatigue, quality of life, and comorbidities in patients with MS.

Methods: Patients with relapsing-remitting MS or clinically isolated syndrome treated with interferon beta-1b were followed over two years. The primary objective was to investigate correlations between sleep quality (PSQI), fatigue (MFIS), and functional health status (SF-36). Secondary objectives were to investigate correlations of sleep quality and daytime sleepiness (ESS), depression (HADS-D), anxiety (HADS-A), pain (HSAL), and restless legs syndrome (RLS). We applied descriptive statistics, correlation and regression analyses.

Results: 139 patients were enrolled, 128 were available for full analysis. The proportion of poor sleepers (PSQI≥5) was 55.47% at the beginning and 37.70% by the end of the study (106 and 41 evaluable questionnaires, respectively). Poor sleepers performed worse in MFIS, SF-36, ESS, HADS-D, and HADS-A scores. The prevalence of patients with RLS was low (4.5%) and all were poor sleepers. Poor sleep quality was positively correlated with fatigue and low functional health status. These relationships were corroborated by multivariable-adjusted regression analyses. ESS values and poor sleep quality at baseline seem to predict sleep quality at the one-year follow-up. No variable predicted sleep quality at the two-year follow-up.

Conclusions: Our results confirm the high prevalence of poor sleep quality among patients with MS and its persistent correlation with fatigue and reduced quality of life over time. They highlight the importance of interventions to improve sleep quality.

Trial registration: The study was registered at clinicaltrials.gov: NCT01766063 (registered December 7, 2012). Registered retrospectively (first patient enrolled December 6, 2012).

Keywords: Multiple sclerosis, Interferon beta-1b, Sleep quality, Fatigue, Functional health status, Real world

* Correspondence: markus.schuerks@bayer.com
[2]Bayer Vital GmbH, Leverkusen, Germany
Full list of author information is available at the end of the article

Background

Multiple sclerosis (MS) is a chronic inflammatory and degenerative autoimmune disorder affecting more than two million people worldwide [1]. The prevalence is higher in women than in men. MS is a frequent cause of nontraumatic neurological disability in young adults [1].

Comorbid conditions are common in MS and may contribute to disability. Many patients with MS report sleep disorders [2], more frequently than in the general population, with prevalence estimates ranging from 25 to 54% [3]. Poor sleep quality in MS has been associated with negative outcomes, such as decreased quality of life [4], exacerbation rate and disease severity [5], and with other comorbidities such as fatigue, depression, anxiety, and pain [6, 7].

Fatigue is another common symptom in patients with MS and is closely connected with sleep disorders [3, 8]. Treatment of sleep disorders may have the potential to improve fatigue [9–11].

The underlying causes of poor sleep quality and fatigue are not fully understood. Restless legs syndrome (RLS) appears to play an important role since it has consistently been shown to be more common in patients with MS [2, 9, 12] and is associated with poor sleep [8, 13, 14]. The type of MS treatment may also impact sleep and fatigue. Disease-modifying drugs (DMD), such as interferon beta-1b, might affect sleep quality and fatigue, but results in this connection are ambiguous [8, 13, 14].

Available studies are small and have included cohorts of patients on various treatments. Prospective studies on sleep quality and fatigue are lacking.

Hence, we conducted a prospective study investigating sleep quality, fatigue, quality of life, and comorbidities in patients with MS in a real-world setting over the course of two years. In order to exclude influence of various disease modifying drugs, only patients with interferon beta-1b were included.

Methods

Study design

The BETASLEEP study (NCT01766063) was a prospective, observational cohort study in Germany sponsored by Bayer Vital GmbH. Patients were recruited from 35 neurological offices and clinics specializing in the treatment of MS between December 2012 and January 2015. Patients were followed up for a total of 24 months, with documented visits at baseline, 6, 12, 18, and 24 months. Detailed information about the data collection process and training of investigators is provided in the Additional file 1.

Eligibility

Eligible patients had relapsing-remitting MS (RRMS) or clinically isolated syndrome (CIS), were at least 18 years

old, and had an EDSS (expanded disability status scale) score ≤ 5. Furthermore, patients had to be on treatment with interferon beta-1b. Treatment duration was to be not more than six months and the treatment had to be tolerated by the patient according to their attending physician. All patients provided their written informed consent to participate in the study.

Objectives

Primary objectives were to investigate correlations between sleep quality, fatigue, and functional health status. Secondary objectives were to investigate correlations of sleep quality and daytime sleepiness, depression, anxiety, pain, and RLS.

Outcome variables

Primary outcome variables were sleep quality assessed with the Pittsburgh Sleep Quality Index (PSQI), fatigue assessed with the Modified Fatigue Impact Scale (MFIS), and functional health status assessed with the Short Form 36 (SF-36). Secondary outcome variables were daytime sleepiness measured with the Epworth Sleepiness Scale (ESS), depression and anxiety assessed with the Hospital Anxiety and Depression Scale (HADS), pain measured with the Hamburg Pain Adjective List (HSAL, Hamburger Schmerz Adjektiv Liste), and the severity of RLS assessed through the International RLS Study Group (IRLSSG) rating scale. Detailed information about the questionnaires is provided in the Additional file 1.

Statistical analyses

Statistical analyses were performed using SAS version 9.4 (SAS Institute Inc., Cary, NC). All analyses were exploratory. Continuous variables were described by sample statistics and categorical variables by frequency tables displaying the number of patients as well as percentages. The analyses were performed for the total population and stratified by baseline PSQI score (< 5, ≥ 5).

Correlations between the primary outcome variables and between sleep quality and the secondary outcome variables were calculated using Spearman rank correlation. Analyses were performed at baseline and all follow-up visits.

To further investigate the impact of potential confounders on the correlations, we also performed multivariable-adjusted regression analyses at baseline controlling for age, gender, EDSS score, and duration of disease.

In order to determine potential baseline predictors of poor sleep quality (PSQI≥5) at 12 and 24 months, we first performed univariate logistic regression for the dependent variable (PSQI< 5 vs. PSQI≥5). Second, we employed a stepwise selection procedure with an entry level of $p = 0.5$ and a stay level of $p = 0.1$. The following independent covariates were considered: gender (female, male), age (years), BMI (kg/m^2), type of MS (CIS, RRMS), baseline EDSS score (<3, ≥ 3), baseline PSQI score (<5, ≥ 5), MS duration (months), duration of interferon beta-1b treatment (<3 months, ≥ 3 months), previous sleep disorder (no, yes), baseline ESS score, baseline HADS depression and anxiety scores (<8, ≥ 8), and concomitant medication (no, yes) until initial visit.

For primary outcome variables, missing data were not imputed. Questionnaires were scored according to standard rules based on available instructions. For the regression models in secondary analyses, missing values in the questionnaire scores were either replaced by the mean or median of the available values (continuous data) or a separate category was created (categorical data).

In order to account for decreasing sample size, we performed sensitivity analyses among patients with available data at each visit.

Results

Patient disposition

From December 2012 to January 2015 a total of 139 patients were enrolled into the study, 128 patients were available for full analysis. A flow chart describing patient disposition is provided in Additional file 2. 45.5% of all patients completed the study. Of the patients who discontinued participation in the study, 35.3% were lost to follow up, 23.5% withdrew consent to participate in the study, 13.7% switched to another medication, and 27.5% discontinued study participation for other reasons.

Baseline characteristics

Baseline characteristics are summarized in Table 1. The median age of the sample was 41 years (range 19–70 years; mean 41.5; SD = 11.3), and 71.1% were female. 89.1% had RRMS, while 10.9% had CIS. The median duration of disease was 6.9 months (range 0.1–315.1 months). The median EDSS was 2 (range 0–5). Some differences in gender and disease duration were seen between the good and the poor sleepers.

Sleep quality

At the initial visit, the mean PSQI score was 7.31 (SD = 4.36; median 6; range 1–18). Among 128 patients (106 patients had evaluable PSQI questionnaires) 55.47% indicated poor sleep quality (Table 2, Additional file 3). The mean and median PSQI scores at the final visit were lower (mean 6.71; SD = 4.11; median 5; range 1–18), with 37.70% of 61 patients (41 patients with evaluable PSQI questionnaires) indicating poor sleep quality.

In the sensitivity analysis considering only patients with PSQI scores at all visits ($n = 28$), the mean PSQI score at baseline was 6.75 (SD = 3.95; median 5; range

1–14), and 57.14% of patients indicated poor sleep quality. At the final visit, the mean PSQI was 6.29 (SD = 3.61; median 5; range 1–16), and 53.57% of patients indicated poor sleep quality.

Health status course

At the initial visit, the mean MFIS score was 32.4 (SD = 20.3; median 34; range 0–76; Fig. 1). Poor sleepers had a higher MFIS score (mean 39.4; SD = 18.8; median 43; range 2–76) than good sleepers (mean 20.2; SD = 15.2; median 18; range 0–51). The differences between poor and good sleepers were apparent at each visit. The sensitivity analysis among participants with available data at each visit confirmed these findings.

Poor sleepers also performed worse than good sleepers in the mean SF-36 physical (PCS) and mental component scores (MCS; Fig. 1). These differences could be observed at each visit. In the sensitivity analysis, the differences between poor sleepers and good sleepers in the PCS were less pronounced, while the differences in the MCS were confirmed.

With respect to the ESS, HADS depression, and HADS anxiety scores, poor sleepers performed worse at each visit (Fig. 1).

The prevalence of RLS in the sample was low (4.48% [$n = 6$] at initial visit, 6.56% [$n = 4$] at final visit); all patients diagnosed with RLS were poor sleepers (Table 3). Likewise, the number of patients with reported chronic pain was low, hence the low number of HSAL scores (Table 3).

The MS Functional Composite was lower in poor sleepers throughout the study and the EDSS score was higher at most visits (Table 3).

Correlations of sleep quality and other comorbidities

There was a strong positive correlation between the PSQI and MFIS total scores at baseline and all follow-up visits, with correlation coefficients ranging from 0.62 to 0.71 (nominal $p < 0.0001$ at all time points; Table 4, Additional file 4). Moderate to strong positive correlations were also found between the PSQI and MFIS physical subscale ($r_s = 0.58$–0.67; nominal $p < 0.0001$ at all time points), MFIS cognitive subscale ($r_s = 0.56$–0.67; nominal $p < 0.0001$ at all time points), and MFIS psychological functioning subscale ($r_s = 0.56$–0.65; nominal $p < 0.0001$ at all time points; Table 4, Additional file 4).

Strong to moderate negative correlations at all visits were found between the PSQI total score and the SF-36 PCS ($r_s = -0.51$–-0.63; nominal $p < 0.0001$ at all time points) and the SF-36 MCS ($r_s = -0.47$–-0.78; nominal $p < 0.0001$ at all time points; Table 4, Additional file 4).

Weak to moderate positive correlations were found between the PSQI total score and ESS ($r_s = 0.27$–0.55; nominal p between 0.005 and < 0.0001), and between

Table 1 Baseline characteristics and scores

Characteristic	All Patients	Good sleepers (PSQI< 5)	Poor sleepers (PSQI≥5)
Age, years	$N = 128$	$N = 35$	$N = 71$
Mean (SD)	41.5 (11.3)	40.4 (11.8)	41.3 (10.7)
Median (range)	41.0 (19–70)	41.0 (19–61)	41.0 (19–65)
Gender, n (%)	$N = 128$	$N = 35$	$N = 71$
Women	91 (71.1)	21 (60.0)	53 (74.7)
Men	37 (28.9)	14 (40.0)	18 (25.4)
Diagnosis, n (%)	$N = 128$	$N = 35$	$N = 71$
RRMS	114 (89.1)	31 (88.6)	62 (87.3)
CIS	14 (10.9)	4 (11.4)	9 (12.7)
Duration of disease, months	$N = 113$	$N = 32$	$N = 61$
Mean (SD)	43.0 (71.6)	30.9 (63.8)	45.6 (74.3)
Median (range)	6.9 (0.1–315.1)	6.9 (0.3–262.3)	6.3 (0.1–315.1)
EDSS, median (range)	$N = 128$	$N = 35$	$N = 71$
	2.0 (0–5)	2.0 (0–5)	2.0 (0–5)
MFIS	$N = 122$	$N = 35$	$N = 71$
Mean (SD)	32.38 (20.33)	20.20 (15.24)	39.38 (18.78)
Median (range)	34.0 (0.0–76.0)	18.0 (0.0–51.0)	43.0 (2.0–76.0)
SF-36 physical component score	$N = 113$	$N = 33$	$N = 67$
Mean (SD)	44.56 (11.35)	50.86 (8.37)	41.80 (11.41)
Median (range)	46.53 (16.50–64.06)	53.00 (22.67–64.06)	41.21 (16.50–60.67)
SF-36 mental component score	$N = 113$	$N = 33$	$N = 67$
Mean (SD)	41.74 (13.28)	47.84 (9.98)	38.27 (13.31)
Median (range)	44.39 (12.44–63.82)	50.96 (22.76–63.82)	39.54 (12.44–59.53)
HADS-D	$N = 128$	$N = 35$	$N = 71$
HADS-D ≥ 8, n (%)	29 (22.66)	2 (5.71)	25 (35.21)
HADS-A	$N = 128$	$N = 35$	$N = 71$
HADS-A ≥ 8, n (%)	41 (32.03)	4 (11.43)	32 (45.07)
ESS	$N = 118$	$N = 35$	$N = 68$
Mean (SD)	8.03 (4.54)	6.69 (4.26)	8.88 (4.71)
Median (range)	8.0 (0.0–16.0)	6.0 (0.0–14.0)	9.0 (1.0–16.0)

Subgroups of good sleepers (PSQI< 5) and poor sleepers (PSQI≥5) do not add up to $N = 128$ (100%) due to missing PSQI baseline values

PSQI Pittsburgh Sleep Quality Index, *SD* standard deviation, *RRMS* relapsing-remitting multiple sclerosis, *CIS* clinically isolated syndrome, *EDSS* Expanded Disability Status Scale, *MFIS* Modified Fatigue Impact Scale, *SF-36* Short Form 36, *HADS* Hospital Anxiety and Depression Scale, *ESS* Epworth Sleepiness Scale

PSQI total score and HADS anxiety subscale ($r_s = 0.51$–0.56; nominal p between 0.0002 and < 0.0001; Table 4, Additional file 4). Moderate to strong positive correlations were found between the PSQI total score and HADS depression subscale ($r_s = 0.44$–0.60; nominal p between 0.0001 and < 0.0001; Table 4, Additional file 4).

The strengths of correlations among all primary and secondary outcome measures are visualized in Fig. 2.

Further investigations using multivariable-adjusted linear regression analyses controlling for age, gender, EDSS score, and duration of disease supported the significant relationships seen in the correlation analysis (Additional file 5). An impact of duration of disease on PSQI scores was seen

in most of these models. The influence of the questionnaire score was always the stronger one.

Predictors of poor sleep quality

In univariate logistic regression analysis, poor sleep quality (PSQI≥5) at the one-year follow-up was associated with higher BMI (odds ratio [OR] 1.122, 95% confidence interval [CI] 1.004–1.254), poor sleep quality at baseline (OR 6.270, 95% CI 2.211–17.784), baseline ESS scores (OR 1.200, 95% CI 1.066–1.351), depression at baseline (OR 4.833, 95% CI 1.001–23.344), and anxiety at baseline (OR 3.741, 95% CI 1.217–11.338). Poor sleep quality at the two-year follow-up was predicted by age (OR

Table 2 Course of sleep quality throughout the study

Patients	Baseline visit	6-month visit	12-month visit	18-month visit	24-month visit
All patients, N	128	109	96	65	61
Patients with evaluable questionnaires, N	106	90	82	51	41
PSQI mean (SD)	7.31 (4.36)	6.37 (3.99)	6.43 (4.03)	6.45 (4.48)	6.71 (4.11)
PSQI median (range)	6.0 (1.0–18.0)	5.5 (1.0–20.0)	5.0 (1.0–18.0)	5.0 (0.0–18.0)	5.0 (1.0–18.0)
Proportion of patients with PSQI≥5 (95% confidence interval)	55.47 (46.43–64.25)	46.79 (37.17–56.59)	50.00 (39.62–60.38)	49.23 (36.60–61.93)	37.70 (25.61–51.04)
Sensitivity analysis, N	28	28	28	28	28
PSQI mean (SD)	6.75 (3.95)	6.43 (4.26)	6.00 (3.22)	6.21 (4.07)	6.29 (3.61)
PSQI median (range)	5.0 (1.0–14.0)	4.0 (1.0–18.0)	5.5 (2.0–14.0)	5.0 (1.0–18.0)	5.0 (1.0–16.0)
Proportion of patients with PSQI≥5 (95% confidence interval)	57.14 (37.18–75.54)	46.43 (27.51–66.13)	57.14 (37.18–75.54)	64.29 (44.07–81.36)	53.57 (33.87–72.49)

PSQI Pittsburgh Sleep Quality Index, *SD* standard deviation

1.073, 95% CI 1.009–1.141), poor sleep quality at baseline (OR 4.500, 95% CI 1.06–19.111), and anxiety at baseline (OR 8.727, 95% CI 1.623–46.935).

In multivariate logistic regression using a stepwise selection procedure, baseline ESS values (OR 1.190, 95% CI 1.039–1.362) and poor sleep quality at baseline (OR 5.980, 95% CI 1.914–18.68) were identified as possible predictors for sleep quality at the one-year follow-up. No variable predicted sleep quality at the two-year follow-up.

Discussion

In the BETASLEEP study, more than half of the patients reported poor sleep quality (PSQI≥5) at baseline, while the proportion was only 37.7% (95% CI 25.61–51.04%) after two years. Poor sleep quality was correlated with fatigue, low functional health status, and high scores of daytime sleepiness, depression, and anxiety.

The proportion of poor sleepers reported at the beginning of our study (55.5%) is comparable to that reported in other studies in Germany [14, 15], confirming the high prevalence of poor sleep among patients with MS. In a prospective study by Kotterba et al. among 73 patients with RRMS or CIS, the proportion of poor sleepers was ~ 50% [14]. In a recent cross-sectional study by Rupprecht et al. among 2062 MS patients irrespective of disease course poor sleep quality was present in 54 to 60% of patients [15]. This proportion is higher than what was recently reported in the general population. A study among 9284 people from a German community sample showed poor sleep quality in 36% of participants [16]. The smaller proportion of poor sleepers at the end of our study compared to the beginning may be due to the decreasing number of participants with evaluable PSQI questionnaire results over the course of the study. On the other hand a stable course of disease during interferon beta-1b may reduce fears concerning the development of the disease and improve sleep quality.

The cross-sectional study by Rupprecht et al. [15] further found that depression (96%), anxiety (88%), and fatigue (45%) were the most common comorbidities. In our study, depression was only present in 15.4 to 22.7% and anxiety was only present in 25.0 to 34.9% of patients. HADS-D scores in our study ranged from 3.92 to 4.91, and HADS-A scores ranged from 4.72 to 6.28. A large study among 4516 MS patients from the UK [17] found higher values for HADS-D (7.73) and HADS-A (8.03). In a German study by Kleiter et al. [18], values for HADS-D (3.7) and HADS-A (5.3) were slightly lower than in our study. The low average EDSS values in our study could be one explanation for a lower prevalence of depression and anxiety.

The study by Rupprecht et al. [15] identified anxiety and fatigue as predictors of poor sleep, while medication showed no effect. Furthermore, in the study by Kotterba et al. [14], poor sleep and fatigue were correlated. Our study confirmed the correlation of poor sleep and fatigue, as well as the association of poor sleep and anxiety. Both fatigue and poor sleep quality have repeatedly been shown to negatively affect quality of life in MS patients [4, 19, 20]. In the present study, fatigue and poor sleep were also associated with reduced quality of life assessed with the SF-36.

In contrast to poor sleep, excessive daytime sleepiness was only reported by between 26.4 and 36.4% of our patients. This finding is consistent with previous findings showing presence of excessive daytime sleepiness in around a quarter of MS patients [14].

MS treatment may influence sleep quality. Available results on the effects of interferon beta-1b on sleep quality are mixed. Some studies report negative effects [19, 21], others beneficial [22] or no effect on sleep quality [6]. In animals, it was shown that interferon type I receptors affect the sleep wake cycle [23]. In order to minimize potential differences in medication effects, only patients who had been treated with interferon beta-1b (Betaferon®) for

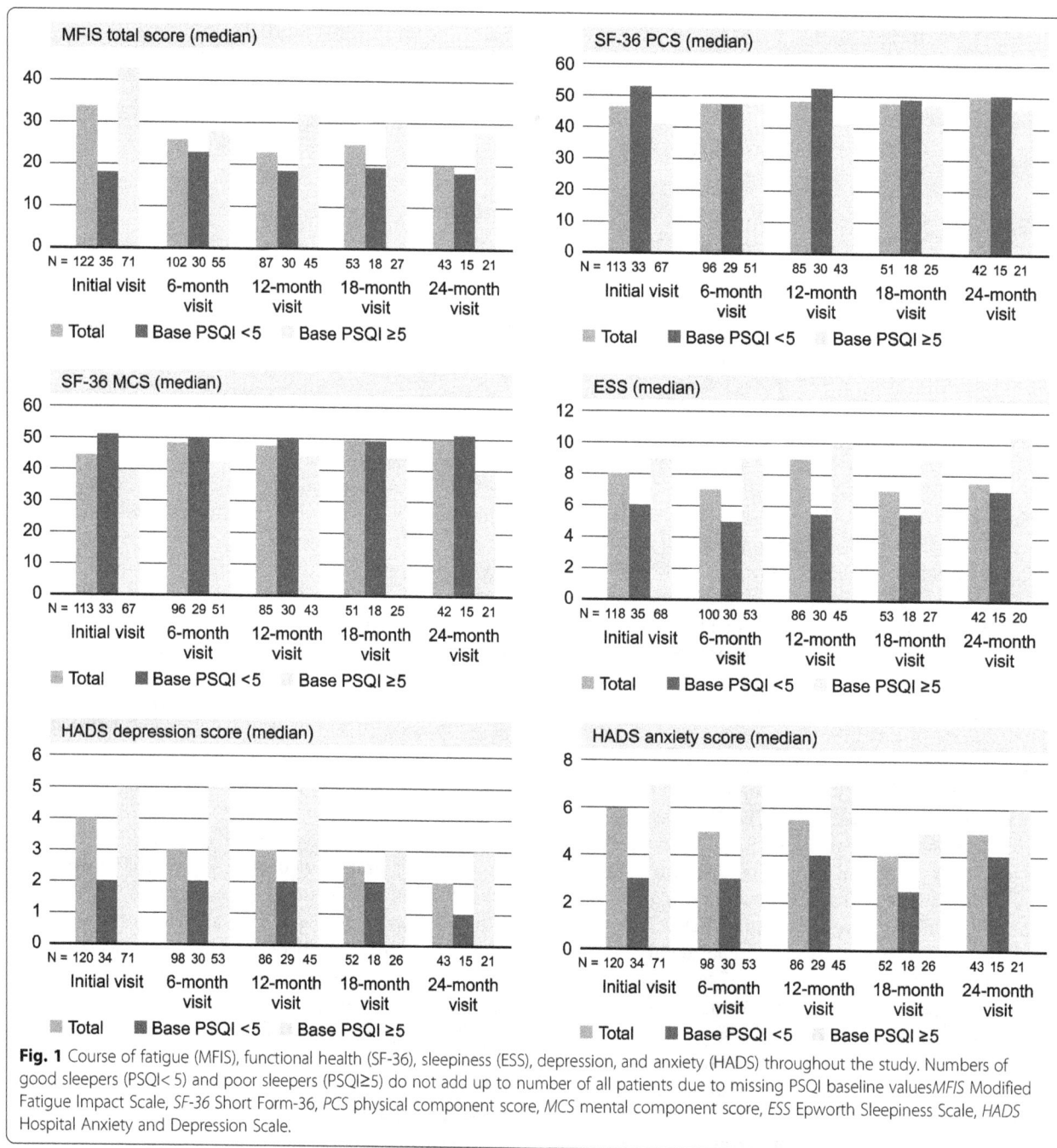

Fig. 1 Course of fatigue (MFIS), functional health (SF-36), sleepiness (ESS), depression, and anxiety (HADS) throughout the study. Numbers of good sleepers (PSQI< 5) and poor sleepers (PSQI≥5) do not add up to number of all patients due to missing PSQI baseline values *MFIS* Modified Fatigue Impact Scale, *SF-36* Short Form-36, *PCS* physical component score, *MCS* mental component score, *ESS* Epworth Sleepiness Scale, *HADS* Hospital Anxiety and Depression Scale.

less than six months and who had tolerated the treatment, were included in the study. Treatment tolerance was required in order to reduce the number of patients prematurely stopping the study.

In the present study, RLS was reported in 2.75 to 6.56% of patients. This proportion is much lower compared to other studies, where diagnosis of RLS was mostly based on questionnaires (prevalence of 14.4 to 57.5%; [2]) and standardized questionnaire-based interviews (prevalence of 32%; [18]). In contrast, in the present study, RLS was assessed by treating physicians based on their evaluation in routine clinical practice. When physicians diagnosed RLS in a patient, the severity was estimated with the IRLSSG. However, treating physicians might not have routinely asked for RLS symptoms. Thus, it is likely that RLS is underreported. The short duration of disease might have further contributed to the low prevalence of RLS in the present study. RLS increases with age in the general population and with disease duration and severity in MS (14). In the presented study patients are mildly impaired and in an early stage of the disease.

Table 3 Course of symptom severity, restless legs syndrome, and pain throughout the BETASLEEP study

Characteristic	Baseline visit			6-month visit			12-month visit			18-month visit			24-month visit		
	All Patients	Good sleepers (PSQI<5)	Poor sleepers (PSQI≥5)	All Patients	Good sleepers (PSQI<5)	Poor sleepers (PSQI≥5)	All Patients	Good sleepers (PSQI<5)	Poor sleepers (PSQI≥5)	All Patients	Good sleepers (PSQI<5)	Poor sleepers (PSQI≥5)	All Patients	Good sleepers (PSQI<5)	Poor sleepers (PSQI≥5)
EDSS	$N=128$	$N=35$	$N=71$	$N=90$	$N=26$	$N=50$	$N=75$	$N=25$	$N=40$	$N=50$	$N=16$	$N=27$	$N=49$	$N=17$	$N=25$
Median (range)	2.0 (0.0–5.0)	2.0 (0.0–5.0)	2.0 (0.0–5.0)	2.0 (0.0–6.5)	2.0 (0.0–4.0)	2.0 (0.0–6.5)	2.0 (0.0–6.5)	1.5 (0.0–4.5)	2.0 (0.0–6.5)	2.0 (0.0–6.5)	1.5 (0.0–4.5)	2.0 (0.0–6.5)	2.0 (0.0–5.0)	1.5 (0.0–5.0)	2.0 (0.0–5.0)
MSFC	$N=93$	$N=26$	$N=55$				$N=54$	$N=18$	$N=31$				$N=31$	$N=8$	$N=17$
Median (range)	0.11 (−3.46–1.49)	0.21 (−1.01–0.69)	0.08 (−3.46–1.49)				0.20 (−1.13–0.87)	0.26 (−0.76–0.87)	0.22 (−1.13–0.80)				0.17 (−1.52–0.99)	0.20 (−0.46–0.73)	0.17 (−1.52–0.99)
RLS, evaluable patients (N)	$N=128$	$N=35$	$N=67$	$N=109$	$N=33$	$N=59$	$N=96$	$N=31$	$N=50$	$N=65$	$N=20$	$N=34$	$N=61$	$N=20$	$N=31$
n (%)	5 (3.9)	0	4 (6.0)	3 (2.8)	0	2 (3.4)	4 (4.2)	0	2 (4.0)	1 (1.5)	0	1 (2.9)	2 (3.3)	0	2 (6.5)
HSAL	$N=7$	$N=1$	$N=5$	$N=6$	$N=1$	$N=3$	$N=5$	$N=1$	$N=2$	$N=4$	$N=1$	$N=2$	$N=3$	$N=0$	$N=2$
Median (range)	111.0 (18–193)	18.0 (18–18)	111.0 (38–193)	42.5 (0–151)	0.0 (0–0)	50.0 (6–133)	48.0 (0–89)	0.0 (0–0)	62.5 (48–77)	61.5 (0–109)	0.0 (0–0)	61.5 (30–93)	124.0 (26–137)	–	75.0 (26–124)

Numbers of good sleepers (PSQI<5) and poor sleepers (PSQI≥5) do not add up to number of all patients due to missing PSQI baseline values

PSQI Pittsburgh Sleep Quality Index, EDSS Expanded Disability Status Scale, RLS restless legs syndrome, MSFC Multiple Sclerosis Functional Composite, SD standard deviation, HSAL Hamburg Pain Adjective List

Table 4 Correlations between the primary and secondary outcome variables

	Baseline visit						12-month visit						24-month visit					
	PSQI (total score)			MFIS (total score)			PSQI (total score)			MFIS (total score)			PSQI (total score)			MFIS (total score)		
	N	r_s	p	N	r_s	p	N	r_s	p	N	r_s	p	N	r_s	p	N	r_s	p
PSQI (total score)	–	–		106	**0.62**	<.0001	–	–		82	**0.68**	<.0001				41	**0.66**	<.0001
MFIS (total score)	106	**0.62**	<.0001	–	–		82	**0.68**	<.0001	–	–		41	**0.66**	<.0001	–	–	
SF-36																		
Physical component score (PCS)	100	−0.54	<.0001	113	−0.72	<.0001	81	−0.63	<.0001	85	−0.75	<.0001	40	−0.61	<.0001	42	−0.72	<.0001
Mental component score (MCS)	100	−0.47	<.0001	113	−0.68	<.0001	81	−0.57	<.0001	85	−0.81	<.0001	40	−0.78	<.0001	42	−0.78	<.0001
ESS score	103	0.27	0.0049				82	0.55	<.0001				40	**0.49**	0.0011			
HADS anxiety	105	0.56	<.0001				81	0.51	<.0001				41	**0.53**	0.0002			
HADS depression	105	**0.60**	<.0001				81	0.44	<.0001				41	**0.55**	0.0001			
HSAL score	6	**0.93**	0.0045				5	**0.97**	0.0021				3	**1.00**	.			
IRLSSG score	4	**0.50**	0.5828				3	**0.50**	.				2	**1.00**	.			

Strong correlations are highlighted in **bold numbers**. *PSQI* Pittsburgh Sleep Quality Index, *MFIS* Modified Fatigue Impact Scale, *SF-36* Short Form-36, *ESS* Epworth Sleepiness Scale, *HADS* Hospital Anxiety and Depression Scale, *HSAL* Hamburg Pain Adjective List, *IRLSSG* International Restless Legs Symptom Study Group

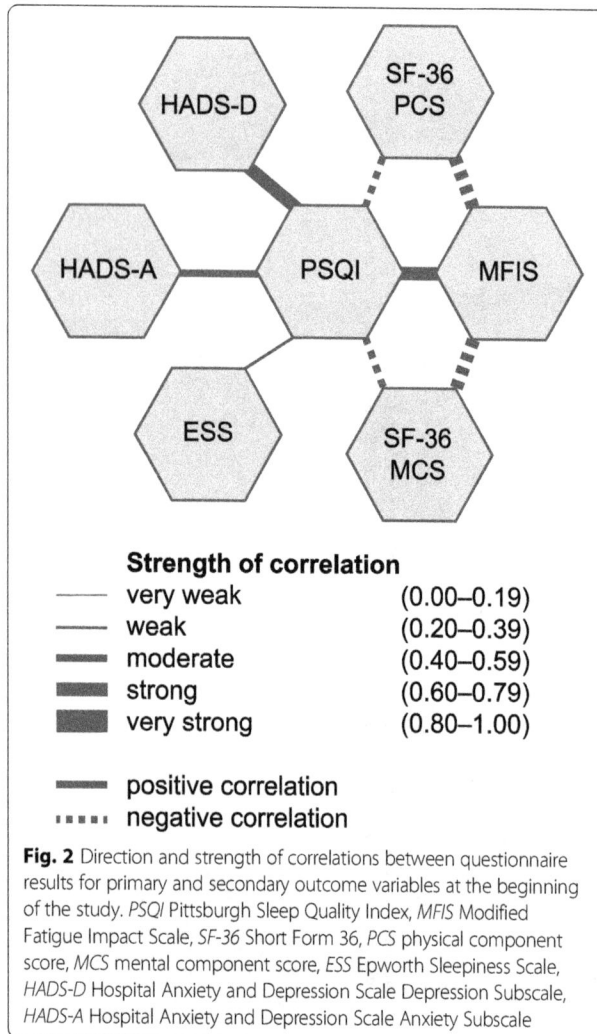

Strength of correlation

——	very weak	(0.00–0.19)
——	weak	(0.20–0.39)
══	moderate	(0.40–0.59)
▬▬	strong	(0.60–0.79)
▬▬	very strong	(0.80–1.00)

▬▬ positive correlation

▪▪▪▪▪ negative correlation

Fig. 2 Direction and strength of correlations between questionnaire results for primary and secondary outcome variables at the beginning of the study. *PSQI* Pittsburgh Sleep Quality Index, *MFIS* Modified Fatigue Impact Scale, *SF-36* Short Form 36, *PCS* physical component score, *MCS* mental component score, *ESS* Epworth Sleepiness Scale, *HADS-D* Hospital Anxiety and Depression Scale Depression Subscale, *HADS-A* Hospital Anxiety and Depression Scale Anxiety Subscale

One of the advantages of our study is the prospective observational study design investigating sleep quality in German MS patients over two years, thus allowing a real-world picture to be drawn. Furthermore, key characteristics and results from questionnaires suggest that participants in the BETASLEEP study are comparable to other cohorts of patients with relapsing forms of MS with a similar functional health status [24] and a slightly lower level of depression and anxiety [17].

Limitations include the lack of a control group. The results therefore allow no conclusion regarding a possible treatment effect. However, the study was not designed to compare the effect of different medications on the course of sleep quality and fatigue, but rather to investigate sleep quality and fatigue under stable treatment conditions. The ideal situation would have been to prospectively investigate the natural course in untreated patients, which however is not possible due to ethical concerns. Further, obstructive sleep apnea was not excluded in patients. Given the observational study design reflecting real-world activities, such screening was not possible. Additional limitations include the low number of participants with RLS and chronic pain, precluding a reliable evaluation of the impact of these conditions on sleep quality and fatigue. Also, a considerable amount of patients was lost to follow-up. This might be due to the observational nature of the study, reflecting the real-world process in patient care. In addition, the patients were only mildly impaired and potentially observable changes may only occur over longer periods of time. Also we cannot draw any conclusion regarding the course of patients who are more severely affected. Finally, we used a forward selection procedure to identy potential predictors of poor sleep quality, which is prone to type I error. Given that the performed analyses are exploratory we wanted to make sure that we do not miss a potential predictor. This could have been the case with backward stepwise selection, for example, which sometimes drops variables that would be significant when added to the final reduced model.

Conclusion

Taken together, our study confirms the high prevalence of poor sleep quality among patients with MS, which can also be seen in our cohort treated with interferon beta-1b over 2 years. Poor sleep quality was correlated with greater fatigue, lower functional health, and more depression and anxiety. The results highlight the importance of interventions targeted at improving sleep quality in patients with MS.

Abbreviations

BMI: Body mass index; CI: Confidence interval; CIS: Clinically isolated syndrome; DMD: Disease modifying drug; EDSS: Expanded disability status scale; ESS: Epworth Sleepiness Scale; HADS: Hospital Anxiety and Depression Scale; HSAL: Hamburg Pain Adjective List; IRLSSG: International RLS Study Group; MCS: Mental component score; MFIS: Modified fatigue impact scale; MS: Multiple sclerosis; OR: Odds ratio; PCS: Physical component score; PSQI: Pittsburgh Sleep Quality Index; RLS: Restless legs syndrome; RRMS: Relapsing remitting multiple sclerosis; SD: Standard deviation

Acknowledgements

The authors wish to thank Sebastian Karl, medizinwelten-services GmbH, for his support in writing this paper.

Funding

The study was funded by Bayer Vital GmbH, Leverkusen, Germany. TN, MD, PB, TG, CN, and MS are former or current employees of Bayer and were involved in the design of the study and collection, analysis, and interpretation of data and in writing the manuscript as indicated in the section Authors' contributions.

Authors' contributions

SK, PB, TG, MS were responsible for the concept and design of the study. TN, MS were responsible for study coordination and conduct. CN, MS were responsible for the data analysis. SK, TN, CN, MD, MS interpreted the data. All authors contributed to and critically reviewed the manuscript during its development and approved the final version of the manuscript for submission.

Consent for publication

Not applicable.

Competing interests

SK received study grants from Bayer Vital GmbH and BiogenIdec, personal compensation as a speaker from Bayer Vital GmbH, BiogenIdec, UCB, Pfizer, and Novartis. TN, MD and MS are full-time employees of Bayer Vital GmbH. MS previously served as an associate editor to BMC Neurology. PB is a full-time employee of Bayer Consumer Care AG. TG is a former employee of Bayer Vital GmbH and currently a consultant to Bayer Vital GmbH. CN is a full-time employee of Bayer AG.

Author details

Klinik für Geriatrie, Klinikum Leer gemeinnützige GmbH, Leer, Germany. Bayer Vital GmbH, Leverkusen, Germany. ³Bayer AG, Wuppertal, Germany. Bayer Consumer Care AG, Basel, Switzerland.

References

1. Browne P, Chandraratna D, Angood C, Tremlett H, Baker C, Taylor BV, et al. Atlas of multiple sclerosis 2013: a growing global problem with widespread inequity. Neurology. 2014;83(11):1022–4.
2. Marrie RA, Reider N, Cohen J, Trojano M, Sorensen PS, Cutter G, et al. A systematic review of the incidence and prevalence of sleep disorders and seizure disorders in multiple sclerosis. Mult Scler. 2015;21(3):342–9. (Houndmills, Basingstoke, England)
3. Barun B. Pathophysiological background and clinical characteristics of sleep disorders in multiple sclerosis. Clin Neurol Neurosurg. 2013;115(1):S82–5.
4. Lobentanz IS, Asenbaum S, Vass K, Sauter C, Klosch G, Kollegger H, et al. Factors influencing quality of life in multiple sclerosis patients: disability, depressive mood, fatigue and sleep quality. Acta Neurol Scand. 2004; 110(1):6–13.
5. Fleming WE, Pollak CP. Sleep disorders in multiple sclerosis. Semin Neurol. 2005;25(1):64–8.
6. Neau JP, Paquereau J, Auche V, Mathis S, Godeneche G, Ciron J, et al. Sleep disorders and multiple sclerosis: a clinical and polysomnography study. Eur Neurol. 2012;68(1):8–15.
7. Cameron MH, Peterson V, Boudreau EA, Downs A, Lovera J, Kim E, et al. Fatigue is associated with poor sleep in people with multiple sclerosis and cognitive impairment. Mult Scler Int. 2014;2014:5.
8. Krupp LB, Serafin DJ, Christodoulou C. Multiple sclerosis-associated fatigue. Expert Rev Neurother. 2010;10(9):1437–47.
9. Veauthier C, Paul F. Sleep disorders in multiple sclerosis and their relationship to fatigue. Sleep Med. 2014;15(1):5–14.
10. Veauthier C, Radbruch H, Gaede G, Pfueller CF, Dorr J, Bellmann-Strobl J, et al. Fatigue in multiple sclerosis is closely related to sleep disorders: a polysomnographic cross-sectional study. Mult Scler. 2011;17(5):613–22. (Houndmills, Basingstoke, England)
11. Cote I, Trojan DA, Kaminska M, Cardoso M, Benedetti A, Weiss D, et al. Impact of sleep disorder treatment on fatigue in multiple sclerosis. Mult Scler. 2013;19(4):480–9. (Houndmills, Basingstoke, England)
12. Li Y, Munger KL, Batool-Anwar S, De Vito K, Ascherio A, Gao X. Association of multiple sclerosis with restless legs syndrome and other sleep disorders in women. Neurology. 2012;78(19):1500–6.
13. Lanza G, Ferri R, Bella R, Ferini-Strambi L. The impact of drugs for multiple sclerosis on sleep. Mult Scler. 2017;23(1):5–13. (Houndmills, Basingstoke, England)
14. Kotterba S, Schwenkreis P, Schölzel W, Haltenhof C. Fatigue and sleep problems in patients with relapsing-remitting multiple sclerosis (RRMS) under treatment with interferon β-1b. Klin Neurophysiol. 2016;47(03):136–41.
15. Rupprecht S, Witte OW, Schwab M, for the SLEEP-MS Study Group. SLEEP-MS: Prevalence of Sleep Disturbances, Fatigue, Anxiety and Depression in Multiple Sclerosis. Presentation at the 90 Congress of the German Society of Neurology. Leipzig; 2017.
16. Hinz A, Glaesmer H, Brahler E, Loffler M, Engel C, Enzenbach C, Hegerl U, Sander C. Sleep quality in the general population: psychometric properties of the Pittsburgh sleep quality index, derived from a German community sample of 9284 people. Sleep Med. 2017;30:57–63.
17. Jones KH, Jones PA, Middleton RM, Ford DV, Tuite-Dalton K, Lockhart-Jones H, et al. Physical disability, anxiety and depression in people with MS: an internet-based survey via the UK MS register. PLoS One. 2014;9(8):e104604.
18. Kleiter I, Lang M, Jeske J, Norenberg C, Stollfuss B, Schurks M. Adherence, satisfaction and functional health status among patients with multiple sclerosis using the BETACONNECT(R) autoinjector: a prospective observational cohort study. BMC Neurol. 2017;17(1):174.
19. Boe Lunde HM, Aae TF, Indrevag W, Aarseth J, Bjorvatn B, Myhr KM, et al. Poor sleep in patients with multiple sclerosis. PLoS One. 2012;7(11):e49996.
20. Amato MP, Ponziani G, Rossi F, Liedl CL, Stefanile C, Rossi L. Quality of life in multiple sclerosis: the impact of depression, fatigue and disability. Mult Scler. 2001;7(5):340–4. (Houndmills, Basingstoke, England)
21. Mendozzi L, Tronci F, Garegnani M, Pugnetti L. Sleep disturbance and fatigue in mild relapsing remitting multiple sclerosis patients on chronic immunomodulant therapy: an actigraphic study. Mult Scler J. 2009;16(2):238–47.
22. Pokryszko-Dragan A, Bilinska M, Gruszka E, Biel L, Kaminska K, Konieczna K. Sleep disturbances in patients with multiple sclerosis. Neurological Sci. 2013; 34(8):1291–6.

11

Circadian rhythms of migraine attacks in episodic and chronic patients: a cross sectional study in a headache center population

Marina de Tommaso[*] and Marianna Delussi

Abstract

Background: Migraine is considered a disease with diurnal and 24 h pattern, though the existence of a prevalent circadian rhythm associated to migraine frequency and severity is still not clear. This observational cross-sectional study aimed to:

1. Assess the circadian rhythm of migraine attacks onset in a large patients' population selected in a headache center and including episodic and chronic migraine 2. Analyze the principal characteristic of the different onset time groups 3. Verify if migraine features, particularly those associated to chronic and disabling migraine, could be discriminant factors for time of onset group.

Methods: We selected 786 consecutive migraine outpatients, who correctly completed the headache diaries for 3 consecutive months and who fulfilled the diagnosis of migraine without aura-MO, migraine with typical aura alone or associated to migraine without aura - MO/MA and chronic migraine – CM. For the time of headache onset, we considered four time slots, from 6 to 12 am (morning), from 1 to 6 pm (afternoon), from 7 to 11 pm (evening), from 12 pm to 5 am (night), and an additional category named "any time". Each time slot included the 60 min preceding the next one (e.g. an onset at 12.30 am was included in 6–12 am time slot). We evaluated in all patients the pericranial tenderness, anxiety and depression tracts, headache-related disability, sleep features, quality of life, allodynia and fatigue.

Results: We scored a total of 16,578 attacks, distributed in the entire day. The most of patients, including CM, satisfied the criteria for the "any time" onset. Night onset was significantly less represented in the MA/MO group. Patients with prevalent night onset were significantly older, with longer migraine history and shorter sleep duration. Age and illness duration were the variables discriminating the different onset time groups.

Conclusions: The most of migraine patients do not report a specific circadian profile of attacks occurrence. Frequent migraine, severe disability, psychopathological tracts as well as central sensitization signs, do not match with a specific circadian rhythm of attacks onset. Night onset migraine seems to be an age related feature, emerging in the course of the disease.

Keywords: Migraine, Circadian rhythm, Central sensitization, Clinical correlation

* Correspondence: marina.detommaso@uniba.it
Applied Neurophysiology and Pain Unit, Basic Medical Science, Neuroscience and Sensory System-SMBNOS-Department, Policlinico General Hospital, Bari Aldo Moro University, Giovanni XXIII Building, Via Amendola 207 A, 70124 Bari, Italy

Background

Migraine is considered a disease with diurnal and 24 h pattern [1]. The periodicity of migraine was frequently demonstrated in observational studies [2–5]. Fox et al. [2], reported prevalent morning onset between 6 to 9 am, though a high number of acute headache episodes occurred along all day, with some nocturnal cases [2]. Alstadhaug et al. [3, 4] described a wide distribution of time of occurrence [4]. A recent study based on general population, assessed the circadian periodicity of migraine patients [5]. In this large database, attacks of migraine frequently occurred early in the morning, characterizing patients with early chronotype. A recent study described the circadian rhythm of migraine patients, who used a on-smartphone headache diary. This could be a reliable and handful method to assess migraine features [6]. In this study, both migraine and not migraine headache occurred preferentially in the early morning, though many acute headache episodes occurred during other hours, including night [6]. These studies spotted a prevalent morning onset of migraine, but the correlation between circadian rhythm and clinical phenotype, as migraine frequency and disability, might be worthy of further evaluation. No study included chronic migraine, possibly because the assessment of headache onset is difficult to spot in patients with persistent and even continuous pain. The recent classifications [7, 8] request at least 8 typical migraine attacks in 1 month, to confirm the diagnosis of Chronic Migraine. If patients are requested to distinguish acute migraine from continuous headache, they could also indicate migraine onset time. Another unclear point is the possible association between circadian rhythm and symptoms of central sensitization as allodynia and pericranial tenderness [9, 10].

This observational cross-sectional study aimed to:

1. Assess the circadian rhythm of migraine attacks onset in a large patients' population collected in our headache-centre and including episodic and chronic migraine.
2. Analyse the principal characteristic of the different onset time groups.
3. Verify if migraine features could be discriminant factors for time of onset group, focusing in particular those associated to chronic and disabling migraine, as pericranial tenderness, allodynia, sleep time, anxiety and depression tracts.

Methods

Study population

Study population included outpatients who came for the first time to the Bari Policlinico General Hospital - Applied Neurophysiology and Pain Unit, in the time between January 2015 – January 2017. Upon the first access to the booking desk, the hospital staff gave patients the headache diary. All patients were invited to fill the headache diary for 3 months, and to present it at their next visit date. We decided to include only patients at their first access to our Unit, because one exclusion criteria was the use of preventive treatment for migraine, which we generally used to suggest during the first visit.

Data collection

The hospital staff requested the patients to complete the hourly chart of headache, reporting: the time of onset of each migraine attack, the quality (throbbing, oppressive, penetrating) and location of headache, the intensity of headache in a scale from 1 (slight) to 3 (intense), the presence of prodromal and aura symptoms, the presence of nausea, vomiting, phono/photo-phobia, and drugs used for single attacks. A sample of original hourly chart and diary of headache can be seen in the supplementary section (Additional file 1: Figure S1, Additional file 2: Figure S2). They also requested to fill the questionnaire of allodynia [11, 12], adapted in the Italian version, for each migraine attack (Additional file 1: Figure S1) [13, 14]. Inclusion criteria were: 1) the diagnosis of migraine without aura-MO (code 1.1), migraine with typical aura-MA (code 1.2.1), migraine with typical aura and migraine without aura MO/MA (code 1.2.1 plus 1.1) and chronic migraine – CM (code 1.3) [7]; 2) age between 18 and 75; 3) at least two migraine attacks in the 3 months; 4) the correct compilation of the hourly chart of headache, with at least the presence of aura symptoms, and the allodynia questionnaires. Exclusion criteria were: general medical and/or other neurological or psychiatric diseases, the use of central nervous system-active drugs or preventive treatment for primary headache, the diagnosis of "probable" migraine, according to classification criteria [7].

Many patients did not report in a complete and precise way the information required, like intensity of headache, vegetative symptoms and use of symptomatic drugs. We did not include these data in the final analysis. For all patients and specially CM, we used these data to confirm the diagnosis, according to the current classification [7, 8].

Clinical assessment

Two neurologists with clinical experience in headache, put the diagnosis of migraine based on headache characteristics and frequency, in the 3 months preceding the first visit, according with the International Headache Society criteria. The medical staff revised the diagnosis retrospectively, considering the most recent criteria [8]. The composition of study population remained exactly the same, as the new diagnostic criteria for migraine did not change from the previous version [7]. During the first visit, patients underwent the clinical assessment that we described in previous studies [13, 15]. First, the neurologists checked the frequency of migraine, and the averaged number of days with headache/month during the last 3 months, then considered headache intensity and the vegetative and or aura symptoms, to confirm migraine diagnosis. They confirmed the presence of acute allodynia symptoms from the allodynia questionnaire [11, 12]. We classified a patient as allodynic if he/she reported at least one symptom included in the questionnaire in over the 50% of the migraine episodes.

For the time of headache onset, we considered four time slots, from 6.00 to 12.00 am (morning), from 1.00 to 6.00 pm (afternoon), from 7.00 to 11.00 pm (evening), from 12.00 pm to 5.00 am (night), and an additional category named "any time". Each time slot included the 60 min preceding the next one (e.g. an onset at 12.30 am was included in 6–12 am time slot). We thus included each patient in a specific time of onset category, based on the 50% of his/her migraine attacks occurrence. Alternatively, if migraine attacks happened in different day times, the patient was included into the "any time" category.

We evaluated in all patients the total tenderness score (TTS), following the procedure described by Langermark and Olesen [16]. We also evaluated anxiety and depression tracts using the depression –self rating depression scale (SDS)- and anxiety -self-rating anxiety scale (SAS)- scales, which we applied in large primary headaches groups [13, 14]. They are reliable tools to detect these symptoms in a general non-psychiatric patient population [17, 18]. According to previous studies [13, 14] we applied the Italian version of the MIDAS score to all type of headaches [19], to quantify headache-related disability.

All patients reported on interview their sleep features, according to the Medical Outcomes Study (MOS) [20], on a scale we previously applied in large headache populations [13, 14]. For the present analysis, we considered the sleep quantity score (MOS2); lower scores indicated worse sleep problems, referring to hours of sleep for night in the last week.

We evaluated the patients' quality of life using The Short-form 36 Questionnaire (SF-36), with the computation of Physical and Mental Health score (PH and MH) [21].

Ethical approval

The Ethical Committee of Bari Policlinico General Hospital approved the study. All patients signed an informed consent for the inclusion of their data in the study.

Statistical analysis

Preliminary descriptive analysis of the sample. We summarized the quantitative continuous variables (age, duration, frequency, SAS, SDS, TTS, MOS2, PH and MH sub scores of SF36) with mean and standard deviation, and where necessary, with median and also the 25th and 75th

percentile (MIDAS). We summarized the categorical variables (sex, presence or absence of fatigue and allodynia) with absolute frequencies and percentages.

The statistical analysis included the chi-square to test for the categorical variables, the variance analysis (ANOVA) and the Kruskal Wallis' non-parametric test for the quantitative continuous variables. We used the Bonferroni post-hoc test. The statistical significance level was fixed at alpha < 0.05.

To satisfy the aim 1) we applied the chi square test to verify the distribution of migraine patients into the different time of onset categories. For aim 2) we thus performed a MANOVA analysis, with a complete factorial Type III model, comparing continuous variables (age, duration, frequency, SAS, SDS, TTS, MOS2, PH and MH sub scores of SF36) among onset time categories, followed by a post-hoc Bonferroni test. Using the chi square test, we evaluated the distribution of patients with or without allodynia and fatigue among the different onset times.

To satisfy the aim 3), we applied a step way discriminant analysis with Wilks lambda model ($p < 0.05$ to entry, p 0, 10 to exclude), to establish if time of onset category could predict clinical features, as age, duration and frequency of migraine, anxiety and depression scores, quality of life, pericranial tenderness, allodynia, sleep time.

We used the Statistical Package for Social Science (SPSS) version 24 software.

Results

Demographic and clinical characteristics

Among a total of 1250 patients who came at the time of visit booking, we considered data from 786 cases (Fig. 1). Two hundred and twenty patients did not correctly complete the diaries and the hourly chart, 30 reported less than 2 migraine attacks, 73 were under CNS active drugs, 141 patients did not fulfil the diagnostic criteria, including those with mixed diagnosis, as chronic patients with associated Medication Overuse Headache (Fig. 1). In fact, the initial number of CM patients was 290, including 150 patients with an adjunctive diagnosis of Medication Overuse Headache (cod 8.2) [7]. After 3 months of drugs withdrawal and detoxification, 94 of them reverted into episodic migraine, so we excluded their data from the final analysis, which included 196 CM patients.

Considering that few migraine patients presented exclusively with migraine with aura episodes (10 patients), we merged MA and MO/MA patients in a unique group.

The 786 patients enrolled for the study, were all born and resided in Southern Italy. They reported in total 16,578 attacks on their diaries. Females prevailed in all group. CM patients were older than the other patients were. Duration of illness was also longer in CM patients, as compared to other groups (Table 1).

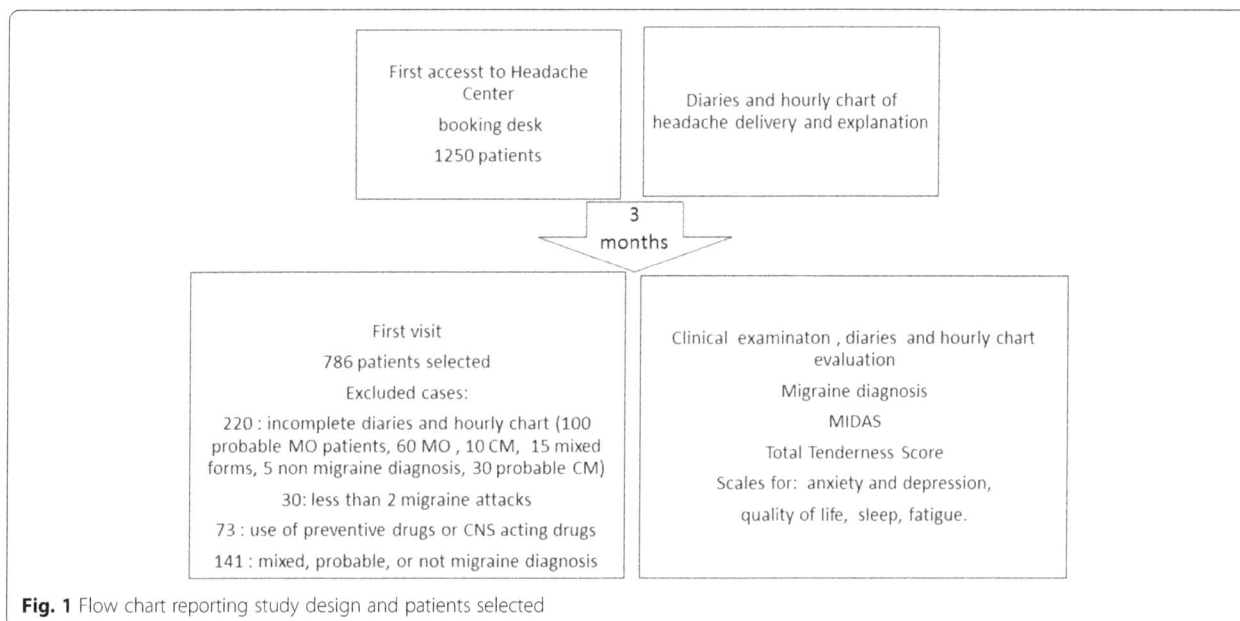

Fig. 1 Flow chart reporting study design and patients selected

Table 1 Demographic and clinic characteristics of migraine patients

	MO		CM		MO + MA		
	N	%	n	%	N	%	
	538	68.4	196	24.9	52	6.6	
Males	123	22.9	23	11.7	10	20	Chi square 0.011
Females	415	77.1	173	88.3	42	80	
	Mean	SD	mean	SD	Mean	SD	One way Anova
Age (years)	37.41*	12.457	42.49*^°	14.656	34.62^	13.45	0.0001
Duration (years)	15.03*	12.87	18.05*	12.599	14.38	11.38	0.008
Frequencies (day/headache/month)	7.64*	6.43	23.35*migraine days 10.15	14.83 3.43	7.7^	6.9	0.0001
SAS	34.06*	7.82	39.12*^°	10.02	32.8^	8.66	0.0001
SDS	32.7*	8.4	38.04*^°	11.018	31.4^	8.45	0.001
TTS	3.86*	4.44	7.02*^	6.037	5.45	5.36	0.0001
MOS2	6.54*	1.35	6.122*^°	1.6284	6.79^	1.13	0.001
PH	36.23	8.71	34.43	8.846	36.94	9.86	n.s.
MH	39.55	7.85	36.56°^	7.044	41.45^	9.99	0.0001
	Median	25°-75°	Median	25°-75°	Median	25°-75°	Kruskal Wallis
MIDAS	6.7*	1.3–16	23.3*^°	8.5–44	3.7^	3–8.5	0.0001

The *p* values are reported for the statistical tests applied. Results of post-hoc Bonferroni test: *CM vs MO; ^CM vs MA; °CM vs MO + MA *p* < 0.05
MO Migraine without aura
CM Chronic Migraine
MO + MA Migraine without aura + migraine with aura
SAS Self Administered Zung Anxiety Scale
SDS Self Administered Zung Depression Scale
TTS Total Tenderness Score
PH SF36 Physical Health score
MH SF 36 Mental Health score

Chronic migraine patients presented with higher anxiety and depression scores, as compared to the other groups. Pericranial tenderness score was also higher in CM patients, as compared to episodic migraine without aura and migraine with aura. Mental quality of life score was also lower in chronic patients, compared to migraine with aura patients and mixed forms. The hours of sleep were also fewer in CM patients, as compared to the remainder migraine patients. In addition, the MIDAS scores, which were summarized as median and percentiles, indicated a more severe disability in CM patients (Table 1).

Fatigue characterized a minority of episodic migraine patients, and around the half of chronic migraine subjects. The presence of allodynia prevailed in all migraine groups, but it was more severe in CM patients compared to episodic migraine without aura and migraine with aura groups (Additional file 3: Table S1).

Time of onset

The distribution of the single migraine attacks covered the entire day, with two peaks of migraine frequency at 10 am and 10 pm. A consistent number of attacks occurred in the night, with a peak around middle night (Fig. 2). However, the number of attacks during night were less than in the morning, afternoon and evening hours, so the distribution was not uniform (Fig. 2).

Most of patients satisfied the criteria for the "any time" category, as they did not report a constant time of migraine onset across their attacks (Table 2). The distribution into the different time of onset slots was similar in CM compared to episodic migraine groups. Few patients with aura symptoms reported a prevalent night onset. The comparison of distribution into the different onset time slots between patients presenting or not with aura symptoms, was significant for a lower percentage of night onset patients in the MO/MA group (MO/MA 9%, CM and MO: 25, 7% chi square 16, 3 p 0.003).

Clinical characteristics of time of onset groups

Patients with presence of fatigue and allodynia symptoms were similarly distributed among different onset time slots (Additional file 3: Table S2 and Additional file 3: Table S3).

The MANOVA analysis, indicated that the onset time groups, were significant different for the included variables (Roy Square DF 10 $p < 0.0001$). Age, duration of illness and sleep time, showed significant differences among onset time groups (Fig. 3). Patients with prevalent night onset, were older than the other groups, excluding morning onset patients, and reported a longer migraine duration as compared to the "anytime" group. The night onset patients had a shorter sleep, as compared to morning and anytime onsets groups. Patients with morning onset were also older than those with evening and afternoon onset (Fig. 3). The other variables, including allodynia, frequency of headache and quality of life scores, were similar among onset time groups.

The MIDAS scores were also similar among the different onset time slots (chi square 3.48 p 0.54).

Discriminant analysis

The step way discriminant analysis, indicated age and illness duration as discriminant variables (Table 3; Additional file 3: Table S4). The discriminant matrix correctly classified into time of onset groups the 27.6% of patients. The night onset group had the best accuracy, with 46% of correct classification.

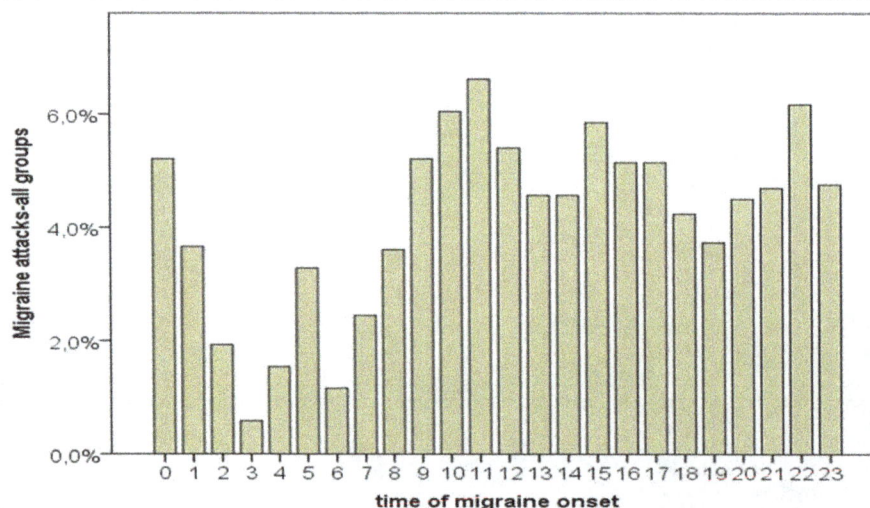

Fig. 2 Circadian rhythm of migraine attacks in the 786 patients. The 16.578 attacks were divided among the 24 h. The distribution was not uniform, for a reduction of the attacks in the night hours. (Bootstrap, Tukey estimator 4.49, distorsion – 0.03)

Table 2 The distribution of patients in the five categories of migraine time of onset

			MO	MO + MA	CM	total
Time of migraine onset	MORNING	n	48	9	23	80
		%	8.9%	17.3%	11.9%	10.2%
	AFTERNOON	n	37	5	13	55
		%	6.9%	9.6%	6.7%	7.0%
	EVENING	n	6	1	3	10
		%	1.1%	1.9%	1.5%	1.3%
	NIGHT	n	136	5	51	192
		%	25.2%	9.6%	26.3%	24.4%
	ANY TIME	n	312	32	104	449
		%	57.9%	61.5%	53.6%	57.1%

Subsets of diagnosis were not different from each other at level 0, 05. The "any time" group included the most of patients. Chi Square test: 24, 64; DF 8; *p* 0.02

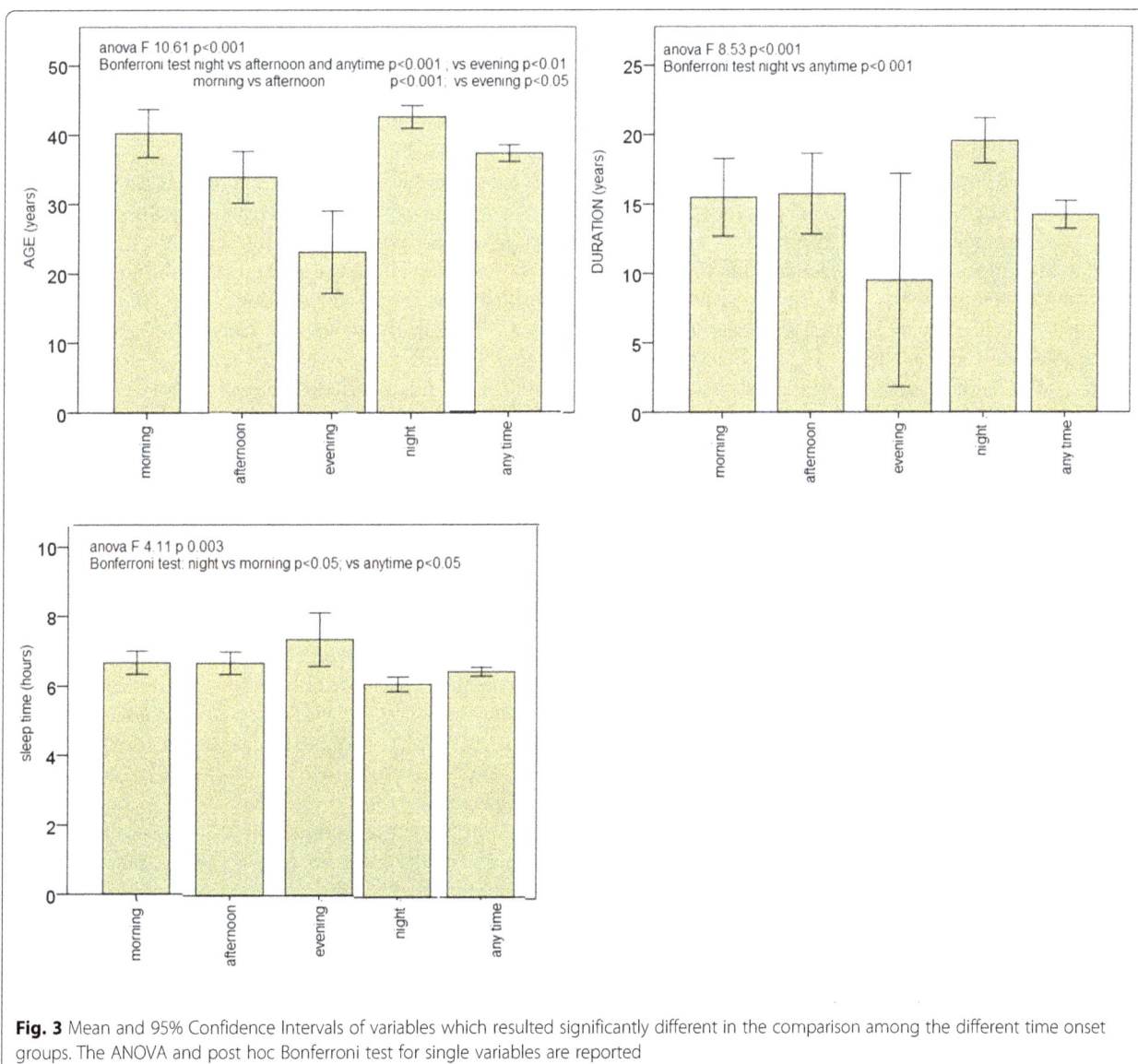

Fig. 3 Mean and 95% Confidence Intervals of variables which resulted significantly different in the comparison among the different time onset groups. The ANOVA and post hoc Bonferroni test for single variables are reported

Table 3 Results of step way discriminant analysis for the onset time groups

Included variables[b,c]

step	Included	Wilks Lambda				F			
		Statistic	df1	df2	df3	Statistic	df1	df2	Sig.
1	AGE	.942	1	4	711	10.962	4	711.000	.000
2	DURATION	.918	2	4	711	7.749	8	1420.000	.000

The variables initially introduced were age, duration, frequency of migraine, sleep duration (MOS score), anxiety and depression scores (SAS and SDS), SF36 quality of life subscores (PH and MH), Total tenderness score, allodynia total score
a. maximal step number 20
b. inclusion significance for F 0.05
c. exclusion significance for F 0.10

Discussion

The main result of this observational study in a population selected at headache centre, indicates that the most of migraine patients, including chronic migraine, do not report a constant circadian rhythm of their attacks. In addition, we did not find an association between a specific circadian recurrence of attack and clinical features. Patients with prevalent night onset were older and reported a longer history of migraine. The following paragraphs deal with the detailed discussion of the results.

Concerning the general clinical characteristics of migraine patients, we confirmed the severity of chronic migraine in comparison to episodic patients. CM patients showed more severe anxiety and depression tracts, short sleep time and clear signs of central sensitization, as pericranial tenderness and allodynia [14, 22, 23]. This is confirmative of numerous studies indicating chronic migraine as an invalidating disorder [24].

The inclusion of chronic patients in the study of the circadian rhythm of migraine, is quite difficult considering that headache is often continuous. However, the accurate description of headache characteristics is necessary to individuate the number of migraine attacks, according to recent classifications [7, 8].

Basing on the present population enrolled in our headache centre, the morning onset group included the 10% of patients, less than in previous studies, where the attacks were distributed during the daytime [2–6]. We assigned each patient to a time onset category in an arbitrary way, using the criterion of the 50% of attacks onset, which may be questionable. The different modalities of division in times slots, could explain some differences related to previous studies. In fact we considered the early morning interval from 6 to 12 am, while other studies included the night hours from 0 to 6 [5]. In any case, the preferential time of migraine onset was indicated around the 6 am [4], a time that we included in the morning time slot.

Observing the daily distribution of single migraine attacks, they were disseminated according to a multiphasic circadian rhythm profile, similar to what described by

Soriani et al. [25]. Based on this distribution, single attacks did not appear to start very frequently in the early morning.

The type of population selected, headache centre patients vs general population, the modality of data collection, hourly charts vs interview, and the number of patients, seems crucial to explain the divergence with previous studies [2–6]. A comparison between the subjective report of migraine onset and the hourly chart should be useful in the same population. In addition, the geographic, climatic and ethnic characteristics of populations seem another important point, which can profoundly change migraine phenotype. Studies conducted in Italian populations, reported an hourly distribution similar to that emerging by present data, with the exception of night occurrence, which may be age-related [25] (see below).

Our study tried for the first time to establish the circadian profile of migraine attacks in CM patients, and to clarify if chronicity and severity of migraine is associated to specific time of onset categories. No particular circadian rhythm characterized CM patients compared to episodic patients, suggesting that the time of migraine onset could not be a factor associated to the chronic form.

We selected few migraine with aura patients and merged pure migraine with aura and mixed forms in a unique group. The rare presence of night onset attacks may be due to the modality of aura presentation, probably favoured by morning light condition. Few studies dealt with the preferential time of migraine with aura onset. Sunlight could be a trigger for migraine with aura [26]; this could explain the rarity of night onset. In any case, the possibility that migraine aura could start during night without wakening the patient, is an intriguing question. In this case, patients could only report migraine, which occurred after the wake up. A higher number of migraine with aura attacks could have resolved this question.

Our migraine patients reported a higher number of attacks in the night time, in respect to previous studies [2–6]. In addition, considering the time distribution of single migraine attacks and the circadian profile attributed to single patients, most of the night attacks characterized patients with the specific night circadian rhythm. This means that night onset recurs frequently in the same patient, and seems not to occur occasionally. Migraineurs with prevalent night occurrence were older than the others, with the exclusion of morning group. Despite the mean age of the included patients was similar to that of patients reported in other studies [2–6], our MO and CM groups included a high number of over 40 patients. The study by van Oosterhout et al., which included older patients [5], indicated a prevalent migraine occurrence in the time slot 0–6, according to our results. The study of Soriani et al. on circadian rhythms in juvenile migraine [25], reported a low frequency of nocturnal attacks, suggesting that the night occurrence may concur with age-related changes of sleep features. In fact, Alstadhaug et al. [4] described the association between night occurrence of migraine and insomnia. Accordingly, our night-onset patients, showed a reduction of sleep time that confirmed the association previously described [4]. The consideration of other sleep features was beyond the aims of this study, but it would be worthy of further consideration, especially for patients with specific night – onset profile.

In this study, we evaluated for the first time if the characteristics of chronic migraine, as high frequency of attacks and signs of central sensitization, as pericranial tenderness and allodynia, could identify a specific circadian profile. The results are substantially negative in this sense, as frequency of migraine was similar among the different onset time groups, as well as pericranial tenderness and allodynia. As regard to allodynia, the most of migraine patients were classified as allodynic, according to previous studies of our group [14, 15], and other researchers [27–29]. The distribution of allodynic and not allodynic patients was similar among the different circadian categories, so allodynia did not emerge as a peculiar characteristic of a specific circadian profile.

The presence of fatigue characterized a minority of episodic migraine patients, and more than 50% of chronic migraine. A recent study on fatigue in migraine patients, reported an association with poor quality of life, headache intensity, age and insomnia, all symptoms characterizing chronic migraine [14]. In the subgroup of fatigued patients, patients with any time onset prevailed, which could confirm that the presence of fatigue, though relevant especially in chronic patients, is substantially independent from a specific circadian occurrence.

Anxiety and depression tracts were similar in the different circadian categories. Ohayon et al. [30] evaluated the symptoms associated to morning headache in general population and found that anxiety and depression were the most significant associated factors. Our data could not confirm the association between anxiety and depression tracts and the morning migraine. Again, the method of data collection seems crucial for the results. Probably the most of patients have a subjective impression of a circadian prevalence of their attacks. Anxious subjects can emphasize the occurrence of morning headache, because they could dedicate attention to the headache episodes that can influence the quality of the entire day. For these reasons, anxious and depressed persons can give special relevance to morning headaches, so the collection of data from dairies seem important to reduce possible biases.

Quality of life and migraine disability was also similar among the different circadian occurrence times. This is a further confirmation that we could not individuate an onset time of migraine characterizing the more disabled migraine patients.

Age and migraine duration were the only discriminating features among the different circadian profiles. The night-onset migraine is thus a characteristic of older patients with a long migraine history, and could be considered a age related change of migraine phenotype.

The disruption of sleep rhythm linked to aging, could cause night onset migraine in older patients. The role of hypothalamus in migraine attacks onset is going into increasing consideration [31]. The suprachiasmatic nucleus (SCN) of the hypothalamus functions as the master pacemaker to initiate daily synchronization according to the photoperiod. With aging, circadian desynchronization occurs with sleep symptoms and progressive change of sleep-wake behaviour [32, 33]. These age-related modifications could have an important impact on neurodegeneration [33]. The clinical feature of migraine in old patients, needs to be taken into consideration in the global management of diseases linked to aging [34].

Study limitations

The major limit of the study is the consistency of diaries. We included a high number of data, and we are basing our conclusions on the reliability of what patients reported, which may be questionable. Electronic diaries, included those on smartphones supports [6, 35] seem handy, especially for the notification of onset time; however, also in this case, the reliability of the data is not for granted. We would have also introduced further data in our database, such as the symptomatic treatments use, or the intensity of single migraine attacks and vegetative symptoms. Unfortunately, many diaries did not report these data in a complete way, so we decided not to include them in the final analysis, and to utilize these to confirm the diagnosis [7, 8]. Another limit regards the selection of outpatients from a headache-centre, with a possible bias as compared to general population. Most of the studies on circadian rhythm reported data from selected migraine groups [2, 3, 25], and one study was on a large Dutch people database [5]. Further studies need to be accomplished for the confirmation of present data in general Italian population.

Another potential cause of divergent results from previous studies, was the type of clinical assessment, based on scales for anxiety, depression and sleep largely applied in our hospital, though not of common use in migraine. In any case, the SAS and SDS are validated for detection of psychopathological tracts in general population and useful when the presence of psychiatric diagnosis is an exclusion criteria [17, 18]. The Medical Outcomes Study (MOS) is also of general use in patients with chronic pain [20], and we previously applied it in large headache populations [13, 14].

Another problem was the consistency of data of smaller groups, especially for patients with aura.

However, conclusions about the circadian rhythm of migraine considered as a whole, with the inclusion of chronic patients, seem robust, taking also into consideration previous studies [2, 3, 6].

Conclusions

Based on present data, the most of migraine patients do not report a specific circadian profile of attacks occurrence. High headache frequency, severe disability, psychopathological tracts as well as central sensitization signs, do not match with a specific circadian rhythm of attacks onset. Data of migraine with aura occurrence are presently not definitive, and worthy of further studies. The night onset migraine could be considered an age- related change occurring in the course of the disease. The present results would be considered, in light of population way of selection as well as ethnic and geographic characteristics.

Additional files

Additional file 1: Headache Diary: Sample of original hourly chart pag.1. (TIF 119 kb)

Additional file 2: Headache Diary: Sample of original hourly chart pag. 2. (TIF 133 kb)

Additional file 3: Table S1. Presence and severity of fatigue and allodynia in the migraine subgroups. The results of statistical test are reported as p values. **Table S2.** Presence of allodynia in the migraine subgroups and onset time slots. **Table S3.** Presence of fatigue in the onset time slots. **Table S4.** Discriminant analysis Variables ordered basing on absolute dimension of intra function correlation. (DOCX 20 kb)

Abbreviations
CM: Chronic Migraine; MAF: Multidimensional Assessment of Fatigue; MH: SF 36 Mental Health score; MH: SF36 Physical Health score; MO: Migraine with aura; MO: Migraine without aura; MOS: Medical Outcome Studies; PH: SF36 Physical Health score; SAS: Self-Administered Zung Anxiety Scale; SDS: Self-Administered Zung Depression Scale; SF-36: Short-form 36 Questionnaire (), with the computation of; TTS: Total Tenderness Score

Funding
The study was supported by Bari University Research funds.

Authors' contributions
MDT: study design, clinical assessment, manuscript preparation. MD: statistical analysis, clinical assessment, manuscript preparation. Both authors read and approved the final manuscript.

Competing interests
The authors declare that they have no competing interests.

References
1. Smolensky MH, Portaluppi F, Manfredini R, Hermida RC, Tiseo R, Sackett-Lundeen LL, Haus EL. Diurnal and twenty-four hour patterning of human diseases: acute and chronic common and uncommon medical conditions. Sleep Med Rev. 2015;21:12–22.
2. Fox AW, Davis RL. Migraine chronobiology. Headache. 1998;38(6):436–41.
3. Alstadhaug K, Salvesen R, Bekkelund S. 24-hour distribution of migraine attacks. Headache. 2008;48(1):95–100.
4. Alstadhaug K, Salvesen R, Bekkelund S. Insomnia and circadian variation of attacks in episodic migraine. Headache. 2007;47(8):1184–8.
5. van Oosterhout W, van Someren E, Schoonman GG, Louter MA, Lammers GJ, Ferrari MD, Terwindt GM. Chronotypes and circadian timing in migraine. Cephalalgia. 2017;1:333102417698953. https://doi.org/10.1177/0333102417698953.
6. Park JW, Cho SJ, Park SG, Chu MK. Circadian variations in the clinical presentation of headaches among migraineurs: a study using a smartphone headache diary. Chronobiol Int. 2017;28:1–9.
7. Headache Classification Subcommittee of International headache Society. The international classification of headache disorders, 2nd edition. Cephalalgia. 2004;24(Suppl. 1):24–36.
8. Headache Classification Committee of the International Headache Society (IHS). The International Classification of Headache Disorders, 3rd edition. Cephalalgia. 2018;38(1):1–211.
9. Buchgreitz L, Lyngberg AC, Bendtsen L, et al. Frequency of headache is related to sensitization: a population study. Pain. 2006;123:19–27.
10. Burstein R, Yarnitsky D, Goor-Aryeh I, et al. An association between migraine and cutaneous allodynia. Ann Neurol. 2000;47:614–24.
11. Jakubowski M, Silberstein S, Ashkenazi A, Burstein R. Can allodynic migraine patients be identified interictally using a questionnaire? Neurology. 2005;65:1419–22.
12. Ashkenazi A, Silberstein S, Jakubowski M, et al. Improved identification of allodynic migraine patients using a questionnaire. Cephalalgia. 2007;27:325–9.
13. de Tommaso M, Federici A, Serpino C, Vecchio E, Franco G, Sardaro M, Delussi M, Livrea P. Clinical features of headache patients with fibromyalgia comorbidity. J Headache Pain. 2011;12(6):629–38.
14. de Tommaso M, Delussi M, Vecchio E, et al. Sleep features and central sensitization symptoms in primary headache patients. J Headache Pain. 2014;15:64.
15. de Tommaso M, Sciruicchio V, Delussi M, Vecchio E, Goffredo M, Simeone M, Barbaro MGF. Symptoms of central sensitization and comorbidity for juvenile fibromyalgia in childhood migraine: an observational study in a tertiary headache center. J Headache Pain. 2017;18(1):59.
16. Langermark M, Olesen J. Pericranial tenderness in tension headache. a blind, controlled study. Cephalalgia. 1987;7:249–55.
17. Zung WWK. A self-rating depression scale. Arch Gen Psychiatry. 1995;12:63–70.
18. WWK Z. SAS, self-rating anxiety scale. In: Guy W, editor. ECDEUAssessment manual for psychopharmacology, revised edition. Rockville: Maryland; 1976. p. 337–40.
19. D'Amico D, Mosconi P, Genco S, Usai S, Prudenzano AM, Grazzi L, Leone M, Puca FM, Bussone G. The migraine disability assessment (MIDAS) questionnaire: translation and reliability of the Italian version. Cephalalgia. 2001;21:947–52.
20. Hays RD, Stewart A. Sleep measures. In: Stewart A, Ware J, editors. Measuring functioning and well-being: the medical outcomes study approach. Durham: Duke University Press; 1992. p. 235–59.
21. McHorney CA, Ware JE, Raczek AE. The MOS 36-item short-form health survey (SF-36): II. Psychometric and clinical tests of validity in measuring physical and mental health constructs. Med Care. 1993;31:247–63.
22. Ashina S, Lipton RB, Bendtsen L, Hajiyeva N, Buse DC, Lyngberg AC, Jensen R. Increased pain sensitivity in migraine and tension-type headache coexistent with low back pain: a cross-sectional population study. Eur J Pain. 2018; https://doi.org/10.1002/ejp.1176.
23. de Tommaso M, Sciruicchio V. Migraine and central sensitization: clinical features, main comorbidities and therapeutic perspectives. Curr Rheumatol Rev. 2016;12(2):113–26.
24. Lantéri-Minet M, Duru G, Mudge M, Cottrell S. Quality of life impairment, disability and economic burden associated with chronic daily headache, focusing on chronic migraine with or without medication overuse: a systematic review. Cephalalgia. 2011;31(7):837–50.
25. Soriani S, Fiumana E, Manfredini R, Boari B, Battistella PA, Canetta E, Pedretti S, Borgna-Pignatti C. Circadian and seasonal variation of migraine attacks in children. Headache. 2006;46(10):1571–4.
26. Hauge AW, Kirchmann M, Olesen J. Characterization of consistent triggers of migraine with aura. Cephalalgia. 2011;31(4):416–38.
27. B B, Ekizoglu E, Karli N, Kocasoy-Orhan E, Zarifoglu M, Saip S, Siva A, Ertas M. Characterization of Migraineurs having allodynia: results of a large population-based study. Clin J Pain. 2016;32(7):631–5.
28. Lipton RB, Munjal S, Buse DC, Bennett A, Fanning KM, Burstein R, Reed ML. Allodynia is associated with initial and sustained response to acute migraine treatment: results from the American migraine prevalence and prevention study. Headache. 2017;57(7):1026–40.
29. T T, T H, K H. Characterization of migraineurs presenting interictal widespread pressure hyperalgesia identified using a tender point count: a cross-sectional study. J Headache Pain. 2017;18(1):117.

30. Ohayon MM. Prevalence and risk factors of morning headaches in the general population. Arch Intern Med. 2004;164(1):97–102.

31. Akerman S, Holland PR, Goadsby PJ. Diencephalic and brainstem mechanisms in migraine. Nat Rev Neurosci. 2011;12:570–84.

32. Liu F, Chang HC. Physiological links of circadian clock and biological clock of aging. Protein Cell. 2017;8(7):477–88.

33. Musiek ES, Holtzman DM. Mechanisms linking circadian clocks, sleep, and neurodegeneration. Science. 2016;354(6315):1004–8.

34. Feleppa M, Fucci S, Bigal ME. Primary headaches in an elderly population seeking medical Care for Cognitive Decline. Headache. 2017;57(2):209–16.

35. Franco G, Delussi M, Sciruicchio V, Marani W, De Rocco L, de Tommaso M. P011 the use of electronic pain diaries via telemedicine for managing chronic pain. J Headache Pain. 2015;16(Suppl 1):A190.

12

Pooling data from different populations: should there be regional differences in cerebral haemodynamics?

Angela S. M. Salinet[1,2,3]* (iD), Ronney B. Panerai[4,5], Juliana Caldas[1,6], Ricardo C. Nogueira[1], Adriana B. Conforto[1], Manoel J. Texeira[1], Edson Bor-Seng-Shu[1] and Thompson G. Robinson[4,5]

Abstract

Background: Though genetic and environmental determinants of systemic haemodynamic have been reported, surprisingly little is known about their influences on cerebral haemodynamics. We assessed the potential geographical effect on cerebral haemodynamics by comparing the individual differences in cerebral blood flow velocity (CBFv), vasomotor tone (critical closing pressure- CrCP), vascular bed resistance (resistance-area product- RAP) and cerebral autoregulation (CA) mechanism on healthy subjects and acute ischaemic stroke (AIS) patients from two countries.

Methods: Participants were pooled from databases in Leicester, United Kingdom (LEI) and São Paulo, Brazil (SP) research centres. Stroke patients admitted within 48 h of ischaemic stroke onset, as well as age- and sex-matched controls were enrolled. Beat-to-beat blood pressure (BP) and bilateral mean CBFv were recorded during 5 min baseline. CrCP and RAP were calculated. CA was quantified using transfer function analysis (TFA) of spontaneous oscillations in arterial BP and mean CBFv, and the derived autoregulatory index (ARI).

Results: A total of 100 participants (50 LEI and 50 SP) were recruited. No geographical differences were found. Both LEI and SP AIS participants showed lower values of CA compared to controls. Moreover, the affected hemisphere presented lower resting CBFv and higher RAP compared to the unaffected hemisphere in both populations.

Conclusions: Impairments of cerebral haemodynamics, demonstrated by several key parameters, was observed following AIS compared to controls irrespective of geographical region. These initial results should encourage further research on cerebral haemodynamic research with larger cohorts combining different populations.

Keywords: Cerebral haemodynamics, Acute stroke, Ischaemic stroke, Cerebral autoregulation, Transcranial Doppler ultrasound

Background

Cerebral haemodynamic abnormalities may be useful early clinical markers in the development of age-related neurodegenerative disorders with vascular aetiologies [1], in determining an increased risk of stroke among healthy and diseased populations [2], and in predicting stroke prognosis [3, 4]. Due to its clinical relevance, in recent years, polling cerebral haemodynamic data from different international research centres has become, an attractive option to generate larger study cohorts, enhancing the statistical power and the generalizability of study results [5, 6]. Understanding to what extent regional differences affect cerebrovascular function is a key to planning international collaborative research and also to improve understanding of regional differences in treatment effectiveness and worldwide patient outcomes.

Health has multi-factorial determinants, including social, cultural, economic and environmental factors, genetic variation, and the quality of healthcare available [5]. Different continents have different health conditions, especially considering marked socioeconomic, ethnical and health care disparities. Moreover, recent studies have reported significant differences between continents in the

* Correspondence: salinetangela@gmail.com
[1]Neurology Department, School of Medicine, University of São Paulo, São Paulo, SP, Brazil
[2]Biomedical Engineering, Engineering, Modelling and Applied Social Sciences Centre, Federal ABC University, Sao Bernardo do Campo, Sao Paulo, Brazil
Full list of author information is available at the end of the article

prevalence of cardiovascular risk factors, such as diabetes mellitus [7, 8], hypertension [9], smoking [10] and hyperlipidaemia [11]. Nevertheless, little information on the possible international regional differences in cerebral haemodynamics is available.

Therefore, with the aim of pooling individual subjects data from different regions in an on-going international collaborative research study of cerebral haemodynamic changes following acute ischaemic stroke (AIS), we investigated systemic and cerebral haemodynamic parameters in healthy older and AIS populations derived from two different regional research centre databases in the United Kingdom and Brazil. Data from these two regions were chosen in order to ensure the homogeneity of the measurement settings and reduce the interference of other confounding factors (e.g. transcranial Doppler inter-operator reliability), as only one researcher (AS) collected and analysed the data.

Methods

Participants

Participants recruited by the same researcher (AS) using a standardized data collection and analysis protocol were included; participants from Leicester, United Kingdom (LEI) [12, 13] and Sao Paulo, Brazil (SP) were investigated. Stroke participants were consecutively recruited either from the Hyperacute Stroke Unit at the University Hospitals of Leicester NHS Trust (LEI) or from the emergency room at the Hospital das Clinicas of São Paulo (SP). Inclusion criteria were acute anterior circulation ischaemic stroke (< 48 h from stroke onset) confirmed by a single acute ischaemic brain lesion on magnetic resonance image (MRI) and/or computerized tomography (CT). Exclusion criteria comprised: (1) presence of intracranial or subarachnoid haemorrhage on CT or MRI; (2) significant ipsilateral carotid artery disease (> 50% stenosis); (3) absence of sufficient bilateral temporal bone window for insonation of the middle cerebral artery (MCA); (4) history of myocardial infarction within 6 months or other neurological disorder. Neurological impairment was assessed with the NIH Stroke Scale (NIHSS) on patient admission [14]. Age- and sex-matched healthy control subjects with no history of stroke or transient ischaemic attack, diabetes mellitus, hypercholesterolemia or carotid artery stenosis were also recruited from departmental staff and their relatives. All participants provided written informed consent in accordance with the Declaration of Helsinki; the Nottingham Research Ethics Committee 1 (LEI) and Ethics Committee of the Hospital das Clinicas (SP) approved the studies.

Research protocol

As previously described [12, 13], measurements were performed with subjects in the supine position with slight elevation of the upper body. CBF velocity (CBFv) was measured in both MCAs by insonation through the temporal bone window with 2-MHz transducers attached to a head frame using a transcranial Doppler ultrasound (TCD) (Viasys Companion III; Viasys Healthcare and Doppler box, DWL for LEI and SP databases, respectively). Continuous non-invasive beat-to-beat blood pressure (BP) recording was performed with arterial volume clamping of the digital artery (Ohmeda 2300; Finapres, Louisville, CO, USA) with the subject's hand (left for control and unaffected hand-side for stroke group) positioned at heart level. End-tidal CO_2 ($EtCO_2$) was monitored using an infrared capnograph (Capnocheck Plus and MX-200 and Transmai for LEI and SP database, respectively) during nasal expiration. After stable values had been established, the servomechanism of the Finapres device was turned off and a data segment of 5 min baseline was recorded to assess systemic and cerebral haemodynamic parameters.

Data were simultaneously recorded onto a data acquisition system (PHYSIDAS, Department of Medical Physics, University Hospitals of Leicester and Doppler Box, DWL for LEI and SP databases, respectively) for subsequent off-line analysis.

Data analysis

All signals were visually inspected and narrow artefacts (< 100 ms) were removed by linear interpolation. CBFv channels were subjected to a median filter and all signals were low-pass filtered with a cut-off frequency of 20 Hz. The R–R interval was then automatically marked from the ECG and continuous heart rate (HR) plotted against time. Mean BP and CBFv values were calculated for each cardiac cycle. The end of each expiratory phase was detected in the $EtCO_2$ signal, linearly interpolated, and resampled with each cardiac cycle. The instantaneous relationship between BP and CBFv was used to estimate critical closing pressure (CrCP) and resistance area product (RAP) for each cardiac cycle using the first harmonic method, as described in Panerai [15]. Beat-to-beat data were spline interpolated and resampled at 5 samples s^{-1} to produce signals with a uniform time-base.

Dynamic cerebral autoregulation (CA) represents the transient relationship between BP (stimulus or input) and CBF (response or output), and was calculated by transfer function analysis (TFA), using the parameters gain, phase and coherence, and autoregulatory index (ARI), as previously described [16, 17]. Gain and phase reflect the relative amplitude and temporal relationship between the changes in BP and CBFv over a specified frequency range, respectively. Low gain indicates intact CA, whereas low phase (oscillations of CBFv and BP are synchronous) impaired CA. Coherence represents the fraction of output power that can be linearly explained by input power. Similarly to a correlation coefficient, it ranges from zero to 1. In the absence of a linear relationship, low signal-to-noise ratio, or other variables contributing to output changes, coherence will approach zero and will reduce the reliability of gain and phase estimates. These parameters were then averaged for the very-low frequency (VLF, 0.02–0.10 Hz), low frequency (LF, 0.10–0.25 Hz) and high frequency (0.25–0.40 Hz) ranges. Inverse FFT was then applied to the TFA, converting data back into the time domain, to calculate the CBFv step response. ARI was assigned to each recording by using the best least squares fit between the CBFv step response and one of the 10 model ARI curves proposed by Tiecks et al. [18]. Values of ARI = 0 represent absence of CA, while ARI = 9 corresponds to best-observed autoregulation. ARI was calculated for each participant for both hemispheres at baseline.

Statistical analysis

Data were analysed using commercially available statistical software (SPSS 18.0, Chicago, IL). Shapiro-Wilk test was adopted to identify parameters that did not fit a normal distribution, which were then log transformed and tested again for normality. Inter-group differences were tested using χ^2 test for categorical data and Student's t-test for continuous variables. Within the stroke and control groups, intra-individual differences in CBFv,

coherence, gain, phase and ARI, between LEI and SP centres were tested using two-way ANOVA with Tukey's post hoc test comparisons performed when appropriate. In addition, Levene's test was used to assess the equality of variances between the populations' variances. Levels of $p < 0.05$ were considered statistically significant. The minimum sample size in each group was calculated by the formula described by Brodie et al. [19]: $44.6/\Delta ARI^2$ (where ΔARI is the expected change in ARI) with 80% power at $\alpha = 0.05$.

Results

A total of 100 participants were recruited from both centres, corresponding to 25 AIS patients and 25 age- and sex-matched control subjects from each centre. Baseline demographic and clinical data are described in Tables 1 and 2, respectively. No significant differences were seen in baseline demographic data, though African ethnicity, dyslipidaemia, cardiomyopathy and atrial fibrillation were more frequent in SP, and sub-surgical carotid artery stenosis (< 50%) more frequent in the LEI stroke population (Table 1). Stroke patients received medication according to local guidelines for secondary prevention at the time of assessment, with the most common antihypertensive treatment including: beta-blockers (LEI = 14 (56%) /SP = 13 (52%)), angiotensin converting enzyme inhibitors (LEI = 11 (44%)/SP = 12 (48%)), diuretics

Table 1 Baseline characteristics of the stroke and control participants by geographical population

Variables	Stroke		Controls	
	LEI (n = 25)	SP (n = 25)	LEI (n = 25)	SP (n = 25)
Age, years	60.6 (15.8)	62.4 (11.8)	61.1 (9.9)	60.7 (10.0)
aNIHSS	11.5 (6.6)	14.3 (5.9)	NA	NA
Sex, n (%)				
Female	10 (40)	12 (48)	10 (40)	11 (44)
Male	15 (60)	13 (52)	15 (60)	14 (56)
Ethnicity, n (%)				
Caucasian	20 (80)	15 (60)	23 (92)	22 (88)
African	4 (16)	9 (36)*	2 (8)	3 (12)
Natives	0	1(4)	0	0
Asian	1(4)	0	0	0
Diabetes, n (%)	2 (8)	4 (16)	0	0
Hypertension, n (%)	6 (24)	10 (40)	2 (8)	0
Dyslipidemia, n (%)	0	4 (16)*	0	0
ICA stenosis, n (%)	4 (16)*	0	0	0
HIV, n (%)	1 (4)	0	0	0
AF, n (%)	0	6 (24)*	0	0
Cardiomyopathy, n (%)	0	3 (12)*	0	0

Data are mean (standard deviation) or n (%)
LEI Leicester, *UK* SP, Sao Paulo, Brazil, *aNIHSS* admission National Institutes of Health Stroke Scale, *ICA* internal carotid artery, *HIV* human immunodeficiency virus, *AF* atrial fibrillation
*$p < 0.02$ for comparisons between LEI and SP

Table 2 Stroke characteristics by region

	LEI ($n = 25$)	SP ($n = 25$)
Stroke Side, n (%)		
Left	11 (44)	12 (48)
Right	14 (56)	13 (52)
Stroke aetiology, n (%)		
CE	14 (56)	18 (72)
LAA	3 (12)	0
SVD	7 (28)*	0
SOE	0	0
SUE	1 (4)	7 (28)*
Stroke type, n (%)		
PACS	14 (56)	15 (60)
TACS	4 (16)	10 (40)*
LACS	7 (28)*	0
Thrombolysis, n (%)	5 (20)	9 (36)

Data are presented as n (%)

LEI Leicester, *UK* SP, São Paulo, Brazil, *CE* cardiac embolism, *LAA* large-artery atherosclerosis, *SVD* small vessel disease, *SOE* stroke of other determined aetiology, *SUE* stroke of undetermined aetiology, *PACS* partial anterior circulation stroke, *TACS* total anterior circulation stroke, *LACS* lacunar circulation stroke

*$p < 0.02$ for comparisons between LEI and SP

(LEI = 10 (40%) /SP = 7 (28%)). Statin therapy was prescribed to three LEI and two SP patients.

Compared to LEI stroke patients, SP patients were more likely to have total anterior circulation stroke syndrome and stroke of undetermined aetiology, and less likely to have had a lacunar stroke and small-vessel disease aetiology, though there were no differences in thrombolysis rates (Table 2). No differences between

time of stroke onset and haemodynamics assessment was found (LEI = 42.0(5.9) and SP = 39.3(7.6) hours).

After confirming a lack of significant inter-hemispheral difference, cerebral haemodynamic parameters (CBFv, CrCP, RAP, ARI, gain, phase and coherence) from the right and left hemispheres in control subjects were merged, as performed previously [13]. Table 3 gives the results of Levene's tests for equality of variances between LEI and SP populations. The results indicate that the population variances across regions are equivalent.

Compared to control subjects, stroke patients had significantly higher mean arterial BP, and significantly reduced CBFv in the affected, but not unaffected, hemisphere at the time of assessment (Table 4). RAP was significantly higher in the affected hemisphere than both the unaffected hemisphere in stroke patients, and control subjects (Table 4). No significant geographical differences were seen in either systemic or cerebral haemodynamic parameters for both stroke patients and control subjects (Table 4).

With respect to CA parameters, compared to control subjects, coherence was significantly increased in both the affected and unaffected hemispheres of AIS patients for both LF and HF ranges (Table 5). In addition, both phase in the VLF range and ARI were significantly reduced in the affected and unaffected hemispheres of AIS compared to control subjects (Table 5). No significant regional differences were observed, except for gain in the HF range between the affected and unaffected hemisphere in SP patients, which was not found in LEI patients (Table 5). Univariate ANCOVA adjusted for stroke aetiology and subtypes of the cerebral haemodynamics parameters also did not revealed any differences between regions (Table 6).

Table 3 Levene's test (statistics based on means) of variances equality between LEI and SP (geographical region) and stroke and control participants (participants type)

	Geographical Region		Participants Type	
	F	p value	F	p value
CBFv, cm.s^{-1}	0.721	0.399	0.195	0.662
CrCP, mm Hg	4.276	0.080	3.153	0.091
RAP, mmHg.s.cm^{-1}	1.496	0.230	2.231	0.120
Coherence VLF range	2.099	0.493	2.443	0.407
Coherence LF range	1.727	0.610	1.987	0.540
Coherence HF range	0.929	0.703	1.592	0.622
Normalized gain VLF range, % mm Hg^{-1}	0.331	0.901	0.486	0.838
Normalized gain LF range, % mm Hg^{-1}	0.297	0.882	3.089	0.567
Normalized gain HF range, % mm Hg^{-1}	3.921	0.098	3.444	0.612
Phase VLF range, radians	2.982	0.801	2.491	0.475
Phase LF range, radians	2.001	0.712	1.984	0.399
Phase HF range, radians	2.665	0.723	2.091	0.523
ARI	0.078	0.762	0.510	0.950

CBFv Cerebral blood flow velocity, *CrCP* Critical closing pressure, *RAP* Resistance Area Product, *VLF, LF, HF* Very low, low and high frequency ranges, respectively

Table 4 Systemic and cerebral hemodynamic parameters in stroke and control participants by region

Variables	Stroke Patients				Controls	
	SP (n = 25)		LEI (n = 25)		SP (n = 25)	LEI (n = 25)
	AH	UH	AH	UH		
MAP, mmHg	109.2 (5.7)#		103.0 (5.5)#		90.0 (6.1)	89.2 (3.9)
CBFv, cm.s^{-1}	47.5 (6.3)#	55.1 (5.8)	41.7 (2.4)*	45.03 (2.8)	60.3(11.6)	53.8 (5.5)
CrCP, mm Hg	18.2 (6.7)	18.0 (4.6)	19.4 (5.0)	17.0 (5.5)	14.2 (4.47)	15.5 (8.0)
RAP, mmHg.s.cm^{-1}	1.97 (0.32)*#	1.76 (0.25)#	2.25 (0.23)*#	1.77 (0.17)#	1.56 (0.27)	1.65 (0.60)

Data are presented as mean (SD)

LEI Leicester, UK SP, Sao Paulo, Brazil, AH affected hemisphere, UH unaffected hemisphere, MAP Mean arterial pressure, CBFv Cerebral blood flow velocity, CrCP Critical closing pressure, RAP Resistance Area Product

*p < 0.01, Tukey's post-hoc test for comparisons between stroke affected and unaffected hemispheres

#p < 0.05, Tukey's post-hoc test for comparisons between controls and stroke participants (same geographical region)

Discussion

Main findings

To the best of our knowledge, this is the first study to compare CA in participants from different geographical regions with marked environmental and socio-economic differences. These pooled analyses suggest no geographical differences in key, commonly measured cerebral haemodynamic parameters, including CBFv, CrCP, RAP and ARI. Overall, and in keeping with previous studies, impairment of cerebral haemodynamic parameters was reported in stroke compared to control participants, particularly in the affected hemisphere. Importantly, no geographical regional differences were found.

Clinical relevance

Recognizing similarities and differences in the cerebral haemodynamics in healthy subjects and stroke has public health and clinical implications for several cardiovascular outcomes. Haemodynamic abnormalities may be useful early clinical markers in the development of age-related vascular neurodegenerative disorders. Describing cerebral haemodynamic changes and their regulation in different geographical populations may help understand differences across age and ethnicities, as well as the potential generalizability of clinical studies results.

Impairment of CBFv and CA has a direct and major impact on secondary brain injury and clinical outcomes [3, 4], as well as on planning effective therapeutic strategies that consider BP management and early mobilization protocols. In line with previous studies, our results showed a deterioration of important haemodynamic parameters in the acute phase of ischaemic stroke, particularly reduced phase and ARI values compared to controls [3, 20–23]. Moreover, no significant alteration in gain between groups was found [6, 20]. Though TFA became a popular approach for assessment of dynamic CA, very few acute stroke studies

Table 5 Dynamic CA parameters in stroke and control participants by geographical region

Variables	Stroke Patients				Controls	
	SP (n = 25)		LEI (n = 25)		SP (n = 25)	LEI (n = 25)
	AH	UH	AH	UH		
Coherence VLF range	0.65 (0.19)	0.64 (0.14)	0.61 (0.14)	0.59 (0.14)	0.52 (0.16)	0.48 (0.11)
Coherence LF range	0.68 (0.23)#	0.73 (0.19)#	0.68 (0.17)#	0.71 (0.15)#	0.56 (0.18)	0.58 (0.15)
Coherence HF range	0.72 (0.18)#	0.77 (0.10)#	0.69 (0.17)#	0.67 (0.16)#	0.52 (0.21)	0.51 (0.15)
Normalized gain VLF range, % mm Hg^{-1}	1.26 (0.57)	1.17 (0.66)	0.94 (0.33)	0.91 (0.34)	1.01 (0.39)	1.19 (0.43)
Normalized gain LF range, % mm Hg^{-1}	1.32 (0.48)	1.22 (0.46)	1.35 (0.44)	1.26 (0.69)	1.45 (0.83)	1.49 (0.78)
Normalized gain HF range, % mm Hg^{-1}	1.50 (0.74)*	1.36 (0.51)	1.36 (0.54)	1.28 (0.55)	1.35 (0.63)	1.40 (0.58)
Phase VLF range, radians	0.53 (0.42)#	0.78 (0.39)#	0.58 (0.50)#	0.70 (0.49)#	0.88 (0.35)	0.87 (0.41)
Phase LF range, radians	0.30 (0.45)	0.25 (0.38)	0.30 (0.35)	0.31 (0.39)	0.48 (0.19)	0.45 (0.41)
Phase HF range, radians	0.09 (0.29)	0.10 (0.25)	0.11 (0.40)#	0.17 (0.21)#	0.05 (0.21)	0.01 (0.28)
ARI	4.8 (2.3)#	4.9 (2.0)#	5.1 (1.8)#	5.0 (1.1)#	5.9 (1.5)	5.5 (1.2)

Data are presented as mean (SD)

LEI Leicester, UK SP, Sao Paulo, Brazil, AH affected hemisphere, UH unaffected hemisphere, ARI Autoregulatory Index, VLF, LF, HF Very low, low and high frequency ranges, respectively

*p < 0.01, Tukey's post-hoc test for comparisons between stroke affected and unaffected hemispheres

#p < 0.05, Tukey's post-hoc test for comparisons between controls and stroke participants

Table 6 ANCOVA and ANOVA results for comparison of cerebral haemodynamics parameters between geographical regions (stroke only)

	MS		F-statistic		p-Value	
	ANCOVA	ANOVA	ANCOVA	ANOVA	ANCOVA	ANOVA
CBFv, cm.s^{-1}	3.2	8.6	0.7	0.9	0.83	0.42
CrCP, mm Hg	2.5	3.0	5.2	4.8	0.60	0.81
RAP, mmHg.s.cm^{-1}	4.9	3.0	6.1	1.8	0.10	0.24
Coherence VLF range	5.7	9.2	3.2	4.5	0.31	0.19
Coherence LF range	3.8	4.4	2.9	4.3	0.44	0.31
Coherence HF range	3.1	5.3	2.3	3.6	0.56	0.29
Normalized gain VLF range, % mm Hg^{-1}	14.0	5.1	5.2	1.4	0.07	0.33
Normalized gain LF range, % mm Hg^{-1}	8.1	4.5	0.9	2.3	0.30	0.12
Normalized gain HF range, % mm Hg^{-1}	7.8	4.4	5.5	1.2	0.21	0.40
Phase VLF range, radians	4.2	2.5	0.2	0.1	0.90	0.90
Phase LF range, radians	6.7	1.8	0.2	0.4	0.80	0.90
Phase HF range, radians	5.5	1.4	1.0	0.2	0.80	0.30
ARI	1.5	1.9	4.5	3.9	0.51	0.77

The analysis of covariance (ANCOVA) model included stroke aetiology and subtypes as covariates
ANOVA analysis of variance, *MS* mean square, *AH* affected hemisphere, *UH* unaffected hemisphere, *VLF, LF, HF* Very low, low and high frequency ranges, respectively
p-value for ANOVA (geographical interaction) and ANCOVA controlled for stroke aetiology and subtype

have reported the use of coherence estimates [3, 22]. These previous studies failed to find raised coherence values in acute stroke, but an analogous parameter (the squared correlation coefficient) was found to be increased bilaterally after the first 48 h of stroke onset, suggesting worsening of CA [23].

The importance and novelty of our results, however, stem from the similarities of the haemodynamic responses from research centres in both UK and Brazil, irrespective of the participant group (stroke or healthy controls). Despite the potential differences in dietary habits and lifestyles, and particularly in SP participants, higher prevalence of uncontrolled hypertension and widespread use of over-the-counter medications, cerebral haemodynamic parameters were not significantly different in our study. The authors believe that the outcome of this paper will strengthen the argument in favour of multicentre and multinational collaborative studies of the impact of cerebral haemodynamics in stroke and other conditions, such as sepsis and traumatic brain injury.

Environment effects on cerebral haemodynamics

Since differences in CBF and its control mechanisms between European and South American populations have not been previously reported, it is difficult to assess consistency with other studies in the literature. A previous TCD study of healthy young participants ($n = 20$) in Germany and Hong Kong described no CBFv differences in the posterior cerebral arteries at rest and during cerebral activation [24]. Nevertheless, slower initial haemodynamic

responses to visual activation paradigms were described in the Asian group that may be related to deficits in the nitric oxide system. Previous studies have also compared cerebral haemodynamic responses between South Asian and Caucasian participants, but the results were inconsistent. In a United Kingdom-based study, resting MCA CBFv and cerebrovascular resistance parameters (Pourcelot's resistive index and Gosling's pulsatility index) were significantly higher, and CA impaired in South Asian participants [25]. By contrast, no difference in the same parameters of CBFv and cerebrovascular resistance was found in another recent study of Canadian-based South Asians and Caucasians [26].

Disparities in cardiovascular and cerebrovascular health and mortality among populations have been well documented [27, 28], but poorly understood. Studies have shown that the prevalence and mortality from hypertensive heart disease, stroke, and renal disease are higher among individuals of African compared to Caucasian descent [29]. Moreover, intracranial atherosclerosis is highly prevalent among patients with Asian, Hispanic, and African ancestry [30].

The present study did not demonstrate significant geographical differences in cerebral haemodynamic parameters between UK and Brazilian populations, with exception of gain at high frequency band. Immink and colleagues (2005) found an increase in gain only at higher frequencies in MCA-only stroke group. This may be the reason for the difference between regions, as SP comprised MCA infarcts only, whereas seven lacunar strokes were included in the LEI group (Table 2). Though recommended by the Cerebral Autoregulation Network (CARNet) [31], there is limited information in the literature on CA status in the complete frequency dependence of coherence, gain and phase in the range 0.02–0.40 Hz. While the TFA parameters changes in VLF and LF ranges are familiar, very little is known about the behaviour of the BP/CBFv system at frequencies higher than 0.25 Hz. In the TFA model, phase and gain are considered two different aspects of a high-pass filter that acts primarily in the VLF and LF ranges. At high frequencies, CA is considered less relevant and CBFv changes are associated with heart stroke volume beat-to-beat variability. More clinical studies are necessary to investigate the clinical importance of investigating CA in the higher frequency band, taking advantage of the work that has already been done. A further finding of the present study related to the responses of cerebrovascular resistance mechanisms, derived from a two-parameter model: RAP-CrCP. Levene's test revealed a marginal difference in CrCP between geographical regions, with a tendency to higher values in LEI participants. Further research is needed to assess the clinical value of this finding.

Standardized protocol

The experimental design of previous cerebral haemodynamic studies has been inconsistent, making it difficult to compare results directly [32, 33]. Furthermore, there have been no previous CA studies in either older or stroke populations in Brazil. In contrast, in the UK, some studies have previously described the haemodynamic responses to spontaneous BP fluctuations, carbon dioxide modulations and brain activation paradigms in both populations [12, 13, 34, 35]. More recently, the Department of Cardiovascular Sciences at the University of Leicester (Leicester, UK) has constructed a large database incorporating recordings from a series of separate studies performed in the same laboratory, using similar protocols, operator training and equipment [36]. They have presented normative values for cerebral haemodynamic parameters in a large healthy population indicating parameters that may help distinguish between normal and abnormal CA.

The present study was only possible due to the development of standardized data collection and analysis that provided a robust approach for the systematic evaluation of CBFv and its main regulatory mechanisms [37]. Similar to the Leicester normative study [36], all data collected in this study were acquired with similar study protocols and laboratory set-up, albeit with minor differences in the equipment used, and most importantly, without observer variability since all recordings were performed by only one researcher (AS). This avoids inter-observer variability in the study protocol (particularly concerning the TCD data), and it consequently increases the reproducibility of study reports.

Study limitations

This study has limitations, including the use of non-invasive measurements of CBF and BP. Another limitation to consider is stroke patients received medication according to local guidelines for secondary prevention at the time of assessment. Though patients were on vasoactive therapy at time of assessment, no significant difference between populations was found. Although TFA and the ARI index can be regarded as the most widely used approach for assessment of dynamic CA, it is important to note that neither can be regarded as a 'gold standard'. Future studies are needed to replicate our findings using alternative approaches such as time-domain analysis or the Mx index [12]. Finally, the sample size is relatively small, and is unlikely to be representative enough to ensure robust conclusions. Therefore, the authors strongly advocate a large multicentre validation study with larger sample size to explore further the possibility of regional geographical influences on cerebral haemodynamics, and possible mechanisms to support any differences.

Conclusion

In conclusion, our results showed no significant differences in selected cerebral haemodynamic parameters between two different socio-economical geographical regions. In both research centres, acute ischaemic stroke depressed key measures of CA compared to a healthy older control population. These findings encourage further larger international studies of cerebral haemodynamic changes following AIS by pooling individual subject's data from different regions.

Abbreviations

AIS: Acute ischaemic stroke; ARI: Autoregulatory index; BP: Blood pressure; CA: Cerebral autoregulation; CBF: Cerebral blood flow; CBFv: Cerebral blood flow velocity; CrCP: Critical closing pressure; CT: Computerized tomography; EtCO$_2$: End-tidal CO$_2$; HR: Heart rate; LEI: Leicester; MCA: Middle cerebral artery; MRI: Magnetic resonance image; NHISS: NIH Stroke Scale; RAP: Resistance area product; SP: Sao Paulo; TCD: Transcranial doppler ultrasound; TFA: Transfer function analysis

Acknowledgements

Authors acknowledge Dr. João Loures Salinet Junior for his contribution in the data analysis and revising the manuscript. TGR is an NIHR Senior Investigator.

Funding

The work was supported by the Brazilian Ministry of Education (Grant number 0411-10-8) and São Paulo Research Foundation (Grant number 2014/04955–8).

Authors' contributions

ASMS, RBP and TGR made a substantial contribution to the concept and design; ASMS, JC, RBP made the acquisition of data or analysis and interpretation of data; ASMS, TGR, RBP drafted the article; JC, RBP, RCN, TGR, ABC, MJT, EBSS revised it critically for important intellectual content; and ASMS, JC, RBP, RCN, TGR, ABC, MJT, EBSS approved the final version to be published.

Pooling data from different populations: should there be regional differences in cerebral...

109

Competing interests

The authors declare that they have no competing interests.

Author details

[1]Neurology Department, School of Medicine, University of São Paulo, São Paulo, SP, Brazil. [2]Biomedical Engineering, Engineering, Modelling and Applied Social Sciences Centre, Federal ABC University, Sao Bernardo do Campo, Sao Paulo, Brazil. [3]Faculty of Physiotherapy, Ibirapuera University, São Paulo, Brazil. [4]Department of Cardiovascular Sciences, Cerebral Haemodynamics in Ageing and Stroke Medicine Research Group, University of Leicester, Leicester, UK. [5]NIHR Leicester Biomedical Research Centre, University of Leicester, Leicester, UK. [6]Critical Care Unit Hospital São Rafael, Salvador, Brazil.

References

1. Keage HAD, Churches OF, Kohler M, Pomeroy D, Luppino R, Bartolo ML, Elliotta S. Cerebrovascular function in aging and dementia: a systematic review of transcranial Doppler studies. Dement Geriatr Cogn Dis Extra. 2012; 2:258–70.
2. Derdeyn CP, Grubb RL Jr, Powers WJ. Cerebral hemodynamic impairment: methods of measurement and association with stroke risk. Neurology. 1999; 53:251–61.
3. Castro P, Serrador JM, Rocha I, Sorond F, Azevedo E. Efficacy of cerebral autoregulation in early ischemic stroke predicts smaller infarcts and better outcome. Front Neurol. 2017;8:113–23.
4. Reinhard M, Rutsch S, Lambeck J, Wihler C, Czosnyka M, Weiller C, et al. Dynamic cerebral autoregulation associates with infarct size and outcome after ischemic stroke. Acta Neurol Scand. 2012;125:156–62.
5. The Nuffield Council on Bioethics. The ethics of research related to healthcare in developing countries. London: Nuffield Council on Bioethics; 2002.
6. Hedman K, Alm A. A pooled data analysis of three randomised, doublemasked six-month clinical studies comparing the intraocular pressure reducing effect of latanoprost and timolol. European J Ophthalmol. 2000;2:94–104.
7. Danaei G, Finucane MM, Lu Y, et al. National, regional, and global trends in fasting plasma glucose and diabetes prevalence since 1980: systematic analysis of health examination surveys and epidemiological studies with 370 country-years and 2.7 million participants. Lancet. 2011;378:31–40.
8. Guariguata L, Whiting DR, Hambleton I, et al. Global estimates of diabetes prevalence for 2013 and projections for 2035. Diabetes Res Clin Pract. 2014; 103:137–49.
9. Danaei G, Finucane MM, Lin JK, et al. National, regional, and global trends in systolic blood pressure since 1980: systematic analysis of health examination surveys and epidemiological studies with 786 country-years and 5.4 million participants. Lancet. 2011;377:568–77.
10. Ng M, Freeman MK, Fleming TD, et al. Smoking prevalence and cigarette consumption in 187 countries, 1980-2012. JAMA. 2014;311:183–92.
11. Farzadfar F, Finucane MM, Danaei G, et al. National, regional, and global trends in serum total cholesterol since 1980: systematic analysis of health examination surveys and epidemiological studies with 321 country-years and 3.0 million participants. Lancet. 2011;377:578–86.
12. Salinet ASM, Robinson TG, Panerai RB. Effects of cerebral ischemia on human neurovascular coupling, CO2 reactivity, and dynamic cerebral autoregulation. J Appl Physiol. 2015;118:170–7.
13. Salinet ASM, Robinson TG, Panerai RB. The longitudinal evolution of cerebral blood flow regulation after acute ischaemic stroke. Cerebrovasc Dis Extra. 2014;4:186–97.
14. Lyden P, Brott T, Tilley B, Welch KMA, Mascha EJ, Levine S, et al. Improved reliability of the NIH stroke scale using video training. Stroke. 1994;25:2220–6.
15. Panerai RB. The critical closing pressure of the cerebral circulation. Med Eng Phys. 2003;25:621–32.
16. Katsogridakis E, Bush G, Fan L, Birch AA, Simpson DM, Allen R, Potter JF, et al. Detection of impaired cerebral autoregulation improves by increasing arterial blood pressure variability. J Cereb Blood Flow Metab. 2013;33:519–23.
17. Meel van den ASS, Simpson DM, Wang LJY, Zhang R, Tarumi T, Rickards CA, et al. Between Centre variability in transfer function analysis, a widely used method for linear quantification of the dynamic pressure-flow relation: the CARNet study. Med Eng Physics. 2014;36:620–7.
18. Tiecks FP, Lam AM, Aaslid R, Newell DW. Comparison of static and dynamic cerebral autoregulation measurements. Stroke. 1995;26:1014–9.
19. Brodie FG, Atkins ER, Robinson TG, Panerai RB. Reliability of dynamic cerebral autoregulation measurement using spontaneous fluctuations in blood pressure. Clin Sci. 2009;116:513–20.
20. Ma H, Guo Z-N, Liu J, Xing Y, Zhao R, Yang Y. Temporal course of dynamic cerebral autoregulation in patients with Intracerebral hemorrhage. Stroke. 2016;47:674–81.
21. Eames PJ, Blake MJ, Dawson SL, Panerai R, Poter J. Dynamic cerebral autoregulation and beat to beat blood pressure control are impaired in acute ischaemic stroke. J Neurol Neurosurg Psychiatry. 2002;72:467–72.
22. Immink RV, van Montfrans GA, Stam J, Karemaker JM, Diamant M, van Lieshout JJ. Dynamic cerebral autoregulation in acute lacunar and middle cerebral artery territory ischemic stroke. Stroke. 2005;36:2595–600.
23. Reinhard M, Wihler C, Roth M, Harloff A, Niesen WD, Timmer J, Weiller C, Hetzel A. Cerebral autoregulation dynamics in acute ischemic stroke after rtPA thrombolysis. Cerebrovasc Dis. 2008;26:147–55.
24. Hao Q, Wong LK, Lin WH, Leung TW, Kaps M, Rosengarten B. Ethnic influences on neurovascular coupling: a pilot study in whites and Asians. Stroke. 2010;41:383–94.
25. Bathula R, Hughes AD, Panerai RB, Potter JF, AS MGT, Tillin T, et al. South Asians have adverse cerebrovascular haemodynamics, despite equivalent blood pressure, compared with Europeans. This is due to their greater hyperglycaemia. Int J Epidemiol. 2011;40:1490–8.
26. Booth HP, Prevost AT, Gulliford MC. Severity of obesity and management of hypertension, hypercholesterolemia and smoking in primary care: population-based cohort study. J Hum Hypetens. 2015;2:1–6.
27. Sheth T, Nair C, Nargundkar M, Anand S, Yusuf S. Cardiovascular and cancer mortality among Canadians of European, south Asian and Chinese origin from 1979 to 1993: an analysis of 1.2 million deaths. CMAJ. 1999;161:132–8.
28. Rambihar VS, Rambihar SP, Rambihar VS. Race, ethnicity, and heart disease: a challenge for cardiology for the 21st century. Am Heart J. 2010;159:1–14.
29. Burt VL, Whelton P, Roccella EJ, Brown C, Cutler JA, Higgins M, et al. Prevalence of hypertension in the US adult population. Results from the third National Health and nutrition examination survey, 1988-1991. Hypertension. 1995;25:305–13.
30. Mille E, Levin J, Brendel M, Zach C, Barthel H, Sabri O. Etal. Cerebral glucose metabolism and dopaminergic function in patients with Corticobasal syndrome. J Neuroimaging. 2016;27:1–7.
31. Claassen JA, Meel-van den Abeelen AS, Simpson DM, Panerai RB, International Cerebral Autoregulation Research Network (CARNet). Transfer function analysis of dynamic cerebral autoregulation: a white paper from the International Cerebral Autoregulation Research Network. J Cereb Blood Flow Metab. 2016;36:665–80.
32. van Beek AH, Claassen JA, Rikkert MG, Jansen RW. Cerebral autoregulation: an overview of current concepts and methodology with special focus on the elderly. J Cereb Blood Flow Metab. 2008;28:1071–85.
33. Aries M, Elting JW, De Keyser J, Kremer BPH, Vroomen P. Cerebral autoregulation in stroke a review of Transcranial Doppler studies. Stroke. 2010;41:12–20.
34. Saeed NP, Panerai RB, Horsfield MA, Robinson TG. Does stroke subtype and measurement technique influence estimation of cerebral autoregulation in acute ischaemic stroke? Cerebrovasc Dis. 2013;35:257–61.
35. Minhas JS, Syed NF, Haunton VJ, Panerai RB, Robinson TG, Mistri AK. Is dynamic cerebral autoregulation measurement using transcranial Doppler ultrasound reproducible in the presence of high concentration oxygen and carbon dioxide? Physiol Meas. 2016;37:673–82.
36. Patel P, Panerai RP, Haunton V, Katsogridakis E, Saeed NP, Salinet ASM, et al. The Leicester cerebral haemodynamics database: normative values and the influence of age and sex. Physiol Meas. 2016;37:1485–99.
37. Giller CA, Bowman G, Dyer H, Mootz L, Krippner W. Cerebral arterial diameters during changes in blood pressure and carbon dioxide during craniotomy. Neurosurgery. 1993;27:737–41.

13

Current approaches for the management of Parkinson's disease in Chinese hospitals: a cross-sectional survey

Gang Wang[†] (ID), Hai-Lun Cui[†], Jun Liu, Qin Xiao, Ying Wang, Jian-Fang Ma, Hai-Yan Zhou, Jing Pan, Yu-Yan Tan, Sheng-Di Chen[*] and on behalf of the Chinese Movement Disorders Society

Abstract

Background: Chinese guidelines for management of Parkinson's disease (PD) have been issued and updated regularly since 2006. We undertook a cross-sectional survey to evaluate the impact of the latest edition (2014) on current approaches to the management of PD based on previous pilot works.

Methods: Seven hundred and seventeen participants, divided into 3 groups (GPs, Neurologists, and Specialists), recruited from 138 randomly chosen hospitals from 30 cities across China, participated by completing the questionnaire describing their current approaches before and after the guidelines were issued.

Results: Considerable discrepancies in management were apparent across the three categories, with different selection of first-choice medication for PD patients. There were also variations in management of concurrent psychiatric symptoms and dementia. Notably, over 50% of participants reported improvements in PD recognition and management by following the guidelines.

Conclusions: The increasing use of Chinese clinical practice guidelines for PD management is having a positive impact on the optimization of care, which in turn offers important economic benefits.

Keywords: Parkinson's disease, Surveys and questionnaires, Guideline, Disease management

Background

Being one of the most common neurodegenerative disease worldwide, Parkinson's disease (PD), with its high prevalence and incidence among aged people, carries a huge economic burden in China and presents with some unique features in Chinese population [1]. To address the aging crisis, the Chinese Parkinson's Disease & Movement Disorders Society (CMDS), Neurology Branch of Chinese Medical Association has consecutively issued three versions of management guidelines for PD since 2006 [2–4]. Drawing upon four eminent guidelines globally ahead, which were formulated respectively by the Movement Disorder Society (MDS) [5], the American Academy of Neurology (AAN) [6–9], the European Federation of Neurological Societies (EFNS) [10], and the UK's National Institute for Health and Care Excellence (NICE) [11]—the CMDS guidelines aim to guide the general direction of PD treatment in order to improve the current management standards in China. A key unique individualized treatment recommendation was the principles of dosage titration and a satisfactory clinical effect with a low dose, i.e., "low and slow", should be followed to avoid acute adverse reactions and to reduce the incidence of long-term motor complications, as important therapeutic strategies in optimizing and standardizing treatment. Specifically, we recommend the principles of medication should be aiming at an optimal status for working and living quality, rather than full-dosage administration [12].

Aiming to acquire the real situation of PD treatment in China, in 2011 we conducted a pilot survey and the results showed significant differences in treatment options and an obvious variation before and after referring of PD guidelines among GPs, general neurologists and

* Correspondence: ruijincsd@126.com

[†]Gang Wang and Hai-Lun Cui contributed equally to this work.

Department of Neurology& Institute of Neurology, Ruijin Hospital affiliated to Shanghai Jiaotong University School of Medicine, No.197, Rui Jin Er Road, Shanghai 200025, China

movement disorders specialists [13]. Given the relatively small sample size of enrolled doctors involved previously, we launched a national survey at a larger scale and specify our research on the latest edition of the PD guideline, hoping to update our awareness of current PD management in China and measure the impact of the latest version (2014). Thus, this survey would evaluate the status quo and shed new light on the future control and management of PD.

Methods
Recruitment

This cross-sectional survey on doctors was performed between December 2015 and February 2016. One hundred and thirty-eight hospitals of different levels were chosen randomly from 30 cities across China. We enrolled 717 doctors in the survey and classified them into three categories: (1) GPs—most belong to general physicians; (2) General neurologists—who specialize in general neurology other than movement disorders; (3) Movement disorders specialists—neurologists with a specific focus on movement disorders, who regularly attend the movement disorders clinics. Among the chosen hospitals, 96% were ranked as tertiary hospitals according to the current grading measures issued by the PRC National Health and Family Planning Commission, which classes hospitals as tertiary if they are characterized by comprehensive multiple functions with specialization in all-purpose high-quality medical services and academic researches across different areas.

Research content

We asked enrolled doctors to complete a 96-item questionnaire covering all aspects of PD, including relevant methods on PD management, and the various therapeutic options they offered to patients. The questionnaire was designed by two of the authors (Dr. Gang Wang and Dr. Sheng-Di Chen) with approval from the Research Ethics Committee, Ruijin Hospital affiliated to Shanghai Jiao Tong University School of Medicine, Shanghai, China. The study included three stages, as following:

Stage1: Background Acquirement: We gathered demographic information from the participants enrolled in the study in order to examine the distribution of the samples. We also assessed the level of understanding on a general basis in order to obtain an overall standard of recognition with regard to PD among the participants.

Stage 2: Differences in PD therapy according to varied clinicians, levels of hospital and city: We questioned participants with detailed and targeted questions on the different medications they tended to offer PD patients

who presented with various symptoms. In order to evaluate the whole situation on a more comparable and meticulous basis, we classified the participants into three categories: by clinicians (GPs/Neurologist/Specialist), level of hospital, and hierarchy of city they worked in (as defined by the general economic status of the city).

Stage 3: Guideline's impact on PD recognition and treatment: Finally, we attempted to investigate the disparity in the understanding and therapeutic methods of PD via the intervention of the latest version CMDS Guidelines (2014) and observed the changes in doctors on how they viewed and dealt with PD after adopting the guideline. The comparison of the two phrases (before and after the release of the guidelines) would be beneficial for the future training of the physicians in the management of PD.

Statistical analysis

All statistics were evaluated and addressed by members of an independent third party, with no underlying competing interests involved. Categorical variables were displayed by frequencies and percentages. The raw data analysis was based on contingency tables. All statistical analyses were performed using SAS version 9.4 software. Chi-square test was used for statistical analysis, and a P-value < 0.05 was considered significant.

Results
Demographics

A total of 717 (Male: female = 43%: 57%) participants were enrolled and mostly aged between 35 and 60 years (66%). Six hundred eighty-four participants (96.2%) were doctors of tertiary hospitals. As for the clinician types, 54% of them were general neurologists, with 28% of specialists in PD, others (18%) were GPs. Among all, 70.4% had no academic memberships, while 17.9% were members of CMDS in China. We also investigated the general level of CME of PD among physicians from various departments. Notably, there were significant differences ($p < 0.05$) in their familiarity with PD guidelines, exchange of academic experience, and level of research for PD.

Differences in PD therapy according to various clinicians, hospitals and cities

With each of the three categories, we sought participants' opinions on the same set of therapeutic measures. Across various clinicians, there was a lack of consensus on several treatment issues, such as the first choice of medication for patients without cognitive decline, management on wearing off phenomenon, peak-dose dyskinesia and morning dystonia (see Table 1). They also thought differently on the management of PD with dementia and/or psychiatric symptoms. When faced with

Table 1 Preferred medication for PD patients under specific circumstances among doctors of different specialties

Items	Total ($n = 711$)[a]	General physicians ($n = 130$)	General neurologists ($n = 381$)	Movement disorders specialists ($n = 200$)	χ^2	P value
Age < 65 years without cognitive impairment						
Levodopa	185 (26.0%)	25 (19.2%)	106 (27.8%)	54 (27.0%)	3.8551	0.1455
Dopamine agonists	333 (46.8%)	38 (29.2%)	177 (46.5%)	118 (59.0%)	28.0886	< 0.0001
MAO-B inhibitors	164 (23.1%)	20 (15.4%)	86 (22.6%)	58 (29.0%)	8.3434	0.0154
Benzhexol	49 (6.9%)	4 (3.1%)	25 (6.6%)	20 (10.0%)	6.0243	0.0492
Amantadine	101 (14.2%)	13 (10.0%)	55 (14.4%)	33 (16.5%)	2.7671	0.2507
Levodopa + COMT inhibitors	95 (13.4%)	19 (14.6%)	48 (12.6%)	28 (14.0%)	0.4386	0.8031
Age > 65 years without cognitive impairment						
Levodopa	345 (48.5%)	42 (32.3%)	187 (49.1%)	116 (58.0%)	20.9235	< 0.0001
Dopamine agonists	180 (25.3%)	22 (16.9%)	99 (26.0%)	59 (29.5%)	6.7851	0.0336
MAO-B inhibitors	101 (14.2%)	15 (11.5%)	62 (16.3%)	24 (12.0%)	2.8932	0.2354
Benzhexol	32 (4.5%)	5 (3.9%)	19 (5.0%)	8 (4.0%)	0.4558	0.7962
Amantadine	69 (9.7%)	8 (6.2%)	44 (11.6%)	17 (8.5%)	3.6800	0.1588
Levodopa + COMT inhibitors	145 (20.4%)	22 (16.9%)	82 (21.5%)	41 (20.5%)	1.2648	0.5313
Wearing off phenomenon						
Add levodopa dose	127 (17.9%)	15 (11.5%)	67 (17.6%)	45 (22.5%)	6.4953	0.0389
Adjust protein diet	181 (25.5%)	18 (13.9%)	87 (22.8%)	76 (38.0%)	27.1973	< 0.0001
Switch from standard levodopa to CR levodopa	260 (36.6%)	30 (23.1%)	140 (36.8%)	90 (45.0%)	16.3361	0.0003
Add COMT inhibitors or MAO-B inhibitors	326 (45.9%)	48 (36.9%)	163 (42.8%)	115 (57.5%)	16.5500	0.0003
Recommend surgical treatment	83 (11.7%)	7 (5.4%)	35 (9.2%)	41 (20.5%)	22.3837	< 0.0001
Peak-dose dyskinesia						
Reduce levodopa dose, add its frequency	296 (41.6%)	7 (28.5%)	156 (40.9%)	103 (51.5%)	17.3687	0.0002
Reduce levodopa dose, add dopamine agonists	319 (44.9%)	33 (25.4%)	168 (44.1%)	118 (59.0%)	36.1891	< 0.0001
Reduce levodopa dose, add COMT inhibitors	249 (35.0%)	33 (25.4%)	129 (33.9%)	87 (43.5%)	11.8497	0.0027
Reduce levodopa dose, add MAO-B inhibitors	204 (28.7%)	23 (17.7%)	101 (26.5%)	80 (40.0%)	21.0749	< 0.0001
Add amantadine	182 (25.6%)	20 (15.4%)	85 (22.3%)	77 (38.5%)	26.7639	< 0.0001
Switch from CR levodopa to standard levodopa	110 (15.5%)	16 (12.3%)	43 (11.3%)	51 (25.5%)	21.4792	< 0.0001

[a]six participants supply insufficient data and not included in the present table

psychiatric symptoms in advanced stage patients, most of the PD specialties (62.0%) would reduce or stop the anti-PD medication, while only 33.08% of GPs would copy the same strategy ($\chi^2(N = 711) = 26.4027$, $p < 0.0001$). However, regardless of their clinician types, most of the participants agreed on the usage of MAO-B inhibitors, which they prescribed for 25–50% of their PD patients to alleviate their symptoms. Nevertheless, there was disagreements about which type of PD might benefit more from MAO-B inhibitors, and an extremely significant disparity ($p < 0.0001$) on familiarity with the use of disease-modifying/neuroprotective therapy ($\chi^2(N = 711) = 42.9005$, $p < 0.0001$), Rivastigmine for PDD patients ($\chi^2(N = 711) = 20.2759$, $p < 0.0001$), and antipsychotics for psychiatric symptoms managements ($\chi^2(N = 711) = 21.8987$, $p < 0.0001$).

With regard to different class of hospital, we found that all participating hospitals were in agreement on most of the questions, including the treatment of PD patients aged < 65 years without cognitive decline, management of wearing off phenomenon, peak-dose dyskinesia and morning dystonia. They also shared similar opinions on treatment strategies for mental disorder and psychiatric symptoms. Some of them had slight differences in treating constipation and held opposite views on continuous dopaminergic stimulation (CDS). But there were no significant differences in the usage of MAO-B inhibitors and the management of Restless legs syndrome (RLS).

Regarding to financial status of the cities in which the participants were working, we discovered that most of the questions we devised received similar responses—that is, no significant differences in PD treatment and understanding were found among the cities we investigated.

Guideline's impact on PD recognition and treatment

Prominent changes have been found. 68.3% of participants agreed with a "low and slow" and dosage titration method as the PD medication principle. In addition to different clinical feature of each patient, 77.7% of participants stressed the necessity of taking ages into account. Specifically, for the treatment of patients aged > 65 years, the top three preferred therapies before the guidelines were levodopa (75.7%), dopamine agonists and MAO-B inhibitors; 29.1% would consider trying a combination of levodopa and catechol-O-methyl transferase (COMT) inhibitors, which have superseded MAO-B inhibitors as the third most common option after the guidelines issued. Patients with wearing off phenomenon were likely to receive more doses of levodopa (52.9%) before the guidelines were issued; now, they would be given COMT inhibitors and MAO-B inhibitors (66.9%) instead. Most participants agreed with a 200-300 mg per day as the recommended starting dose for levodopa treatment. Memantine has been acknowledged as one of the preferred options (57.9%) for treating Parkinson's disease with dementia (PDD) (χ^2 ($N = 717$) = 21.1521, $p < 0.0001$) (see Table 2).

We tallied the general satisfaction on the updated guidelines at the end of our investigation. More than 95% of the respondents confirmed its efficiency and application value. Importantly, 36.1% of participants reported a 25–50% of improvement in PD recognition, and 73.5% of them responded ≥25% increased accuracy in diagnosis. These findings reflect the benefit of the wider use of the guidelines.

Discussion

The purpose of this investigation is to determine at what level our neurologists are on the PD recognition and therapeutic methods. The current situation in China concerning PD management is that this disease is not only treated in neurological department, but non-neurology as well. What's more, the attending doctors are not simply limited to PD professions, but general neurologist of no PD-treating experience, or even physicians of other departments also. We deem it necessary to gain a thorough and validated situation of status quo on how the PD treatment is really carried out in China and the differences in therapeutic level among doctors of distinguished backgrounds. Supposing that the results of this survey shows significant differences in PD recognition and treatment methods, it is hopefully an optimal guidance for further reformation and improvement in this particular field.

During stage 1, we gathered information of participants involved in this study and classified their backgrounds. Female doctors made up of 57% of the total, and 66% of the samples were in the age group of 35–60 years. With 78% of them selected in first-tier or quasi

first-tier cities and 98% worked in tertiary class hospitals, we could determine that this study is highly representative in large public hospitals among capital cities with integrated financial and economic centers in China. During stage 2, we asked the participants to fill in the questionnaire which contains clinical tendency on PD and their personal understanding on certain therapy. We found that the most notable discrepancies came from the feedbacks given by doctors of different specialties. Among which, highly significant differences were seen not only in guideline reference, academic exchanging, researching experience, but were not rare in detailed diagnostic methods like Madopar loading test on suspected patients and MRI application. Situations like these further substantiate our hypothesis that PD treatment in China have not been completely standardized so far. When compared on the ground of distinguished levels of hospitals and cities, we discovered minor differences, indicating the fact that the diagnostic and therapeutic level among hospitals and cities are generally similar, with no significant differences exposed. During stage 3, we discovered an inspirational phenomenon that the treating methods and PD recognition have prominently ameliorated after referring to the CMDS guidelines. Moreover, symptoms presented on PD patients have been significantly improved as well, as over half of the doctors surveyed reported improvements in their patients. Specifically, 36.8% of the participants confirmed an over 50% of improvements during clinical practice; while 62.1 and 63.1% of participants affirmed a reduction in patients with wearing off phenomenon and peak-dose dyskinesia, respectively. In short, the guideline is markedly beneficial to reasonable PD medications strategy, and hopefully, its dissemination will greatly enhance the standard of our PD management.

Compared to the guidelines issued before represented by MDS, etc., CMDS guidelines has a relatively short history. When first issued in 2006, it has been updated regularly and remained one of the young members among the family of PD guidelines worldwide. Its localization strategy in optimizing and standardizing management of PD, especially its emphasis about "low and slow", have covered a large range of patients in need, and is conducive to disease management in a prolonged period [5, 6]. Inspirationally, we found that the clinical guideline is already helping the standardization of practice via improving the level of clinicians. It not only improved the diagnostic accuracy, but decreased the motor complications as well, which is in consistent with another study we have done recently [6].

However, since the survey was performed on doctors from tertiary class hospitals only, with no data gathered from the patients, we have not drawn any objective statistics that could directly show the improvement of the

Table 2 The impact of PD guidelines reference on the selection of medication under specific circumstances

Items	Overall (n = 717)	Haven't read the PD guidelines (n = 57)	Have read the PD guidelines (n = 660)	χ^2	P value
Age < 65 years without cognitive impairment					
Levodopa	185 (25.8%)	5 (8.8%)	180 (27.3%)	9.3807	0.0022
Dopamine agonists	334 (46.6%)	4 (7.0%)	330 (50.0%)	38.9561	< 0.0001
MAO-B inhibitors	164 (22.9%)	2 (3.5%)	162 (24.6%)	13.1620	0.0003
Benzhexol	49 (6.8%)	0 (0.0%)	49 (7.4%)	4.5422	0.0331
Amantadine	101 (14.1%)	1 (1.8%)	100 (15.2%)	7.7814	0.0053
Levodopa + COMT inhibitors	95 (13.3%)	1 (1.8%)	94 (14.2%)	7.1189	0.0076
Age > 65 years without cognitive impairment					
Levodopa	345 (48.1%)	7 (12.3%)	338 (51.2%)	31.8549	< 0.0001
Dopamine agonists	181 (25.2%)	3 (5.3%)	178 (27.0%)	13.1001	0.0003
MAO-B inhibitors	101 (14.1%)	3 (5.3%)	98 (14.9%)	3.9834	0.0460
Benzhexol	32 (4.5%)	0 (0.0%)	32 (4.9%)	2.8927	0.0890
Amantadine	69 (9.6%)	2 (3.5%)	67 (10.2%)	2.6620	0.1028
Levodopa + COMT inhibitors	145 (20.2%)	1 (1.8%)	144 (21.8%)	13.0918	0.0003
Wearing off phenomenon					
Add levodopa dose	127 (17.7%)	3 (5.3%)	124 (18.8%)	6.5847	0.0103
Adjust protein diet	182 (25.4%)	2 (3.5%)	180 (27.3%)	15.6441	< 0.0001
Switch from standard levodopa to CR levodopa	261 (26.4%)	3 (5.3%)	258 (39.1%)	25.9346	< 0.0001
Add COMT inhibitors or MAO-B inhibitors	327 (45.6%)	5 (8.8%)	322 (28.8%)	33.8682	< 0.0001
Recommend surgical treatment	83 (11.6%)	0 (0.0%)	83 (12.6%)	8.1066	0.0044
Peak-dose dyskinesia					
Reduce levodopa dose, add its frequency	297 (41.4%)	5 (8.8%)	292 (44.2%)	27.2061	< 0.0001
Reduce levodopa dose, add dopamine agonists	319 (44.5%)	7 (12.3%)	312 (47.3%)	26.0137	< 0.0001
Reduce levodopa dose, add COMT inhibitors	251 (35.0%)	5 (8.8%)	246 (37.3%)	18.7324	< 0.0001
Reduce levodopa dose, add MAO-B inhibitors	206 (28.7%)	4 (7.0%)	202 (30.6%)	14.2578	0.0002
Add amantadine	182 (25.4%)	2 (3.5%)	180 (27.3%)	15.6441	< 0.0001
Switch from CR levodopa to standard levodopa	110 (15.3%)	0 (0.0%)	110 (16.7%)	11.2216	0.0008
PD with psychosis (advanced stage)					
Reduce levodopa dose	147 (20.5%)	2 (3.5%)	145 (22.0%)	10.9712	0.0009
Add antipsychotics	321 (44.8%)	11 (19.3%)	310 (47.0%)	16.2481	< 0.0001
PD with visual hallucination and delirium during treatment (ineffective with drug adjustment)					
Clozapine	267 (37.2%)	13 (22.8%)	254 (38.5%)	5.5181	0.0188
Olanzapine	301 (42.0%)	22 (38.6%)	279 (42.3%)	0.2911	0.5895
Quetiapine	301 (42.0%)	9 (15.8%)	292 (44.2%)	17.4394	< 0.0001
Risperidone	85 (11.9%)	3 (5.3%)	82 (12.4%)	2.5749	0.1086
PD with depression					
Tricyclic antidepressants	59 (8.2%)	8 (14.0%)	51 (7.7%)	2.7645	0.0964
SSRIs, e.g. sertraline	487 (67.9%)	39 (68.4%)	448 (67.9%)	0.0071	0.9329
Pramipexole	420 (58.6%)	20 (35.1%)	400 (60.6%)	14.0811	0.0002
PD with dementia (PDD)					
Huperzine A	82 (11.4%)	1 (1.8%)	81 (12.3%)	5.7312	0.0167
Donepezil	346 (48.3%)	13 (22.8%)	333 (50.5%)	16.0620	< 0.0001
Rivastigmine tartrate	275 (38.4%)	7 (12.3%)	268 (40.6%)	17.8047	< 0.0001

Table 2 The impact of PD guidelines reference on the selection of medication under specific circumstances *(Continued)*

Items	Overall (n = 717)	Haven't read the PD guidelines (n = 57)	Have read the PD guidelines (n = 660)	χ^2	P value
Memantine	397 (55.4%)	15 (26.3%)	382 (57.9%)	21.1521	< 0.0001
Traditional Chinese Medicine (TCM), e.g. ginkgo leaf	82 (11.4%)	1 (1.8%)	81 (12.3%)	5.7312	0.0167
PD with periodical limb movement syndrome (PLMS) or restless legs syndrome (RLS)					
Levodopa	153 (21.3%)	6 (10.5%)	147 (22.3%)	4.3130	0.0378
Dopamine agonists	376 (52.4%)	6 (10.5%)	370 (56.1%)	43.6187	< 0.0001
Amantadine	17 (2.4%)	0 (0.0%)	17 (2.6%)	1.5038	0.2201
Benzodiazepines	94 (13.1%)	3 (5.3%)	91 (13.8%)	3.3472	0.0673

effectiveness of PD management and the health condition on patients' perspective. Further researches need to be conducted in order to make up for this deficiency.

Conclusions

In general, the CMDS guidelines has demonstrated a clear impact on therapeutic strategies for PD, and the clinical management of PD in China could be improved considerably if the deficiencies revealed in this study could be effectively addressed. Hopefully, the wider dissemination of the CMDS guidelines will greatly enhance the standard of China's PD management continuatively in the long run.

Abbreviations
AAN: American Academy of Neurology; CDS: Continuous dopaminergic stimulation; CMDS: Chinese Parkinson's Disease & Movement Disorders Society; EFNS: European Federation of Neurological Societies; GPs: General practitioners; MAO-B: Monoamine oxidase BCOMT: catechol-O-methyl transferase; MDS: Movement Disorder Society; NICE: UK's National Institute for Health and Care Excellence; PD: Parkinson's disease; PDD: Parkinson's disease with dementia; RLS: Restless legs syndrome

Funding
This work was supported by the National Natural Science Foundation of China [grant numbers 91332107] and the Shanghai Municipal Education Commission-Gaofeng Clinical Medicine Grant Support [grant numbers 20172001]; Lundbeck China provided the fund for medical editing; and PAREXEL gave the assistance on medical editor.

Authors' contributions
GW and HLC contributed to the drafting of the manuscript; GW and SDC designed the study, analyzed the data and revised the manuscript; others participated in the data collecting and study design. All authors read and approved the final manuscript.

Competing interests
The authors declare that they have no competing interests.

References
1. Wang G, Cheng Q, Zheng R, Tan YY, Sun XK, Zhou HY, Ye XL, Wang Y, Wang Z, Sun BM, et al. Economic burden of Parkinson's disease in a developing country: a retrospective cost analysis in shanghai, China. Mov Disord. 2006;21(9):1439–43.
2. Chen SD. The guideline for management of Parkinson's disease in China. Chin J Neurol. 2006;39:409–12.
3. Chen SD. The guideline for management of Parkinson's disease in China (second edition). Chin J Neurol. 2009;42(5):352–5.
4. Chen SD. The guideline for management of Parkinson's disease in China (third edition). Chin J Neurol. 2014;47(6):428–33.
5. Postuma RB, Berg D, Stern M, Poewe W, Olanow CW, Oertel W, Obeso J, Marek K, Litvan I, Lang AE, et al. MDS clinical diagnostic criteria for Parkinson's disease. Mov Disord. 2015;30(12):1591–601.
6. Miyasaki JM, Shannon K, Voon V, Ravina B, Kleiner-Fisman G, Anderson K, Shulman LM, Gronseth G, Weiner WJ. Practice parameter: evaluation and treatment of depression, psychosis, and dementia in Parkinson disease (an evidence-based review): report of the quality standards Subcommittee of the American Academy of neurology. Neurology. 2006;66(7):996–1002.
7. Pahwa R, Factor SA, Lyons KE, Ondo WG, Gronseth G, Bronte-Stewart H, Hallett M, Miyasaki J, Stevens J, Weiner WJ. Practice parameter: treatment of Parkinson disease with motor fluctuations and dyskinesia (an evidence-based review): report of the quality standards Subcommittee of the American Academy of neurology. Neurology. 2006;66(7):983–95.
8. Suchowersky O, Gronseth G, Perlmutter J, Reich S, Zesiewicz T, Weiner WJ. Practice parameter: neuroprotective strategies and alternative therapies for Parkinson disease (an evidence-based review): report of the quality standards Subcommittee of the American Academy of neurology. Neurology. 2006;66(7):976–82.
9. Montgomery EB Jr. Practice parameter: neuroprotective strategies and alternative therapies for Parkinson disease (an evidence-based review): report of the quality standards Subcommittee of the American Academy of neurology. Neurology. 2007;68(2):164. author reply 164
10. Berardelli A, Wenning GK, Antonini A, Berg D, Bloem BR, Bonifati V, Brooks D, Burn DJ, Colosimo C, Fanciulli A, et al. EFNS/MDS-ES/ENS [corrected] recommendations for the diagnosis of Parkinson's disease. Eur J Neurol. 2013;20(1):16–34.
11. Ryton BA, Liddle BJ. Implementing NICE clinical guidelines on Parkinson's disease. Clin Med(Lond). 2009;9(5):436–40.
12. Chen S, Chan P, Sun S, Chen H, Zhang B, Le W, Liu C, Peng G, Tang B, Wang L, et al. The recommendations of Chinese Parkinson's disease and movement disorder society consensus on therapeutic management of Parkinson's disease. Transl Neurodegener. 2016;5:12.
13. Chen W, Chen S, Xiao Q, Wang G, Chen SD. Current clinical practice for Parkinson's disease among Chinese physicians, general neurologists and movement disorders specialists: a national survey. BMC Neurol. 2012;12:155.

14

Can the health related quality of life measure QOLIBRI- overall scale (OS) be of use after stroke? A validation study

Guri Heiberg[1,2,7*] [iD], Synne Garder Pedersen[1,3], Oddgeir Friborg[4], Jørgen Feldbæk Nielsen[5], Henriette Stabel Holm[5], Nicole Steinbüchel von[6], Cathrine Arntzen[1,3] and Audny Anke[1,2]

Abstract

Background: Brief measures of health-related quality of life (HRQOL) that assess both patient-reported functioning and well-being after stroke are scarce. The objective of this study was to examine reliability and validity of one of these measures, the patient-reported Quality of Life after Brain Injury–Overall Scale (QOLIBRI-OS), in patients after stroke.

Methods: Stroke survivors were examined prospectively using survey methods. Core survey data ($n = 125$) and retest data ($n = 36$) were obtained at 3 and 12 months, respectively. Item properties (distribution, floor and ceiling effects), psychometric properties (reliability and model fit), and validity (correlations with established measures of anxiety, depression and HRQOL) of the QOLIBRI-OS were examined.

Results: Missing responses on the questionnaire were low (0.5%). All items were positively skewed. No floor effects were present, whereas five out of six items showed ceiling effects. The summary QOLIBRI-OS score exhibited no floor or ceiling effects, and had excellent internal consistency (Cronbach's α =0.93). All item-total correlations were high (0.73–0.88). The test-retest reliability of single items varied from 0.74 to 0.91 and was 0.93 for the overall score. The confirmatory factor analysis yielded an excellent fit for a five-item version and provided tentative support for the original six-item version. The convergent validity correlations were in the hypothesized directions, thus supporting the construct validity.

Conclusions: The brief QOLIBRI-OS is a valid and reliable brief health-related outcome measure that is appropriate for screening HRQOL in patients after stroke.

Keywords: QOLIBRI-OS, Stroke, Health related quality of life, Validity

Background

Strokes are associated with complex physical, cognitive and psychosocial consequences that pose challenges to valid long-term outcome assessments [1, 2]. Due to a combination of functional, psychological and social constraints, the use of patients reported outcomes (PROs) to assess progress following treatment is advocated [3, 4]. PROs also seek to ascertain patients' views of the severity of their symptoms and functional status [5].

Generic and disease-specific health related quality of life (HRQOL) instruments assess consequences of health conditions on quality of life comprising psychological, physical, social and daily-life domains [6]. Both generic and disease-specific scales are used following stroke [7–9].

A comprehensive evaluation of the available HRQOL measures found that generic scales had limited value due to their lack of specificity to particular conditions and low responsiveness to change [7]. In the past decade, the use of stroke-specific scales has increased [10].

Stroke-specific HRQOL measures should ideally be reliable, valid, responsive, precise and appropriate as well as feasible, interpretable and easy to complete [3, 11–13]. Examples of these types of measures are the Stroke-Specific Quality of Life (SS-QOL) scale [14] and the Stroke Impact

* Correspondence: guri.heiberg@unn.no
[1]Department of Rehabilitation, University Hospital of North Norway, Tromsø, Norway
[2]Department of Clinical Medicine, Faculty of Health Sciences, University of Tromsø, The Arctic University of Norway, Tromsø, Norway
Full list of author information is available at the end of the article

Scale (SIS) [15], which both have shown good psychometric properties and been translated into several languages [16–18]. Although these scales adequately assess functional problems post-stroke, their comprehensive approach, i.e., inclusion of a large number of items covering multiple domains, reduce their feasibility in research and clinical use, especially for patients with cognitive deficits [19] or fatigue post-stroke [20]. A brief HRQOL measure could be useful for screening or in situations where the workload should be minimal. Additionally, a brief disease-specific version of the SIS with eight items has been developed [21], but this index does not address satisfaction, subjective functioning and subjective health status. Moreover, to compare conditions between patients with different disorders the measure has to be validated for use in several diagnostic groups.

In literature search of a suitable brief instrument assessing well-being, according to patient-reported satisfaction and important functional domains following stroke, the short Quality of Life after Brain injury Overall Scale (QOLIBRI-OS) [22] was identified as a possible option. This instrument was cross-culturally developed in six European countries between 2000 and 2010, and validated in more than 2000 patients after traumatic brain injury (TBI) [23].

The QOLIBRI-OS is a brief TBI-specific HRQOL index that addresses wellbeing and functioning [22]. The psychometric properties for the QOLIBRI-OS after TBI are satisfactory to good and are highly correlated with the 37 QOLIBRI scale (six subscales), indicating that a comparable construct is assessed [22]. The six items of the QOLIBRI-OS assess overall satisfaction with physical function, cognition, emotional status, ability to perform daily activities, personal life and social relationships, and satisfaction with the current situation and future prospects. A confirmatory factor analysis of the scale seem to support uni-dimensionality; however with some reservations as absolute fit seems clearly poorer (i.e., RMSEA = .07) than the relative fit (e.g., CFI = .98) [22]. QOLIBRI-OS has also been validated for patients with aneurysmal subarachnoid haemorrhage [24].

Stroke has important cognitive, emotional and physical clinical consequences that are similar to those of TBI, even though the health conditions differ in pathogenesis [25, 26]. Thus, the aim of this study was to investigate whether the QOLIBRI-OS is uni-dimensional and a reliable and valid measure of HRQOL post-stroke. To investigate its construct validity, we hypothesized positive correlations between the QOLIBRI-OS and the other HRQOL measures and negative correlations between the QOLIBRI-OS and psychological distress. In addition, concurrent relations of the individual QOLIBRI-items with relevant measures were explored.

Methods

This validation study is a part of a larger stroke study consecutively enrolling all patients, who were admitted to the stroke units of the University Hospital of Northern Norway (UNN) between March 2014 and December 2014. The inclusion criteria were in accordance with those of the National Stroke Registry. The exclusion criteria were age below 18 years, residence outside the hospital's region or foreign nationality. Patients with stroke related to brain malignancy, brain trauma or subarachnoid haemorrhage were excluded. A few patients who received acute stroke care in wards other than stroke units, due to the presence of other serious diseases, were also excluded. In total, 161 of 214 eligible patients with ischaemic or haemorrhagic stroke (ICD10 codes I.61 and I.63) consented to participate in the validation study, and 125 finally answered the questionnaire. While the response rate for eligible patients was 56%, the response rate for included consenting patients at 3 months was.

125 /161 = 78%. The flowchart in Fig. 1 shows more information on patient enrolment.

The study was approved by the Norwegian Regional Committee for Medical and Health Research Ethics (2013/ 1472).

Data collection

Patients were recruited during hospitalization in the stroke unit or by telephone within 3 months of discharge. Participants were asked to provide written consent. A local coordinator at all participating hospitals distributed the questionnaires by mail. Self-reported data were collected 3 months after stroke. Incomplete questionnaires were completed by filling in all missing items after an additional telephone interview. When up to two responses on any questionnaire were missing, mean imputation was performed. Questionnaires with more than 2 missing data points were excluded. Test-retest analysis of the QOLIBRI-OS was performed at 12-month follow-up due to the expected stability in functioning post-stroke [27] at this time point. The first 40 participants who answered at 12 months were asked to complete the retest in a 7- to 12-day period. Of these, 36 participants completed and returned the QOLIBRI-OS within the timeframe, which provides a response-rate of 90%. We conducted statistical tests (e.g., Student t- and chi-square tests) comparing the retest group (n = 36) with those not retested (n = 89), but no significant differences in any demographic characteristics or stroke severity emerged.

Demographic and stroke registry data

Information about age, gender, living condition and stroke was collected from the Norwegian Stroke Registry. Questions regarding education, marital status and work status

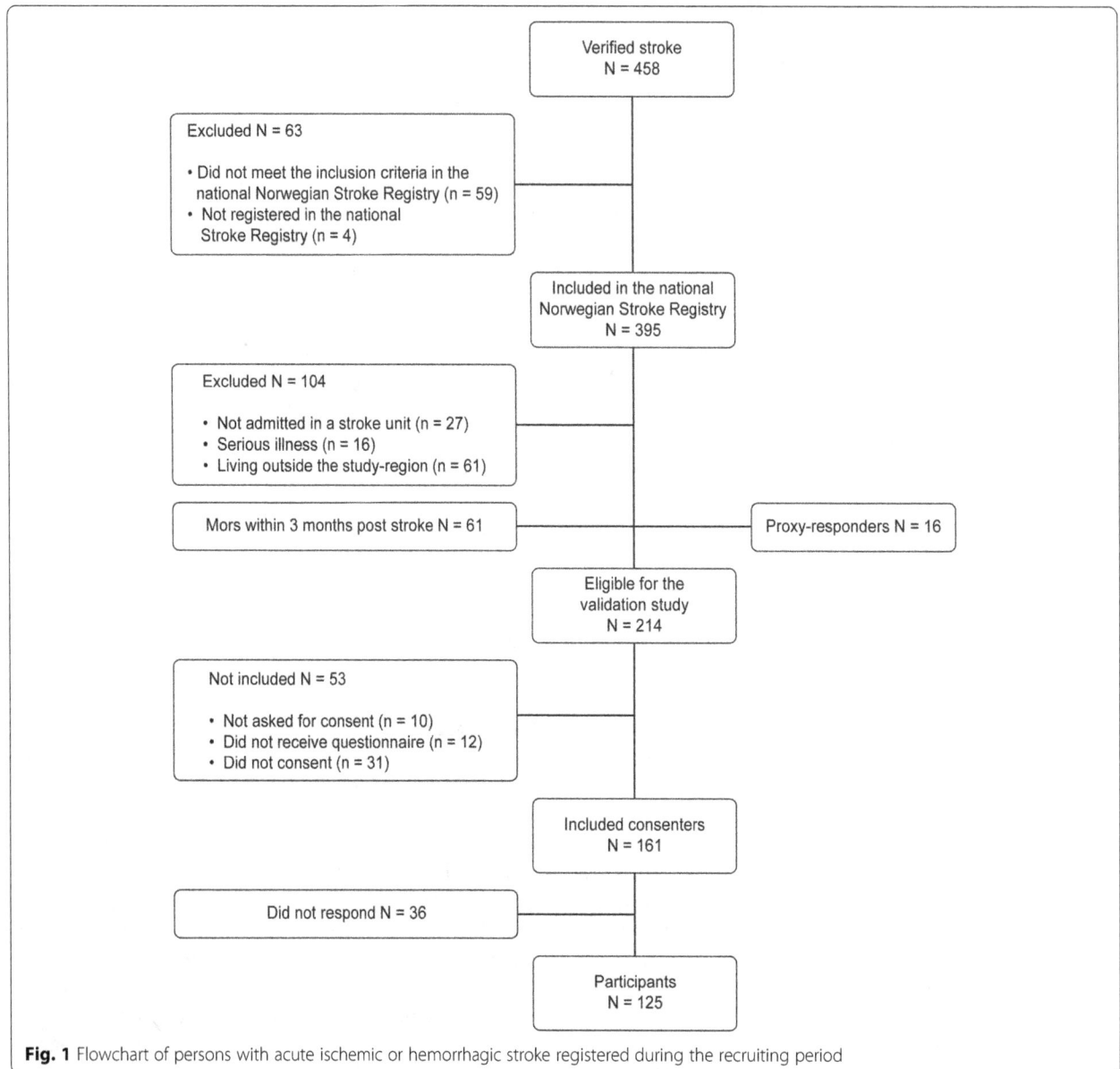

Fig. 1 Flowchart of persons with acute ischemic or hemorrhagic stroke registered during the recruiting period

were included in the mailed questionnaires, or were collected from the medical records after consent. Function was assessed with the Modified Rankin scale (MRS) [28], a clinician-reported measure of global disability widely used to evaluate post-stroke outcomes [28]. The scale consists of six categories assessing the level of independence, ranging from independent to bedridden or death. There is extensive evidence on the validity of the MRS [28]. In our study, the MRS was registered at 3 months after telephone interviews, as part of the national stroke registry registration.

Participants

Sociodemographic and clinical characteristics of the 125 participants are shown in Table 1. The average age was 70.5 years, and 62% were male. Approximately 50% of

patients had less than 11 years of education, and three out of four had retired before stroke.

At 3 months after stroke approximately 75% lived at home without personal assistance. Compared to those who did not respond ($n = 36$), participants were 5 years younger and a larger proportion lived at home at 3 months. The participants and non-responders differed statistically significantly in age, MRS score at 3 months, and proportion living in an institution and in need of assistance. Gender and stroke subtypes were similar in both groups (Table 1).

Comparisons between participants and patients that were eligible for the validation study, but did not participate, were performed only for age and gender for ethical reasons. However, there were no statistically significant

Table 1 Sociodemographic and stroke characteristics of the participants and non-responders

	Participants N = 125	Non-responders N = 36	P-values
Age at time of stroke, Mean (SD)	70.5 (13.1)	75 (13.6)	< 0.05
Gender, n (%)			
Female	48 (38)	16 (44)	
Male	77 (62)	20 (56)	0.34
Stroke subtype, n (%)			
Ischaemic	113 (90)	31 (86)	
Haemorrhagic	12 (10)	5 (14)	0.33
Marital status at time of stroke, n (%)			
Married/cohabitant	80 (64)	16 (45)	
Widowed/single	45 (36)	20 (55)	< 0.05
Education, time of stroke, n (%)			
≤ 10 years (y)	60 (48)	–	
> 10	62 (50)	–	–
Unknown	3 (2)	–	
Living conditions at 3 months, n (%)			
Home, without assistance	92 (73)	12 (33)	
Home, with assistance	23 (19)	14 (39)	< 0.01[a]
Institution/residence for the elderly	10 (8)	10 (28)	
Work status at 3 months, n (%)			
Student/Unemployed/Working fulltime or part-time	23 (18)	3 (8)	0.77
Retired/ Sick-leave	102 (82)	33 (92)	
MRS at 3 months, n (%)			
0–1 no symptoms or significant disability	84 (67)	15 (42)	
2–3 slight or moderate disability	33 (26)	16 (44)	
4–5 severe disability	8 (7)	7 (14)	< 0.05[b]

[a]Significantly more responders than non-responders lived at home without assistance vs. at home with assistance/in institution at 3 months after stroke
[b]Wilcoxon signed rank test

differences in these demographic data between the participants and the patients who refused to participate or between those who, due to a administrate failure, were not contacted.

Measurements

The QOLIBRI-OS comprises six items that assess the degree of overall satisfaction with "Physical Condition", "Cognition", "Emotions", "Ability to Perform Daily Activities", "Personal and Social Life," and "Current Situation and Future Prospects". A Likert scale provides the following five response categories: not at all (score 1), slightly (score 2) moderately (score 3), quite (score 4), very (score 5) for each item [22]. Accordingly, item score range is 1–5 and sum score range 6–30.

Von Steinbuchel et al. [22] arithmetically converted the sum of all items to a percentage scale (0–100). In the present study, both the raw item scores and the overall sum score were used. The QOLIBRI-OS has

demonstrated good internal consistency with a Cronbach's α value of 0.86 in patients after TBI [22] and 0.88 in patients with subarachnoid haemorrhage. [24]. The QOLIBRI full scale (37 items) questionnaire has been examined in a Norwegian study of patients after TBI and showed metric properties supporting the reliability and factor structure. To date, the QOLIBRI-OS (6 items) has not been validated in Norwegian samples. The QOLIBRI-OS was translated into Norwegian in 2008 in accordance with recommended procedures and is used in a longitudinal international observational study (the European Union Study CENTER-TBI-HEALTH. 2013.2.2.1–1). [29, 30] The translation used in our study was slightly modified to improve language fluency, and checked with back translation by a professional translation service. According to a bilingual professional translator the semantic meaning in our Norwegian version express the meaning of the original English version.

The Hospital Anxiety and Depression Scale (HADS), originally published by Zigmond and Snaith in 1983 [31], is a widely used instrument that screens for non-vegetative symptoms of anxiety (seven items) and depression (seven items) [32]. The HADS items are scored from 0 to 3 with higher scores indicating worse symptoms. A cut-off score of 8 indicates a possible diagnosis of anxiety or depression [33]. The total score (HADS-14) can also be used as a global measure of psychological distress [34]. The HADS questionnaire has been applied several times in Norwegian populations [29], also post-stroke [35].

The EuroQol Five Dimensions Questionnaire (EQ-5D) [36] is a three-level generic HRQOL questionnaire comprising 5 items measuring the dimensions of mobility, self-care, ability to perform daily activities, pain/discomfort and anxiety and depression [37]. The levels are rated as 1, 2, or 3, indicating no (1), some (2), and considerable problems (3). Each dimension can be scored separately. The questionnaire includes the EuroQol Visual analogue Scale.

(EQ-VAS), which is a 0–100 visual analogue scale intended to measure actual self-reported health status from worst to best imaginable health [38].

The Stroke Specific Quality of Life (SS-QOL) scale [14] assesses the functional impact of stroke across 12 domains using 49 items and a five-point Likert scale where higher scores indicate better functioning. The SS-QOL measures energy, mood, family roles, language, mobility, self-care, social roles, thinking, personality, and upper extremity function, vision and work/ productivity. A sum score can be extracted from each domain. Separate domain scores are obtained from unweighted average of all items belonging to a particular domain, but the overall SS-QOL score is most often used as the primary outcome. The SS-QOL scale has recently been translated into Norwegian in accordance with recommended procedures [39, 40].

Validation study design

The construct and criterion-related validity of the QOLIBRI-OS were examined in a confirmatory factor analysis and as concurrent correlations with theoretically related measures, respectively.The instruments chosen represent different aspects like stroke specific health related functions in HRQOL-measures, generic health related quality of life instruments, single questions and instruments assessing anxiety and depression. Moreover, the criterion-related measures included in our study are validated in Norwegian samples.The convergent and divergent validity of the QOLIBRI-OS, as one specific type of criterion-related validity, were supported if the Spearman rank-order correlations with the HADS total and anxiety scales were negative and the EQ-5D and SS-QOL were positive. Such correlations were calculated

for both the QOLIBRI-OS total and item scores. The direction of these a priori hypothesised correlations were based on the literature review in the introduction. According to the COSMIN guidelines [41], the overall construct validity is rated positively if the hypothesized relationships are specified in advance and supported in at least 75% of the reported results and based on a minimum of 50 patients.

Correlations above 0.50, between 0.31 and 0.49 and less than 0.30 were considered high, moderate and low, respectively [42]. Based on the literature review, we expected moderate to strong correlations between the QOLIBRI-OS and the criterion measures (see Table 2).The psychometric results from the current study were also used to re-evaluate the content validity of the QOLIBRI-OS, and discuss improvements.

Statistical and psychometric analyses

The Consensus-based Standards for the Selection of Health Measurement Instruments (COSMIN) guidelines [41] were used as guidelines for this validation study. The psychometric classical test theory analyses were conducted in Mplus version 7.4 [43] whereas all other inferential analyses were conducted in IBM SPSS version 23.

Descriptive characteristics

The QOLIBRI-OS items were described in terms of means and distributional properties. The degree of floor and ceiling effects, as defined by more than 15% of responses in the extreme lower or upper categories of the scale, were reported [44].

Uni-dimensionality

A confirmatory factor analysis was conducted to examine the fit of the QOLIBRI-OS as a uni-dimensional model. The maximum likelihood with robust standard errors (MLR) was applied, as the item distributions were non-normal. Model fit was evaluated in terms of the root mean square error of approximation (RMSEA), the standardized root mean square residual (SRMR), the comparative fit index (CFI) and the non-normed fit index (NNFI) [45]. West et al. [45] suggest that RMSEA < 0.05, CFI > 0.95, NNFI > 0.90 and SRMR < 0.06 represent a well-fitting model, while CFI > 0.90, NNFI > 0.85, RMSEA < 0.08, and SRMR < 0.10 indicate a tentatively adequate model.

Reliability

Cronbach's α was used to investigate the internal consistency. A value larger than 0.70 is generally recommended for research purposes (e.g., group comparisons), whereas values above 0.90 is desirable for individual clinical assessment [46]. Correlations between QOLIBRI-OS items and its total score were examined (values > 0.40 are preferable) [44] to identify items contributing poorly to the reliability or the ranking of the patients. Test-retest reliability was evaluated with intra-class correlation coefficients (ICCs) based on a two-way mixed model (i.e., treating items and subjects as fixed and random components, respectively). Both ICC absolute agreement and ICC consistency estimates were extracted for comparison purposes [47]. ICC consistency values > 0.75 was considered as excellent.

Results

Item characteristics and data quality of the QOLIBRI-OS

The degree of missing QOLIBRI-OS data was below 0.5% (Table 3). Single items were moderately positively skewed. The QOLIBRI-OS total score did not show floor or ceiling effects according to the COSMIN criterion we used, whereas a modest ceiling effect (defined as $> 15\%$) was observed in all items with the exception of one ("Physical condition"). All items robustly contributed to the overall QOLIBRI score, with all item-total correlations above 0.4 (ranging between 0.73–0.88).

Confirmatory factor analysis (CFA) of the QOLIBRI-OS

The model fit indicators of the hypothesized one-factor model were not universally good (robust $\chi^2_{df=9} = 21.83$, $p = 0.009$). Although the relative fit indices were good (CFI = 0.972 and NNFI = 0.953), the important non-centrality index (RMSEA = 0.107) was poorer as opposed to the absolute difference in unexplained standardized residuals that were low (SRMR = 0.029). This model thus yielded mixed support. Removing a single item, i.e., item 3 ("Overall, how satisfied are you with your feelings and emotions?"), yielded a model with

excellent universal fit (robust $\chi^2_{df=5} = 3.47$, $p = 0.63$; RMSEA = 0; SRMR = 0.015; CFI = 1.0; NNFI = 1.0).

As shown in Table 3, the ICC of the individual QOLIBRI-OS items were high and ranged from 0.75 to 0.91, whereas the overall score had excellent stability, ICC = 0.93.

Internal consistency of the QOLIBRI-OS overall score was excellent (Cronbach's $\alpha = 0.93$). We also calculated Cronbach's α after removing the item "feelings and emotions".

to observe changes in the internal consistency. In the resulting five-item scale, the Cronbach's α declined from 0.93 to 0.90.

Construct validity

As the results of the CFA were mixed, and as the authors considered the item in question (item 3) important for evaluations of HRQOL after stroke, additional correlation analyses were performed. First, the correlation between the five-item (after removing item 3) and six-item overall QOLIBRI-OS was 0.99. Second, the correlations between the HADS, EQ-VAS and the SS-QOL, and the five-and six-item QOLIBRI-OS yielded almost identical results.

Discussion

The results of this study indicated that the QOLIBRI-OS had excellent internal consistency, with slightly higher values than those reported in comparable studies after TBI and subarachnoid haemorrhage [22, 24]. All item-total correlations were high, and the items thus significantly contributed to a reliable ranking of patients. According to the COSMIN guidelines, floor and ceiling effects should not

Table 2 Construct validity of the QOLIBRI-OS at 3 months after stroke

Items	Measure for comparison	Correlation hypotheses	Spearman's Rho
1 Physical condition	SS-QOL sum mobility	High	0.44[a]
	EQ5D mobility	Moderate	0.31[a]
2 Cognitive function	SS-QOL sum thinking	Moderate to high	0.65[a]
3 Emotions	SS-QOL sum mood	High	0.66[a]
	HADS-total score	Moderate to high, negative	−.70[a]
4 Daily activities	SS-QOL sum work	Moderate to high	0.62[a]
	EQ5D Usual activities	High	0.64[a]
5 Personal and social life	SS-QOL sum social role	Moderate	0.55[a]
	HADS total score	Moderate, negative	−0.61[a]
6 Current situation and future prospects	EQ VAS score	High	0.57[a]
	HADS anxiety scale	High, negative	−0.58[a]
Sum QOLIBRI-OS	HADS total score	High, negative	−0.74[a]
	EQ VAS score	Moderate	0.56[a]
	SS-QOL sum score	High	0.71[a]

EQ5D EuroQol Quality of Life Scale-5D, HADS Hospital Anxiety and Depression Scale, SS-QOL Stroke-Specific Quality of Life Scale
[a]Correlation is significant at the 0.01 level (two-tailed)

exceed 15% [41]. In our study population, the summary QOLIBRI-OS score had no floor or ceiling effects. Modest ceiling effects were observed for the individual items. Stroke populations are very heterogeneous, thus these ceiling effects are difficult to interpret. For instance, certain subgroups are expected to experience few or no cognitive symptoms [48], therefore, the 20% of persons in this study reporting optimal satisfaction with cognitive functioning (item 2) did not necessarily indicate a problem with the scale, but might rather represent a clinical feature of this population [19]. No other studies have specifically investigated ceiling effects for single items in the QOLIBRI-OS, but von Steinbuchel et al. [22] reported a positive skew for all items indicating positive HRQOL in patients with TBI.

The uni-dimensionality of the QOLOBRI-OS received mixed support, as reported by others [49]. Muehlan et al. [49] identified item 5 (personal and social life) as a potentially problematic item after TBI. In the present study the cause of the mixed fit was related to another item (item 3: feelings and emotions). Removing this item led to an excellent model fit for the resulting five-item QOLIBRI-OS. Nevertheless, we retained all items in the final model because the differences in the validity correlations between the six- versus the five-item versions were negligible. Because this item has not been reported as problematic in other studies, and as the model fit of the six-item QOLIBRI-OS in the present study may be considered as fair, future studies should confirm a problem with this particular item before considering its removal. The problem with item 3 could be related to the translation, which differs slightly from the Norwegian CENTER-TBI version. Norwegian language don't differentiate between the terms "«feelings" and "«emotion", hence there was a minor problem in back-translation from Norwegian to English. Therefore a Norwegian replication study containing some changes in wording may be performed, investigating whether the translation of the above mentioned item is inaccurate.

Validity of the QOLIBRI-OS

Analysis of the a priori hypotheses confirmed construct validity. All a priori hypothesis tests, apart from one hypotheses, showed correlations with the selected other measures in the presumed directions and magnitude (Table 2). The correlation between Physical condition and SS-QOL sum mobility was moderate 0.44, though hypothesised to be high.

The COSMIN criteria indicate that construct validity can be supported if the concurrent correlations with other criterion-related variables are in the magnitude and direction hypothesized or predetermined by the authors. The present results uniformly fulfilled the COSMIN criteria [44]. The lowest correlation was observed between the "satisfaction with physical condition" item and the EQ-5D "mobility" question; this finding is not surprising, as the EQ-5D assesses walking ability in isolation, thus overlooking upper arm function and general health [38]. The highest correlation was observed in a negative relationship between item 3 on the QOLIBRI-OS, "satisfaction with feelings and emotions", and the HADS total score, which assesses psychological distress [31]; this result is in accordance with previous findings [50]. Emotions contribute substantially to HRQOL, and the high correlation between the QOLIBRI-OS emotion item and mental distress supported maintaining this item, even though the CFA indicated that it might be potentially problematic.

Table 3 Psychometric properties of the QOLIBRI-OS in 125 participants post-stroke: missing, mean values, item-total correlations and floor and ceiling effects. Test-retest reliability in 36 participants

Item N = 125	Missing %	Mean (SD)	Corrected item-total correlation	Floor and ceiling effects (%)	Test-retest reliability N = 36
QOL1: Physical condition	0	3.47 (1.02)	0.74	5.6 12.6	0.81
QOL2: Cognitive function	0	3.58 (1.06)	0.73	2.4 20.0	0.87
QOL3: Emotions	0.8	3.58 (1.08)	0.85	3.2 20.8	0.80
QOL4: Daily activities	1.6	3.75 (1.11)	0.78	4.0 28.8	0.91
QOL 5: Personal and, social life	0	3.62 (1.19)	0.83	7.2 24.8	0.75
QOL 6: Current life and, future prospects	0	3.50 (1.09)	0.88	6.4 17.6	0.84
QOLIBRI-OS sum score	0.4	3.58 (0.93)		0.8 7.2	0.93

Score reliability as test-retest stability

The ICC was tested using both consistency and agreement methods. The results were nearly identical, indicating that the subjects provided rather identical responses. The test-retest stability was particularly high for the overall scale (ICC = 0.93), which is higher than in previously published studies (ICC = 0.81) [22]. This may relate to differences in time periods of assessment. In our study, all participants performed test-retest at 12 months, whereas in former studies of QOLIBRI-OS, test-retest was investigated from 3 months to 15 years post stroke.The test-retest stability of all single items were comparable excellent.

Summarized, the psychometric results of the QOLIBRI-OS administered after stroke in this study are comparable or better than the results determined after TBI and subarachnoid haemorrhage [22, 24].

Can single items be considered individual domains?

The literature is ambiguous about the use of single items [51] to assess HRQOL, as single items are less reliable and valid than sum scores. Nevertheless, other scholars have reported that the reliability of global questions regarding HRQOL might be adequate [52–54].

The EQ-5D [36] has scoring options that include the use of single items. In our study, all of the QOLIBRI-OS items appeared to be uniformly consistent. Means, item-total correlations and test-retest stability varied slightly between items and differed slightly from the results of the total QOLIBRI-OS scale. Moreover, the concurrent validity coefficients of the individual items were high, given the high correlations with criterion-related measures, such as the HADS and SS-QOL. A higher ceiling effect for single items compared to the total score can be expected because of more variation within sum scores. More patients after stroke are expected to have optimal function in one specific aspect assessed by the QOLIBRI-OS, than in all aspects.

Use of QOLIBRI-OS in patients after stroke?

For clinical and research purposes after stroke there is no single preferred choice of outcome measure yet [4]. We performed a literature search in PubMed from 2014 to 2016 and discovered that the MRS was by far the most commonly used outcome measure in stroke research studies published from 2014 to 2016. However, the MRS does not assess the patients' subjective perspectives of their health and wellbeing and is unable to differentiate between physical and cognitive sequelae, which is an important argument for including a patient reported outcome measure (PROM).

However, can the QOLIBRI-OS, which is a brief measure, collect substantial information about important HRQOL domains for patients after stroke? In our opinion, the QOLIBRI-OS assesses the major consequences of stroke. Compared to the SIS [55] the QOLIBRI-OS contains one item measuring satisfaction with physical condition but lacks detailed measurements of strength and hand function. The SS-QOL which has 49 items, also includes domains that assess vision and energy [14]. Both the SIS and SS-QOL address communication. The lack of measurement of communication abilities (speaking and understanding) presents, in our opinion, a weakness of the QOLIBRI-OS for use post-stroke. The lack of a specific communication component is likely due to the fact that the instrument was developed only with generalizing overall questions, and the communication aspect was included in the overall item assessing cognition. In addition, motor activity was assumed to be included in the item assessing satisfaction with the physical condition. However, in stroke, communicative and motoric problems are frequent specific problems [56]. Therefore, we suggest that two additional new items should be developed and added to the QOLIBRI-OS- For instance, an item from the QOLIBRI scale regarding satisfaction with language and communicative skills and one item assessing motor function could be included and the scale should then be re-validated in a comprehensive stroke population. For the time being, however, we recommend the use of the QOLIBRI-OS in patients after stroke because it provides a short, reliable and valid index of HRQOL after stroke.

Strengths and limitations of the study

The strengths of this study are that a major proportion of the unselected stroke population admitted to UNN in 2014 is included. Patients were recruited from stroke units and followed through early rehabilitation, in both hospital and community settings. Of the consenting patients, 78% responded to the main questionnaire, despite the broad inclusion criteria and no exclusion of patients with aphasia or cognitive problems. All patients responded during the same time period post-stroke. The data quality was excellent, and the results were consistent.

A significantly higher portion of non-responders was institutionalized. However, the absolute number of patients with considerable functional deficits post-stroke was low in both groups. A total of 14% of non-responders versus 7% of participants had MRS scores of 4 or 5. This finding may limit the validity of the QOLIBRI-OS in the most severely affected patients post-stroke. Due to Norwegian ethical rules, comparisons between consenters and non-participants are possible for the variables age and gender only, which may limit the representativeness of the results. Furthermore, this study did not evaluate responsiveness to change.

The sample size of 125 patients is less than the first original multinational study of the validity of the QOLIBRI-OS [22], which included 795 patients after

TBI and thus provided more substantial statistical evidence of the psychometric data quality. Our study is consistent with the sample sizes from other validation studies of HRQOL measures [18, 57].

Conclusions

The QOLIBRI-OS is a valid and reliable brief HRQOL measure that is appropriate for application to patients after stroke in research and clinical contexts.

Abbreviations
COSMIN: Consensus-based Standards for the selection of health Measurement Instruments; HADS: The Hospital anxiety and depression scale; HRQOL: Health related quality of life; MRS: Modified Rankin scale; PROM: Patients reported outcome measure; QOLIBRI: Quality of Life after Brain Injury; QOLIBRI-OS: Quality of Life after Brain Injury – Overall Scale; SIS: Stroke Impact Scale; SS-QOL: Stroke Specific Quality of Life

Acknowledgements
The staff of the stroke units in the University Hospital in North Norway recruited patients after stroke and performed a telephone interview at 3 months post-stroke. Ralph Telgmann commented the final version of the manuscript. The publication charges for this article have been funded by a grant from the publication fund of UiT, The Arctic University of Norway.

Funding
Health region North Norway has funded the study. Grant number SFP1175–14.

Authors' contributions
GH, SGP and AA designed this study, analysed the data and were responsible for the overall decision-making in this study. GH and SGP collected all data. AA, OF and NVS contributed with supervision on the use of methods, analysis and interpretation of data. OF, JFN, HH, CA and NVS overlooked statistical analysis and interpretation. GH drafted the manuscript and all authors contributed to critical revision of the article. All authors read and approved the final manuscript.

Competing interests
The authors declare that they have no competing interests.

Author details
[1]Department of Rehabilitation, University Hospital of North Norway, Tromsø, Norway. [2]Department of Clinical Medicine, Faculty of Health Sciences, University of Tromsø, The Arctic University of Norway, Tromsø, Norway. [3]Department of Health and Care Sciences, Faculty of Health Sciences, University of Tromsø The Artic University of Norway, Tromsø, Norway. [4]Department of Psychology, Faculty of Health Sciences, University of Tromsø, the Artic University of Norway, Tromsø, Norway. [5]Hammel Neurorehabilitation Centre and University Research Clinic, Aarhus University, Aarhus, Denmark. [6]Universitäty Medicine, Georg-August-University, Göttingen, Germany. [7]Department of Rehabilitation, University Hospital of North Norway- Harstad, 9480 Harstad, Norway.

References
1. Feigin VL, Forouzanfar MH, Krishnamurthi R, Mensah GA, Connor M, Bennett DA, et al. Global and regional burden of stroke during 1990-2010: findings from the global burden of disease study 2010. Lancet. 2014;383(9913):245–55.
2. Adamson J, Beswick A, Ebrahim S. Is stroke the most common cause of disability? J Stroke Cerebrovasc Dis. 2004;13:171–7.
3. McClimans LM, Browne J. Choosing a patient-reported outcome measure. Theor Med Bioeth. 2011;32:47–60.
4. Kasner SE. Clinical interpretation and use of stroke scales. Lancet Neurol. 2006;5:603–12.
5. Black N. Patient reported outcome measures could help transform healthcare. BMJ. 2013;346:f167.
6. von Steinbuechel N, Petersen C, Bullinger M, Grp Q. Assessment of health-related quality of life in persons after traumatic brain injury--development of the Qolibri, a specific measure. Acta Neurochir Suppl. 2005;93:43–9.
7. Buck D, Jacoby A, Massey A, Ford G. Evaluation of measures used to assess quality of life after stroke. Stroke. 2000;31:2004–10.
8. Owolabi MO. What are the consistent predictors of generic and specific post-stroke health-related quality of life? Cerebrovasc Dis. 2010;29:105–10.
9. Almborg AH, Berg S. Quality of life among Swedish patients after stroke: psychometric evaluation of SF-36. J Rehabil Med. 2009;41:48–53.
10. Carod-Artal FJ. Determining quality of life in stroke survivors. Expert Rev Pharmacoecon Outcomes Res. 2012;12:199–211.
11. Fitzpatrick R, Fitzpatrick R, Davey C, Davey C, Buxton MJ, Buxton MJ, et al. Evaluating patient-based outcome measures for use in clinical trials. Health Technol Assess. 1998;2(i–iv):1–74.
12. Kimberlin CL, Winterstein AG. Validity and reliability of measurement instruments used in research. Am J Heal Syst Pharm. 2008;65:2276–84.
13. McLeod LD, Coon CD, Martin SA, Fehnel SE, Hays RD. Interpreting patient-reported outcome results: US FDA guidance and emerging methods. Expert Rev Pharmacoecon Outcomes Res. 2011;11:163–9.
14. Williams LS, Weinberger M, Harris LE, Clark DO, Biller J. Development of a stroke-specific quality of life scale. Stroke. 1999;30:1362–9.
15. Vellone E, Savini S, Fida R, Dickson VV, Melkus GD, Carod-Artal FJ, et al. Psychometric evaluation of the stroke impact scale 3.0. J Cardiovasc Nurs. 2015;30:229–41.
16. Caël S, Decavel P, Binquet C, Benaim C, Puyraveau M, Chotard M, et al. Stroke impact scale version 2: validation of the French version. Phys Ther. 2015;95:778–90.
17. Petersen C, Morfeld M, Bullinger M. Testing and validation of the German version of the stroke impact scale. Fortschr Neurol Psychiatr. 2001;69:284–90.
18. Muus I, Christensen D, Petzold M, Harder I, Johnsen SP, Kirkevold M, et al. Responsiveness and sensitivity of the stroke specific quality of life scale Danish version. Disabil Rehabil. 2011;33:2425–33.
19. Levine DA, Galecki AT, Langa KM, Unverzagt FW, Kabeto MU, Giordani B, et al. Trajectory of cognitive decline after incident stroke. JAMA. 2015;314:41–51.
20. Duncan F, Wu S, Mead GE. Frequency and natural history of fatigue after stroke: a systematic review of longitudinal studies. J Psychosom Res. 2012; 73:18–27.
21. Jenkinson C, Fitzpatrick R, Crocker H, Peters M. The stroke impact scale: Validation in a UK setting and development of a SIS short form and SIS index. Stroke. 2013;44:2532–5.
22. von Steinbuechel N, Wilson L, Gibbons H, Muehlan H, Schmidt H, Schmidt S, et al. QOLIBRI overall scale: a brief index of health-related quality of life after traumatic brain injury. J Neurol Neurosurg Psychiatry. 2012;83:1041–7.
23. Truelle J-L, Koskinen S, Hawthorne G, Von Wild K, Von Steinbuechel N. Traumatic brain injury quality of life tool: QOLIBRI. Brain Inj. 2012;26:421.
24. Wong GKC, Lam SW, Ngai K, Wong A, Mok V, Poon WS. Quality of life after brain injury (QOLIBRI) overall scale for patients after aneurysmal subarachnoid hemorrhage. J Clin Neurosci. 2014;21:954–6.
25. Nunnari D, Bramanti P, Marino S. Cognitive reserve in stroke and traumatic brain injury patients. Neurol Sci. 2014;35:1513–8.
26. Nortje J, Menon DK. Traumatic brain injury: physiology, mechanisms, and outcome. Curr Opin Neurol. 2004;17:711–8.
27. Guidetti S, Ytterberg C, Ekstam L, Johansson U, Eriksson G. Changes in the impact of stroke between 3 and 12 months post-stroke, assessed with the stroke impact scale. J Rehabil Med. 2014;46:963–8.
28. Banks JL, Marotta CA. Outcomes validity and reliability of the modified Rankin scale: implications for stroke clinical trials - a literature review and synthesis. Stroke. 2007;38:1091–6.
29. Soberg HL, Roe C, Anke A, Arango-Lasprilla JC, Skandsen T, Sveen U, et al. Health-related quality of life 12 months after severe traumatic brain injury: a prospective nationwide cohort study. J Rehabil Med. 2013;45:785–91.
30. Soberg HL, Roe C, Brunborg C, von Steinbüchel N, Andelic N. The Norwegian version of the QOLIBRI–a study of metric properties based on a 12 month follow-up of persons with traumatic brain injury. Health Qual Life Outcomes. 2017;15:14.
31. Zigmond AS, Snaith RP. The hospital anxiety and depression scale (HADS). Acta Psychiatr Scand. 1983;67:361–70.

Can the health related quality of life measure QOLIBRI- overall scale (OS) be of use after stroke? A validation...

125

32. Bjelland I, Dahl AA, Haug TT, Neckelmann D. The validity of the hospital anxiety and depression scale. J Psychosom Res. 2002;52:69–77.

33. Oyane NMF, Bjelland I, Pallesen S, Holsten F, Bjorvatn B. Seasonality is associated with anxiety and depression: the Hordaland health study. J Affect Disord. 2008;105:147–55.

34. Pallant JF, Tennant A. An introduction to the Rasch measurement model: an example using the hospital anxiety and depression scale (HADS). Br J Clin Psychol. 2007;46(Pt 1):1–18.

35. Sagen U, Vik TG, Moum T, Mørland T, Finset A, Dammen T. Screening for anxiety and depression after stroke: comparison of the hospital anxiety and depression scale and the Montgomery and Åsberg depression rating scale. J Psychosom Res. 2009;67:325–32.

36. Rabin R, De Charro F. EQ-5D: a measure of health status from the EuroQol group. Ann Med. 2001;33:337–43.

37. van Reenen M, Janssen B. EQ-5D-5L User Guide - Basic information on how to use the EQ-5D-5L instrument. Version 21. 2015.

38. Whynes DK. Correspondence between EQ-5D health state classifications and EQ VAS scores. Health Qual Life Outcomes. 2008;6:94.

39. Beaton DE, Bombardier C, Guillemin F, Ferraz MB. Guidelines for the process of cross-cultural adaptation of self-report measures. Spine. 2000;25:3186–91.

40. Pedersen SG, Heiberg GA, Nielsen JF, Friborg O, Stabel HH, Anke A, et al. Validity, reliability and Norwegian adaptation of the stroke-specific quality of life (SS-QOL) scale. SAGE Open Med. 2018;6:2050312117752031. https://doi.org/10.1177/2050312117752031.

41. Mokkink LB, Terwee CB, Patrick DL, Alonso J, Stratford PW, Knol DL, et al. The COSMIN checklist for assessing the methodological quality of studies on measurement properties of health status measurement instruments: an international Delphi study. Qual Life Res. 2010;19:539–49.

42. von Steinbüchel N, Wilson L, Gibbons H, Hawthorne G, Höfer S, Schmidt S, et al. Quality of life after brain injury (QOLIBRI): scale development and metric properties. J Neurotrauma. 2010;27:1167–85.

43. Muthén L, Muthén B. Mplus user's guide. 6th ed; 2012.

44. Terwee CB, Mokkink LB, Knol DL, Ostelo RWJG, Bouter LM, De Vet HCW. Rating the methodological quality in systematic reviews of studies on measurement properties: a scoring system for the COSMIN checklist. Qual Life Res. 2012;21:651–7.

45. West SG, Taylor AB, Wu W. Model fit and model selection in structural equation modeling. In: Handbook of structural equation modeling. New York: Guilford Press; 2012. p. 209–31.

46. Field A. Andy field - discovering statistics using SPSS. 2005.

47. Field AP. Intraclass correlation. Encycl Stat Behav Sci. 2005;2:948–54.

48. Sun J-H, Tan L, Yu J-T. Post-stroke cognitive impairment: epidemiology, mechanisms and management. Ann Transl Med. 2014;2:80.

49. Muehlan H, Wilson L, von Steinbüchel N, von Steinbüchel N. A Rasch Analysis of the QOLIBRI Six-Item Overall Scale. Assessment. 2016;23:124–30.

50. Donnellan C, Hickey A, Hevey D, O'Neill D. Effect of mood symptoms on recovery one year after stroke. Int J Geriatr Psychiatry. 2010;25:1288–95.

51. Loo R. A caveat on using single-item versus multiple-item scales. J Manag Psychol. 2002;17:68–75.

52. Gardner DG, Cummings LL, Dunham RB, Pierce JL. Single-item versus multiple-item measurement scales: an empirical comparison. Educ Psychol Meas. 1998;58:898–915.

53. Hoeppner BB, Kelly JF, Urbanoski KA, Slaymaker V. Comparative utility of a single-item versus multiple-item measure of self-efficacy in predicting relapse among young adults. J Subst Abus Treat. 2011;41:305–12.

54. de Boer AGEM, van Lanschot JJB, Stalmeier PFM, van Sandick JW, Hulscher JBF, de Haes JCJM, et al. Is a single-item visual analogue scale as valid, reliable and responsive as multi-item scales in measuring quality of life? Qual Life Res. 2004;13:311–20.

55. Dunning K, Mulder M, Nijland R. Stroke impact scale. J Physiother. 2011;62:117.

56. Nicholl J, LaFrance WC. Neuropsychiatric sequelae of traumatic brain injury. Semin Neurol. 2009;29:247–55.

57. Siponkoski ST, Wilson L, Von SN, Sarajuuri J, Koskinen S. Quality of life after traumatic brain injury: finnish experience of the qolibri in residential rehabilitation. J Rehabil Med. 2013;45:835–42.

15

Accuracy of seizure semiology obtained from first-time seizure witnesses

Taim A. Muayqil[1][*] , Mohammed H. Alanazy[1], Hassan M. Almalak[2], Hussain Khaled Alsalman[2], Faroq Walid Abdulfattah[2], Abdullah Ibrahim Aldraihem[2], Fawaz Al-hussain[1] and Bandar N. Aljafen[1]

Abstract

Background: Little is known of how accurately a first-time seizure witness can provide reliable details of a semiology. Our goal was to determine how accurately first-time seizure witnesses could identify key elements of an epileptic event that would aid the clinician in diagnosing a seizure.

Methods: A total of 172 participants over 17 years of age, with a mean (sd) of 33.12 (13.2) years and 49.4% female, composed of two groups of community dwelling volunteers, were shown two different seizure videos; one with a focal seizure that generalized (GSV), and the other with a partial seizure that did not generalize (PSV). Participants were first asked about what they thought was the event that had occurred. They then went through a history-taking scenario by an assessor using a battery of pre-determined questions about involvement of major regions: the head, eyes, mouth, upper limbs, lower limbs, or change in consciousness. Further details were then sought about direction of movement in the eyes, upper and lower limbs, the side of limb movements and the type of movements in the upper and lower limbs. Analysis was with descriptive statistics and logistic regression.

Results: One hundred twenty-two (71.4%) identified the events as seizure or epilepsy. The accuracy of identifying major areas of involvement ranged from 60 to 89.5%. Horizontal head movements were significantly more recognized in the PSV, while involvement of the eyes, lateralization of arm movement, type of left arm movement, leg involvement, and lateralization of leg movement were significantly more recognized in the GSV. Those shown the GSV were more likely to recognize the event as "seizure" or "epilepsy" than those shown the PSV; 78 (84.8%) vs 44 (55.7%), (OR 0.22, $p < 0.0001$). Younger age was also associated with correct recognition (OR 0.96, P 0.049). False positive responses ranged from 2.5 to 32.5%.

Conclusion: First-time witnesses can identify important elements more than by chance alone, and are more likely to associate generalized semiologies with seizures or epilepsy than partial semiologies. However, clinicians still need to navigate the witness's account carefully for additional information since routine questioning could result in a misleading false positive answer.

Keywords: Seizure semiology, History, Seizure witness

Backgound

The occurrence of a seizure is a relatively common event that can develop in about 10% of the population [1]. The diagnosis of a seizure or epilepsy relies heavily on the description of the event by a witness. The seizure description of the clinically observed behavioral motor, sensory or psychiatric signs that occur in a pattern or sequence is known as the semiology, understanding the semiology is useful in diagnosis and localization [2–4]. The task of reporting the details of a semiology usually falls on the shoulders of a bewildered bystander, and when it involves a first-time seizure victim, the witness is likely a first-timer as well. Obtaining an appropriate account of events from a witness is a crucial component of the patient assessment, particularly since most seizures do not last long enough to be identified by first responders, and patients are also unable to provide helpful information because they present to the emergency in a post-ictal and confused

* Correspondence: tmuayqil@gmail.com
[1]Division of Neurology, College of Medicine, King Saud University, PO Box 7805 (38), Riyadh 11472, Saudi Arabia
Full list of author information is available at the end of the article

state with no memory of the event [1]. Although assessment tools like routine electroencephalogram or brain imaging can help, they are not always diagnostic [1, 5]. Also, while inquiring about seizure risk factors or looking for clinical signs that suggest a seizure has occurred are important [1, 4], knowing the semiology details provides additional localizing and diagnostic value that can aid in management. For example, recognizing a primary generalized semiology in a young female would raise the suspicion for juvenile myoclonic epilepsy, which is known to respond to certain drugs and worsen with others [1].

The physician carries the responsibility of taking the appropriate history in order to extract useful information. Non-specialists and trainees may be more concrete in their history taking technique, which creates a challenge in obtaining diagnostic information given the wide variability in how witnesses report their experiences. An accurate interpretation of the history is the most important step in patient evaluation [6], and it takes years of experience for a physician to acquire the skills and knowledge to differentiate relevant information from not. Therefore, our goal with this study was to assess the accuracy of the accounts of first time witnesses of seizures when history is obtained through a routine battery of questions that probe common seizure semiology components. First, we identify if a first time seizure witness could recognize the occurrence of an epileptic event; second, we examine what seizure semiology components are recognized and if there will be a difference in responses according to seizure type, after viewing two different seizure semiology videos, one generalized and the other partial.

Methods

Participants

In this experiment, we recruited willing volunteers from the community over 17 years of age by convenience sampling. Recruitment was done between June and August 2017, in Riyadh, Saudi Arabia. Those with a personal or family history of epilepsy or workers of any kind in the healthcare field were excluded from the study. To screen for this, and preserve participant unawareness of what is about to be watched, our question about a personal or family history of epilepsy was embedded within a long list of other neurological conditions. Information was also gathered regarding age, education level, marital status, and place of residence.

Materials

Two different seizure videos obtained from the reference "Manual of Neurological Signs" [7] were used to assess participant responses. Two neurologists and an epileptologist chose the videos based on the clarity of the features to be assessed in the study. The first video showed a generalized tonic-clonic convulsion that had a focal onset. The patient was awake in her bed initially, and then developed a brief stare. This was followed by head deviation upward and to the right, with widely opened eyes that deviated in the same direction. The mouth was open with incoherent vocalization; this was then followed by tonic posturing of upper and lower limbs bilaterally and a subsequent clonic phase. The patient was not awake at the end of the video and did not interact with anyone surrounding her. The whole event lasted 65 s. For brevity, this video was referred to as the generalized seizure video (GSV). The second video showed a different patient who, while asleep, began to develop left sided mouth clonic twitching, followed by head clonic movements to the left and leftward eye deviation. This was then followed by the development of clonic movements of the left arm and leg. The patient did not exhibit any ability to communicate or interact with her surrounding and was not awake at the end. The entire event lasted 45 s. This second video was referred to as the partial seizure video (PSV).

Procedure

Participants were pseudo-randomized at the time of recruitment to balance gender distribution into two groups. Each group was shown one of the two videos and all were asked the same battery of questions. These questions were designed in Arabic by three neurologists (TAM, MHA, and BNJ) and pilot tested on seven individuals matching the target population to check the comprehensibility of the questionnaire and eliminate ambiguous questions. The assessments occurred within the confines of the academic institute and videos were viewed only once per participant on a laptop monitor.

The interviewer first asked an open question at the end of each video on what the viewer thought the event that happened to the patient was. Those that referred to it as epilepsy or seizure were considered correct. Participants were then asked a series of questions about the semiology, these questions were designed without reference to the two videos and not modified according to seizure type. This ensured that both groups were exposed to the same battery of questions in order to mimic all the inquiring that occurs during an actual history-taking scenario. Identification of a feature that was independently identified by all three neurologists or present in the reference's seizure description was considered a correct response. Patients were asked "yes/no" questions on whether there was involvement of the head, eyes, mouth, upper limbs, lower limbs, consciousness, or the presence of vocalization. During this phase of questioning, answers were considered correct if they answered "yes" to any of the above regions that had exhibited epileptic involvement of any kind without going into the specifics of the involvement such as direction or type of abnormal movement. For consciousness, the answer was correct if it was "yes" to *Was there loss of consciousness?"* The answer to the question about vocalization was correct if it was identified as "present" in the GSV and identified as "absent" in the PSV. Participants were also asked if they noticed a focal region where the seizure started (which happened in both videos) or not.

Participants were than asked about details of movements: direction of movement in the main body parts queried (head, eyes, upper and lower limbs), the lateralization of limb movements (right, left or both sides), and the type of movement in the upper and lower limbs (tonic, clonic or both). With regard to questions on the latter, we considered a correct response in the GSV when a participant indicated either tonic or clonic activity. At the end, we inquired about an estimation of how long the event lasted. All participants had to sign consent before starting the interview, and an ethical approval was obtained from the internal review board at the college of medicine at King Saud University.

Analysis

Descriptive statistics were used for assessing demographic features and percentage of individuals with correct responses to any of the queried features. Univariate and multivariate logistic regression analysis was done; identification of the event as a seizure was the dependent variable and the demographic variables of age, sex, marital status and type of seizure shown represented the independent variables. The significance of adding the video type viewed by participants to a model containing only the demographic variables was also tested. Proportions of false positive responses to queries about semiology details were also tabulated. STATA statistical software was used.

Results

Table 1 shows the demographic characteristics and the proportions of correct responses to whether the event was a seizure, and to which body part exhibited involvement for each of the six main shared semiology features in both videos. Only two individuals resided in a rural area. Three individuals requested the videos be stopped before completion at 34 and 36 s for the PSV, and at 75 s for the GSV; their responses were included in the analysis, as the full semiology had developed by the time a stop was requested. Regarding the responses to each video, there was a slight difference in age, with the PSV group being older by about 6 years. The differences in gender, marital status and mean years of education were not significant (Table 2).

Table 2 demonstrates the differences in correct responses to the general questions and to specific involvement of different body regions and types of movements. Generally, the correct identification of semiology components was less in the PSV group, with the exception of head movement along the horizontal axis being significantly more identified in the

Table 1 Demographic distribution and identification of shared seizure features between the two videos

	N = 172
Female	85 (49.42%)
Age, years (SD)	33.12 (13.2)
Years of Education, years (SD)	13.3 (3.9)
Married, yes	93 (54.7%)

Number and percentage of subjects who correctly identified the following features:

• The event was a seizure	122 (71.4%)
• Involvement of head/neck[a]	154 (89.5%)
• Involvement of eyes[a]	108 (63.2%)
• Involvement of mouth[a]	143 (83.1%)
• Involvement of upper limb(s)[a]	142 (83%)
• Involvement of lower limb(s)[a]	118 (68.6%)
• There was loss of consciousness[a]	102 (60%)
• Presence or absence of vocalization[b]	87 (51.2%)
• Starting region of the seizure	143 (86.6%)

[a]Represents a shared feature between both videos. [b] Considered correct if identified vocalization in GSV and identified no vocalization in PSV

PSV. In the GSV, participants were more likely to identify involvement of the eyes, direction of eye movement, lateralization of arm movement, type of movement in the left arm, involvement in a leg, and lateralization of leg movement. Vocalizations were difficult to detect by observers in the GSV 27 (29.7%). More participants identified tonic than clonic movements. In the right upper limb, tonic and clonic movements were identified by 44 (47.8%) and 32 (34.8%), respectively. In the left upper limb, tonic and clonic movements were identified by 44 (47.8%) and 27 (29.4%), respectively. In the right lower limb, tonic and clinic movements were identified by 40 (43.5%) and 32 (34.8%), respectively. In the left lower limb, tonic and clonic movements were identified by 35 (38%) and 25 (27.2%), respectively.

Logistic regression analysis is demonstrated in Table 3. Participants were significantly more likely to identify the event as a seizure or epilepsy depending on the type of seizure viewed, with the GSV more likely to be called a seizure or epileptic event ($p < 0.0001$). Younger individuals were also more likely to identify the event correctly, and this finding just barely reached statistical significance. A hierarchal approach to the logistic regression showed that adding the type of seizure shown improved the prediction of the model containing the demographic variables with likelihood ratio (χ^2) 15.4 and p value of 0.0001.

Finally, we looked at the responses of participants who viewed the PSV to queries about events that did not occur (Table 4). The most frequent false positive response was of seizure involvement on the contralateral

Table 2 Correct responses to each video

	GSV N = 92	PSV N = 80	p Value
Female	42 (45.7%)	43 (53.8%)	0.36
Age	30.1 (10.9)	36.6 (14.6)	0.002
Years of Education	12.9 (3.7)	13.6 (4.2)	0.25
Married	46 (50.5)	47 (59.5)	0.28
Correctly identified:			
• The event as a seizure	78 (84.78%)	44 (55.7%)	< 0.0001
• Involvement of head	79 (89.9%)	75 (93.8%)	0.13
• Vertical head movement	17 (18.5%)	–	–
• Horizontal head movement	29 (31.5%)	55 (68.8%)	< 0.0001
• Involvement of eyes	68 (73.9%)	40 (50%)	0.002
• Direction of eye movement	64 (69.6%)	36 (45%)	0.002
• Involvement of the mouth	75 (81.5%)	68 (85%)	0.68
• Involvement in an arm (s)	78 (84.8%)	64 (80%)	0.43
• Lateralization of arm movement	72 (78.3%)	35 (43.8%)	< 0.0001
• Type of movement (right arm)	76 (82.6%)	–	–
• Type of movement (left arm)	71 (77.2%)	42 (52.5%)	0.001
• Involvement in a leg (s)	76 (82.6%)	42 (52%)	< 0.0001
• Lateralization of leg movement	72 (78.3%)	20 (25%)	< 0.0001
• Type of movements (right leg)	72 (78.3%)	–	–
• Type of movements (left leg)	60 (65.2%)	23 (28.8%)	0.06
• Loss of consciousness	60 (65.9%)	42(53.2%)	0.06
• Vocalizations	27 (29.7%)	–	
• A focal start for the event	72 (78.3%)	71 (88.8%)	0.16
• Duration of seizure	Mean (SD) 97.4 (97.5), Median 60 (Seconds)	Mean (SD) 52.9 (49.1), Median 37.5 (Seconds)	

upper and lower limbs, followed by discriminating tonic from clonic activity.

Discussion

Little attention has been given to the accuracy of reports from first time seizure witnesses thus far. In this study, we have demonstrated that seizure witnesses are able to identify key elements that aid the clinician in considering a seizure diagnosis in the majority of encounters.

These witnesses are also likely to call these events "seizures" or "epilepsy". While we found that first-time witnesses can also recognize the involvement of different body regions, the exact detail of this involvement appears to be more difficult to accurately report. Participants were clearly less assertive about calling the event a seizure when they were shown the PSV, and their detection of its semiology components was also less frequent. These findings suggest that in the mind of the average individual, seizures

Table 3 Logistic regression. The odds of describing the event as a seizure or epilepsy in relation to demographic variables and the seizure video shown

	Univariate		Multivariate: LR (χ^2) 26.4, p = 0.0001	
	OR (95% CI)	p value	OR (95% CI)	p value
Age	0.97 (0.941–0.992)	0.01*	0.96 (0.93–0.9998)	0.049*
Years of education	1.02 (0.938–1.109)	0.65	0.99 (0.896–1.093)	0.83
Male gender	1.25 (0.642–2.423)	0.514	1.21 (0.568–2.597)	0.62
Married	0.79 (0.402–1.545)	0.49	1.95 (0.699–5.433)	0.2
PS Video	0.23 (0.11–0.464)	< 0.0001*	0.22 (0.098–0.481)	< 0.0001*

* Statistically significant result

Table 4 False positive answers for the different movements which did not occur in the PSV

Movement	N = 80
Head movement along vertical axis	7 (8.5%)
Vocalization	2 (2.5%)
Tonic/clonic movements in the right upper limb	26 (32.5%)
Tonic/clonic movements in the right lower limb	18 (22.5%)
Tonic activity left upper limb	15 (18.8%)
Tonic activity left lower limb	14 (17.5)

are a generalized event. We also found that there was a high identification rate of limb and head movements in general, this is corroborated by similar findings obtained in a study that researched experienced seizure witnesses which included relatives, friends or care-givers [8].

Interestingly, the direction of eye movement was more frequently identified in the GSV than the PSV. This is probably because the GSV patient was lying more upright, and the eyes moved both upward and to the side, any of which were considered a correct response, thus increasing the probability of obtaining a correct answer. In the PSV, the patient was on her back during the whole event and had prominent left head deviation and left facial twitching that may have distracted the viewer from seeing the eyes. This is also supported by the fact that, in the same video, eye involvement was recognized less frequently than head and mouth involvement (Table 2.). Similarly, only a third of our first-time seizure witnesses were able to identify the vocalization in the GSV. Although correct identification of vocalization and direction of eye movements have been previously described [3], this too was a finding in experienced witnesses. The videos in our study did not focus on the eyes enough to allow accurate reporting from a novice. We intentionally kept the questioning restricted to gross movements to look for the essential descriptions that would enable physicians to recognize that a seizure had occurred, and because observations of more subtle features like automatisms, lip movements or staring episodes are more difficult to identify [8, 9]. Previous evaluations of experienced seizure witnesses have also showed that different semiologies can be associated with different levels of reporting accuracy [3].

While level of education was previously found to be an important factor in providing semiology details in experienced witnesses [8], it was not significant in our study of first-time witnesses. Younger age being associated with higher odds of calling an event a seizure is probably the result of increasing media and societal awareness that has lead to higher health literacy in younger generations, consistent with the fact that medical knowledge is associated with more accurate seizure descriptions [10]. The

influence of gender was not significant in our study, which is consistent with a previous study that compared descriptions of syncopal with epileptic events and found no influence from gender [11]. Nonetheless, the majority of witnesses in our study recognized involvement of multiple body regions, and their observations were more likely to be correct in a generalized seizure.

There appears to be a small tendency by some participants to falsely describe movements that could lead an assessor to believe it was a generalized event. In fact, false positive responses occurred previously among nine out of 20 participants in a study that looked at the seizure descriptions from volunteers with varying medical backgrounds, [12]. Another study that looked at the accounts of experienced witnesses suggests that inaccuracies are more likely to occur in reporting convulsive than non-convulsive events [3] and, similar to our study, it was highest when addressing limb movements. It seems that while witnesses will recognize limb movements frequently, there is a small trade-off that a small proportion will report inaccurate information. While experienced observers have been found to recall the presence or absence of certain semiology components, they too have mistaken the side of involvement or even believed the involvement to be bilateral [8].

Insistent questioning or restricting the witness to provide a "yes" or "no" response could result in misleading information or even in increasing confidence in the false answer if perpetuated [13–15]. However, witnesses usually do not spontaneously offer all the required information [12], and obtaining a useful account relies on the clinician's skills; going through a battery of routine questions may not be applicable in all situations [16].

In this study, participants described the findings in two videos in a controlled and reassuring environment where no safety concerns are required for the victim. A real-world seizure however is a very dramatic event to a first-time witness; the emotional impact will affect observation details. While accuracy and consistency for recall of witnessed events is addressed frequently in events of a legal nature, witnessed medical conditions and the impact it has on clinical history taking has not been similarly studied. Recollection of emotional events and their sequence has been found to be variable, incomplete, and dependent on the personal consequences of the witness [17, 18]. This is also an important consideration when assessing the perception of lapsed time, while the mean estimated time reported here was higher than the actual, it is probably less than the estimated time provided by witnesses of an actual event.

One advantage to our study design is that we used a battery of standard questions usually used during witness interviews to mimic the actual history taking process, where the physician has to ask questions about events that both did and did not occur, especially since witnesses do not spontaneously provide all the required information without prompting [12]. Some limitations include that participants had to determine loss of consciousness from watching the videos; the segments did not contain any part that specifically assessed consciousness. The assessment of eye direction might have been difficult to determine because they were not the main focus of the camera angles. Reevaluating the ability of the participants to recount the semiologies after a time period from 30 min to 1 hour might offer a more precise mimicry of recounting in clinical settings [11]. The responses we obtained were not confounded by emotional stressors, it is yet to be seen if real world accuracy would be higher or lower than that found here. If anything, this information provides us with the reporting potential of first time witnesses. Since the goal of the study was to focus on what semiology elements would be recalled after witnessing a seizure, further research investigating the reports of first time witnesses to non-epileptic events or more difficult semiology types such as automatisms, could supplement the findings in this study.

Conclusion

In conclusion, the ability to identify major seizure semiology elements by inexperienced witnesses is more than chance alone, based on these results, there is a good chance of obtaining an informative description from first time witnesses that would help diagnose a seizure or even aid in lateralization. However, false positive information may be inadvertently given, especially when inquiring about limb movements, and the clinician still needs to use his or her history taking skills in retrieving the additional information that would support the diagnosis or aid with lateralization.

Abbreviations
GSV: Generalized Seizure Video; PSV: Partial Seizure Video

Acknowledgements
To the College of medicine research center, Deanship of scientific research, King Saud University, Riyadh, Saudi Arabia for supporting this research; In the form of general consulting and feedback.

Authors' contributions
TAM was involved in study conception and design, analysis of results, data interpretation, supervision of data acquisition, and writing the manuscript. MHA, FAH & BNJ were involved in conception, supervision and revision of manuscript. HMM, HKS, FWA & AID were involved in assessment, data management, and drafting of manuscript. All authors read and approved the final manuscript'

Competing interests
The authors declare that they have no competing interests.

Author details
[1]Division of Neurology, College of Medicine, King Saud University, PO Box 7805 (38), Riyadh 11472, Saudi Arabia. [2]College of Medicine, King Saud University, PO Box 7805 (38), Riyadh 11472, Saudi Arabia.

References
1. Gavvala JR, Schuele SU. New-onset seizure in adults and adolescents: a review. JAMA. 2016;316:2657–68.
2. Tufenkjian K, Luders HO. Seizure semiology: its value and limitations in localizing the epileptogenic zone. J Clin Neurol. 2012;8:243–50.
3. Rugg-Gunn FJ, Harrison NA, Duncan JS. Evaluation of the accuracy of seizure descriptions by the relatives of patients with epilepsy. Epilepsy Res. 2001;43:193–9.
4. Nowacki TA, Jirsch JD. Evaluation of the first seizure patient: key points in the history and physical examination. Seizure. 2017;49:54–63.
5. Beghi E. Management of a first seizure. General conclusions and recommendations. Epilepsia. 2008;49(Suppl 1):58–61.
6. Kunze A, Reuber M. The first seizure as an indicator of epilepsy. Curr Opin Neurol. 2018;31:156–61.
7. Morris JG, Grattan-Smith PJ (2015) Manual of Neurological Signs. Oxford University Press; https://doi.org/10.1093/med/9780199945795.001.0001.
8. Heo JH, Kim DW, Lee SY, Cho J, Lee SK, Nam H. Reliability of semiology description. Neurologist. 2008;14:7–11.
9. Benbir G, Demiray DY, Delil S, Yeni N. Interobserver variability of seizure semiology between two neurologist and caregivers. Seizure. 2013;22:548–52.
10. Ristic AJ, Draskovic M, Bukumiric Z, Sokic D. Reliability of the witness descriptions of epileptic seizures and psychogenic non-epileptic attacks: a comparative analysis. Neurol Res. 2015;37:560–2.
11. Thijs RD, Wagenaar WA, Middelkoop HA, Wieling W, van Dijk JG. Transient loss of consciousness through the eyes of a witness. Neurology. 2008;71: 1713–8.
12. Mannan JB, Wieshmann UC. How accurate are witness descriptions of epileptic seizures? Seizure. 2003;12:444–7.
13. Patihis L, Frenda SJ, LePort AK, Petersen N, Nichols RM, Stark CE, McGaugh JL, Loftus EF. False memories in highly superior autobiographical memory individuals. Proc Natl Acad Sci U S A. 2013;110:20947–52.
14. Pezdek K, Sperry K, Owens SM. Interviewing witnesses: the effect of forced confabulation on event memory. Law Hum Behav. 2007;31:463–78.
15. Wells G, Olson E. Eyewitness testimony. Annu Rev Psychol. 2003;54:277–95.
16. Haidet P, Paterniti DA. "Building" a history rather than "taking" one: a perspective on information sharing during the medical interview. Arch Intern Med. 2003;163: 1134–40.
17. Brown R, Kulik J. Flashbulb memories. Cognition. 1977;5:73–99.
18. Smeets T, Candel I, Merckelbach H. Accuracy, completeness, and consistency of emotional memories. Am J Psychol. 2004;117:595–609.

16

Feasibility trial of an early therapy in perinatal stroke (eTIPS)

Anna Purna Basu[1,2]* (iD), Janice Pearse[3], Rose Watson[4], Pat Dulson[5], Jessica Baggaley[1], Blythe Wright[6], Denise Howel[4], Luke Vale[4], Dipayan Mitra[7], Nick Embleton[5] and Tim Rapley[8]

Abstract

Background: Perinatal stroke (PS) affects up to 1/2300 infants and frequently leads to unilateral cerebral palsy (UCP). Preterm-born infants affected by unilateral haemorrhagic parenchymal infarction (HPI) are also at risk of UCP. To date no standardised early therapy approach exists, yet early intervention could be highly effective, by positively influencing processes of activity-dependent plasticity within the developing nervous system including the corticospinal tract. Our aim was to test feasibility and acceptability of an "early Therapy In Perinatal Stroke" (eTIPS) intervention, aiming ultimately to improve motor outcome.

Methods: Design: Feasibility trial, North-East England, August 2015–September 2017. Participants were infants with PS or HPI, their carers and therapists. The intervention consisted of a parent-delivered lateralised therapy approach starting from term equivalent age and continuing until 6 months corrected age. The outcome measures were feasibility (recruitment and retention rates) and acceptability of the intervention (parental questionnaires including the Warwick-Edinburgh Mental Wellbeing Scale (WEBWMS), qualitative observations and in-depth interviews with parents and therapists). We also reviewed clinical imaging data and undertook assessments of motor function, including the Hand Assessment for Infants (HAI). Assessments were also piloted in typically developing (TD) infants, to provide further information on their ease of use and acceptability.

Results: Over a period of 18 months we screened 20 infants referred as PS/HPI: 14 met the inclusion criteria and 13 took part. At 6 months, 11 (85%) of those enrolled had completed the final assessment. Parents valued the intervention and found it acceptable and workable. There were no adverse events related to the intervention. We recruited 14 TD infants, one of whom died prior to undertaking any assessments and one of whom was subsequently found to have a condition affecting neurodevelopmental progress: thus, data for 12 TD infants was analysed to 6 months. The HAI was well tolerated by infants and highly valued by parents. Completion rates for the WEBWMS were high and did not suggest any adverse effect of engagement in eTIPS on parental mental wellbeing.

Conclusion: The eTIPS intervention was feasible to deliver and acceptable to families. We plan to investigate efficacy in a multicentre randomised controlled trial.

Trial registration: ISRCTN12547427 (registration request submitted 28/05/2015; retrospectively registered, 30/09/2015).

Keywords: Early intervention, Therapy, Hand function, Infant, Perinatal stroke, Haemorrhagic parenchymal infarction, Parent-delivered therapy, Feasibility trial

* Correspondence: Anna.basu@ncl.ac.uk
[1]Institute of Neuroscience, Newcastle University, Newcastle upon Tyne NE1 7RU, UK
[2]Department of Paediatric Neurology, Newcastle upon Tyne Hospitals NHS Foundation Trust, Newcastle upon Tyne NE7 7DN, UK
Full list of author information is available at the end of the article

Background

Perinatal stroke (PS) is due to an interrupted blood supply to part of the brain before birth or in the first 28 days of life [1]. Perinatal arterial ischaemic stroke affects around 1/2300 term [1, 2] and 7/1000 preterm deliveries [1, 3]. Some infants present with seizures and encephalopathy, whilst others (around 40%) appear asymptomatic in the neonatal period though signs of unilateral cerebral palsy (UCP) emerge over time. Furthermore, not all infants who sustain a perinatal stroke will have an abnormal motor outcome, though up to 60% do have neurological deficits [4]: the risk of developing UCP can be assessed through cranial imaging [5]. Perinatal stroke remains one of the leading causes of UCP, with associated lifelong morbidity affecting function in activities of daily living [6].

Preterm infants with unilateral haemorrhagic parenchymal infarcts (HPI) after grade IV intraventricular haemorrhage (IVH) are also at high risk of developing UCP. In a study from 2006, HPI was observed in 1% of all premature infants with a birthweight of under 2500 g, occurring more frequently in infants with lower birthweight and lower gestational age [7]. 74% of cases of HPI are unilateral [8, 9]. The pathophysiology of HPI differs from that of arterial ischaemic stroke – it is a form of venous infarction due to impaired drainage from veins in the periventricular white matter because of pressure from the intraventricular haemorrhage [10]. In a study by Maitre et al., [9] 67% of patients with unilateral HPI developed cerebral palsy, with UCP being the commonest form. Imaging (including cranial ultrasound) provides some guidance regarding the risk of developing UCP [11], though tractography within the first 4 weeks of life and MRI at term equivalent age may be more accurate [12].

Whilst the pattern of neuronal damage and the nature and scope for reorganisation differ between these two forms of injury [13], both frequently lead to UCP, and for both conditions, options for primary prevention are limited [14, 15]. For symptomatic cases, stem cell therapy and neuroprotection are under investigation as part of acute management [16], but there remains no established approach except symptomatic management. Therapy intervention programmes aiming to improve hand function exist for infants and children with established UCP [17], with evidence of benefit from high-dose constraint-induced movement therapy and bimanual therapy [18]. However, there has been little focus on early therapy intervention in the period between onset of the brain insult and emergence of UCP. This is despite extensive evidence from studies demonstrating ongoing activity-dependent corticospinal tract plasticity [19, 20] which could be modulated during this early time window with the potential for a greater influence on motor outcomes than with later interventions [16]. We have detailed elsewhere the rationale for an early lateralised therapy approach [21].

Prior to undertaking this feasibility trial, we confirmed the lack of a recognised evidence-based alternative early therapy approach to perinatal stroke through a national (UK-based) survey of current practice [22]. Interventions such as early modified constraint-induced movement therapy ("Baby CIMT"), and early intensive bimanual task-specific training, are under investigation outside the UK but do not have definitive evidence of effectiveness to date [23, 24]. In conjunction with key stakeholders, we developed a novel parent-delivered pervasive therapy approach aiming to promote activity of the potentially affected side of the body from as soon as possible after diagnosis. Details of the intervention and the development process have already been published [21]. The aims of this trial were to assess feasibility of the intervention and to pilot the outcome assessments prior to proceeding to a definitive randomised controlled trial.

Objectives

Our primary objectives were:

1) To establish feasibility of delivery and the acceptability of an early parent-delivered home-based therapy intervention in PS/HPI and identify and address potential barriers to implementation.
2) To obtain information on rates of eligibility, consent, participation and retention.
3) To pilot assessments and outcome measures for use in a future trial.

Methods

Trial design

We conducted a feasibility trial of the eTIPS intervention in infants with PS/HPI. All infants with PS/HPI received the intervention, to maximise our experience with delivery at the feasibility stage. We recruited an equal number of typically developing (TD) infants to undertake the assessments, but TD infants did not undertake the eTIPS intervention: the inclusion of TD infants gave us additional information on the ease of use and acceptability of the assessments.

Eligibility criteria for participants

Eligible infants were recruited from four hospitals with level three neonatal units; a further four other hospitals were added as participant identification centres to avoid missing potentially eligible infants. Inclusion criteria were: a) term or preterm infants who sustained a predominantly unilateral stroke (arterial ischaemic, haemorrhagic or haemorrhagic periventricular venous infarction) demonstrated on cranial imaging and identified within the first 3 months of life, b) fully informed parental consent and c) ability and willingness of the parent/carer to adhere to the protocol. Participants were not eligible if they had a) additional significant medical diagnoses which would render the therapy inappropriate or outcomes uninterpretable in relation to the therapy, e.g. known progressive or neurodegenerative disorder or severe visual impairment, b) evidence of significant bilateral intracerebral motor pathology, c) strokes shown radiologically to affect only occipital, prefrontal or temporal areas of the brain (which would not be expected to produce adverse motor outcomes), or d) ongoing involvement in another research study where this was likely to interfere with the interpretation of either study. Initially we had a further exclusion criterion of extreme prematurity (less than 26 weeks gestation), but after discussions with neonatologists in the first 3 months of the study we decided that cases should be considered regardless of gestation, to avoid missing otherwise eligible recruits, and because the incidence of HPI is higher in infants with lower gestational age. Thirteen TD infants (including preterm infants with gestational ages matching those of the infants with HPI) were also recruited to obtain comparative data for exploratory assessments of limb movements, and to pilot the infant massage materials we developed as a potential attentional control, as described below. All TD infants were recruited from the Newcastle site: preterm TD infants were recruited from the neonatal unit through the same procedures as for the infants with PS/HPI, whilst term infants were recruited through postnatal wards and through provision of flyers approved by the ethics committee.

Participant identification and consent procedure

Between August 2015 and January 2017, clinical staff at participating centres and sites identified and approached parents/carers of potential infant participants, providing flyers and information sheets. These materials were developed with the involvement of a parent of a young child with UCP. With parental consent, contact details were forwarded to a member of the eTIPS team, and they were then screened for eligibility to participate in the trial. If eligible, written informed consent was obtained. Parents/carers of infants in the trial were also recruited as participants, so we could capture their experiences regarding the therapy and assessments. We included mothers, fathers and grandparents if actively involved in the infant's care on a regular basis, and allowed more than one such carer to participate per infant. After commencing the trial, we also sought permission to recruit (with parental permission) therapists involved in the clinical care of recruited infants, to capture their views on the approach.

eTIPS intervention

The eTIPS intervention was developed with input from parents of children with UCP and healthcare professionals caring for these children; it is described in our intervention development paper [21]. In summary, it is a parent-delivered, pervasive, lateralised therapy intervention in the first 6 months of life, aiming to improve infant motor outcome. The therapy is incorporated into all day-to-day infant activities (infant holding, feeding, bathing, play) to promote opportunities for active use and stimulation (including the use of massage) of the potentially affected side of the body by adapting the way these activities are undertaken rather than by introducing specific blocks of therapy time into the day. The environment around the infant is also adapted to maximise opportunities to see, reach and grasp for objects on the potentially affected side.

All infants with PS/HPI received the eTIPS intervention in addition to usual National Health Service care. The intervention began when medically stable but not before term-equivalent age, and continued until 6 months of age (or for preterm infants, 6 months corrected age). At the baseline visit, parents were given education and materials covering all aspects of the eTIPS approach, including the rationale for the approach. The materials comprised a pictorial manual tailored to the side of the stroke, a DVD with videos demonstrating the desired behaviours, and password protected access to a website hosting the same materials. The manual included an introductory section ("Why have I been given this manual?") with an overview of the approach. Subsequent sections (e.g. Day to Day Care, and Play) provided examples for parents of how to promote opportunities for, and encourage, active pre-reaching or reaching and grasping on the potentially affected side during everyday activities. Much of this consisted of very straightforward suggestions e.g. presenting suitable toys to the potentially affected side during play sessions. The manual (and parent education) also included some information on the developmental context, and on parent-infant interaction (for example, advice regarding reading and responding to infant cues).

Monthly visits (usually at home, occasionally in hospital depending on circumstances), interim telephone calls (at least monthly) and fortnightly texts from the eTIPS team provided ongoing opportunities to reinforce messages regarding the intervention, troubleshoot and support families including provision of positive feedback and encouragement. During these visits, assessments were also undertaken as described below.

Materials provided to parents of TD infants

Parents of TD infants were also provided with a manual, and videos providing guidance on a baby massage program, accessible through a website with password protected access. The materials were developed as a possible attentional control for use in a future trial. Baby massage has been successfully used in this context in a previous trial [24].

Assessments

Table 1 shows the schedule of assessments for infants with PS/HPI and TD infants. TD infants underwent the same assessments as infants with PS/HPI, except for the Pediatric Stroke Outcome Measure, eTIPS feasibility questionnaire, and questionnaires/interviews with therapists.

Feasibility and acceptability of the eTIPS approach were assessed through qualitative analysis of in-depth interviews undertaken in the last month of the intervention, as well as from researcher observations recorded after undertaking visits. Acceptability and feasibility of the intervention to the families involved were the key requirement for progression to a subsequent randomised trial. Interviews with carers of TD infants focused on feasibility and acceptability of trial procedures, including experiences with baby massage and assessments. We obtained feedback from therapists involved in the clinical care of infants recruited to the eTIPS study, through a questionnaire about their practice and an in-depth interview.

Just after trial commencement we requested approval to include an eTIPS feasibility questionnaire to be completed 1 month after initiating the intervention and at the final visit by parents of infants with PS/HPI. The questionnaire was adapted from feasibility questionnaires used by Ferre et al. [25] and Wallen et al. [26]; its design was informed by Normalisation Process Theory [27]. The questionnaire had two parts. Part A contained 8 questions (answered using a 5-point Likert scale) regarding how easy or difficult the participant found the eTIPS approach. Part B had 3 questions, each answered on a continuous rating scale from 0 to 10, regarding the extent to which the approach became a familiar, normal part of the daily routine.

We also added two short questionnaires for completion by both parents 1 month after entry into the study and at the final visit, which would capture any effects on parental coping and wellbeing. The Parenting Sense of Competence scale (PSOC) and the Warwick-Edinburgh Mental Well-being Scale (WEMWBS) are fully validated and have excellent psychometric properties. The PSOC is a quick (5 min) 16-point questionnaire using a 6 point Likert scale to examine parental confidence and satisfaction with parenting, which has been studied in parents of healthy infants and children throughout the age range 0–18 years and has adequate psychometric properties [28–30]. The WEMWBS scale is validated for the measurement of mental wellbeing [31]. It is short (14 items each on a 1–5 Likert scale), quick to score (under 5 min), and contains statements phrased positively. Participants complete the scale based on their thoughts and feelings over the previous 2 weeks. Whilst there is no cut-off for low levels of mental wellbeing, mean scores in a study in Scotland were 50.7 (95% CI 50.3–51.1) [31].

Hand assessment for infants (HAI)

The HAI [32] is an assessment of the quality of goal-directed unimanual and bimanual actions in infants age 3–12 months with unilateral CP. A validation paper has been published [33] and the assessment is being actively used in current research [24, 34, 35]. It comprises a 10 to 15-min semi-structured play session which is video recorded. The assessment is then formally scored on 17 items each with a three-point rating scale based on the manual abilities of each hand separately (12 items; raw score range 0–24 for each hand) and bimanual hand use (5 items). The final "Both Hands" score is expressed on a scale from 0 to 100 units, with higher scores representing better hand function: it has been validated by a Rasch-model analysis. An asymmetry score is also generated. In our study, the HAI was undertaken at 3, 4, 5 and 6 months.

Table 1 Schedule of assessments

	BASELINE	1 M	2 M	3 M	4 M	5 M	6 M
Review imaging	x						
PSOM	**x**			**x**			**x**
AIMS	x		x		x		x
GMs	x	x	x	x			
HAI				x	x	x	x
Accelerometry (during GMs/HAI)	x	x	x	x	x	x	x
Qualitative observations		x			x	x	
In-depth interviews						x	
PSOC		x					x
WEBWMS		x					x
eTIPS Feasibility Questionnaire		**x**					**x**
Questionnaire for therapists		**x**					
Telephone interview with therapists						**x**	

Those in bold were undertaken for infants with PS/HPI only

Paediatric stroke outcome measure (PSOM)

Clinical assessments at baseline, 3 and 6 m were undertaken with the PSOM [36] - the only disease-specific measure of neurological outcome after paediatric stroke [37]. The PSOM is valid, reliable and completed in around 15 min [36].

General movements assessments (GM)

This is a Gestalt classification of the quality of spontaneous infant movements whilst in a quiet, alert state and supine, scored from a 3–5-min-long video recording. In high-risk infants the test has a high sensitivity and specificity for prediction of cerebral palsy [38]. GM assessments were undertaken monthly until age 4 months.

Alberta infant motor scale (AIMS)

This 58-item test, taking under 5 min to complete, is validated for the assessment of motor performance of infants from birth to 18 months; scores can be compared against the trajectory for typically developing term and preterm infants [39–41]. The assessment was performed at birth, 2, 4 and 6 months.

Accelerometry

Lightweight (7 g) 3-axis wireless accelerometers (WAX9, Axivity, Newcastle upon Tyne, UK) were secured at the wrists and ankles of the infants during the HAI and GM assessments using soft straps, to obtain exploratory data. We established, through examining video footage of assessments with and without accelerometers in situ, that infant limb movements were not qualitatively affected by this procedure. In addition to the formal GM assessments, accelerometry data synchronised to video data of infant movements in supine was collected at each visit up to and including 6 months. Results of the accelerometry analysis will be reported separately.

Piloting of healthcare resource use data collection forms

Data collection forms on healthcare resource use, modelled on the UK working party cost questionnaire [42] were piloted in all families in the study at the 3 and 6 month visits.

Rationale for sample size

As this was a feasibility study, a sample size calculation was not performed [43]. The sample size was chosen pragmatically based on the expected number of cases in the recruitment area within the pre-specified recruitment period. A sample size of 12 affected infants, supplemented by interviews with a similar number of parents of TD infants, was expected to be adequate to reach data saturation regarding the emergence of themes from the qualitative interviews [44].

Data analysis

Qualitative data analysis was theoretically informed by Normalisation Process Theory [27]. This provides a framework upon which to consider factors influencing the incorporation into routine practice ("normalisation") of complex interventions. We used the same approach for the intervention development stage [21]. All analysis was conducted according to the standard procedures of rigorous qualitative analysis [45]. We used procedures from first-generation grounded theory (coding, constant comparison, memoing) [46], from analytic induction (deviant case analysis) [47] and from constructionist grounded theory (mapping) [48]. We undertook independent coding and cross checking, and a proportion of data was analysed collectively in 'data clinics' where the research team shared and exchanged interpretations of key issues emerging from the data. Pseudonyms were used for all participant names in the transcripts and in any quotes used.

Descriptive statistics were used to summarise quantitative data on rates of eligibility, consent, recruitment and retention; summary statistics were also included for assessment and outcome measures.

Results

Figure 1 shows the flow diagram for participants with PS/HPI. Twenty infants were screened and 14 found to be eligible. Of these, one parent of a preterm infant declined to participate and 13 families were enrolled (6 PS; 7 HPI). Two other parents of preterm infants withdrew from the study, so 11 families were followed up to the 6-month assessment. One parent who withdrew expressed a feeling of being overwhelmed by visits from healthcare professionals and the other felt that participation caused her to dwell excessively on her infant's medical problems. Interestingly, this latter parent made contact several months later, asking to be re-enrolled in the study to participate in the interview. During the in-depth interview, she commented that she had continued to follow the eTIPS approach after study withdrawal.

We also approached and screened 14 TD infants. One preterm (23-week gestation) TD infant died of a respiratory infection prior to undertaking any assessments. Another TD infant was excluded due to the subsequent identification of a medical condition affecting eligibility; thus, we could analyse data for 12 TD infants to age 6 months.

Participant enrolment started in August 2015 and was completed in January 2017 for infants and carers and for therapists by June 2017.

Table 2 shows the demographic and clinical characteristics for each group. There were 4 missed/cancelled visits in TD infants (three at 5 months and one at 4 months) but none in the infants with HPI and only one missed/cancelled visit in an infant with PS (at 5 months, which included the qualitative interview). This was inevitable due

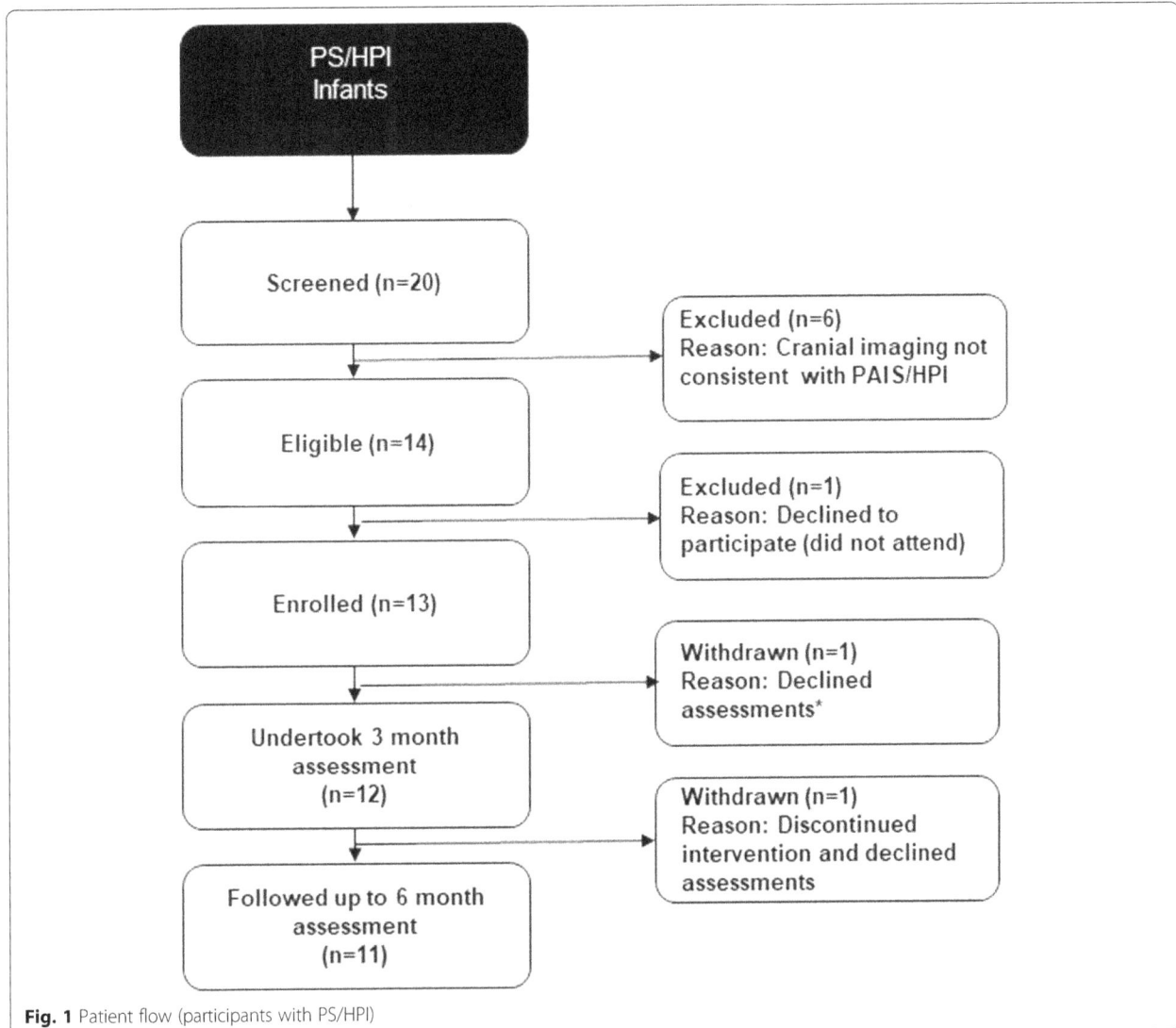

Fig. 1 Patient flow (participants with PS/HPI)

Table 2 Baseline demographic and clinical characteristics for each group

		PS	HPI	TD
Number		6	7	13
Number Term-born		5	0	8
Gestational age for preterm infants (weeks)	Median	35 ($n = 1$)	27	31
	Range	n/a	23–30	24–35
Birthweight (g) for preterm infants	Median	2575 ($n = 1$)	786	1361
	Range		550–1300	740–1644
Number of males		2	6	5
Parents/carers recruited (M, F, GM, GF)		6, 6, 1, 0	7, 5, 0, 1	13, 12, 0, 0
Side of brain lesion (L, R, N/A)		3, 3	4, 3	N/A

M mother, *F* father, *GM* grandmother, *GF* grandfather

to the personal circumstances of the infant and family at the time.

Feasibility and acceptability

Table 3 summarises the results of the eTIPS feasibility questionnaire.

Eleven families with an infant with PS/HPI took part in in-depth interviews (six with only the mother; five with both parents), as did thirteen families with a TD infant (twelve with only the mother, one with both parents), and six therapists, who between them were supporting ten of the infants with PS/HPI. From the interviews, we gained a number of insights. Firstly, parents were very willing to enter the study to make sure that they had done everything they could to help their child's future:

> like it took us like five minutes to decide 'cause I was like, "If we don't do it and he is left with obvious like damage then we, we would always think, 'What if we'd done that, that thing and it might've made it better?'" (Helen).

In addition to this they felt that there was a very low risk of harm to and that 'this is less invasive, this trial' (Barney), in comparison to others they were offered at the time as well as seeming to hold face validity:

> and I know it isn't backed up yet 'cause it is a trial, but this feels more like, er, "Surely this has got to work". It feels like there's more science behind it (Barbara).

The high-quality materials were appreciated by the families: 'It's not a cheap piece of paper or a cheap, you

know, stapled sheets of paper together, it's a full-on book' (Selina), as was the layout and format. Although at first they reported that the size of the manual looked a little daunting, they quickly came to appreciate that the information was simple and easy to follow:

> It wasn't really too bad once you start looking through the book you... At first, yes, it does sound like a hell of a lot. Once you start looking through the book, it's sort of like really easy to integrate into day-to-day things that you do with, with the child (Belinda).

The eTIPS approach integrated into family life relatively easily, particularly when parents had been given information before leaving the hospital. It quickly became a normal and pervasive part of their everyday interactions with their child:

> It is second nature now as we did it this way from coming home from hospital, it's routine, we don't have to think about it (Emma).

Parents of TD infants were comfortable with the use of infant massage; some were also attending baby massage classes independently.

As well as learning from the eTIPS materials, parents also modelled researcher behaviours in interactions with their children. In particular, parents were often inspired by observing the Hand Assessment for Infants and sourced similar toys to those used in the assessment. Feedback from the team regarding the HAI assessment helped parents to understand how to focus on specific

Table 3 eTIPS Feasibility Questionnaire

Item	Description	Mother 1 m	Mother 6 m	Father 1 m	Father 6 m
	Number in section A	12	11	9	7
A1	I understand the purpose of eTIPS	5 (4–5)	5 (4–5)	5 (4–5)	5 (4–5)
A2	I understand the types of things eTIPS requires me to do with my child	5 (4–5)	5 (4–5)	5 (4–5)	5 (4–5)
A3	I can see the potential value of eTIPS for my child	5 (4–5)	5 (4–5)	5 (4–5)	5 (4–5)
A4	I can easily fit eTIPS into my day	5 (3–5)	5 (4–5)	5 (3–5)	4 (3–5)
A5	It is easy to carry out the eTIPS approach with my child	5 (2–5)	5 (4–5)	4 (3–5)	4 (4–5)
A6	Using eTIPS disrupts my relationship with my child	0.5 (1–3)	1 (1–2)	2 (1–3)	1 (1–2)
A7	Sufficient training is provided for me to use eTIPS with my child	4.5 (3–5)	5 (2–5)	5 (3–5)	4 (3–5)
A8	My child tolerates eTIPS well	4.5 (3–5)	4 (4–5)	4 (4–5)	5 (4–5)
	Number in section B	11	11	9	7
B1	When you use eTIPS, how familiar does it feel?	6.97 (1.91)	9.14 (0.84)	5.71 (2.44)	7.69 (1.76)
B2	Do you feel eTIPS is currently a normal part of your day/time with your child?	6.95 (1.90)	9.36 (0.81)	6.24 (2.07)	7.81 (2.07)
B3	Do you feel eTIPS will become a normal part of your day/time with your child?	9.13 (1.29)	9.45 (0.82)	9.26 (0.78)	8.97 (0.94)

A 5 point Likert scale was used: 1 = "strongly disagree"; 2 = "disagree"; 3 = "neither agree nor disagree"; 4 = "agree"; 5 = "strongly agree". Median values for each of items A1–8, with minimum and maximum in brackets. For items B1–3, mean and standard deviation are given as these were represented as a continuous scale (0–10), with increasing scores representing increasing familiarity with/perceived normality of the approach

developmentally appropriate areas of practice with their infant. Parents were also appreciative of the positive reinforcement they received from the eTIPS team and of the positive interactions with their infants during visits. The assessments were also considered acceptable, though one parent felt uncomfortable with the use of accelerometers.

Parents were prepared to alter their behaviours and the environment around their child to fit in with the eTIPS approach. Siblings also became involved:

> She [the mother] tells them [siblings] to stand on the side where the yellow rattle is so even the quite young ones can understand that and go and stand on that side and sing to him and things (Researcher observation).

Parents rightly did not feel restricted to the suggestions in the manual for promoting activity of the potentially affected side: there were many examples of parents being resourceful and innovating or generalising the eTIPS approach to fit in with their lives. This included methods they had found to encourage others to approach and interact with their infant from the affected side, e.g. by considering the positioning of their infant's pram or crib within the environment. They also felt that the eTIPS approach was a positive factor in their interactions with their infants:

> I never used to get smiles or anything like that. And I think all the eTIPS and stuff, and the playing, and stuff like that, and the different toys, I think that... And obviously I've been getting more smiles. Everyone gets them, apart from me. And I'll get upset. But I think, like, this has helped him interact with me. (Fiona).

Therapists agreed with the approach and could understand the science/evidence behind it. Therapists reported demonstrating therapy activities and leaving advice for families to work on specific activities between sessions as part of their normal practice. They liked the eTIPS materials and felt they assisted them in teaching the families without having to spend a lot of time pre-preparing personalised therapy plans. They appreciated the pervasiveness of the approach and felt that it would lead to better outcomes.

> Yeah, erm, I really don't think the approach is too different, like I said, to anything that I would do anyway. I suppose it's just more structured and a lot more information for parents. But, that's what you want. We go in once a week maximum. It's no good us just doing something with them once a week. You know, it needs to be done all the time. (Nicola).

The idea of integrating the therapy into daily activities as opposed to being a separate 'therapy session' was also seen as useful by therapists:

> 'Cause, what I always say to any parent, is when I give them their programme, I always put, "Integrate this into your daily play. Don't make it, right, now we're doing your physio." (Nicola).

The regular communication between the eTIPS team and families was acceptable to all. There was variation in how families responded to text messages and phone calls. Some replied regularly and gave the team updates about their infant, while some families rarely responded but when questioned did not want the messages to stop. They appreciated that the team were available for specific questions and support.

> I like the texts as well, but, er, I, I like that fact that you just keep in touch consistently, because then... And I've got all the numbers as well, so if anything happens I know that you're just at the end of the phone. (Deirdre).

Maintaining this communication also reinforced the importance of eTIPS, their involvement in it and the research team's commitment:

> It [text messages and phone calls] makes us feel, me and Samuel, and, and dad, important that, you know, again it isn't just a paper exercise....that we have actually got full involvement in something which is hopefully going to be making a difference. (Selina).

Infants sustained no adverse events related to the eTIPS intervention: no injuries were reported from the activities undertaken and no infant developed a preference for the hand contralateral to the side of the brain affected by the lesion.

Assessments

It was possible to undertake the required assessments within the context of a 1 h visit, fitting them around the infant's needs and parental requests for information and support.

Figure 2 shows the individual 0–100 HAI scores for the group. For the 11 affected infants with HAI data at 6 months, the mean Both Hands Score was 58.5 HAI units (s.d. 19.1). Change scores for the HAI from 3 to 6 months were available for 12 TD and 10 affected infants. For TD infants, the mean change score was 32.4 HAI units (s.d. 17.1 units; 95% CI 21.5 to 43.3). For infants with stroke the mean change score was 27.2 HAI units (s.d. 8.5 units; 95% CI 21.1 to 33.3). At age 6 months the mean

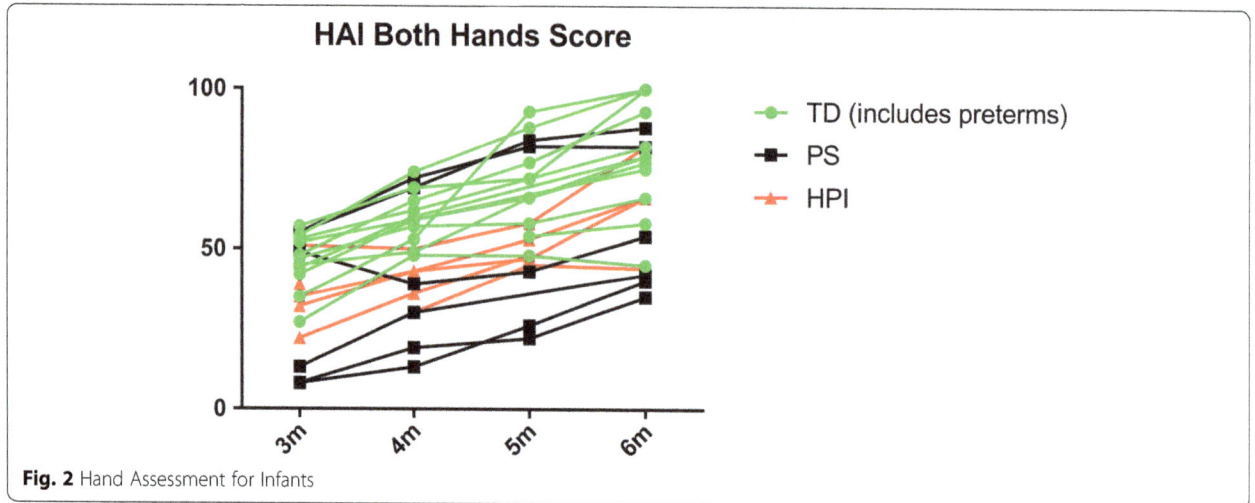

Fig. 2 Hand Assessment for Infants

asymmetry index in the affected group was 35.5% (95% CI 12.8–58.1); for TD infants, it was 5.2% (95% CI -2.0 to 12.3). Table 4 summarises findings in relation to the other assessments piloted. In addition, multiple improvements to the healthcare resource use data collection forms were made in response to feedback and evidence of need for improved clarity. Table 5 summarises the neuroimaging

findings in relation to the HAI Both Hands scores at 6 months.

Discussion
The eTIPS intervention was, in general, extremely well received and appreciated by families, and fitted into their everyday lives. This is likely to be due in part to the

Table 4 Summary of findings from other assessments piloted

Assessment	Findings	Implications for future trial
HAI	Assessments generally enjoyed by infants and perceived as valuable by parents in demonstrating their infant's abilities, identifying challenges to work on and modelling strategies.	Valuable assessment, worth the training required for therapists to undertake and score. Resource implications: need to video and upload assessments for later scoring.
PSOM	Useful clinical proforma though in the context of the other data collected (HAI, GMs and AIMS), the motor summary scores were not required, and the cognitive, behavioural and language scores were more suited to older infants.	Useful for summarising longer term outcomes and for comparison with other infants with PS/HPI. The HINE would be another option.
GM	Straightforward to undertake, video record and score. Two infants showed fidgety movements (predictive of good motor outcome) by 4 m which were not seen at 3 m.	Provides early indicator of likely normal vs. abnormal motor outcome. For centralised scoring, video upload to a central server is required.
Accelerometry	Time-consuming and at times technically challenging; one parent uncomfortable with use. Analysis complex.	Valuable exploratory data but current approach unsuitable for RCT given resources required.
AIMS	Easy to obtain and score. AIMS at 6 m were 25th centile or above for all except one TD term infant (10–25 centile) but lower for preterm TD and PS/HPI infants (one exception with small cortical infarct and good outcome).	Useful to describe early gross motor function which impacts hand use. However, abnormal motor patterns seen in infants with evolving neurology could distort scores.
WEBWMS	All returned questionnaires were fully completed. Two mothers of TD infants at baseline and two at 6 m failed to return questionnaires. Questionnaires from fathers were less frequently returned (3 TD missing at start and end; 3 PS/HPI missing at end). Change scores did not suggest any adverse effect of eTIPS on parental mental wellbeing: PS/HPI maternal change score 2.2 (95% CI -3.9 to 8.3; $n = 10$). TD maternal change score − 3.2 (95% CI -9.4 to 3.0, $n = 10$); higher scores represent better mental wellbeing.	Questionnaire return rate optimised by sending out forms prior to visit, bringing spare forms and collecting them during the visit. Extra vigilance required to obtain questionnaires from fathers.
PSOC	Questionnaire return rate same as WEBWMS but multiple non-completed items which qualitative data suggested were due to reluctance to answer questions perceived as sensitive, as well as initial failure of some fathers to complete the reverse of the form.	An alternative and positively framed questionnaire addressing aspects of parental sense of competence could be used, e.g. Family Empowerment Scale.

Table 5 Imaging findings and HAI Both Hands scores at 6 months

No.	Imaging	Side (brain)	Lesion type	Description	6 m HAI Both Hands
1	CrUSS, MRI	Right	Infarct	Right cerebral cortex & PLIC; left occipital lobe infarct	35
2	MRI	Right	Infarct	MCA territory infarct involving cortex, PLIC & corticospinal tracts	42
3	MRI	Left	Infarct	Left frontoparietal; small left posterior parietal & tiny right frontal subcortical lesion	88
4	CT, MRI	Left	Infarct	Segmental MCA territory infarct involving frontal & parietal lobes.	54
5	CrUSS, MRI	Left	Infarct	Anterior circulation infarct affecting cortical & subcortical structures	82
6	CT, MRI	Right	Infarct, SAH, IVH	Extensive MCA territory infarct involving cortical & subcortical structures, basal ganglia & corticospinal tract	40
7	CrUSS	Right	HPI	Frontal lobe	45
8	CrUSS	Left	HPI	Frontoparietal	n/a
9	CrUSS	Right	HPI	Adjacent to body of lateral ventricle	66
10	CrUSS	Right	HPI	Adjacent to body of lateral ventricle, extending to temporal lobe	44
11	CrUSS	Left	HPI	Left periventricular	66
12	CrUSS	Left	HPI	Left frontoparietal	n/a
13	CrUSS	Left	HPI	Frontotemporal	82

CrUSS Cranial Ultrasound, *PLIC* Posterior limb of internal capsule, *MCA* middle cerebral artery

involvement of parents and therapists throughout the intervention development process and the use of Normalisation Process Theory [21]. It was important to ensure that parents felt capable of delivering the intervention and were not overburdened or stressed by it; our results support this finding. A supportive, problem-solving approach from the eTIPS team is likely to have influenced this positive outcome: parent-delivered therapy is underpinned by therapists who empower, motivate and support families to deliver effective interventions (Lord et al., under submission).

Therapists were also supportive of the eTIPS approach; this is important in terms of future implementation of the approach. An issue relevant to our planned randomised controlled trial is the need to train therapists at remote sites on the eTIPS approach and assess the fidelity of their delivery of parental training and supervision. Commitment of local teams to the endeavour will be important and we plan to provide centralised support as well as training. We are currently developing a training package, which will itself be piloted prior to use. Central video-based review of selected sessions can be a useful method for assessment of intervention fidelity.

We found the HAI to be a very valuable assessment. Parents were engaged with the assessment and infants enjoyed taking part; researchers could use the HAI to help parents to know what developmental skills to focus on next and how to help the child to develop those skills. It was clear that for parents, the changes in hand function seen from visit to visit were meaningful and important. The HAI gives a detailed summary of hand function not currently available in this age group through any other measure.

Regarding our inclusion criteria, we had hoped to include some infants with presumed perinatal stroke (who typically present with emerging signs of motor problems after the first months of life), by allowing infants aged up to 3 months to enter the trial. However, we did not recruit any such infants, presumably because they had not come to medical attention by this point. Therefore, for a future randomised trial it would be appropriate to restrict recruitment age to 1 month corrected or less, to maximise and standardise the duration of subsequent intervention. We also recruited infants with varying degrees of brain injury, and this also has relevance to our future recruitment strategy. Of the infants with infarcts, the two infants with only cortical and subcortical lesions had excellent motor outcomes, though one of these infants had a 13% difference in hand function on the HAI score which was clinically noticeable. Similarly, infants with extensive lesions also involving the basal ganglia and corticospinal tract had more marked motor involvement in our study. Given the likelihood of a good motor outcome in infants with radiological sparing of the basal ganglia and corticospinal tract and conversely the high likelihood of hemiparesis with involvement of these structures in addition to a cortical/subcortical lesion [5], we will aim in future to include only infants with infarcts predicted to have a moderate or high risk of an abnormal motor outcome. Prompt centralised reporting of imaging findings will be necessary to ensure this. We also intend to explore the relationship between imaging findings and outcome as part of a mechanistic evaluation.

The influence of initial radiological findings on motor outcome in infants with HPI was less clear based on cranial ultrasound, as predicted from the literature [11, 12]; imaging with MRI in this latter group is not part of standard practice and would need to be incorporated into a trial protocol. Importantly, the existence of a relationship between initial imaging findings and motor outcome should not preclude attempts to improve outcome through intervention.

The retention rate in our trial was high. A few mothers of preterm infants struggled with the overall burden of care for those infants due to other morbidity related to their prematurity, making it harder for them to take on additional commitments related to the research. Based on their feedback we would see this as reflecting an increased need for support of these parents rather than a reason to exclude preterm infants from the intervention per se. With preterm infants, there may be an advantage in starting parent training in eTIPS before the infant is discharged from hospital, to offset some of this burden. Overall, parents in both the PS and HPI groups felt that their infants benefitted from the approach. Whilst one parent of a preterm infant disengaged from eTIPS assessments because she felt she was dwelling excessively on her infant's medical problems as a result, she continued to deliver the eTIPS approach. This highlights a challenge faced by researchers in delivering an intervention such as eTIPS: parents need to understand the rationale for the intervention, which includes an awareness that their infant is at risk of developing a motor disability which the intervention aims to mitigate against. Assessments, whilst essential, may augment anxiety in parents as they seek to determine whether any signs of motor disability have emerged. This is a strong argument for rationalising the assessment profile to key time points in the planned future definitive trial, for encouraging parents to see the progress their infants have made and for providing emotional support.

The assessments piloted were in the most part suitable for use in a large-scale trial. The main exception to this was the PSOC for which parents often omitted to provide answers for certain items. Findings from qualitative data analysis indicated that parents found some of the questions sensitive and were wary of providing written answers. We included the questionnaire because we wanted to be able to demonstrate in a trial that parenting confidence was not adversely affected by participation. However, our qualitative data findings indicate that parents generally found participation a positive experience and the WEBWMS suggested that parental wellbeing did not decline. One option would be to include a parental empowerment scale such as the Psychological Empowerment Scale [49] (though this frames questions to parents as if they have already acknowledged their child to have a disability, which is inappropriate for parents of such young infants) or the Family Empowerment Scale [50], though

another (preferred) option would be simply to omit the PSOC without replacement. Similarly, although the Pediatric Stroke Outcome Measure (PSOM) allows comparison of motor outcomes to those of other infants with PS, the Hammersmith Infant Neurological Examination (HINE) would be a useful addition given its psychometric properties [51].

To progress to a randomised controlled trial one further issue to be addressed was that of randomisation. As we needed to maximise feedback regarding the trial materials, we did not randomise infants in the feasibility trial. However, since completing the trial we conducted a workshop with 8 parents (4 couples) who took part, to obtain their views on randomisation. Parents felt strongly that their infants had benefited from the eTIPS approach; through discussion they understood that a randomised trial would be necessary to provide definitive evidence regarding benefit. Knowing that infants in the standard care arm of the trial would still receive regular therapist review meant that all parents agreed that eTIPS should proceed to a randomised controlled trial.

Conducting a randomised controlled trial of a behaviour change intervention will have its challenges, not least in terms of avoidance of contamination, for which we have plans in place [52]. Issues such as competitive therapy bias have affected previous therapy trials by reducing the difference between the interventions provided to the intervention and control group [53]. Cluster randomisation is one way to avoid such problems, but has the disadvantage of introducing potential bias due to differences in other aspects of care between clusters. Another option is to have a group of trial therapists who oversee the intervention and a separate group who oversee standard care. Many UK sites will be required, and therapists may be employed by different organisations (and therefore sites) from the recruiting clinicians for any one infant: the trial will require expert input from a clinical trials manager to assist with these issues. However, our positive experiences regarding this feasibility trial indicate that we should proceed.

Conclusions

The eTIPS intervention was feasible to deliver and acceptable to families and therapists. We plan to investigate efficacy of this parent-delivered early intervention in a multicentre randomised controlled trial.

Abbreviations

AIMS: Alberta infant motor scale; CIMT: Constraint-induced movement therapy; CrUSS: Cranial ultrasound; eTIPS: Early therapy in perinatal stroke; GM: General movements; HAI: Hand assessment for infants; HINE: Hammersmith infant neurological examination; HPI: Haemorrhagic parenchymal infarction; MCA: middle cerebral artery; PLIC: Posterior limb of internal capsule; PS: Perinatal stroke; PSOC: Parenting sense of competence scale; PSOM: Pediatric stroke outcome measure; TD: Typically developing; UCP: Unilateral cerebral palsy; WEBWMS: Warwick-Edinburgh Mental Wellbeing Scale

Acknowledgements

Thanks to Claire Marcroft for reviewing assessments to confirm inter-observer reliability; and to Niina Kolehmainen for helpful initial discussions. We would like to thank steering group meeting attendees, led by Rob Forsyth and including several PPI representatives.

(Nicola Spoors, Fliss Hunter-Nott, Johanna Smith), PIs at sites (Ruppa Geethanath, Shalabh Garg, Chidambara Harikumar), and all infants, their families and therapists who participated in the research.

Funding

The feasibility trial was funded through the National Institute for Health Research, Newcastle Healthcare Charity and the Tiny Lives Charity. The funders had no role in the design of the study, the collection, analysis or interpretation of data, the writing of the report, or the decision to submit the article for publication. Dr. Anna Basu is funded through a National Institute of Health Research Career Development Fellowship. The views expressed are those of the authors and not necessarily those of the NHS, the National Institute for Health Research, or the Department of Health.

Authors' contributions

APB conceived and designed the study as CI, contributed to data acquisition, undertook data analysis and interpretation, drafted and critically revised the manuscript. JP contributed substantially and critically to the intervention development, undertook data acquisition, processing, analysis and interpretation, and critically revised the manuscript. RW undertook data acquisition, undertook and analysed the qualitative interviews and other qualitative data, and drafted the qualitative data sections of the manuscript as well as critically revising the manuscript. PD contributed substantially to data analysis and interpretation and critically reviewed the manuscript. JB contributed substantially to the development of the intervention materials, data collection and analysis, and critically revised the manuscript. BW contributed substantially to data collection, analysis of the questionnaire data, and critically revised the manuscript. DH advised on data analysis and interpretation, and critically revised the manuscript. LV supervised the development and piloting of the healthcare usage questionnaires and critically revised the manuscript. DM reviewed, reported on and interpreted cranial imaging and critically revised the manuscript. NE contributed to the study design, was PI at the lead site, advised on and assisted with patient identification, and critically revised the manuscript. TR contributed to the study design and contributed substantially to the qualitative data analysis as well as critically revising the manuscript. All authors read and approved the final manuscript.

Consent for publication

Not applicable

Competing interests

The authors declare that they have no competing interests.

Author details

[1]Institute of Neuroscience, Newcastle University, Newcastle upon Tyne NE1 7RU, UK. [2]Department of Paediatric Neurology, Newcastle upon Tyne Hospitals NHS Foundation Trust, Newcastle upon Tyne NE7 7DN, UK. [3]Therapy Services, Newcastle upon Tyne Hospitals NHS Foundation Trust, Newcastle upon Tyne NE7 7DN, UK. [4]Institute of Health and Society, Newcastle University, Newcastle upon Tyne NE2 4AX, UK. [5]Newcastle Neonatal Service, Newcastle upon Tyne Hospitals NHS Foundation Trust, Newcastle upon Tyne, UK. [6]Human Biosciences, Northumbria University, Newcastle upon Tyne NE1 8ST, UK. [7]Department of Neuroradiology, Newcastle upon Tyne Hospitals NHS Foundation Trust, Newcastle upon Tyne NE7 7DN, UK. [8]Department of Social Work, Education and Community Wellbeing, Northumbria University, Coach Lane Campus West, Newcastle upon Tyne NE7 7XA, UK.

References

1. Raju TN, Nelson KB, Ferriero D, Lynch JK. Ischemic perinatal stroke: summary of a workshop sponsored by the National Institute of Child Health and Human Development and the National Institute of Neurological Disorders and Stroke. Pediatrics. 2007;120(3):609–16.
2. Schulzke S, Weber P, Luetschg J, Fahnenstich H. Incidence and diagnosis of unilateral arterial cerebral infarction in newborn infants. J Perinat Med. 2005;33(2):170–5.
3. Benders MJ, Groenendaal F, Uiterwaal CS, de Vries LS. Perinatal arterial stroke in the preterm infant. Semin Perinatol. 2008;32(5):344–9.
4. Sreenan C, Bhargava R, Robertson CM. Cerebral infarction in the term newborn: clinical presentation and long-term outcome. J Pediatr. 2000;137(3):351–5.
5. Husson B, Hertz-Pannier L, Renaud C, Allard D, Presles E, Landrieu P, Chabrier S. Motor outcomes after neonatal arterial ischemic stroke related to early MRI data in a prospective study. Pediatrics. 2010;126(4):912–8.
6. van der Slot WM, Roebroeck ME, Landkroon AP, Terburg M, Berg-Emons RJ, Stam HJ. Everyday physical activity and community participation of adults with hemiplegic cerebral palsy. Disabil Rehabil. 2007;29(3):179–89.
7. Bassan H, Feldman HA, Limperopoulos C, Benson CB, Ringer SA, Veracruz E, Soul JS, Volpe JJ, du Plessis AJ. Periventricular hemorrhagic infarction: risk factors and neonatal outcome. Pediatr Neurol. 2006;35(2):85–92.
8. Bassan H, Benson CB, Limperopoulos C, Feldman HA, Ringer SA, Veracruz E, Stewart JE, Soul JS, Disalvo DN, Volpe JJ, et al. Ultrasonographic features and severity scoring of periventricular hemorrhagic infarction in relation to risk factors and outcome. Pediatrics. 2006;117(6):2111–8.
9. Maitre NL, Marshall DD, Price WA, Slaughter JC, O'Shea TM, Maxfield C, Goldstein RF. Neurodevelopmental outcome of infants with unilateral or bilateral periventricular hemorrhagic infarction. Pediatrics. 2009;124(6): e1153–60.
10. Volpe JJ. Brain injury in premature infants: a complex amalgam of destructive and developmental disturbances. Lancet Neurol. 2009;8(1):110–24.
11. Roze E, Kerstjens JM, Maathuis CG, ter Horst HJ, Bos AF. Risk factors for adverse outcome in preterm infants with periventricular hemorrhagic infarction. Pediatrics. 2008;122(1):e46–52.
12. Roze E, Benders MJ, Kersbergen KJ, van der Aa NE, Groenendaal F, van Haastert IC, Leemans A, de Vries LS. Neonatal DTI early after birth predicts motor outcome in preterm infants with periventricular hemorrhagic infarction. Pediatr Res. 2015;78(3):298–303.
13. Staudt M. Reorganization after pre- and perinatal brain lesions. J Anat. 2010;217(4):469–74.
14. Lynch JK, Nelson KB. Epidemiology of perinatal stroke. Curr Opin Pediatr. 2001;13(6):499–505.
15. Kirton A, Armstrong-Wells J, Chang T, Deveber G, Rivkin MJ, Hernandez M, Carpenter J, Yager JY, Lynch JK, Ferriero DM. Symptomatic neonatal arterial ischemic stroke: the international pediatric stroke study. Pediatrics. 2011;128(6):e1402–10.
16. Basu AP. Early intervention after perinatal stroke: opportunities and challenges. Dev Med Child Neurol. 2014;56(6):516–21.
17. Basu AP, Pearse J, Kelly S, Wisher V, Kisler J. Early intervention to improve hand function in hemiplegic cerebral palsy. Front Neurol. 2015;5:281. https://doi.org/10.3389/fneur.2014.00281.
18. Sakzewski L, Ziviani J, Boyd RN. Efficacy of upper limb therapies for unilateral cerebral palsy: a meta-analysis. Pediatrics. 2014;133(1):e175–204.
19. Eyre J, Taylor J, Villagra F, Smith M, Miller S. Evidence of activity-dependent withdrawal of corticospinal projections during human development. Neurology. 2001;57:1543–54.
20. Eyre JA. Corticospinal tract development and its plasticity after perinatal injury. Neurosci Biobehav Rev. 2007;31(8):1136–49.
21. Basu AP, Pearse JE, Baggaley J, Watson RM, Rapley T. Participatory design in the development of an early therapy intervention for perinatal stroke. BMC Pediatr. 2017;17(1):33.
22. Marcroft C, Tstutsumi A, Pearse JE, Dulson P, Embleton ND, Basu AP: Current therapeutic management of perinatal stroke with a focus on the upper limb: a cross sectional survey of UK physiotherapists and occupational therapists. Phys Occup Ther Pediatr (in press).
23. Novak I, Morgan C, Adde L, Blackman J, Boyd RN, Brunstrom-Hernandez J, Cioni G, Damiano D, Darrah J, Eliasson AC, et al. Early, accurate diagnosis and early intervention in cerebral palsy: advances in diagnosis and treatment. JAMA Pediatr. 2017;
24. Eliasson AC, Nordstrand L, Ek L, Lennartsson F, Sjostrand L, Tedroff K, Krumlinde-Sundholm L. The effectiveness of baby-CIMT in infants younger than 12 months with clinical signs of unilateral-cerebral palsy; an explorative study with randomized design. Res Dev Disabil. 2017;72:191–201.
25. Ferre CL, Brandao MB, Hung YC, Carmel JB, Gordon AM. Feasibility of caregiver-directed home-based hand-arm bimanual intensive training: a brief report. Dev Neurorehabil. 2015;18(1):69–74.

26. Wallen M, Ziviani J, Naylor O, Evans R, Novak I, Herbert RD. Modified constraint-induced therapy for children with hemiplegic cerebral palsy: a randomized trial. Dev Med Child Neurol. 2011;53(12):1091–9.

27. Murray E, Treweek S, Pope C, MacFarlane A, Ballini L, Dowrick C, Finch T, Kennedy A, Mair F, O'Donnell C, et al. Normalisation process theory: a framework for developing, evaluating and implementing complex interventions. BMC Med. 2010;8:63.

28. Gilmore L, Cuskelly M. Factor structure of the parenting sense of competence scale using a normative sample. Child Care Health Dev. 2009;35(1):48–55.

29. Johnston C, Mash EJ. A measure of parenting satisfaction and efficacy. J Clinical Child Psychol. 1989;18(2):167–75.

30. Gibaud-Wallston J, Wandersman LP. Development and utility of the parenting sense of competence scale. Toronto, Canada: American Psychological Association; 1978.

31. Tennant R, Hiller L, Fishwick R, Platt S, Joseph S, Weich S, Parkinson J, Secker J, Stewart-Brown S. The Warwick-Edinburgh mental well-being scale (WEMWBS): development and UK validation. Health Qual Life Outcomes. 2007;5:63.

32. Krumlinde-Sundholm L, Sicola E, Ek L, Guzzetta A, Sjöstrand L, Cioni G. A E: the hand assessment for infants, a new test for measuring use of hands and possible asymmetry in infants 3–10 months of age. Dev Med Child Neurol. 2015;57:54–5.

33. Krumlinde-Sundholm L, Ek L, Sicola E, Sjostrand L, Guzzetta A, Sgandurra G, Cioni G, Eliasson AC. Development of the hand assessment for infants: evidence of internal scale validity. Dev Med Child Neurol. 2017;59(12):1276–83.

34. Eliasson AC, Sjostrand L, Ek L, Krumlinde-Sundholm L, Tedroff K. Efficacy of baby-CIMT: study protocol for a randomised controlled trial on infants below age 12 months, with clinical signs of unilateral CP. BMC Pediatr. 2014;14:141.

35. Guzzetta A, Boyd RN, Perez M, et al. UP-BEAT (Upper Limb Baby Early Action–observation Training): protocol of two parallel randomised controlled trials of action–observation training for typically developing infants and infants with asymmetric brain lesions. BMJ Open. 2013;3: e002512. https://doi.org/10.1136/bmjopen-2012-002512.

36. Kitchen L, Westmacott R, Friefeld S, MacGregor D, Curtis R, Allen A, Yau I, Askalan R, Moharir M, Domi T, et al. The pediatric stroke outcome measure: a validation and reliability study. Stroke. 2012;43(6):1602–8.

37. Engelmann KA, Jordan LC. Outcome measures used in pediatric stroke studies: a systematic review. Arch Neurol. 2012;69(1):23–7.

38. Bosanquet M, Copeland L, Ware R, Boyd R. A systematic review of tests to predict cerebral palsy in young children. Dev Med Child Neurol. 2013;55(5): 418–26.

39. Darrah J, Redfern L, Maguire TO, Beaulne AP, Watt J. Intra-individual stability of rate of gross motor development in full-term infants. Early Hum Dev. 1998;52(2):169–79.

40. Darrah J, Piper M, Watt MJ. Assessment of gross motor skills of at-risk infants: predictive validity of the Alberta infant motor scale. Dev Med Child Neurol. 1998;40(7):485–91.

41. Pin TW, Eldridge B, Galea MP. Motor trajectories from 4 to 18 months corrected age in infants born at less than 30 weeks of gestation. Early Hum Dev. 2010;86(9):573–80.

42. Thompson S, Wordsworth S. An annotated cost questionnaire for completion by patients. UK working party on patient costs. HERU discussion paper. University of Aberdeen Aberdeen. 2001. http://www.dirum.org/instruments/details/28.

43. Eldridge SM, Chan CL, Campbell MJ, Bond CM, Hopewell S, Thabane L, Lancaster GA, group pc. CONSORT 2010 statement: extension to randomised pilot and feasibility trials. BMJ. 2016;355:i5239.

44. Francis JJ, Johnston M, Robertson C, Glidewell L, Entwistle V, Eccles MP, Grimshaw JM. What is an adequate sample size? Operationalising data saturation for theory-based interview studies. Psychol Health. 2010;25(10):1229–45.

45. Rapley T. Some Pragmatics of Qualitative Data Analysis. In: Qualitative Research: Theory, Method & Practice. London: Sage Publications Ltd.; 2010. p. 273–90.

46. Glaser BG. The constant comparative method of qualitative analysis. Soc Probl. 1965;12:436–45.

47. Seale C. Quality in Qualitative Research. Qual Inq 1999. 1999;5:465–78.

48. Charmaz K. Constructing grounded theory: a practical guide through qualitative analysis. London: Sage Publications; 2006.

49. Akey TM, Marquis JG, Ross ME. Validatieon of scores on the psychological empowerment scale: a measure of empowerment for parents of children with a disability. Educ Psychol Meas. 2000;60(3):419–38.

50. Singh NN, Curtis WJ, Ellis CR, Nicholson MW, Villani TM, Wechsler HA. Psychometric analysis of the family empowerment scale. J Emot Behav Disord. 1995;3(2):85–91.

51. Maitre NL, Chorna O, Romeo DM, Guzzetta A. Implementation of the Hammersmith infant neurological examination in a high-risk infant follow-up program. Pediatr Neurol. 2016;65:31–8.

52. Basu AP, Pearse JE, Rapley T. Publishing protocols for trials of complex interventions before trial completion - potential pitfalls, solutions and the need for public debate. Trials. 2017;18(1):5.

53. Rodgers H, Mackintosh J, Price C, Wood R, McNamee P, Fearon T, Marritt A, Curless R. Does an early increased-intensity interdisciplinary upper limb therapy programme following acute stroke improve outcome? Clin Rehabil. 2003;17(6):579–89.

17

Trends in stroke outcomes in the last ten years in a European tertiary hospital

Emilio Rodríguez-Castro[1,2], Iria López-Dequit[1,2], María Santamaría-Cadavid[1,2], Susana Arias-Rivas[1,2], Manuel Rodríguez-Yáñez[1,2], José Manuel Pumar[1,3], Pablo Hervella[1], Esteban López-Arias[1], Andrés da Silva-Candal[1], Ana Estany[4], María Piñeiro-Lamas[5], Tomás Sobrino[1], Francisco Campos[1], Manuel Portela[1,6], Manuel Vázquez-Lima[7], José Castillo[1,8]* and Ramón Iglesias-Rey[1,8]* (iD)

Abstract

Background: Studying the impact of demographic changes and progress in the management of stroke patients is necessary in order to organize care structures for the coming years. Consequently, we analyzed the prognostic trends of patients admitted to the Stroke Unit of a tertiary hospital in the last ten years.

Methods: The University Clinical Hospital of Santiago de Compostela is the referral hospital for stroke in a catchment area that accounts for 16.5% of the population of Galicia. Data from patients admitted to the Stroke Unit were registered prospectively. A multinomial logistic regression was performed to determine the influence of new trends in demographic factors and in the management of patients with acute stroke. For the expected trend of progression, a 2008–2011 and 2012–2017 time series model was made by selecting the most appropriate model.

Results: In the last 10 years, the age of stroke onset has only increased in women (from 74.4 ± 2.2 years in 2008 to 78.8 ± 2.1 years in 2017; $p = 0.037$), and the same happens with the severity of neurological symptoms (ischemic stroke (IS), $p < 0.0001$; from 14 [10, 19] in 2008 to 19 [15, 26] in 2017), with a higher percentage of cardioembolic strokes (40.7% vs. 32.2% of cardioembolic strokes in women vs. men, $p < 0.0001$). In a multiple linear regression model, hospital improvement was mainly associated with the use of reperfusion treatment (B 53.11, CI 95% 49.87, 56.36, $p < 0.0001$). A differentiated multinomial logistic regression analysis conducted for the whole sample with ischemic strokes in the two time periods (2008–2011 and 2012–2017) showed no differences in the influence of factors associated with higher morbidity and mortality. The modeling of time series showed a distinct falling trend in mortality, with a slight increase in good outcome as well as morbidity in both ischemic and hemorrhagic stroke.

Conclusions: Our results showed that mortality decreased in the entire sample; however, although outcome at discharge improved in ischemic stroke, severe disability also increased in these patients. Importantly, this tendency towards increased morbidity seems to be confirmed for the coming years.

Keywords: Ischemic stroke, Intracerebral hemorrhage, Mortality, Morbidity

Background

In the last decades, there have been important changes in the management of acute stroke. These changes include modifications in the care chain of these patients [1–3], due to better diagnostic processes [4] and new therapeutic targets [5–8]. In the same line, other strategies as the incorporation of multidisciplinary and specialized Stroke Units (24-h neurology and interventional neuroradiology attention) [9], the protocolization of hemodynamic [10], thrombolytic [11] and endovascular recanalization treatments [12], as well as the creation of specific neurology wards and telemedicine systems [13] have provided improvements in patient care. This situation has led to a new paradigm in the appreciation of the emergency standard of care and to an improved knowledge of the patient with stroke, both in healthcare structures and by the public at large [14].

* Correspondence: jose.castillo.sanchez@sergas.es;
ramon.iglesias.rey@sergas.es
[1]Clinical Neurosciences Research Laboratory, Health Research Institute of Santiago de Compostela (IDIS), Santiago de Compostela, Spain
Full list of author information is available at the end of the article

The new healthcare scenario has been accompanied by more effective and more generalized primary prevention measures [15, 16]. However, in a context of deep demographic changes, the age-standardized incidence of stroke in Europe and developed countries is increasing and it seems that it will continue to do so in the next decades [17–19].

Galicia is a Spanish region on the northwest of the Iberian Peninsula, with a total population of 2,707,700 inhabitants concentrated mainly on the coastal areas (population density of 92.5 inhabitants/km^2). Life expectancy at birth is 82.6 years and has increased by 5 years since 1981.

The percentage of aging (population over the age of 65 divided by population younger than 15 multiplied by 100) of Galicia is 151.9%. In the public network hospitals of Galicia, stroke admissions account for 2.35% of the total hospitalization. This rate has remained stable for the last five years and is similar for both sexes [20].

Therefore, the analysis of the impact of all these changes on the clinical results obtained should provide valuable data to further organize health system structures and improve management protocols. For this purpose, we analyzed the trend in the progress of patients admitted to a specialized Stroke Unit of a tertiary hospital (Galicia) in the last ten years.

Methods

Study population and patient characteristics

The University Clinical Hospital of Santiago de Compostela serves a catchment area of 447,699 people (16.5% of the total Galician population), plus 18–22% referred from other health centers. The center has a Stroke Unit and provides 24-h neurology and interventional neuroradiology attention (Fig. 1).

Since October 2004, we have prospectively included patients with ischemic stroke (IS) and non-traumatic intracerebral hemorrhage (ICH) admitted to the Stroke Unit of the University Clinical Hospital of Santiago de Compostela in the BICHUS registry. We would like to note that the present study was conducted using the last 10-year data (From September 2007 to September 2017). This research was conducted in accordance with the Declaration of Helsinki of the World Medical Association

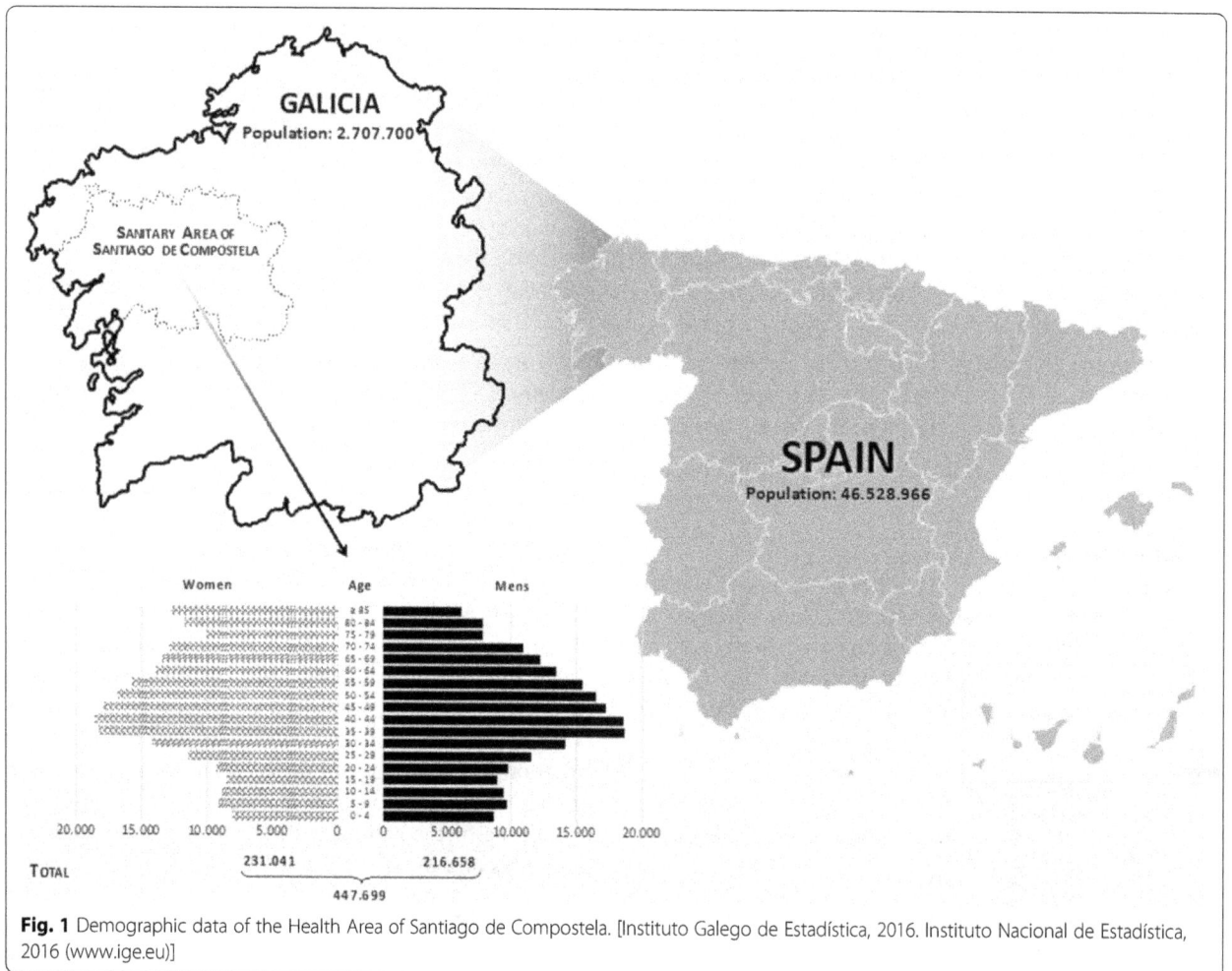

Fig. 1 Demographic data of the Health Area of Santiago de Compostela. [Instituto Galego de Estadística, 2016. Instituto Nacional de Estadística, 2016 (www.ige.eu)]

(2008) and approved by the Ethics Committee of Galicia (EC). Written informed consent was obtained from each patient or from their relatives after full discussion of the procedures.

Clinical variables

The variables of our registry included stroke date, latency time from the stroke onset and care in the Emergency Department, and whether it was a wake-up stroke. Demographic data, previous modified Rankin scale (mRS) [21] and vascular risk factors were included. Data of previous carotid disease and processes of carotid revascularization were also collected, and in the case of patients with a previous transient ischemic attack (TIA), the time between TIA and stroke, as well as the coincidence or not with topography.

The clinical variables collected were: National Institute of Health Stroke Scale (NIHSS) [22] on admission, at 48 h and at discharge, mRS at discharge and at 3 months, and maximum axillary temperature within the first 24 h.

Blood sample measurements were: glucose levels at admission, glycated hemoglobin, white blood cell, red blood cell and platelets count, fibrinogen, C-reactive protein, total and fractionated cholesterol, triglycerides, proBNP, D-vitamin, and cholecalciferol. Neuroimaging variables in ischemic stroke were: baseline infarct volume (DWI-lesion) and final ischemic lesion volume (a second CT between 4th–7th day) and, existence and type of hemorrhagic transformation. In hemorrhagic stroke we collected basal hematoma volume (CT) and hematoma and edema volume (second CT between 4th–7th day). We evaluated the neurological progress during hospitalization according to the following formula: (NIHSS on admission - NIHSS on discharge) / NIHSS on admission) × 100. Patients who died during hospitalization were given a zero score. The mRS at 3 ± 1 months was assessed face-to-face in 3151 patients and by telephone in 1731. Accredited expert neurologists assessed both scales (ER-C, IL-D, MS-C, SA-R, MR-Y). The etiological diagnosis of IS was performed according to TOAST criteria [23]. Non-traumatic ICH was classified into hypertensive, amyloid, related to antiplatelets / anticoagulants and undetermined [24, 25]. We also recorded whether patients were treated by telemedicine, type of reperfusion therapy and complications during the acute phase.

Clinical data were available of all patients, laboratory variables in 87% of cases and neuroimaging variables in 73% of patients.

Statistical analysis

From September 2007 to September 2017; 6129 patients were included. Patients who: suffered from transient ischemic attack (512), were transferred to other hospital during the acute phase (42), died for causes other than vascular (39), had non-confirmed stroke diagnosis (85), were referred from other hospital after acute phase management (94) and were lost to follow-up at 3 months (475) were excluded. Finally, 4882 patients (3921 with IS and 961 with ICH) were considered valid for the analysis.

Results were expressed as percentages, mean and standard deviation or median and 25–75% percentiles, and the differences were determined by the chi-square, t-student or Mann-Whitney-Wilcoxon tests. The distribution of the same variable in the 10 years of the study was analyzed using ANOVA test. The relationship between the two variables was determined by Pearson or Spearman coefficients, depending on the nature of the variable.

In 2012, endovascular treatment was implemented as the standard of care in our hospital, so we compared 2008–2011 and 2012–2017 periods to determine the influence of new trends in the management of patients with acute stroke. First, a bivariate multinomial logistic regression (MLR) was performed, testing the significance of each of the variables considered as candidates from a clinical approach. Next, a multivariate analysis was proposed, using the MLR technique. At this point, the variables whose p-values of the likelihood ratio contrast were > 0.20 were discarded. Strategy was repeated until finding the definitive set of variables that integrated all those that were significant ($p < 0.05$) for the variable mRS at 3 months. Three models were constructed following this methodology and differentiating IS from ICH: using all data (model 1), using data from the 2008–2011 period (model 2) and using data from the 2012–2017 period (model 3). To determine the influence of variables in the in-hospital improvement we performed a multiple linear regression model adjusted for those variables that reached statistical significance $p < 0.05$ in univariate analysis [IBM SPSS Statistics software v19.0].

The expected trend in patient progress for the next few years at 3 months after a stroke – categorized as good outcome (mRS ≤ 2), morbidity (mRS > 2 and ≤ 5) and mortality (mRS = 6) – was estimated by time series model. A time series trend model was made by selecting the most appropriate one (from a list of 5 possible models) through Schwarz Information Criteria (SBIC) and Akaike Information Criteria (AIC). Once the time series trend was estimated, the residual component was analyzed. To determine whether the residual series was white noise or not, graphic tests, the tests of Ljung-Box and Durbin-Watson were performed. In the cases where the residual series were not white noise, this residual component was modeled through autoregressive and moving averages models (AR, MA or ARMA). Once the models are adjusted, the forecasts are calculated as the sum of the forecasts of both components. In the cases where the residual series are white noise, their forecast will be zero [R statistical software v3.2.21].

Results

Demographic, clinical and progress characteristics of the sample analyzed

The mean age was 71.9 ± 13.9 years; 55.3% were male and 44.7% female. The pyramid of age and sex distribution can be seen in Fig. 2a (80.3% IS and 19.7% ICH). The IS subtypes were classified as: 23.6% atherothrombotic, 36.5% cardioembolic, 7.9% lacunar, 30.9% indeterminate and 1.1% of rare causes. Of ICH, 48.9% were hypertensive, 6.7% amyloid, 13.6% antiplatelet/anticoagulant, and 30.8% undetermined (26.7%) or due to unusual causes (4.1%).

8.9% of patients were wake-up stroke (9.9% of IS and 4.7% of ICH), and in the rest, the latency time between the symptoms onset and hospital arrival was 218.9 ± 177.2 min (219.8 ± 168.1 min in IS and 215.0 ± 210.8 min in the ICH). 1.6% of patients were treated in another hospital by a telemedicine system.

Of the whole sample analyzed, 62.5% of patients presented with hypertension, 23.4% had diabetes, 15.6% were smokers, 12.5% had alcoholic habit, 34.6% hyperlipidemia, 18.8% atrial fibrillation, 16.4% carotid disease (13.4% ipsilateral, 1.4% contralateral and 1.6% bilateral) and 4.5% had suffered a previous transitory ischemic attack, 3 ± 4.6 days before. The NIHSS score on admission was 13 [8, 19] and percentage of hospital improvement was $28.9 \pm 44.7\%$. At 3 months, 52.2% had a good outcome and mortality was 15.6%.

Since 2015, the age of stroke patients admitted has shown a progressive increase, especially significant in women (Fig. 2b). The percentage of wake-up stroke did not change in the 10-year analyzed (10.7 vs. 9.8%, $p = 0.071$), and there was a significant reduction in time between stroke onset and hospital arrival (269.8 ± 225.5 min in 2008 and 202.1 ± 201.3 min in 2017, $p < 0.0001$).

The severity of neurological symptoms determined by NIHSS on admission has increased progressively ($p < 0.0001$) in patients with IS (14 [10, 19] in 2008 to 19 [15, 26] in 2017), and has remained stable ($p = 0.176$)

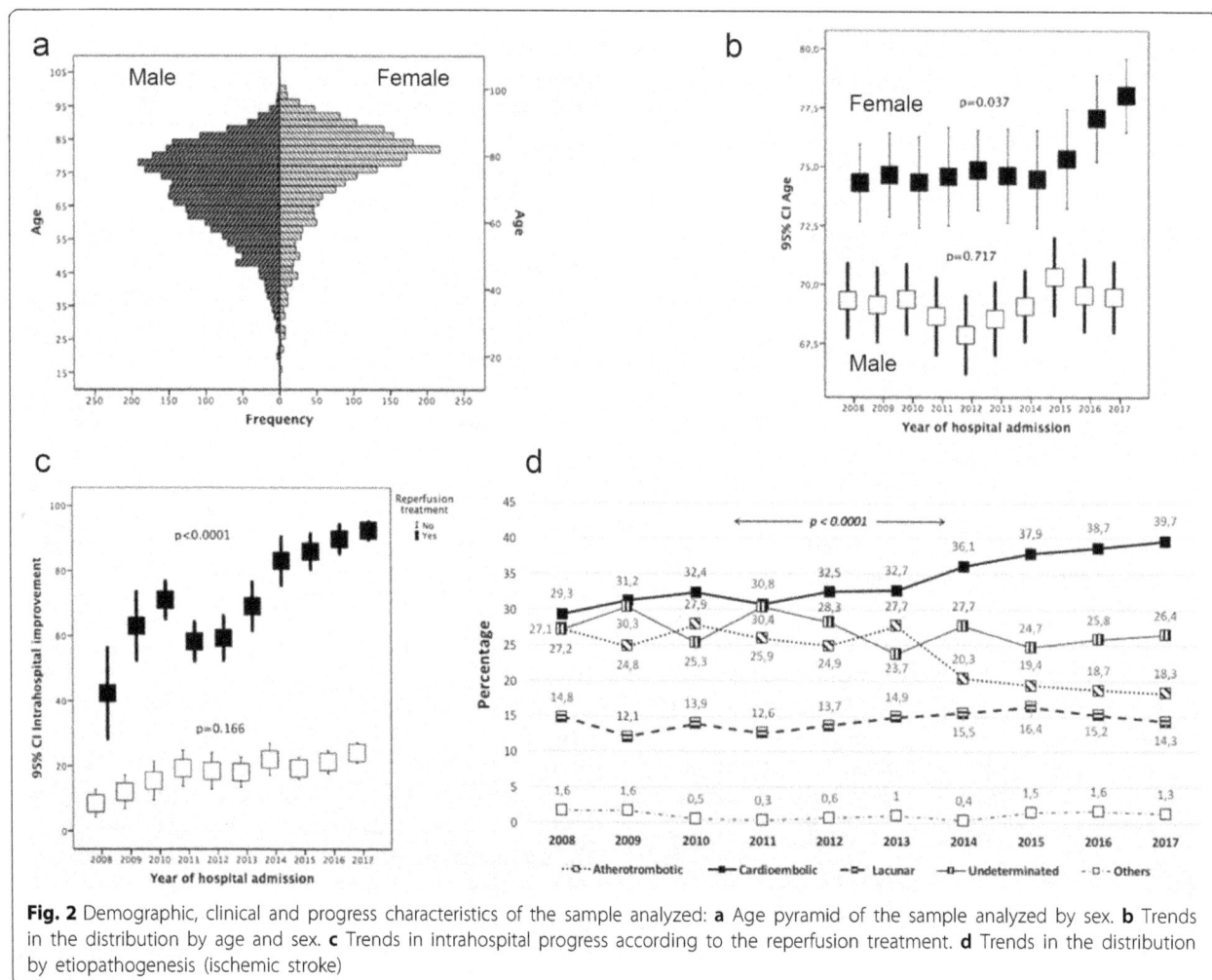

Fig. 2 Demographic, clinical and progress characteristics of the sample analyzed: **a** Age pyramid of the sample analyzed by sex. **b** Trends in the distribution by age and sex. **c** Trends in intrahospital progress according to the reperfusion treatment. **d** Trends in the distribution by etiopathogenesis (ischemic stroke)

in ICH (14 [9, 18] to 15 [8, 22]). Hospital improvement has shown a marked increase since 2009 in IS ($p < 0.0001$) and has remained stable ($p = 0.302$) in ICH. The improvement in IS was associated with the increase in reperfusion therapies, from 9.1% in 2008 to 28.8% in 2107 (Fig. 2c).

In the years under analysis, the trend in the global distribution of the IS and the ICH has remained stable ($p = 0.602$). However, among the IS there has been an increase in cardioembolic stroke origin (29.3% to 39.7% in 10 years). Patients with cardioembolic stroke were older (age in atherothrombotic 69.3 ± 13.7, cardioembolic 75.2 ± 13.3, lacunar 67.1 ± 13.4, undetermined 70.7 ± 14.2, unusual causes 56.5 ± 16.2 years, $p < 0.0001$) and tended to be women (40.7% vs. 32.2% of cardioembolic strokes in women vs. men, $p < 0.0001$) (Fig. 2d). The etiology of the ICH has remained stable ($p = 0.286$).

In a multiple linear regression model, hospital improvement was mainly associated with the use of reperfusion therapy (B 53.11, CI 95% 49.87, 56.36, $p < 0.0001$), but a positive trend in patient progress has also been found in the last ten years (B 0.88, 95% CI 0.32, 1.43, $p = 0.002$).

Trends in the development of the incidence of factors that modify the risk of stroke

Classical risk factors, such as arterial hypertension ($p = 0.648$), tobacco ($p = 0.931$), alcohol use ($p = 0.550$) and hyperlipidemia ($p = 0.193$), showed no variation in the last ten years. The incidence of diabetes has decreased ($p = 0.036$) from 27.6% in 2008 to 21.5% in 2017 (Fig. 3a). Fig. 3b shows the progress of heart diseases, peripheral arterial disease and the administration of preventive drugs. The incidence of atrial fibrillation ($p < 0.0001$) and a history of coronary disease ($p < 0.0001$) have significantly increased. Peripheral arterial disease ($p = 0.264$) and previous carotid disease ($p = 0.438$, not shown in the graph) did not show any differences. The

administration of antiplatelet drugs has not been modified ($p = 0.642$), but a progressive increase in the percentage of patients with oral anticoagulation was observed ($p < 0.0001$; 7.2% in 2008 to 13.2% in 2017).

Trends in mortality, morbidity and good outcome at 3 months

Mortality at 3 months has decreased in all groups of patients ($p = 0.016$). In the IS mortality decreased from 15.4% in 2008 to 9.8% in 2017 (atherothrombotic from 6.0 to 4.7%, cardioembolic from 16.8 to 10.7%, lacunar from 1.6 to 0.8%, undetermined from 10.3 to 6.4%, others from 14.3 to 11.2%). Mortality in ICH decreased from 31.6% in 2008 to 26.6% in 2017. Morbidity at 3 months remained stable in ICH ($p = 0.709$) and IS ($p = 0.087$), except in the subgroup of patients who received reperfusion therapy ($p < 0.0001$). Similarly, all IS groups have also experienced a trend in progress towards a good outcome ($p = 0.028$, 48.8% in 2007 to 55.3% in 2017) with the exception of the ICH ($p = 0.392$). The administration of reperfusion therapy is not only associated with a decrease in mortality, common to all patients with IS, but also with a notable increase in good outcome and a marked decrease in morbidity (Fig. 4a-b).

Influence of clinical variables on the outcome at 3 months in 2008–2011 and 2012–2017 periods

In the multinomial logistic regression study conducted for the whole sample with ischemic stroke, age, stroke on awakening, higher axillary temperature on admission, baseline blood glucose > 110 mg/dL and a higher white blood cell count were independent factors associated with higher morbidity and mortality. When we analyzed the patients admitted in 2008–2011 and 2012–2017 periods separately, we could see differences in the factors associated with greater morbidity and mortality. The

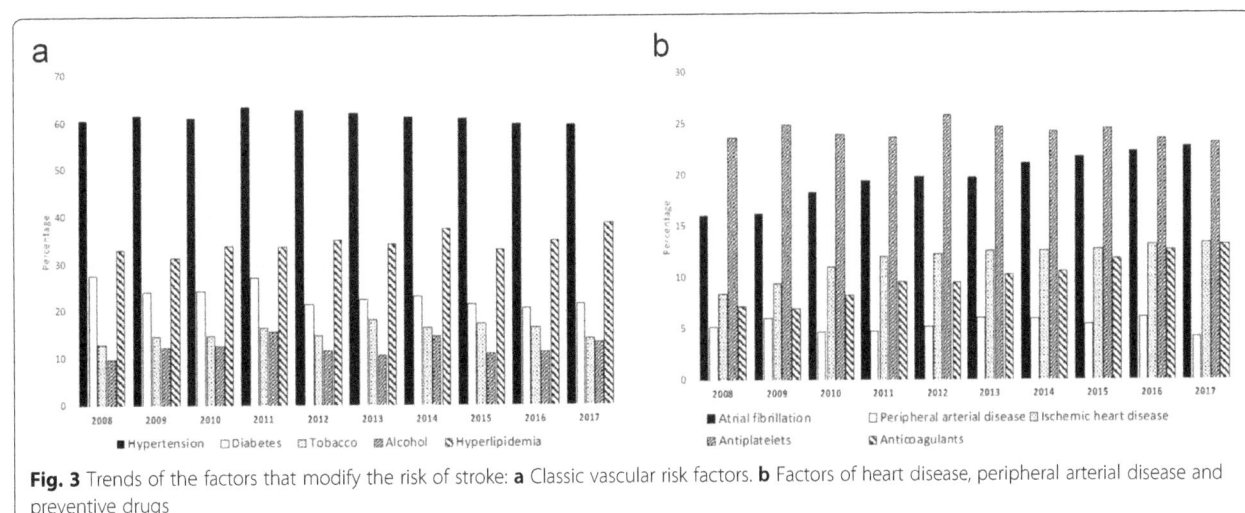

Fig. 3 Trends of the factors that modify the risk of stroke: **a** Classic vascular risk factors. **b** Factors of heart disease, peripheral arterial disease and preventive drugs

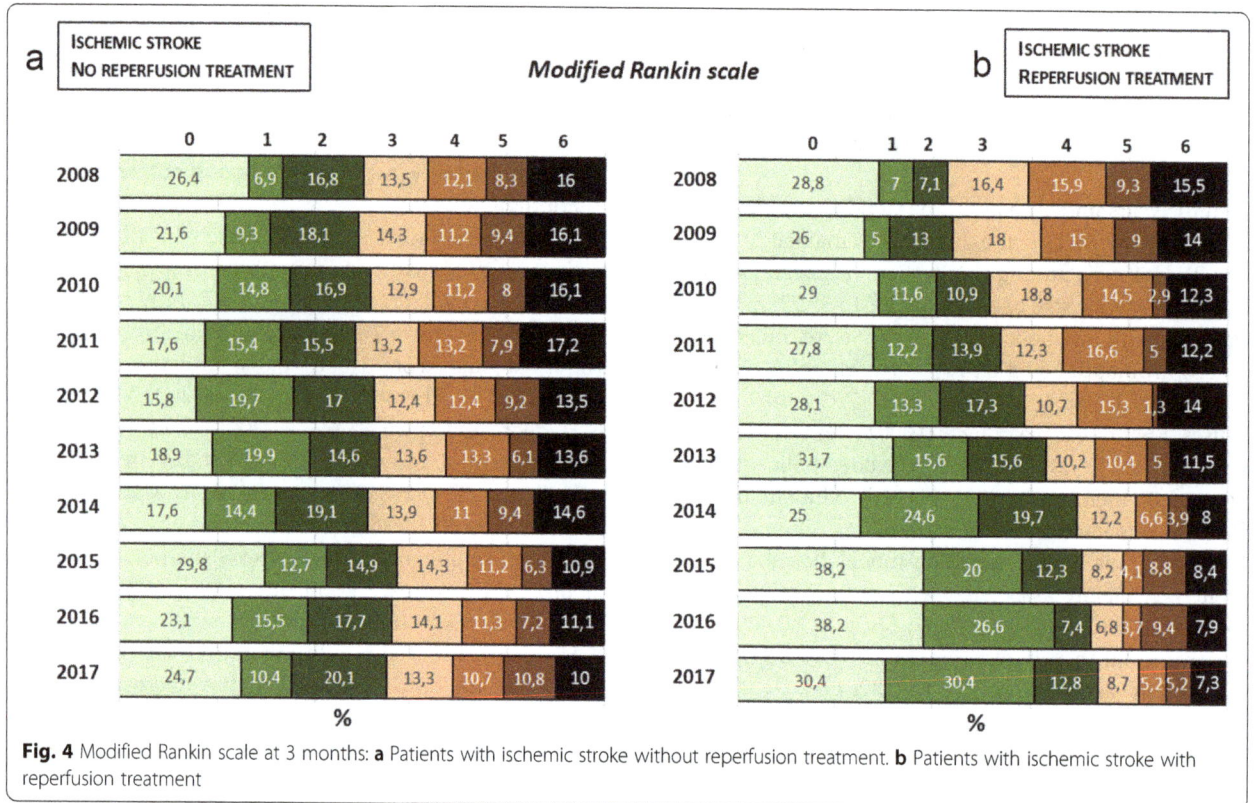

Fig. 4 Modified Rankin scale at 3 months: **a** Patients with ischemic stroke without reperfusion treatment. **b** Patients with ischemic stroke with reperfusion treatment

influence of the diagnostic type and the volume of the ischemic lesion has disappeared in recent years (Table 1).

In the global population of patients with intracerebral hemorrhage, age and baseline hematoma volume were the only factors associated with greater morbidity and mortality; hyperthermia was associated with mortality and elevated fibrinogen levels with increased morbidity (Table 1). Differentiated multinomial logistic regression analysis in the two time periods did not show differences in the influence of factors associated with higher morbidity and mortality (Table 1).

Estimation of the forecast trend

Time series model allowed us to establish the prognostic progress of patients admitted to our center, given that the current diagnostic and therapeutic procedures have not been substantially modified. In these circumstances, the marked tendency towards decreased mortality (Ljung-Box's test $p = 0.2124$, Dubin-Watson's test $p = 0.7659$) can be verified, with a slight increase in good outcome (Ljung-Box's test $p = 0.2444$, Dubin-Watson's test $p = 0.0141$), as well as morbidity (Ljung-Box's test $p = 0.8284$, Dubin-Watson's test $p = 0.1007$) in the coming years (Fig. 5). Given its statistical weight, this trend is more linked to patients with IS than with intracerebral hemorrhage.

Discussion

Our results showed remarkable changes in the demography and clinical progress in the 10-year follow-up, which explain the modification in the management of patients with acute cerebrovascular disease. The first modification observed is the rise in the age of stroke presentation that affects women exclusively. This demographic trend may influence comorbidity, the intensity of neurological involvement, access to certain treatments and prognostic evolution. The increase in the incidence of the first stroke, especially in women, has already been confirmed [17, 26–29], in previous literature although it was associated with those geographical areas with a marked aging process [30].

Increase in the age of stroke presentation is likely to be the cause of the greater severity of the neurological symptoms at admission (Spearman coefficient = 0.272; $p < 0.0001$, data not shown in the results), but despite this, a progressive hospital improvement is seen in patients with IS, especially in those who received reperfusion therapies. This trend is not seen in patients with ICH.

The 60-min reduction in the time interval between onset of symptoms and specialized care in the emergency department in the last 10-year is undoubtedly a reflection of the change in the social and health attitude towards stroke. Over the last decade, there has been developed in Spain a specialized press and television advertising campaign about stroke symptoms and 'time is

Table 1 Multinomial logistic regression: Influence of the clinical, biochemical and neuroimaging variables on the outcome variables (morbidity and mortality) at 3 months from stroke onset

	Ischemic stroke				Intracerebral hemorrhage			
	Morbidity		Mortality		Morbidity		Mortality	
	OR (95% CI)*	p	OR (95% CI)*	p	OR (95% CI)*	p	OR (95% CI)*	p
WHOLE SAMPLE								
Age (year)	1.03 (1.02–1.04)	<0.001	1.06 (1.05–1.07)	<0.001	1.01 (0.99–1.03)	0.148	1.04 (1.02–1.06)	0.001
Stroke on awakening	1.35 (1.06–1.72)	0.014	1.57 (1.06–2.37)	0.024				
Maximum axillary temperature - first 24 h (°C)	1.51 (1.33–1.71)	<0.001	2.22 (1.06–2.37)	<0.001	1.32 (0.97–1.79)	0.076	1.92 (1.37–2.68)	<0.001
Baseline glycemia (mg/dL)	1.00 (1.00–1.00)	<0.001	1.00 (1.00–1.00)	<0.001	1.00 (1.00–1.00)	0.019	1.00 (1.00–1.00)	0.065
Fibrinogen (mg/dL)	1.11 (1.09–1.14)	<0.001	1.23 (1.19–1.28)	<0.001				
White blood cells (×10³/mL)					1.03 (1.02–1.04)	<0.001	1.05 (1.04–1.06)	<0.001
Baseline volume of hematoma (mL)					1.02 (0.99–1.05)	0.079	1.05 (1.02–1.09)	0.001
PERIOD 2008–2011								
Age (years)								
Maximum axillary temperature - first 24 h (°C)	1.20 (0.86–1.64)	0.280	2.37 (1.47–3.82)	<0.001				
Baseline glycemia (mg/dL)	1.00 (1.00–1.00)	0.001	1.00 (1.00–1.01)	0.047	1.00 (1.00–1.00)	0.043	1.00 (1.00–1.00)	0.123
Fibrinogen (mg/dL)								
C-reactive protein (mg/L)	1.11 (1.05–1.17)	<0.001	1.22 (1.14–1.31)	<0.001				
TOAST:								
- Lacunar	0.29 (0.13–0.64)	0.002	1.14 (0.13–9.90)	0.905				
- Cardioembolic + Indeterminate	1.32 (0.90–1.93)	0.153	3.08 (1.48–6.40)	0.003				
- Atherothrombotic + Others	ref.		ref.					
Ischemic injury volume in 2nd CT (mL)	1.04 (1.03–1.05)	<0.001	1.05 (1.04–1.06)	<0.001				
Baseline hematoma volume (mL)					1.03 (1.01–1.05)	0.001	1.08 (1.05–1.10)	<0.001
PERIOD 2012–2017								
Age (years)	1.04 (1.03–1.05)	<0.001	1.07 (1.05–1.09)	<0.001	1.01 (0.97–1.04)	0.679	1.05 (1.01–1.10)	0.025
Maximum axillary temperature - first 24 h (°C)	1.12 (1.08–1.15)	<0.001	1.24 (1.17–1.30)	<0.001				
Baseline glycemia (mg/dL)	1.00 (1.00–1.00)	0.019	1.00 (1.00–1.00)	<0.001				
Fibrinogen (mg/dL)	1.12 (1.08–1.15)	<0.001	1.24 (1.17–1.30)	<0.001	1.00 (1.00–1.01)	0.015	1.00 (0.99–1.00)	0.177
White blood cells (×10³/mL)								
Baseline hematoma volume (mL)					1.03 (1.01–1.06)	0.001	1.05 (1.03–1.07)	<0.001
Edema volume in 2nd CT (mL)					1.02 (0.98–1.05)	0.290	1.04 (1.00–1.07)	0.047

*Adjusted OR. Good outcome was considered the reference category to calculate the ORs (CI 95%)

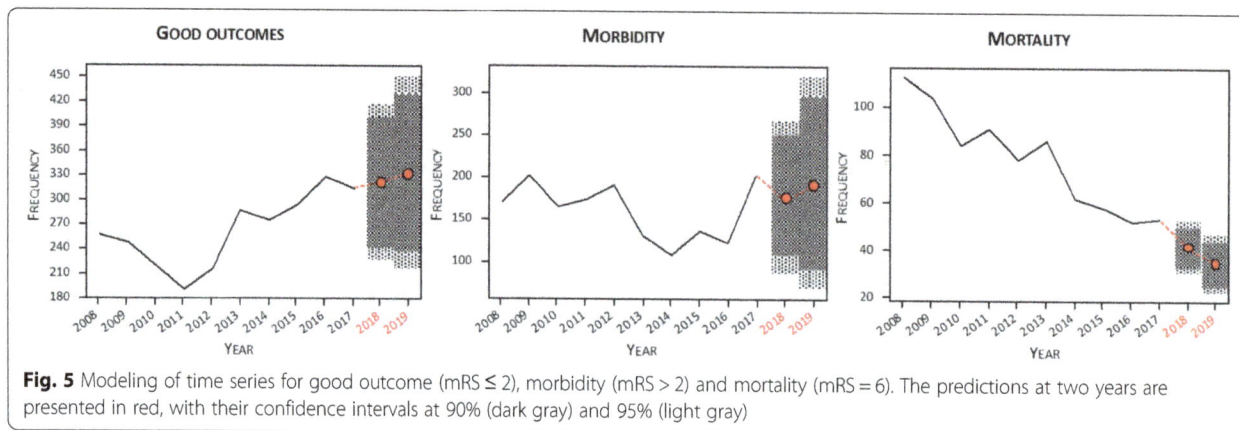

Fig. 5 Modeling of time series for good outcome (mRS ≤ 2), morbidity (mRS > 2) and mortality (mRS = 6). The predictions at two years are presented in red, with their confidence intervals at 90% (dark gray) and 95% (light gray)

brain' concept. The main objective was to inform and sensitize patient's families and medical services care about the importance of rapidly hospital patient's transfer. This shortening of the admission time and the speed in healthcare contribute to the rise in the percentage of reperfusion therapies, despite the increase in the age of the population served. The increase in patients treated within the therapeutic window for reperfusion therapies has been the objective achieved by the structural and functional modification developed in the stroke care systems [3, 30–32], although in some cases the total time has not improved [3].

The distribution of the etiological types of intracerebral hemorrhages has remained stable in the last ten years, but in ischemic strokes an increase in cardioembolic strokes has occurred, compensated by a decrease in atherothrombotic ones. This tendency has been reported in other studies in populations with similar characteristics [33–35], but not in younger populations [36].

This increase is not due to an improvement in the identification of embolic sources, since the proportion of undetermined strokes remains stable, but it may be associated with the increase in the age of the population and the greater proportion of elderly women (with more atrial fibrillation). Although the prescription of anticoagulants has increased (from 7.2% in 2008 to 13.2% in 2017), this increase has not been sufficient, since the percentage of patients with atrial fibrillation who do not take anticoagulants has increased (45.0% in 2008 to 58.1% in 2017) but remains significantly below the recommendations of European guidelines [37] and the figures reported for other populations [16].

In contrast to other publications [36], the incidence of risk factors has not changed significantly, with the exception of the decrease in diabetes mellitus and the increase in ischemic heart disease. This paradox could be explained by the marked aging of the population who has had a stroke. The increase in age can explain that the risk factors condition in the first-place coronary

disease and that diabetes conditions other vascular diseases in younger ages. The change of attitude in the management of patients with stroke in recent decades has been associated with a progressive trend towards a better prognosis in IS, with a reduction in mortality and improvement of good outcome [18, 29], also found in ICH patients. However, in a meta-analysis that included the 1980–2008 period, the prognosis of ICH remained stable [38].

Reperfusion therapy is the main factor responsible for the change in prognosis and attitude in the management of acute IS [39]. Consequently, we analyzed separately (before and after endovascular treatment was implemented as the standard of care in our hospital in 2012) the factors that could influence the stroke prognosis. In the two time periods, we did not find clear differences of the influence of modifiable factors on morbidity and mortality. The temperature and blood glucose control should condition a decrease or loss of the relationship between these parameters and the prognosis, but we only noted a decrease in temperature and mortality (from an adjusted OR of 2.37 in 2008–2011 to 1.24 in 2012–2017).

Of particular importance for the planning of stroke care in the coming years is the behavior of patients who suffered from significant disabilities (mRS 3, 4 5). In our study, mortality decreases, but the increase in good prognosis is hampered by the tendency to increase morbidity in the coming years. The expected increase in age in the population means that the proportion of patients with ischemic stroke who will not be able to benefit from reperfusion treatment will increase. This rise in morbidity will increase the health expenditure caused by stroke care. The absence of effective treatment for the ICH will aggravate this perspective. It should also be noted that the ICH mortality decrease cannot be associated with a specific factor, however, intensive blood-pressure control, temperature and blood glucose were carried out. Likewise, in recent years the dicumarinics have been replaced by new dependent non-vitamin K anticoagulants (only in a very few cases subjected to clinical trials with anticoagulants).

Our study has some strengths: it encompasses the vast majority of stroke patients treated in a geographical area of half a million inhabitants, with a homogeneous population and minimal immigration. The data were obtained and included by the same neurologists trained in cerebrovascular diseases and all patients were managed under the same protocol. Nevertheless, our study also shows some weaknesses; a relatively short follow-up time (3 months) as a consequence of clinical guidelines. The health area studied belongs to the Atlantic provinces of Galicia consisting mainly of urban and coastal population, but with little rural population. The sample used may be insufficient to establish associations and trends with a strong statistical value. Finally, we consider that the demographic change could make difficult the possible modification of the outcomes of patients in coming years, but future studies should take into account the negative evolution of patients with reperfusion treatment that is not effective [40], the new strategies for combining thrombolytic and endovascular therapies, as well as the analysis of patients from different world regions.

Conclusion

We found that the age of the stroke patients admitted has increased, especially in women. Hospital improvement has been progressive in the IS, despite a greater severity of patients, and an increase in cardioembolic stroke patients. This trend was not found in patients with ICH. No differences were observed between the incidence of the risk factors and the trend in the poor outcome in the different time periods analyzed. In our study, mortality decreased in the entire sample, but the improvement in the prognosis of patients with IS was negatively compensated by the tendency to an increase in all patients with stroke who had serious sequelae. Our data indicate morbidity is likely to increase in the coming years.

Abbreviations

AIC: Akaike Information Criteria; AR, MA or ARMA: Autoregressive and moving averages models; CT: Computed tomography; DWI: Diffusion weighted image; EC: Ethics Committee; ICH: Intracerebral hemorrhage; IS: Ischemic stroke; MLR: Multinomial logistic regression; mRS: Modified Rankin scale; NIHSS: National institute of Health Stroke Scale; ProBNP: pro-Brain Natriuretic Peptide; SBIC: Schwarz Information Criteria; TIA: Transient ischemic attack

Funding

Spanish Ministry of Economy and Competitiveness (SAF2014–56336-R and SAF2017–84267-R), Xunta de Galicia (Consellería Educación [Regional Ministry-Education]: GRC2014/027), Instituto de Salud Carlos III (PI17/00540 and PI17/01103), Spanish Research Network on Cerebrovascular Diseases RETICS-INVICTUS-PLUS (RD16/0019) and by the European Union FEDER program. T. Sobrino (CPII17/00027) and F. Campos (CP14/00154) are recipients of research contracts from Miguel Servet Program of Instituto de Salud Carlos III. Sponsors did not participate in study design, collection, analysis, or interpretation of the data.

Authors' contribution

JC and RI-R designed and coordinated the study, participated in the analyzed the data and manuscript preparation. ER-C, IL-D, MS-C, SA-R, MR-Y and JMP collected the data, and have been involved in the statistical analysis. MP, AE, MP-L and MV-L have been involved in the statistical analysis, interpretation and processed data. ADS-C, EL-A, PH, TS and FC participated in the data analysis, statistical treatment, and have been involved in revising the manuscript for important intellectual content. All authors have critically read and approved the submitted manuscript.

Competing interests

The authors report no conflicts of interest.

Author details

[1]Clinical Neurosciences Research Laboratory, Health Research Institute of Santiago de Compostela (IDIS), Santiago de Compostela, Spain. [2]Stroke Unit, Department of Neurology, Hospital Clínico Universitario, Santiago de Compostela, Spain. [3]Department of Neuroradiology, Hospital Clínico Universitario, Santiago de Compostela, Spain. [4]Unit of Methodology of the Research, Health Research Institute of Santiago de Compostela (IDIS), Santiago de Compostela, Spain. [5]Consortium for Biomedical Research in Epidemiology and Public Health, Instituto de Salud Carlos III, Madrid. Health Research Institute of Santiago de Compostela, Santiago de Compostela, Spain. [6]Health Area Management of Santiago de Compostela, Servicio Galego de Saúde, Santiago de Compostela, Spain. [7]Emergency Department, Hospital do Salnés, Pontevedra, Vilagarcía de Arousa, Spain. [8]Clinical Neuroscience Research Laboratory (Hospital Clínico Universitario), Rúa Travesa da Choupana, s/n, 15706 Santiago de Compostela, Spain.

References

1. Dávalos A, Castillo J, Martínez-Vila E. For the cerebrovascular disease study Group of the Spanish Society of neurology. Delay in neurological attention and stroke outcome. Stroke. 1995;26:2233–7.
2. Castillo J, Dávalos A, Marrugat J, Noya M. Timing for fever-related brain damage in acute ischemic stroke. Stroke. 1998;29:2455–60.
3. Puy L, Lamy C, Canaple S, Arnoux A, Laine N, Iacob E, et al. Creation of an intensive care unit and organizational changes in an adult emergency department: impact on acute stroke management. Am J Emerg Med. 2017; 35:716–9.
4. Dávalos A, Blanco M, Pedraza S, Leira R, Castellanos M, Pumar JM, et al. The clinical-DWI mismatch. A new diagnostic approach to the brain tissue at risk of infarction. Neurology. 2004;62:2187–92.
5. Demaerschalk BM, Kleindorfer DO, Adepye OM, Demchuck AM, Fugate JE, Grotta JC, et al. Scientific rationale for the inclusion and exclusion criteria for intravenous alteplase in acute ischemic stroke: a statement for healthcare professionals from the American Heart Association/American Stroke Association. Stroke. 2016;47:581–641.
6. Bellwald S, Weber R, Dobroxky T, Norddemeyer H, Jung S, Dadisury J, et al. Direct mechanical intervention versus bridging therapy in stroke patients elegible for intravenous thrombolysis: A pooled analysis of 2 registries. Stroke. 2017; https://doi.org/10.1161/STROKEAHA.117.018459.
7. Fischer U, Kaesmacher J, Mendes Pereira V, Chapor t R, Siddiqui AH, Froehler MT, et al. Direct mechanical thrombectomy versus combined intravenous and mechanical thrombectomy in large-artery anterior circulation stroke: a topical review. Stroke. 2017;48:2912–8.
8. Cao Y, Wang S, Sun W, Dai Q, Li W, Cai J, et al. Prediction of favorable outcome by percent improvement in patients with acute ischemic stroke treated with endovascular stent thrombectomy. J Clin Neurosci. 2017;38: 100–5.
9. Fens M, Vluggen T, van Haastregt JC, Verbunt JA, Beusmans GH, van Heugten CM. Multidisciplinary care for stroke patients living in the community: a systematic review. J Rehabil Med. 2013;45:321–30.
10. Sen A, Miller J, Wilkie H, Moyer M, Lewandowski C, Nowak R. Continuous hemodynamic monitoring in acute stroke: an exploratory analysis. West J Emerg Med. 2014;15:345–50.
11. Elmaraezy A, Abushouk AI, Saad S, Eltoomy M, Mahmoud O, Hassan HM, et al. Desmoteplase for acute ischemic stroke: a systematic review and metaanalysis of randomized controlled trials. CNS Neurol Disord Drug Targets. 2017;16:789–99.

12. Badhiwala JH, Nassiri F, Alhazzani W, Selim MH, Farrokhyar F, Spears J, et al. Endovascular thrombectomy for acute ischemic stroke: a meta-analysis. JAMA. 2015;314:1832–43.
13. Baratloo A, Rahimpour L, Abushouk AI, Safari S, Lee CW, Abdalvand A. Effects of telestroke on thrombolysis times and outcomes: a meta-analysis. Prehosp Emerg Care. 2018;22:472–84.
14. Segura T, Vega G, López S, Rubio F, Castillo J. On behalf of the cerebrovascular disease study Group of the Spanish Society of neurology. Public perception of stroke in Spain. Cerebrovasc Dis. 2003;16:21–6.
15. Lip G, Freedman B, De Caterine R, Potpara TS. Stroke prevention in atrial fibrillation: past, present and future. Comparing the guidelines and practical decision making. Thromb Haemost. 2017;117:1230–9.
16. Mochalina N, Isma N, Svensson PJ, Själander A, Carlsson M, Juhlin T, et al. Ischemic stroke rates decline in patients with atrial fibrillation as anticoagulants uptake improves: a Swedish cohort study. Thromb Res. 2017; 158:44–8.
17. Feigin VL, Forouzanfar MH, Krishnamurthi R, Mensah GA, Connor M, Bennett DA, et al. Global and regional burden of stroke during 1990-2010: findings from the global burden of Disiase study 2010. Lancet. 2014;383:245–54.
18. Béjot Y, Bailly H, Duriewr J, Giroud M. Epidemiology of stroke in Europe and trends for the 21st century. Presse Med. 2016;45:e391–8.
19. Lecoffre C, de Peretti C, Gabet A, Grimaud O, Woimant F, Giroud M, et al. National trends in patients hospitalized for stroke and stroke mortality in France, 2008 to 2014. Stroke. 2017;48:2939–45.
20. IGE://www.ige.eu. Instituto Galego de Estadística, 2015.
21. Bonita R, Beaglehole R. Modification of Rankin scale: recovery of motor function after stroke. Stroke. 1988;19:1497–500.
22. Montaner J, Álvarez-Sabín J. NIHSS stroke scale and its adaptation to Spanish. Neurologia. 2006;21:192–202.
23. Adams HP Jr, Bendixen BH, Kapelle LJ, Biller J, Love BB, Gordon DL, et al. Classification of subtype of scute ischemic stroke. Definitions for use in a multicenter clinical trial. TOAST. Trial of org 10172 in acute stroke treatment. Stroke. 1993;24:35–41.
24. Meretoja A, Strbian D, Putaala J, Curtze S, Haapaniemi E, Mustanoja S, et al. SMASH-U: a proposal for etiologic classification of intracerebral hemorrhage. Stroke. 2012;43:2592–7.
25. Martí-Fábregas J, Prats-Sánchez L, Martínez-Domeño A, Camps-Renom P, Marín R, Jiménez-Xarrié E, et al. The H-ATOMIC criteria for the etiologic classification of patients with intracerebral hemorrhage. PLoS One. 2017:11 e0156992.
26. Powles J, Kirov P, Feschieva N, Stanoev M, Atanasova V. Stroke in urban and rural population in north-East Bulgaria: incidence and case fatality findings from a "hot pursuit" study. BMC Public Health. 2002;2:24.
27. Kelly PJ, Crispino G, Sheehan O, Kelly L, Marname M, Merwick A, et al. Incidence, event rates, and early outcome of stroke in Dublin, Ireland: the Noth Dublin population stroke study. Stroke. 2012;43:2042–7.
28. Tsivgoulis G, Patousi A, Pikilidou M, Birbilis T, Katsanos AH, Mantatzis M, et al. Stroke incidence and outcomes in Northeasteren Greece. The Evros stroke registry. Stroke. 2018; 49:288 295.
29. Feigin VL, Lawes CM, Bennett DA, Barker-Collo SL, Parag V. Worldwide stroke incidence and early case fatality reported in 56 population-based studies: a systematic review. Lancet Neurol. 2009;8:355–69.
30. Fonarow GC, Smith EE, Saver JL, Reeves MJ, Bhatt DL, Grau-Sepúlveda MV, et al. Timeliness of tissue-type plasminogen activator therapy in acute ischemic stroke: patients characteristics, hospital factors, and outcomes associated with the door-to-imaging times within 60 minutes. Circulation. 2011;123:750–8.
31. Fonarow CG, Zhao X, Smith EE, Saver JL, Reeves MJ, Bhatt DL, et al. Door-to-needle times for tissue plasminogen activator administration and clinical outcomes in acute ischemic stroke before and after a quality improvement initiative. JAMA. 2014;311:1632–40.
32. Nardetto L, Giometto B, Moretto G, Mantoan D, Saia M. Hub-and-spoke stroke network in the Veneto region: a retrospective study investigating the effectiveness of the stroke pathway and trends over time. Neurol Sci. 2017; 38:2117–21.
33. Kolominsky-Rabar PL, Weber M, Gefeller O, Neundoerfer B, Heuschmann PU. Epidemiology of ischemic stroke subtypes according to TOAST criteria: incidence, recurrence, and long-term survival in ischemic stroke subtype: a population-based study. Stroke. 2001;32:2735–40.
34. Hajat C, Heuschmann PU, Coshall C, Padayachee S, Chambers J, Rudd AG, et al. Incidence of aetiological subtypes of stroke in a multiethnic population based study: the South London stroke register. J Neurol Neurosurg Psychiatry. 2011;82:527–33.
35. Leyden JM, Kleining TJ, Newbury J, Castle S, Canefield J, Anderson CS, et al. Adelaide stroke incidence study: declining stroke rates but many preventable cardioembolic strokes. Stroke. 2013;44:1226–31.
36. Krishnamurthi RV, Barker-Collo S, Parag V, Parmar P, Witt E, Jones A, et al. Stroke incidence by major pathological type and ischemic subtypes in the Auckland regional community stroke studies. Changes between 2002 and 2011. Stroke. 2018;49:3–10.
37. Kirchhof P, Benussi S, Kotecha D, Ahlsson A, Atar D, Casadei B, et al. Guidelines for the management of atrial fibrillation developed in collaboration with EACTS. Eur Heart J 2016. 2016;37:2893–962.
38. van Asch CJ, Luitse MJ, Rinkel GJ, van der Tweel I, Algra A, Klijn CJ. Incidence, case fatality, and functional outcome of intracerebral haemorrhage over time, according to age, sex, and ethnic origin: a systematic review and meta-analysis. Lancet Neurol. 2010;9:167–76.
39. Cao Y, Wang S, Sun W, Dai W, Li W, Cai J, et al. Prediction of favorable outcome by percent improvement in patients with acute ischemic stroke treated with endovascular stent thrombectomy. J Clin Neurosci. 2017;38:100–5.
40. Iglesias-Rey R, Rodríguez-Yáñez M, Rodríguez-Castro E, Pumar JM, Arias S, Santamaría M, et al. Worse outcome in stroke patients treated with rt-PA without early reperfusion: associated factors. Transl Stroke Res. 2018;9:347–55.

18

The effect of occipital nerve field stimulation on the descending pain pathway in patients with fibromyalgia: a water PET and EEG imaging study

Shaheen Ahmed[1], Mark Plazier[2], Jan Ost[3], Gaetane Stassijns[4], Steven Deleye[5], Sarah Ceyssens[5], Patrick Dupont[5], Sigrid Stroobants[6], Steven Staelens[7], Dirk De Ridder[8] and Sven Vanneste[1*] (ID)

Abstract

Background: Fibromyalgia is a chronic disorder characterized by widespread musculoskeletal pain accompanied by fatigue, sleep, memory, and mood problems. Recently, occipital nerve field stimulation (ONS) has been proposed as an effective potential treatment for fibromyalgia-related pain. The aim of this study is to unravel the neural mechanism behind occipital nerve stimulation's ability to suppress pain in fibromyalgia patients.

Materials and methods: Seven patients implanted with subcutaneous electrodes in the C2 dermatoma were enrolled for a Positron Emission Tomography (PET) $H_2^{15}O$ activation study. These seven patients were selected from a cohort of 40 patients who were part of a double blind, placebo-controlled study followed by an open label follow up at six months. The $H_2^{15}O$ PET scans were taken during both the "ON" (active stimulation) and "OFF" (stimulating device turned off) conditions. Electroencephalogram (EEG) data were also recorded for the implanted fibromyalgia patients during both the "ON" and "OFF" conditions.

Results: Relative to the "OFF" condition, ONS stimulation resulted in activation in the dorsal lateral prefrontal cortex, comprising the medial pain pathway, the ventral medial prefrontal cortex, and the bilateral anterior cingulate cortex as well as parahippocampal area, the latter two of which comprise the descending pain pathway. Relative deactivation was observed in the left somatosensory cortex, constituting the lateral pain pathway as well as other sensory areas such as the visual and auditory cortex. The EEG results also showed increased activity in the descending pain pathway. The pregenual anterior cingulate cortex extending into the ventral medial prefrontal cortex displayed this increase in the theta, alpha1, alpha2, beta1, and beta2 frequency bands.

Conclusion: PET shows that ONS exerts its effect via activation of the descending pain inhibitory pathway and the lateral pain pathway in fibromyalgia, while EEG shows activation of those cortical areas that could be responsible for descending inhibition system recruitment.

Trial Registration: This study is registered with ClinicalTrials.gov, number NCT00917176 (June 10, 2009).

Keywords: Positron emission tomography (PET), Occipital nerve stimulation, Fibromyalgia

* Correspondence: sven.vanneste@utdallas.edu
[1]School of Behavioral and Brain Sciences, The University of Texas at Dallas, Richardson, Texas, USA
Full list of author information is available at the end of the article

Background

Fibromyalgia is a pain syndrome characterized by widespread chronic pain in the four quadrants of the body that can be attributed to abnormalities in central pain processing circuits, rather than to damage to or inflammation of peripheral areas [1]. Fibromyalgia is not restricted to pain symptoms alone but also includes non-restorative sleep, fatigue, headaches, and mood disorders [2]. The American College of Rheumatologists (ACR) proposed diagnostic criteria in 1990. In 2010, these criteria were revised taking into account 18 pain areas and as well as other symptoms such as fatigue, memory disturbances, lower abdominal cramps, depressive mood, and headache as diagnostic criteria. The prevalence of fibromyalgia fluctuates between 0.4% up to 9.4% [3]. The economic burden of this disease is extremely high with a health related costs in a United States population up to o $11,049 per patient per year [4, 5]. A plethora of treatments have been trialed in clinical studies. Current treatment methods consist of both pharmacological (e.g. antidepressants, anti-seizure medication, etc.) and non-pharmacological approaches (e.g. exercise therapy, massage therapy, etc.); however, a group of fibromyalgia patients remains refractory with these treatments [6, 7]. Therefore, improvements to current treatments and new treatment approaches must be explored to raise treatment outcomes.

Recently, occipital nerve field stimulation (ONS) has been proposed as a potential treatment intervention for fibromyalgia symptoms [8–12]. ONS via a subcutaneous implanted electrode in the area of the greater occipital nerve was initially introduced to treat intractable headache syndromes and can be performed via a minimally invasive procedure [13]. Interestingly, patients with headache disorders comorbid with fibromyalgia showed improvement not only in headaches but also in pain and fibromyalgia-related symptoms [10]. Since then, ONS has been investigated as a potential treatment and seems to offer a safe and effective treatment option for selected medically intractable patients with fibromyalgia.

The occipital nerves interconnect with the trigeminal nerves and form a continuous network affecting the trigeminal nucleus caudalis and the cervical horn at the C1 and C2 levels, which are collectively called as "trigeminocervical complex" [14–16]. Imaging modalities such as functional Magnetic Resonance Imaging (fMRI) and ^{18}F-fluorodeoxyglucose Positron Emission Tomography (^{18}F-FDG PET) have demonstrated activities in this region of the nervous system during occipital nerve field stimulation [17–20]. An initial fMRI pilot study with a healthy subject undergoing ONS demonstrated that the procedure affects the central nervous system [18]. The predominant areas of activation were in the hypothalamus, thalamus, orbitofrontal cortex, prefrontal cortex, periaqueductal gray area, and cerebellum. A ^{18}F-FDG

PET study in patients with chronic migraine treated with ONS showed increased activity in the anterior cingulate cortex, pulvinar, and cuneus regions—all of which are involved in the affective dimension of pain [20]. Another ^{18}F-FDG PET study on cluster headaches showed that the pregenual anterior cingulate cortex, a major component of the descending pain inhibitory pathway, is involved in the pain-suppressing effects of ONS [17].

The underlying mechanism of fibromyalgia is not known, but there is a possible mechanism contributing to sensitization that relates to increased facilitatory modulation that might go together with dysfunctional inhibitory pathway activity [21]. Two ascending pathways and one descending pathway encode pain from fibromyalgia. The ascending medial pathways encode the motivational/affective components of pain [22, 23], clinically expressed as unpleasantness, while the ascending lateral pathway [23] discriminates the sensory aspects of pain that include localization, intensity, and character of pain. The descending inhibitory pain pathway seems to be involved in decreasing the ongoing pain in a state-dependent manner [24]. Indeed, several neuroimaging studies have shown both structural and functional alterations via connectivity changes that amplify the pain perception in combination with defective inhibition of nociceptive signals [25, 26]. The pregenual anterior cingulate cortex, which plays a critical role in this pain inhibitory pathway, has been found to be altered in fibromyalgia patients [25, 27]. More recent research fine-tunes this concept by considering the underlying pathophysiological mechanism of fibromyalgia as a balance problem between the descending pain inhibitory pregenual anterior cingulate cortex pathway and the pain-detecting dorsal anterior cingulate cortex [19].

The exact mechanism of action that underpins the effect of ONS to treat fibromyalgia-related symptoms is not clear. Therefore, the aim of current study is to investigate how ONS exerts pain inhibition on fibromyalgia patients. Fibromyalgia patients implanted at the greater occipital nerve were scanned using $H_2^{15}O$ – PET to measure regional cerebral blood flow (rCBF). The advantage of using PET instead of fMRI is a reduced risk of electrode migration after implantation along with clearer data that is unaffected by electromagnetic artifacts. In addition, neurophysiological data were also collected. Previous research demonstrated that occipital nerve field tDCS normalizes the imbalance between the pain provoking dorsal anterior cingulate cortex and pain inhibiting pregenual anterior cingulate cortex mainly by modulating the descending pain inhibitory pathway [19]. Based on these previous findings, we expect changes in the descending pain inhibitory pathway during ONS that correlate with a reduction in the pain-related symptoms of fibromyalgia.

Methods

Patients suffering from fibromyalgia were selected by the Department of Physical Medicine and Rehabilitation at the University Hospital Antwerp, Belgium according to the criteria of the ACR-90 [28]; note that the data were collected in 2010, i.e. before the ACR 2010 guidelines. Patients with pathologies mimicking the symptoms of fibromyalgia as well as patients suffering from severe organic or neuropsychiatric comorbidity (except minor depressive disorder or headache) were excluded from participation. None of the patients were suffering from cervicotrigeminal tract radicular symptoms or types of hemicrania.

All patients enrolled in this study were also part of a large, double blind, placebo-controlled clinical trial that is already published [12]. Seven patients agreed to be part of this sub-study. All patients were female with a mean age of 42.34 years (± 4.53 years). All patients were intractable to tricyclic antidepressants (amitriptyline), pain medication, magnesium supplements, physical therapy, and psychological support. All patients agreed to make no changes to their current medication intake, which primarily included the aforementioned medications. All patients gave written informed consent, and the ethical committee of the University Hospital Antwerp, Belgium approved the study.

Surgical procedures

The implantation was performed in an operating room under local anesthesia. After removing a small area of the occipital scalp hair, a 2.6-cm vertical incision was made left of the midline just underneath the occipital protuberance. A Tuohy needle was inserted in the subcutaneous plane and tunneled 5.2 cm directed to the contralateral pinna of the ear. Next, a St. Jude Medical Octrode electrode (St Jude Medical, Plano, TX, USA) was inserted through the Tuohy needle, after which the needle was removed. Just underneath the hairline, the lead was tunneled at a sharp angle (315°) to the contralateral side to exit the skin and was then affixed to the skin by a butterfly anchor with a restraining loop. In order to create a similar strain relief loop, the lead was tunneled to a small subcutaneous pocket at the contralateral cervical area in order. In order to connect to an extension lead from the pocket, the lead was tunneled to the ipsilateral intrascapular area (extension 60 cm, St Jude Medical, Plano, TX, USA). The extension lead was tunneled to a subcutaneous pocket in the gluteal area and connected to an internal pulse generator (Eon mini, St. Jude Medical, Plano, TX, USA).

Stimulation parameters

Patients were stimulated at sub-sensory threshold stimulation for two weeks. This threshold was determined by increasing the amplitude until patients experienced paresthesia and then decreasing the amplitude to 90% of this threshold, with manual pressure overlying the electrode to ascertain no paresthesia would be felt while lying down with pressure on the back of the head.

Clinical outcomes

The primary outcome parameter for the efficacy of treatment is change in Fibromyalgia Impact Questionnaire scores (FIQ). This questionnaire measures the overall impact of fibromyalgia-related symptoms on a patient's quality of life. The maximum score is 100, and a higher score indicates a higher disease burden [29]. This questionnaire was assessed at baseline, after 4-weeks, after 12-weeks, after 18-weeks, and after 24-weeks of treatment. The secondary outcomes are the Pain Vigilance and Awareness Questionnaire (PVAQ), Pain Catastrophizing Scale (PCS), and Numeric Rating Scales (NRS) for both pain and quality of life. The PVAQ measures preoccupation with or attention to pain and is associated with pain-related fear and perceived pain severity [30]. The NRS was used to assess quality of life; a higher NRS score indicates a higher quality of life while living with pain caused by a) fibromyalgia, b) bone pain, c) non-specific pain, or d) headache-related pain. It was used to measure symptom relief and treatment satisfaction. This was performed at baseline, after 4-weeks, after 12-weeks, after 18-weeks, and after 24-weeks of treatment.

Pet

The $H_2^{15}O$ PET scans were acquired with a Siemens Biograph 64 TOF MI PET/computed tomography (Siemens, Knoxville, USA). PET scans were taken during both A) "ON" (active stimulation) and B) "OFF" (stimulation device turned off) conditions. A total of 6 scans (2 conditions × 3 samples) were performed per patient in randomized order. Data acquisition (2 min) started simultaneously with the intravenous bolus injection of 10 mCi $H_2^{15}O$. There was a 15-min interval between 2 successive injections. The data were reconstructed with the Ordered Subsets Expectation Maximization algorithm followed by a 4-mm Gaussian filter to a 200 × 200 × 74 matrix with zoom set equal to 2 resulting in 2 × 2 × 3 mm voxels.

Image preprocessing was performed using PMOD (version 3.3; PMOD Technologies, Switzerland) and included normalization of the PET images to the SPM water template in MNI space followed by smoothing with a 12-mm FWHM Gaussian Kernel. Voxel-based statistical analysis was carried out using the Statistical Parametric Mapping 8 program (SPM8; Institute of Neurology, University College of London, England, U.K.), implemented in Matlab version 2011a (MathWorks Inc., Natick, MA, USA). The SPM analysis included a flexible factorial design with proportional scaling to account for global changes. Two contrasts were analyzed: (1) ON – OFF (activation) and (2) OFF – ON (deactivation) and the resulting T-map data were interrogated at a peak probability level of 0.05 (uncorrected) and an extent threshold of more than > 250 voxels.

EEG

Recordings were obtained in a fully lighted room with each participant sitting upright on a small but comfortable chair. The actual recording lasted approximately five minutes. The EEG was sampled using Mitsar-201 amplifiers (NovaTech http://www.novatecheeg.com/) with 19 electrodes placed according to the standard 10–20 International placement (Fp1, Fp2, F7, F3, Fz, F4, F8, T7, C3, Cz, C4, T8, P7, P3, Pz, P4, P8, O1, O2), analogous to what was done in the normative group. Impedances were checked to remain below 5 kΩ. Data were collected eyes-closed (sampling rate = 500 Hz, band passed 0.15–200 Hz). Recordings were done during stimulation (ON) and without stimulation (OFF). We recorded for 2 min ON followed by 2 OFF and continued this pattern until we had 6 min of data for both conditions.

To remove artifacts related to stimulation, we used an ICA method to specifically select the signal related to the stimulation. Neuling and coworkers recently described this method as a reliable way to remove these specific artifacts [31, 32]. In addition, off-line data were resampled to 128 Hz, band-pass filtered in the range 2–44 Hz, subsequently transposed into Eureka! software [33], plotted, and carefully inspected for manual artifact-rejection. All episodic artifacts including eye blinks, eye movements, teeth clenching, body movement, and ECG artifacts were removed from the stream of the EEG. Average Fourier cross-spectral matrices were computed for frequency bands delta (2–3.5 Hz), theta (4–7.5 Hz), alpha1 (8–10 Hz), alpha2 (10–12 Hz), beta1 (13–18 Hz), beta2 (18.5–21 Hz), beta3 (21.5–30 Hz), and gamma (30.5–44 Hz).

Standardized low-resolution brain electromagnetic tomography (sLORETA; Pascual-Marqui, 2002) was used to estimate the intracerebral electrical sources. As a standard procedure, a common average reference transformation [34] was performed before applying the sLORETA algorithm. sLORETA computes electric neuronal activity as current density (A/m^2) without assuming a predefined number of active sources. The solution space used in this study and associated lead field matrix are those implemented in the LORETA-Key software (freely available at http://www.uzh.ch/keyinst/loreta.htm). This software implements revisited realistic electrode coordinates [35] and the lead field produced by [36] applying the boundary element method on the MNI-152 (Montreal Neurological Institute, Canada). The sLORETA-key

anatomical template divides and labels the neocortical (including hippocampus and anterior cingulate cortex) MNI-152 volume into 6239 voxels of dimension 5 mm^3, based on probabilities returned by the Demon Atlas [37]. The co-registration makes use of the correct translation from the MNI-152 space into the Talairach and Tournoux space.

The methodology used is a non-parametric permutation test. It is based on estimating, via randomization, the empirical probability distribution for the max-statistic under the null hypothesis comparisons [38]. This methodology corrects for multiple testing (i.e. for the collection of tests performed for all voxels and for all frequency bands). Due to the non-parametric nature of this method, its validity does not rely on any assumption of Gaussianity [38]. The significance threshold for all tests was based on a permutation test with 5000 permutations. Comparisons were made between the ON and OFF stimulation conditions. These comparisons were performed on a whole brain by sLORETA statistical contrast maps through multiple voxel-by-voxel comparisons in a logarithm of t-ratio.

Results

Clinical outcome

Clinical data of patients at baseline, after 4-weeks, after 12-weeks, after 18-weeks, and after 24-weeks of treatment are summarized in Table 1. For the primary outcome measure (FIQ), we observe a decrease of 25.84%. For the secondary outcome measure PVAQ, we found a decrease of 34.51%. For the pain complaints, there was a drop of 30.71% for fibromyalgia pain, 35.75% for bone and joint pain, and 30.52% for non-specified pain. In addition, patients reported a 59.24% improvement in quality of life.

PET results

We identified activation (ON – OFF contrast) in the left ventral medial prefrontal cortex, the dorsal lateral prefrontal cortex, the left superior frontal gyrus, the right parahippocampal gyrus, the left inferior temporal gyrus extending into the right fusiform gyrus, and the bilateral anterior cingulate cortex. In addition, deactivation (OFF – ON contrast) was demonstrated in the left somatosensory association cortex, the right lingual gyrus extending into the cuneus, the left precentral gyrus, the left supramarginal gyrus, and the right precuneus (See Table 2 and Fig. 1).

EEG results

A comparison between the ON and OFF stimulation conditions shows a significant increase ($t = 3.65$, $p < .05$) in activity at the pregenual anterior cingulate cortex extending into the ventral medial prefrontal cortex for the theta, alpha1, alpha2, beta1, and beta2 frequency bands

Table 1 Primary and secondary outcomes at baseline and 4-weeks, 12-weeks, 18-weeks, and 24-weeks after baseline

	Baseline	4-weeks	12-weeks	18-weeks	24-weeks	p value
Primary Outcome Measure						
FIQ	59.26[a]	37.16[b]	40.36[b]	42.04[b]	43.95[b]	0.006
Secondary Outcome Measures						
PVAQ	40.57[a]	32.71[b]	26.71[b]	26.71[b]	26.57[b]	0.003
PCS	20.84[a]	10.43[b]	8.86[b]	8.29[b]	10..28[b]	0.006
NRS						
Overall Quality of Life	3.14[a]	6.00[b]	6.14[b]	6.00[b]	5.00[b]	0.01
Overall Fibromyalgia Pain	7.00[a]	4.00[b]	4.29[b]	4.42[b]	4.85[b]	0.001
Overall Bone and Joint Pain	8.00[a]	4.14[b]	5.14[b]	4.86[b]	5.14[b]	0.004
Overall Non-Specified Pain	5.57[a]	4.00[a,b]	3.28[b]	3.42[b]	3.87[b]	0.033

[a], [b] indicate that they are significantly different

during stimulation (see Fig. 2). No effects were obtained for the delta, beta3, or gamma frequency bands.

Discussion

This study aims to better understand the underlying neural effects of occipital nerve field stimulation (ONS) for the treatment of fibromyalgia using $H_2^{15}O$ PET. The therapeutic outcome after 24 weeks of treatment was similar to the outcome in a larger population showing significant decreases in both the perceptual and affective components of pain as well as an improvement in quality of life [12]. Our research demonstrated increased rCBF changes (activation) in the ventral medial prefrontal cortex, dorsal lateral prefrontal cortex, pregenual anterior cingulate cortex, and parahippocampus. In addition, we also observed decreased rCBF (deactivation) in the somatosensory cortex, the ventral lateral prefrontal cortex, and the precuneus during subthreshold stimulation in comparison to no subthreshold stimulation. We also found increased activity in the pregenual anterior cingulate cortex extending into the ventral

medial prefrontal cortex for the theta, alpha1, alpha 2, beta1, and beta2 frequency bands during subthreshold stimulation in comparison to no subthreshold stimulation. In the discussion, we will only focus on the PET findings.

Our results showed increased activity for both $H_2^{15}O$ PET and EEG in the pregenual anterior cingulate cortex extending into the ventral medial prefrontal cortex during ONS in comparison to no stimulation. The pregenual anterior cingulate cortex extending into the ventral medial prefrontal cortex, as well as the periaqueductal gray, parahippocampus, anterior insula, hypothalamus, and rostral ventromedial brainstem are all part of the descending pain inhibitory or antinociceptive pathway [24, 39]. Previous research has shown that this descending pathway is involved in stress-mediated pain inhibition [40] and placebo analgesia [41] and is deficient in pain syndromes such as fibromyalgia [42]. This deficiency in the descending pain pathway could explain why fibromyalgia patients have spontaneous widespread pain all over their body, i.e. the pain results from insufficient spontaneous pain suppression, and is non-topographic. Mechanistically, the rostral- to

Table 2 Statistical Parametric Mapping PET Analysis: regions of activation (ON – OFF) and regions of deactivation (OFF – ON) with $p_{uncorrected} < 0.05$ and k > 250 voxels

Region	Talairach coordinates (x, y, z)			Side	Area	t-value
Activation	−11.80	49.47	0.25	Left	Ventral medial prefrontal cortex	5.27
	−16.18	41.41	43.96	Left	Dorsolateral prefrontal cortex	4.41
	34.29	−17.32	−11.20	Right	Parahippocampus	4.06
	−45.22	−16.39	−17.86	Left	Left inferior temporal gyrus	3.51
	39.86	−39.19	−18.58	Right	Fusiform gyrus	3.51
	0.93	28.21	5.16	Interhemispheric	Pregenual anterior cingulate cortex	3.21
Deactivation	−20.35	−42.47	55.76	Left	Somatosensory cortex	4.60
	17.30	−81.81	−4.98	Right	Visual cortex	3.89
	16.90	6.97	3.88	Left	Ventral lateral prefrontal cortex	3.88
	−62.46	−35.21	21.50	Left	Auditory cortex	3.01
	18.56	−44.19	52.65	Right	Precuneus	2.99

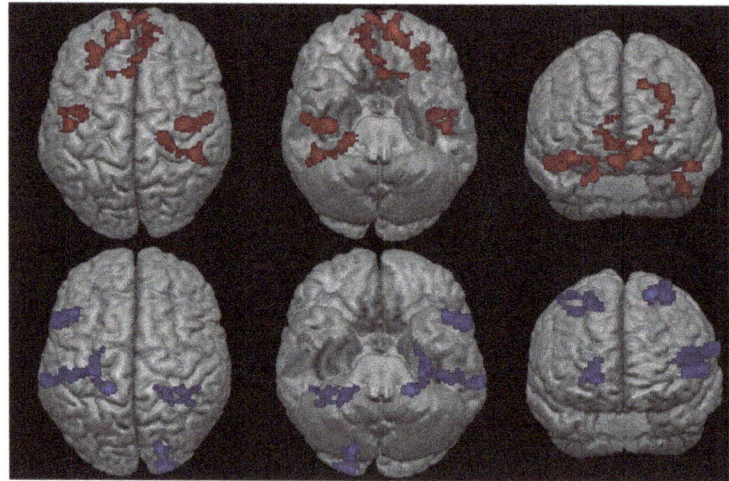

Fig. 1 Pet scan data regions of activation (on - off; red) and regions of deactivation (off - on; blue)

pregenual anterior cingulate cortex is functionally connected to the periaqueductal gray [43], and this resting state functional connectivity between the anterior cingulate cortex and the periaqueductal gray is abnormal in fibromyalgia patients [44]. Furthermore, a direct link between the pregenual anterior cingulate cortex and periaqueductal gray (i.e. main areas of the descending pain pathways) and the C2 area has been shown [45]. This fits with our findings that stimulating the greater occipital nerve modulates the pregenual anterior cingulate cortex extending into the ventral medial prefrontal cortex. The changes seen in the pregenual anterior cingulate cortex activity both on PET and EEG functional imaging during ONS are associated with a decrease in pain complaints. It is therefore very likely that

ONS reverses the dysfunction of the pain inhibition pathway in fibromyalgia, resulting in the pregenual anterior cingulate cortex extending into the ventral medial prefrontal cortex regaining its ability to suppress pain. A recent PET study in patients with cluster headache showed that changes in the pregenual anterior cingulate cortex are involved in the pain-suppressing effect of ONS [46]. This suggests that the pregenual anterior cingulate cortex is involved in pain suppression in a non-specific way, as a similar mechanism is involved in migraine and fibromyalgia related pain.

Increased activity was also observed for the left dorsal lateral prefrontal cortex during ONS in comparison to no stimulation using $H_2^{15}O$ PET. Previous research

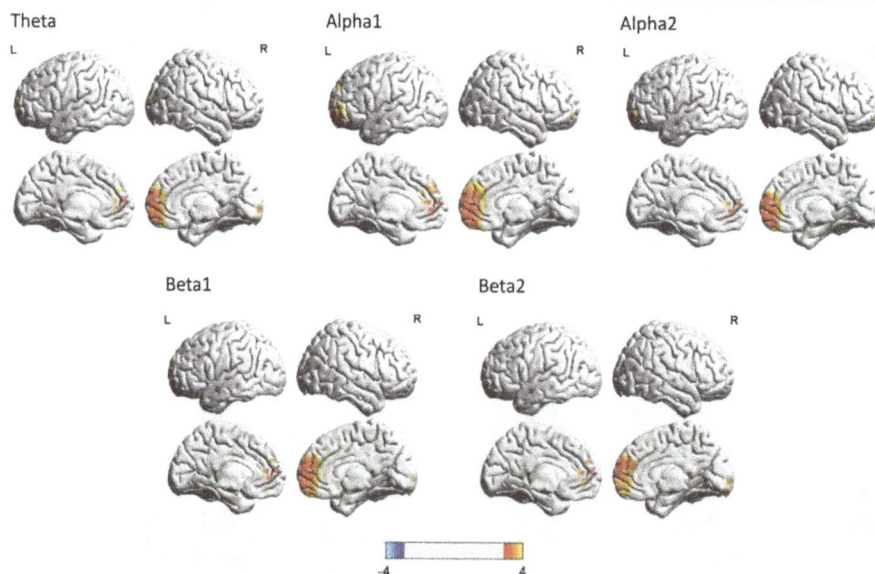

Fig. 2 A comparison between the on and off stimulation conditions show a significant increase in activity at the pregenual anterior cingulate cortex extending into the ventral medial prefrontal cortex for the theta, alpha1, alpha2, beta1, and beta2 frequency bands during stimulation

already demonstrated the involvement of the dorsal lateral prefrontal cortex in cognitive processes [47] such as attention [48, 49], value encoding [50–52], and emotional regulation [53]. Important to the concept of pain, the left dorsal lateral prefrontal cortex has also been associated with regulation of top-down modulation and driving appropriate behavioral responses [54, 55]. Indeed, a recent PET study reported that the dorsal lateral prefrontal cortex plays a role in inhibiting pain [56]. Furthermore, it has been reported that stimulating the left dorsal lateral prefrontal cortex using non-invasive brain stimulation improves attention in patients with cognitive dysfunction. Taken together, these findings lead to the hypothesis that left dorsal lateral prefrontal cortex activation during stimulation inhibits the affective/emotional pain pathway via a top-down mechanism. Other supporting evidence for this effect comes from spinal cord stimulation (SCS) for pain. It has been shown that burst SCS, in contrast to tonic SCS, modulates the affective/motivational/attentional component of pain [57–60], and this is associated with changes in the dorsal anterior cingulate cortex and dorsal lateral prefrontal cortex [58].

Our results also demonstrate increased activation of the parahippocampus during ONS. The parahippocampus is associated with contextual processing and is important in pain processing [61–65]. It has been shown that fibromyalgia is associated with metabolite abnormalities within the right (para)hippocampus that correlate with patient symptoms due to chronic stress [66, 67]. This is consistent with the notion of a generalized aversion/distress network consisting of the parahippocampus, cerebellum, hypothalamus, and subgenual anterior cingulate cortex [68]. Parahippocampal involvement in pain might be due to contextual memory, which can modulate pain via its influence on the descending pain pathway, thereby encoding aversive pain memory [39, 69]. In fibromyalgia, it is known that this contextual pain suppression mechanism is dysfunctional, leading to a subsequent dysregulation of emotional contextual pain suppression [42, 70]. Based on these findings it is hypothesized that the parahippocampal area is a control switch for the involvement of the ascending medial pathway in the affective component of pain and the descending pain inhibitory pathway [71]. Conceptually, stimulation of the greater occipital nerves activates the parahippocampus, which subsequently controls the mobilization of the medial pain and descending inhibitory pathway [72].

Although several papers have reported activity changes in the inferior temporal and fusiform gyri in the pain literature, the exact functional significance of these changes is unknown. It has been hypothesized that these areas are involved in cognitive pain-processing related to

greater vigilance and attention to pain. This is based on recollection of prior pain experience, expectations for future pain, and negative pain appraisal [73]. Interestingly, both anxiety and mental fatigue have been negatively associated with activation of the inferior temporal gyrus/fusiform gyrus [74]. Our data show increased activation during ONS in the inferior temporal and fusiform gyri might be due to reduced anxiety and/or mental fatigue; however, further research is needed to verify this speculation.

We also observed decreased rCBF in the somatosensory, auditory, and visual cortices during ONS in comparison to no stimulation. Previous literature has already suggested an indirect connection between the C2-C3 nerve and these sensory areas [75, 76], and occipital nerve stimulation has been shown to help in the suppression of auditory phantom percepts such as tinnitus [77–79]. The role of the somatosensory cortex as part of the lateral pain pathway responsible for encoding discriminatory/sensory pain information is well known in the pain literature generally [80], but even more specifically in fibromyalgia [81–84]. Our findings suggest that ONS can also modulate the lateral pain pathway, thereby changing the balance between pain input and pain suppression [85], leading to probable restoration of defective intracortical inhibition as we hypothesized [86]. This also confirms a recent study using functional magnetic resonance imaging during ONS that shows alterations in the somatosensory cortex during stimulation in healthy subjects [18].

Another interesting finding is reduced rCBF in the precuneus when the stimulation is turned on. The precuneus extending into posterior cingulate cortex is thought to comprise the functional core of the default mode network, which also includes the bilateral inferior parietal cortices and medial prefrontal cortex. It is known that the default mode network undergoes reorganizational changes and functional connectivity changes during chronic pain in fibromyalgia patients [87]. The default mode network is activated when attention is engaged with thoughts unrelated to pain or mind wandering and deactivated when the attention is focused on pain [88]. Furthermore, it is known that the precuneus extending into the posterior cingulate cortex is activated during pain processing and inactive during (placebo) analgesia [89, 90]. Similarly, ONS reduces rCBF in the precuneus extending into the posterior cingulate cortex in fibromyalgia, leading to pain suppression. Alternatively, it also possible that ONS modifies the pain percept and indirectly modulates the internal model (self-reference) of pain that is associated with fibromyalgia patients. The main hub of the self-referential default mode network is the posterior cingulate cortex [91, 92] that allows adaptation to changes in the environment [93]. Adapting to these changes requires that internal and external stimuli are predicted and compared to the current state of the self. This likely occurs at the posterior cingulate cortex [94–96]. ONS consequently could induce reference resetting due to changes in the precuneus extending into the posterior cingulate—areas of the brain that could obtain an internal reference without pain, analogous to what has been proposed in obesity. Indeed, in food addiction, it has been proposed that the self-referential set point of how much energy was required to maintain a stable energetic milieu interieur critically depends on the posterior cingulate/precuneus, and that the precuneus resets the balance between food input (i.e. dorsal anterior cingulate cortex) and food input suppression (pregenual anterior cingulate cortex) [97]. Even though this is speculation, it is possible that the posterior cingulate cortex's function, as a regulator of the body's adaptation to the external and internal environment, might indeed be analogous for different stimuli, i.e. might be non-specific, similar to the dorsal anterior cingulate cortex, whether for pain or for food.

Conclusion

In this study, we demonstrated the effect of ONS in fibromyalgia patients and specifically its effect on different brain structures. ONS seems to exert an inhibitory effect on structures in the ascending lateral pathways of multiple sensory inputs (such as the somatosensory, visual, and auditory cortices) and medial pain pathways (such as the dorsal lateral prefrontal cortex) that mediate the affective component of pain. ONS also modulates the descending pain pathway by activating the pain-suppressing pregenual anterior cingulate cortex and parahippocampal area. Further functional imaging studies should be performed to evaluate these findings on a larger sample size and with other neuromodulation techniques.

Abbreviations
^{18}F-FDG PET: ^{18}F-fluorodeoxyglucose positron emission tomograph; EEG: Electroencephalogram; FIQ: Fibromyalgia impact questionnaire scores; fMRI: Functional magnetic resonance imaging; NRS: Numeric rating scales; ONS: occipital nerve field stimulation; PCS: Pain catastrophizing scale; PVAQ: Pain vigilance and awareness questionnaire; rCBF: Regional cerebral blood flow; SCS: Spinal cord stimulation

Acknowledgements
The authors thank Christian Davidson for his help in proofreading the manuscript.

Funding
This research was supported by the St. Jude Medical. The funders had no role in study design, data collection and analysis, decision to publish or preparation of the manuscript.

Authors' contribution
Conceived and design the experiments: MP, DDR, JO, GS, SS, SC, PD, SS. Data analysis: SD, SA, SV. Manuscript preparation: SA, SV, DDR. All authors read and approved the final manuscript.

Competing interest
The authors declare that they have no competing interests.

Author details
[1]School of Behavioral and Brain Sciences, The University of Texas at Dallas, Richardson, Texas, USA. [2]Department of Neurosurgery, University Hospital Antwerp, Antwerp, Belgium. [3]BRAI3N, Ghent, Belgium. [4]Department of physical health hand rehabilitation, University Hospital Antwerp, Edegem, Belgium. [5]Department of Cognitive Neurology, UZ Leuven, Leuven, Belgium. [6]Department of nuclear medicine, University Hospital Antwerp, Edegem, Belgium. [7]Molecular Imaging Centre, University of Antwerp, Edegem, Belgium. [8]Department of Surgical Sciences, Dunedin School of Medicine, University of Otago, Dunedin, New Zealand.

References
1. Wolfe F, et al. Aspects of fibromyalgia in the general population: sex, pain threshold, and fibromyalgia symptoms. J Rheumatol. 1995;22(1):151–6.
2. Rahman A, Underwood M, Carnes D. Fibromyalgia. Bmj. 2014;348:g1224.
3. Queiroz LP. Worldwide epidemiology of fibromyalgia. Curr Pain Headache Rep. 2013;17(8):356.
4. Berger A, et al. Patterns of healthcare utilization and cost in patients with newly diagnosed fibromyalgia. Am J Manag Care. 2010;16(5 Suppl):S126–37.
5. Perrot S, et al. Societal and individual burden of illness among fibromyalgia patients in France: association between disease severity and OMERACT core domains. BMC Musculoskelet Disord. 2012;13:22.
6. Sauer K, Kemper C, Glaeske G. Fibromyalgia syndrome: prevalence, pharmacological and non-pharmacological interventions in outpatient health care. An analysis of statutory health insurance data. Joint Bone Spine. 2011;78(1):80–4.
7. Chinn S, Caldwell W, Gritsenko K. Fibromyalgia pathogenesis and treatment options update. Curr Pain Headache Rep. 2016;20(4):25.
8. Marlow NM, Bonilha HS, Short EB. Efficacy of transcranial direct current stimulation and repetitive transcranial magnetic stimulation for treating fibromyalgia syndrome: a systematic review. Pain Practice. 2013;13(2):131–45.
9. Taylor AG, et al. Cranial electrical stimulation improves symptoms and functional status in individuals with fibromyalgia. Pain Management Nursing. 2013;14(4):327–35.
10. Thimineur M, De Ridder D. C2 area neurostimulation: a surgical treatment for fibromyalgia. Pain Med. 2007;8(8):639–46.
11. Plazier M, et al. Peripheral nerve stimulation for fibromyalgia, in Peripheral Nerve Stimulation. Basel: Karger Publishers; 2011. p. 133–46.
12. Plazier M, et al. Occipital nerve stimulation in fibromyalgia: a double-blind placebo-controlled pilot study with a six-month follow-up. Neuromodulation: Technology at the Neural Interface. 2014;17(3):256–64.
13. Weiner RL, Reed KL. Peripheral neurostimulation for control of intractable occipital neuralgia. Neuromodulation: Technology at the Neural Interface. 1999;2(3):217–21.
14. Le Doare K, et al. Occipital afferent activation of second order neurons in the trigeminocervical complex in rat. Neurosci Lett. 2006;403(1):73–7.
15. Goadsby PJ, Knight YE, Hoskin KL. Stimulation of the greater occipital nerve increases metabolic activity in the trigeminal nucleus caudalis and cervical dorsal horn of the cat. Pain. 1997;73(1):23–8.

16. Busch V, et al. Functional connectivity between trigeminal and occipital nerves revealed by occipital nerve blockade and nociceptive blink reflexes. Cephalalgia. 2006;26(1):50–5.

17. Magis D, et al. Occipital nerve stimulation for drug-resistant chronic cluster headache: a prospective pilot study. The Lancet Neurology. 2007;6(4):314–21.

18. Kovacs S, et al. Central effects of occipital nerve electrical stimulation studied by functional magnetic resonance imaging. Neuromodulation: Technology at the Neural Interface. 2011;14(1):46–57.

19. De Ridder D, Vanneste S. Occipital nerve field transcranial direct current stimulation normalizes imbalance between pain detecting and pain inhibitory pathways in fibromyalgia. Neurotherapeutics. 2016:1–18.

20. Matharu MS, et al. Central neuromodulation in chronic migraine patients with suboccipital stimulators: a PET study. Brain. 2004;127(1):220–30.

21. Pujol J, et al. Mapping brain response to pain in fibromyalgia patients using temporal analysis of FMRI. PLoS One. 2009;4(4):e5224.

22. Price DD. Psychological and neural mechanisms of the affective dimension of pain. Science. 2000;288(5472):1769–72.

23. Bushnell MC, Čeko M, Low LA. Cognitive and emotional control of pain and its disruption in chronic pain. Nat Rev Neurosci. 2013;14(7):502–11.

24. Fields H. State-dependent opioid control of pain. Nat Rev Neurosci. 2004; 5(7):565–75.

25. Jensen KB, et al. Overlapping structural and functional brain changes in patients with long-term exposure to fibromyalgia pain. Arthritis Rheum. 2013;65(12):3293–303.

26. Schmidt-Wilcke T, et al. Resting state connectivity correlates with drug and placebo response in fibromyalgia patients. Neuroimage Clin. 2014;6:252–61.

27. Jensen KB, et al. Patients with fibromyalgia display less functional connectivity in the brain's pain inhibitory network. Mol Pain. 2012;8:32.

28. Wolfe F, et al. The American College of Rheumatology 1990 criteria for the classification of fibromyalgia. Report of the multicenter criteria committee. Arthritis Rheum. 1990;33(2):160–72.

29. Bennett R. The fibromyalgia impact questionnaire (FIQ): a review of its development, current version, operating characteristics and uses. Clin Exp Rheumatol. 2005;23(5 Suppl 39):S154–62.

30. McCracken LM. "Attention" to pain in persons with chronic pain: a behavioral approach. Behav Ther. 1997;28(2):271–84.

31. Neuling T, et al. Friends, not foes: magnetoencephalography as a tool to uncover brain dynamics during transcranial alternating current stimulation. Neuroimage. 2015;118:406–13.

32. Neuling T, et al. Faith and oscillations recovered: on analyzing EEG/MEG signals during tACS. Neuroimage. 2017;147:960–3.

33. Congedo, M., EureKa! (version 3.0) [computer software]. Knoxville, TN: NovaTech EEG Inc. freeware available at www.NovaTechEEG. 2002.

34. Pascual-Marqui RD. Standardized low-resolution brain electromagnetic tomography (sLORETA): technical details. Methods Find Exp Clin Pharmacol. 2002;(24 Suppl D):5–12.

35. Jurcak V, Tsuzuki D, Dan I. 10/20, 10/10, and 10/5 systems revisited: their validity as relative head-surface-based positioning systems. Neuroimage. 2007;34(4):1600–11.

36. Fuchs M, et al. A standardized boundary element method volume conductor model. Clin Neurophysiol. 2002;113(5):702–12.

37. Mazziotta JC, et al. A probabilistic atlas of the human brain: theory and rationale for its development. Neuroimage. 1995;2(2):89–101.

38. Nichols TE, Holmes AP. Nonparametric permutation tests for functional neuroimaging: a primer with examples. Hum Brain Mapp. 2002;15(1):1–25.

39. Kong J, et al. Exploring the brain in pain: activations, deactivations and their relation. Pain. 2010;148(2):257–67.

40. Yilmaz P, et al. Brain correlates of stress-induced analgesia. Pain. 2010;151(2): 522–9.

41. Eippert F, et al. Activation of the opioidergic descending pain control system underlies placebo analgesia. Neuron. 2009;63(4):533–43.

42. Jensen KB, et al. Overlapping structural and functional brain changes in patients with long-term exposure to fibromyalgia pain. Arthritis & Rheumatism. 2013;65(12):3293–303.

43. Coulombe MA, et al. Intrinsic functional connectivity of periaqueductal gray subregions in humans. Hum Brain Mapp. 2016;37(4):1514–30.

44. Truini A, et al. Abnormal resting state functional connectivity of the periaqueductal grey in patients with fibromyalgia. Clin Exp Rheumatol. 2016; 34(2 Suppl 96):S129–33.

45. Xie Y-f, Huo F-q, Tang J-s. Cerebral cortex modulation of pain. Acta Pharmacol Sin. 2009;30(1):31–41.

46. Magis D, et al. Central modulation in cluster headache patients treated with occipital nerve stimulation: an FDG-PET study. BMC Neurol. 2011;11:25.

47. Cieslik EC, et al. Is there "one" DLPFC in cognitive action control? Evidence for heterogeneity from co-activation-based parcellation. Cereb Cortex. 2013; 23:2677–789.

48. Vossel S, Geng JJ, Fink GR. Dorsal and ventral attention systems distinct neural circuits but collaborative roles. Neuroscientist. 2014;20(2):150–9.

49. Kouneiher F, Charron S, Koechlin E. Motivation and cognitive control in the human prefrontal cortex. Nat Neurosci. 2009;12(7):939–45.

50. Liu Y, et al. Top-down modulation of neural activity in anticipatory visual attention: control mechanisms revealed by simultaneous EEG-fMRI. Cereb Cortex. 2016;26:517–29.

51. Sokol-Hessner P, et al. Decision value computation in DLPFC and VMPFC adjusts to the available decision time. Eur J Neurosci. 2012;35(7):1065–74.

52. Barbey AK, Koenigs M, Grafman J. Dorsolateral prefrontal contributions to human working memory. Cortex. 2013;49(5):1195–205.

53. Treadway MT, et al. Corticolimbic gating of emotion-driven punishment. Nat Neurosci. 2014;17(9):1270–5.

54. Sallet J, et al. The organization of dorsal frontal cortex in humans and macaques. J Neurosci. 2013;33(30):12255–74.

55. O'Reilly RC. The what and how of prefrontal cortical organization. Trends Neurosci. 2010;33(8):355–61.

56. Lorenz J, Minoshima S, Casey K. Keeping pain out of mind: the role of the dorsolateral prefrontal cortex in pain modulation. Brain. 2003;126(5):1079–91.

57. De Ridder D, et al. Burst spinal cord stimulation for limb and back pain. World neurosurgery. 2013;80(5):642–9.

58. De Ridder D, et al. Burst spinal cord stimulation: toward paresthesia-free pain suppression. Neurosurgery. 2010;66(5):986–90.

59. Courtney P, et al. Improved pain relief with burst spinal cord stimulation for two weeks in patients using tonic stimulation: results from a small clinical study. Neuromodulation: Technology at the Neural Interface. 2015;18(5):361–6.

60. Schu S, et al. A prospective, randomised, double-blind, placebo-controlled study to examine the effectiveness of burst spinal cord stimulation patterns for the treatment of failed back surgery syndrome. Neuromodulation: Technology at the Neural Interface. 2014;17(5):443–50.

61. Aminoff E, Gronau N, Bar M. The parahippocampal cortex mediates spatial and nonspatial associations. Cereb Cortex. 2007;17(7):1493–503.

62. Bar M, Aminoff E, Ishai A. Famous faces activate contextual associations in the parahippocampal cortex. Cereb Cortex. 2008;18(6):1233–8.

63. Bar M, Aminoff E, Schacter DL. Scenes unseen: the parahippocampal cortex intrinsically subserves contextual associations, not scenes or places per se. J Neurosci. 2008;28(34):8539–44.

64. Eichenbaum H, Lipton PA. Towards a functional organization of the medial temporal lobe memory system: role of the parahippocampal and medial entorhinal cortical areas. Hippocampus. 2008;18(12):1314–24.

65. Ranganath C, Ritchey M. Two cortical systems for memory-guided behaviour. Nat Rev Neurosci. 2012;13(10):713–26.

66. Wood PB, et al. Hippocampal metabolite abnormalities in fibromyalgia: correlation with clinical features. J Pain. 2009;10(1):47–52.

67. Wood PB, Ledbetter CR, Patterson JC 2nd. Changes in hippocampal metabolites after effective treatment for fibromyalgia: a case study. Clin J Pain. 2009;25(9):810–4.

68. Moulton EA, et al. Aversion-related circuitry in the cerebellum: responses to noxious heat and unpleasant images. J Neurosci. 2011;31(10):3795–804.

69. De Ridder D, et al. Phantom percepts: tinnitus and pain as persisting aversive memory networks. Proc Natl Acad Sci U S A. 2011;108(20):8075–80.

70. Kamping S, et al. Deficient modulation of pain by a positive emotional context in fibromyalgia patients. Pain. 2013;154(9):1846–55.

71. De Ridder D, Vanneste S. Burst and tonic spinal cord stimulation: different and common brain mechanisms. Neuromodulation. 2016;19(1):47–59.

72. Leknes S, et al. The importance of context: when relative relief renders pain pleasant. Pain. 2013;154(3):402–10.

73. Schwedt TJ, et al. Enhanced pain-induced activity of pain-processing regions in a case-control study of episodic migraine. Cephalalgia. 2014;34(12):947–58.

74. Glass JM, et al. Executive function in chronic pain patients and healthy controls: different cortical activation during response inhibition in fibromyalgia. J Pain. 2011;12(12):1219–29.

75. Wu C, et al. Tinnitus: maladaptive auditory-somatosensory plasticity. Hear Res. 2016;334:20–9.

76. Lambert GA, et al. Effect of cortical spreading depression on activity of trigeminovascular sensory neurons. Cephalalgia. 1999;19(7):631–8.

77. Vanneste S, et al. Transcutaneous electrical nerve stimulation (TENS) of upper cervical nerve (C2) for the treatment of somatic tinnitus. Exp Brain Res. 2010;204(2):283–7.

78. De Ridder D, Vanneste S. Multitarget surgical neuromodulation: combined C2 and auditory cortex implantation for tinnitus. Neurosci Lett. 2015;591:202–6.

79. De Ridder D, et al. Surgical brain modulation for tinnitus: the past, present and future. J Neurosurg Sci. 2012;56(4):323–40.

80. Cagnie B, et al. Central sensitization in fibromyalgia? A systematic review on structural and functional brain MRI. Semin Arthritis Rheum. 2014;44(1):68–75.

81. Friebel U, Eickhoff SB, Lotze M. Coordinate-based meta-analysis of experimentally induced and chronic persistent neuropathic pain. Neuroimage. 2011;58(4):1070–80.

82. Price DD. Neuroscience - psychological and neural mechanisms of the affective dimension of pain. Science. 2000;288(5472):1769–72.

83. Bushnell MC, Ceko M, Low LA. Cognitive and emotional control of pain and its disruption in chronic pain. Nat Rev Neurosci. 2013;14(7):502–11.

84. Pujol J, et al. The contribution of sensory system functional connectivity reduction to clinical pain in fibromyalgia. Pain. 2014;155(8):1492–503.

85. De Ridder D, Vanneste S. Occipital nerve field transcranial direct current stimulation normalizes imbalance between pain detecting and pain inhibitory pathways in fibromyalgia. Neurotherapeutics. 2016.

86. Lim M, et al. Disinhibition of the primary somatosensory cortex in patients with fibromyalgia. Pain. 2015;156(4):666–74.

87. Baliki MN, et al. Functional reorganization of the default mode network across chronic pain conditions. PLoS One. 2014;9(9):e106133.

88. Kucyi A, Davis KD. The dynamic pain connectome. Trends Neurosci. 2015; 38(2):86–95.

89. Amanzio M, et al. Activation likelihood estimation meta-analysis of brain correlates of placebo analgesia in human experimental pain. Hum Brain Mapp. 2013;34(3):738–52.

90. Benedetti F, Amanzio M. Mechanisms of the placebo response. Pulm Pharmacol Ther. 2013;26(5):520–3.

91. Svoboda E, McKinnon MC, Levine B. The functional neuroanatomy of autobiographical memory: a meta-analysis. Neuropsychologia. 2006;44(12): 2189–208.

92. Buckner RL, Andrews-Hanna JR, Schacter DL. The brain's default network: anatomy, function, and relevance to disease. Ann N Y Acad Sci. 2008;1124:1–38.

93. Pearson JM, et al. Posterior cingulate cortex: adapting behavior to a changing world. Trends Cogn Sci. 2011;15(4):143–51.

94. De Ridder D, et al. The brain, obesity and addiction: an EEG neuroimaging study. Sci Rep. 2016;6:34122.

95. Bzdok D, et al. Subspecialization in the human posterior medial cortex. Neuroimage. 2015;106:55–71.

96. Leech R, Sharp DJ. The role of the posterior cingulate cortex in cognition and disease. Brain. 2014;137(Pt 1):12–32.

97. De Ridder D, et al. Allostasis in health and food addiction. Sci Rep. 2016;6: 37126.

19

Hydrogel coils versus bare platinum coils for the endovascular treatment of intracranial aneurysms

Tao Xue[1†], Zhouqing Chen[1†], Weiwei Lin[2], Jiayi Xu[3], Xuming Shen[4*] and Zhong Wang[1*] (iD)

Abstract

Background: Recent studies have shown conflicting results regarding the effect of hydrogel coils for treating intracranial aneurysm compared to bare platinum coils. We implemented a meta-analysis to assess the value of hydrogel coils in intracranial aneurysm treatment.

Methods: The MEDLINE, EMBASE, and Cochrane Library databases were searched for randomized controlled trials (RCTs) which had evaluated hydrogel coils versus bare platinum coils for intracranial aneurysms.

Results: We pooled 1526 patients from 4 RCTs with the mean follow-up time of more than 16 months. Hydrogel coils had reductions on mid-term recurrence (RR 0.78, 95% CI 0.65 to 0.94, $P = 0.008$) and residual aneurysm (RR 0.71, 95% CI 0.57 to 0.88, $P = 0.002$), but didn't show any significant differences in other favorable outcomes such as functional recovery, mortality and so on. In the subgroup analysis, we found that second-generation hydrogel coils might exhibit potential impacts on increasing mid-term complete occlusion (RR 1.26, 95% CI 1.07 to 1.48, $P = 0.005$) and decreasing residual aneurysm neck. (RR 0.54, 95% CI 0.34 to 0.86, $P = 0.010$).

Conclusions: Hydrogel coils showed no significant efficacy on functional recovery but exhibited a lower rate of recurrences and residual aneurysms in patients with intracranial aneurysms.

Keywords: Hydrogel coils, Bare platinum coils, Endovascular treatment, Intracranial aneurysms, Meta-analysis

Background

Worldwide, intracranial aneurysm, as a life-threatening disease with a high morbidity and mortality rate, brings great economic burdens to both the society and the patient [1]. Intracranial aneurysm is the third most common type of stroke, after ischemic stroke and hypertensive cerebral hemorrhage, which plays the most important role in subarachnoid hemorrhage [2].

Before 1990, neurosurgical operations were the only option for patients with intracranial aneurysm [3]. At 1992, Guglielmi detachable platinum coils(GDC) were introduced as an endovascular treatment which provided patients with an additional treatment option [4–6]. Endovascular coil emblization eventually became the preferred modality for many patients, due to better clinical outcomes than neurosurgical clipping in some patients with intracranial aneurysm demonstrated in ISAT(International Subarachnoid Aneurysm Trial) [7]. Although endovascular treatment is a less invasive procedure than neurosurgical aneurysm clipping, patients with endovascular treatment have a higher rate of aneurysm remnant, recurrence and retreatment than patients treated by clipping, in spite of the overall incidence is low [8–11]. Hence, there still exists a need for improvement in methods of embolization to reduce incomplete occlusion, recurrence, retreatment and post-treatment adverse events [4, 12, 13].

* Correspondence: szdx519@163.com; wangzhong761@163.com
†Tao Xue and Zhouqing Chen contributed equally to this work.
4Department of Neurosurgery, Taicang Affiliated Hospital of Soochow University, Suzhou 215400, Jiangsu Province, China
1Department of Neurosurgery & Brain and Nerve Research Laboratory, The First Affiliated Hospital of Soochow University, 188 Shizi Street, Suzhou 215006, China
Full list of author information is available at the end of the article

Hydrogel embolic system(HES) is made up of platinum coils covered with cross-linked material, which can absorb much water without dissolving, and presents both liquid-like and solid-like softening behaviors [4, 14]. Therefore, it may provide better efficacy and safety in endovascular treatment. The first-generation hydrogel-coated coils (hydro-Coil; MicroVention, Inc., Tustin,CA) [15] were assessed in some clinical trials to compare the clinical outcomes of hydrogel coils and bare platinum coils. These clinical trials include HELPS (Hydrocoil Endovascular aneurysm occLusion and Packing Study) [16] and Poncyljusz's RCT [17]. HELPS demonstrated that hydrogel coils have a reduction of adverse events and recurrence among intracranial aneurysm patients [18]. In contrast, Poncyljusz's RCT concluded that hydrogel coils were equally as effective as bare platinum coils [17]. Later, the second-generation hydrogel (Hydrosoft, HydroFrame[3D], MicroVention, Inc) was developed, which was softer, contained less hydrogel, and expanded slower than the first-generation one [19]. In 2018, GREAT(German-French Randomized Endovascular Aneurysm Trial) was established, and some researchers found that compared to bare platinum coils, hydrogel coils decrease the rate of unfavorable outcome events, recurrence, retreatment, morbidity mortality, and need for retreatment in small- and medium-sized intracranial aneurysms [19, 20]. Containing both types of hydrogel coils, PRET 2017(Patients prone to Recurrence after Endovascular Treatment) illustrated that there were no significant differences between hydrogel coils group and bare platinum coils group [21].

Based on the above-mentioned results from previous clinical studies and trials, the efficacy and safety of hydrogel coils treatment for intracranial aneurysm are unclear. Several issues still need to be resolved, including whether or not the use of hydrogel coils reduces incomplete occlusion, complications, adverse events, recurrence, retreatment, morbidity, mortality, etc. We present a meta-analysis of pooled data from previous clinical trials to investigate the value of hydrogel coils treatment for intracranial aneurysm and to explore the potential factors that might influence the efficacy and safety of hydrogel coils.

Methods

Study protocol

A research protocol was drafted following the Cochrane Collaboration format at the beginning of the project [22].

Eligibility criteria

The inclusion criteria were as follows: (a) Type of study: RCT; (b) Language restriction: only available in English; (c) Participating patients: patients with intracranial aneurysms; (d) Intervention: Hydrogel coils or bare platinum coils; (e) Outcomes: complete occlusion, residual neck and residual aneurysm on DSA, excellent outcome (mRS score = 0) and favorable outcome (mRS score = 0–2) based on mRS score, periprocedural complications, major recurrence, retreatment and adverse events. The exclusion criteria were as follows: (a) Types of study: retrospective studies, cohort studies, case reviews and case reports; (b) Control: positive control.

Information sources and search strategy

Three main databases: EMBASE, MEDLINE and Cochrane Library were systematically searched by three authors (TX, ZC and JX). The search strategy was a combination of the variables "coil" AND "intracranial aneurysm" for MEDLINE. Only studies that match the titles and abstracts were searched. The search strategy of Cochrane Library and EMBASE were similar to that search strategy of MEDLINE. In addition, two investigators (TX and ZC) ensured all relevant studies included in the study. They independently manually screened the list of references from the RCTs and systematic reviews.

Study selection and data collection

Two reviewers (TX and ZC) independently assessed all study records from systematic search in systematic reviews and reference lists of RCTs and electronic database on the previously mentioned the eligbility criteria. After the rigorous selection and evaluation of the literature by the two reviewers, the data were extracted from the included RCTs as follows: basic information for included RCTs, inclusion, exclusion criteria, study design and outcome assessments (Table 1).

Risk of Bias

The risk of bias plot was based on the Review Manager 5.2 software for individual studies. We applied the unified standard of the Cochrane Collaboration to assess the risk of bias of RCTs, which included: selection bias, performance bias, detection bias, attrition bias, reporting bias, and other potential biases.

Summary measures and synthesis of results

The data was assessed by STATA (Version 12.0) software. The risk ratio (relative risk [RR]; 95% confidence interval [CI]) was analyzed using dichotomous outcomes and calculated using a random effect model. Heterogeneity was estimated by the I^2 statistic. The I^2 statistic as follows: $I^2 < 30\%$ means "low heterogeneity"; $I^2 = 30$ to 50% denotes "moderate heterogeneity"; $I^2 > 50\%$ represents "substantial heterogeneity". Subgroup analyses were implemented to detect different generations hydrogel coils and ruptured rate of aneurysm at baseline. Explore the stability of the consolidated results using sensitivity analysis. A P value of less than 0.05 was considered to be significant and two-tailed tests were implemented for all analyses.

Hydrogel coils versus bare platinum coils for the endovascular treatment of intracranial...

167

Table 1 Characteristics of the Included Studies and Outcome Events

Trials	GREAT 2018 (DRKS00003132)	PRET 2017 (NCT00626912)	Poncyljusz's RCT 2014 (EURR-6928)	HELP 2011 (ISRCTN30531382)
Regions	22 centers in 2 countries	25 centers in 6 countries	1 centers in 1 country	24 centers in 7 countries
Publication	Stroke	Am J Neuroradiol	European Journal of Radiology	Lancet
Inclusion Criteria	Ruptured or unruptured IAs; WFNS grade: 0–3; Age: 18–75 years; IA size: 4-12 mm in diameter; Endovascular occlusion is deemed possible; Neurointerventionist is content to use either HC or BPC.	Ruptured or unruptured IAs; WFNS grade: 0–3; Age: > 18 years; Life expectancy: > 2 years Endovascular occlusion is considered possible by both coils; Neurointerventionist is satisfied with using either HC or BPC but not other type.	Only unruptured IAs; Endovascular occlusion is considered possible by both coils; Neurointerventionist is satisfied with using either HC or BPC but not other type.	Ruptured or unruptured IAs; Previously untreated IAs; Not pregnant; WFNS grade: 0–3; Age: 18–75 years; IA size: 2-25 mm in maximum diameter; Endovascular occlusion is deemed possible; Neurointerventionist is content to use either HC or BPC.
Exclusion Criteria	Patients already randomized in this trials; Pre-treated IA by coiling or clipping; More than one IAs need to be treated at the same treatment episode.	Other IAs requiring to be treated at the same treatment episode; Presence of AVM; Absolue contraindication to endovascular treatment.	Ruptured IAs; Intolerance to heparin or resistance to antiplatelet therapy, coagulopathies and abnormal platelet outcome.	Patients already randomized in this trials; More than one IAs need to be treated at the same treatment episode.
Study Design	Second-generation hydrogel coil (HydroSoft and/or HydroFrame) vs. Bare platinum coil	First or Second-generation hydrogel coil vs. Bare platinum coil	Hydrogel-coated coil vs. Bare platinum coil	First-generation hydrogel coil vs. Bare platinum coil
Efficacy outcomes	Complete occlusion, residual neck and residual aneurysm at periprecedure and 6–18 months; Recurrence, retreatment and mRS responese at 6–18 months.	Complete occlusion, residual neck and residual aneurysm at periprecedure; Recurrence, retreatment and mRS responese at 18 months.	Complete occlusion, residual neck and residual aneurysm at periprecedure and 12 months; Recurrence, retreatment and mRS responese at 12 months.	Complete occlusion, residual neck and residual aneurysm at periprecedure and 18 months; Recurrence, retreatment and mRS responese at 18 months.
Safety outcomes	Thromboembolic complications, coil migration, peforation, etc. at periprecedure; AEs, SAEs and death at periprocedure and 6-18 months.	Thromboembolic complications, hydrocephalus, peforation, etc. at periprecedure; AEs, SAEs and death at periprocedure and 18 months.	Thromboembolic complications, hydrocephalus, cerebral edema, etc. at periprocedure; AEs and death at periprocedure and 12 months.	Thromboembolic complications, artery occlusion, peforation, etc. at periprecedure; AEs and death at periprocedure and 18 months.

GREAT German-French Randomized Endovascular Aneurysm Trial, *PRET* Patients prone to Recurrence after Endovascular Treatment, *HELP* Hydrocoil Endovascular aneurysm occLusion and Packing Study, *WFNS* World Federation of Neurosurgeons Societies, *IA* Intracranial aneurysm, *AEs* Adverse Events, *SAEs* Severe Adverse Events, *AVM* arteriovenous malformation, *HC* hydrogel coil, *BPC* Bare platinum coil

Results

A total of 1256 titles and abstracts were identified through MEDLINE, EMBASE, and Cochrane Library (Fig. 1). After removing the duplicates and irrelevant records, 28 full-text articles were assessed for eligibility. Additionally, 24 articles were excluded as a result of the limitation of publication types: 5 multiple reports on one RCT, 3 post-hoc analysis, 2 meta-analysis, 2 comments, 7 reviews and 5 clinical trials. Ultimately, four RCTs containing 1526 patients (hydrogel, $n = 767$; bare, $n = 759$) were included in qualitative synthesis (Fig. 1). The main characteristics of the included studies are listed in Table 1.

Outcomes analysis

All 4 RCTs [16, 17, 19, 21] enrolling 1526 patients were pooled for the analysis of periprocedural and mid-term outcome respectively from two aspects of efficacy and safety.

Periprocedural efficacy and safety outcome

There were no significant differences observed in the numbers of patients with initial complete occlusion after endovascular treatment (RR 1.02, 95% CI 0.93 to 1.13, $P = 0.679$; Fig. 2A) between the hydrogel coil and bare platinum coil groups. Compared with bare platinum coils, hydrogel coils showed no significant differences in preventing periprocedural events, including: failed procedure (RR 1.97, 95% CI 0.68 to 5.76, $P = 0.213$, Fig. 2B), coil migration (RR 1.53, 95% CI 0.83 to 2.82, $P = 0.168$, Fig. 2C), perforation (RR 1.25, 95% CI 0.54 to 2.94, $P = 0.603$, Fig. 2D), hydrocephalus (RR 1.16, 95% CI 0.71 to 1.91, $P = 0.555$, Fig. 3A) and thromboembolic complications (RR 0.74, 95% CI 0.49 to 1.12, $P = 0.148$, Fig. 2E). The numbers of periprocedural residual aneurysm neck (RR 0.88, 95% CI 0.76 to 1.02, $P = 0.098$, Fig. 2F) and residual aneurysm (RR 1.20, 95% CI 0.98 to 1.46, $P = 0.080$, Fig. 2G) were also similar in the two groups; In addition, morbidity (RR 1.95, 95% CI 0.76 to 5.01, $P = 0.167$, Fig. 3B) or mortality (RR 1.03, 95% CI 0.26 to 4.16, $P = 0.962$, Fig. 3C) also showed no significant difference. The heterogeneity of periprocedural mortality is 63.8% with a P value of 0.063 (Fig. 3C). To detect the source of this statistical heterogeneity, a sensitivity analysis was performed. The sensitivity analysis

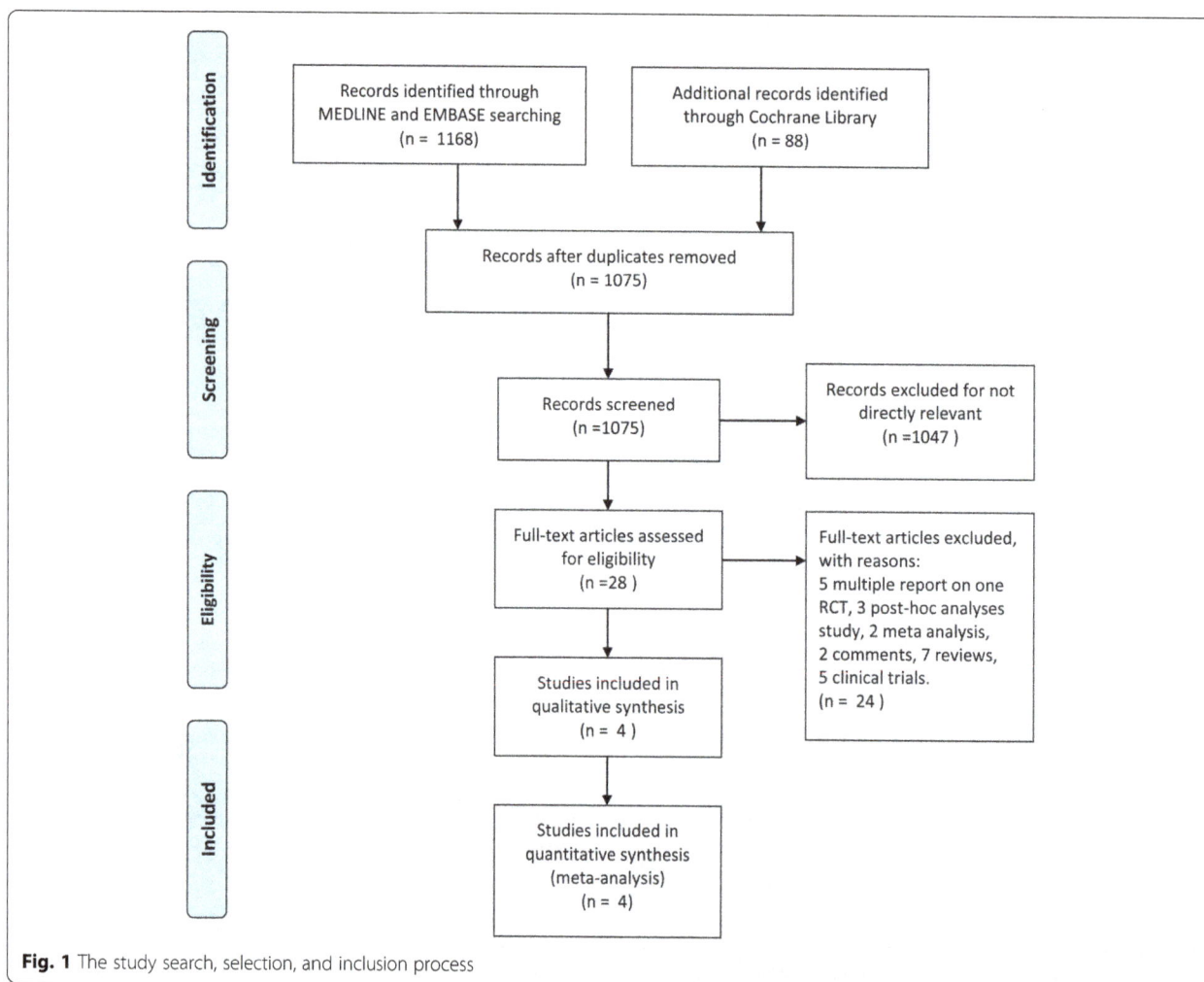

Fig. 1 The study search, selection, and inclusion process

showed that all of the consolidated results were stable (Additional file 1: Figure S1).

Mid-term efficacy outcome

Although no significant differences exist in the numbers of mid-term complete occlusion (RR 1.13, 95% CI 0.98 to 1.31, $P = 0.094$; Fig. 4A), no intracranial aneurysms recurrences in DSA (RR 1.06, 95% CI 0.99 to 1.13, $P = 0.106$; Fig. 4B) and excellent functional outcome (mRS score = 0) (RR 0.96, 95% CI 0.91 to 1.01, $P = 0.150$; Fig. 4C) for both groups, bare platinum coils group have an advantage over hydrogel coils group in patients' good functional outcome(RR 0.97, 95%CI 0.94 to 1.00, $P = 0.046$, Fig. 4D), which is defined as the follow-up mRS score from 0 to 2. The heterogeneity of mid-term complete occlusion is 49.6% with a P value of 0.138(Fig. 4A). To detect the source of the statistical heterogeneity, a sensitivity analysis was performed. The sensitivity analysis showed that all of the consolidated results were stable (Additional file 1: Figure S2).

Mid-term safety outcome

Patients in the hydrogel coils group have a lower rate of mid-term residual neck (RR 0.70, 95% CI 0.49 to 1.01, $P = 0.054$; Fig. 5A), residual aneurysm (RR 0.71, 95% CI 0.57 to 0.88, $P = 0.002$; Fig. 5B) and major recurrence (RR 0.78, 95% CI 0.65 to 0.94, $P = 0.008$; Fig. 5C) than that of the bare platinum coils group. However, this was accompanied by no reduction in the need for retreatment (RR 0.92, 95% CI 0.61 to 1.37, $P = 0.675$; Fig. 5D), stroke (RR 0.97, 95% CI 0.49 to 1.93, $P = 0.934$; Fig. 5E), morbidity (RR 1.11, 95% CI 0.73 to 1.69, $P = 0.615$; Fig. 5E) and mortality (RR 1.49, 95% CI 0.58 to 3.86, $P = 0.411$; Fig. 5G) after hydrogel coil treatment compared to bare coil treatment. The heterogeneity of Mid-term mortality is 62.0% with P value of 0.072 (Fig. 5G). To detect the source of this statistical heterogeneity, sensitivity analysis was performed. The sensitivity analysis showed that all of the consolidated results were stable (Additional file 1: Figure S3).

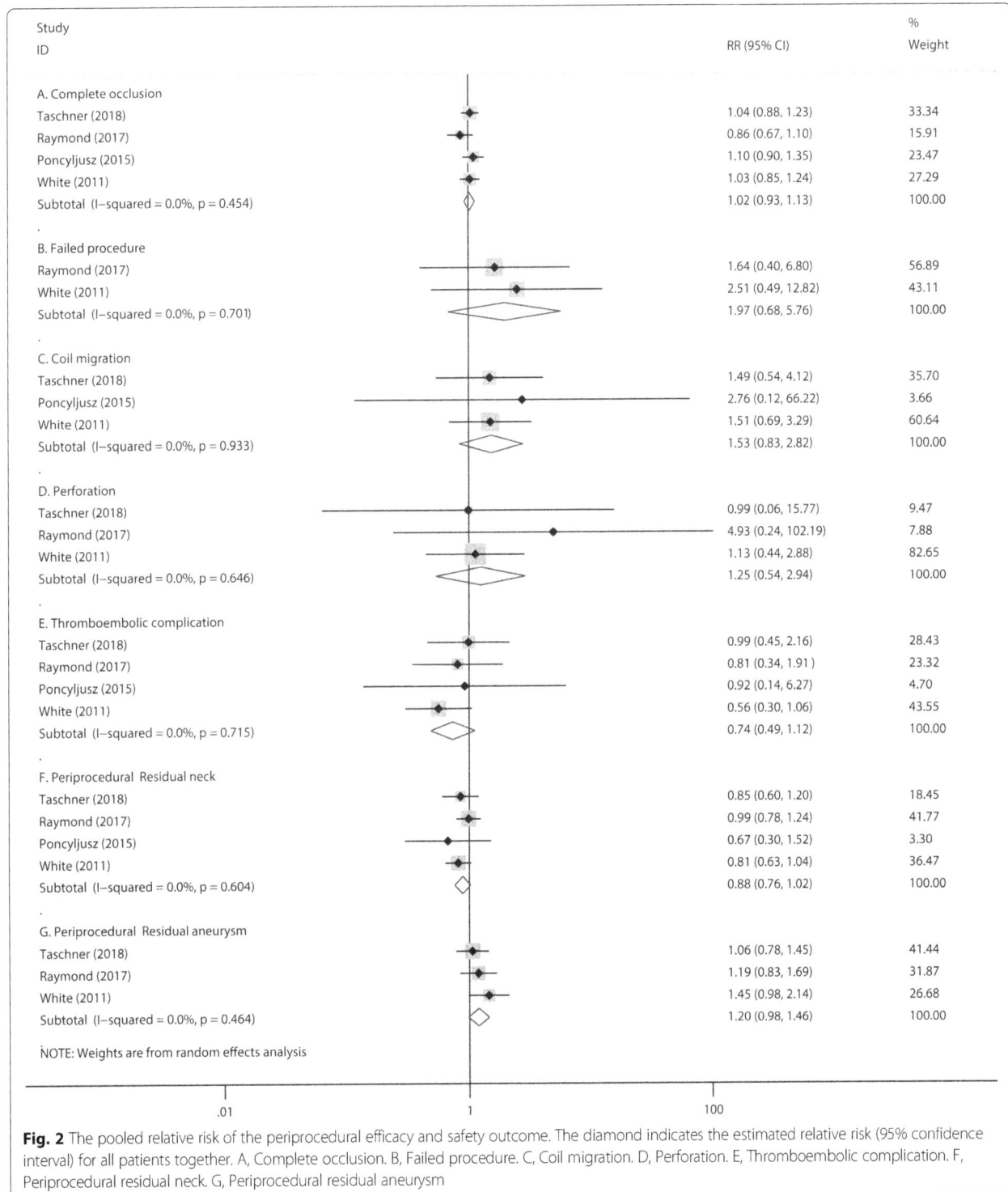

Fig. 2 The pooled relative risk of the periprocedural efficacy and safety outcome. The diamond indicates the estimated relative risk (95% confidence interval) for all patients together. A, Complete occlusion. B, Failed procedure. C, Coil migration. D, Perforation. E, Thromboembolic complication. F, Periprocedural residual neck. G, Periprocedural residual aneurysm

Subgroup analysis

Subgroup analyses were implemented to assess the influence of different generations of hydrogel coils and ruptured rate of aneurysm at baseline. Second-generation hydrogel coils were more effective in mid-term complete occlusion (RR 1.26, 95% CI 1.07 to 1.48, $P = 0.005$; Table. 2) and had a lower rate of residual neck (RR 0.54, 95% CI 0.34 to 0.86, $P = 0.010$; Table. 2). For high ruptured rate subgroup, in which each trial's proportion of ruptured aneurysms was more than 30%, intracranial aneurysms were more likely to be occluded completely by hydrogel coils than bare platinum coils (RR 1.21, 95% CI 1.07 to 1.38, $P = 0.002$; Table. 2). The sensitivity analysis demonstrated that all the consolidated statistics were stabilized.

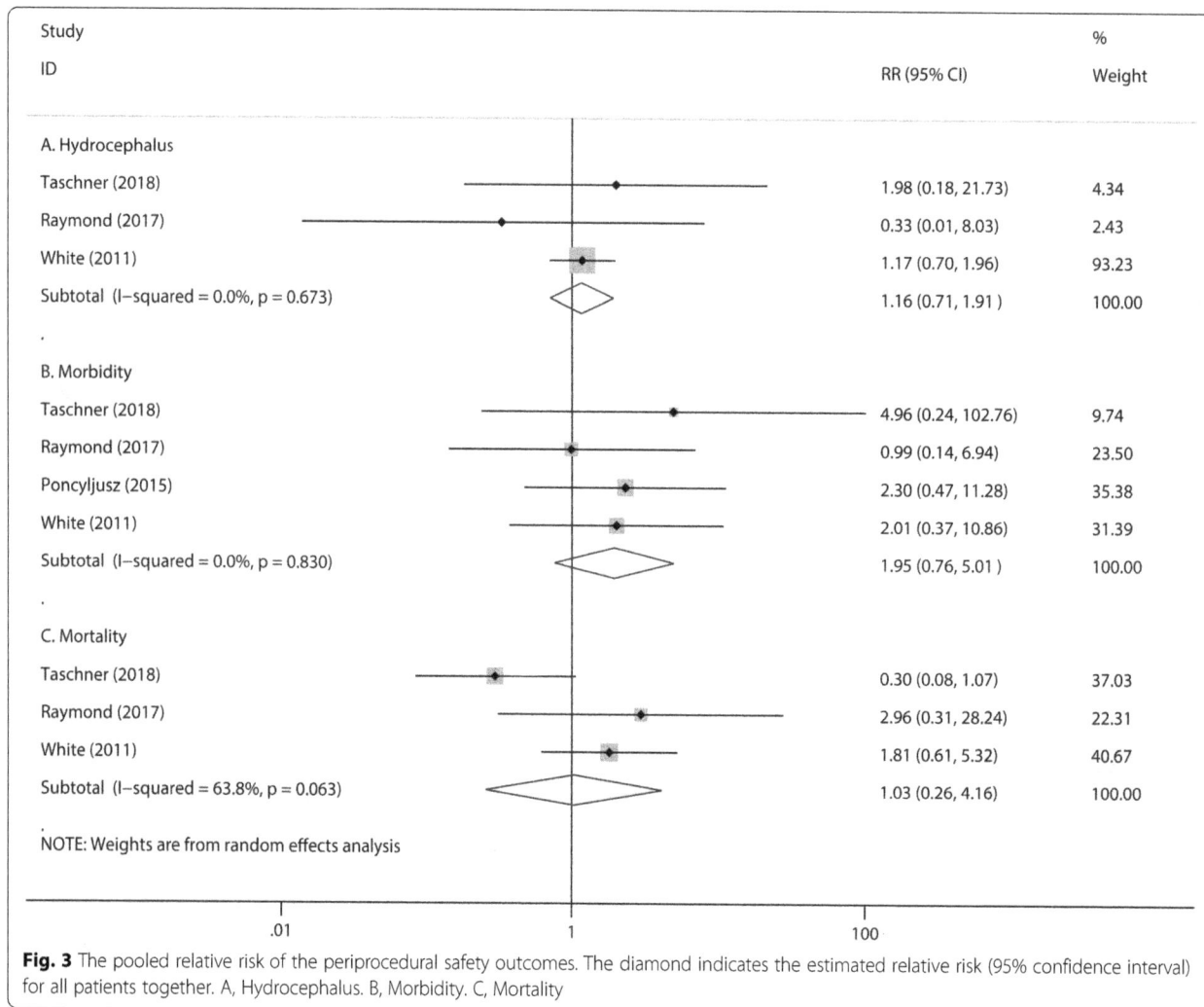

Fig. 3 The pooled relative risk of the periprocedural safety outcomes. The diamond indicates the estimated relative risk (95% confidence interval) for all patients together. A, Hydrocephalus. B, Morbidity. C, Mortality.

Risk of Bias in included studies

The details of the risk bias for all studies were shown in Fig. 6. There were two clinical trials that have a higher risk of bias in allocation concealment. For the blinding of participants and personnel, the risk of bias was high in one study and the other three trials were unclear. For the blinding of outcome assessment, the risk of bias was high in one study and unclear risk of bias in another trial. For incomplete outcome data, the risk of bias was unclear in one trial. Apart from these four items, there were no high or unclear risk of bias in any of the other items was observed.

Discussion

Hydrogel coils embolization for intracranial aneurysm might be superior to bare platinum coils in mid-term outcome based on the evidence from our current meta-analysis. We discovered that hydrogel coils had no distinct benefit in periprocedural efficacy and safety outcomes, including initial post-operational complete occlusion,

residual aneurysm neck, residual aneurysm, failed procedure, coil migration, perforation, thromboembolic complication, hydrocephalus, morbidity and mortality, which was in accordance with other studies [4, 9, 16, 17, 19, 21, 23, 24].

Hydrogel coils had a tendency of decreasing mid-term residual aneurysm neck ($P = 0.054$) and exhibited valid preventions from the mid-term residual aneurysm ($P = 0.002$). Meanwhile, as a potential tendency of a favorable outcome, no significant differences in the numbers of mid-term complete occlusion were detected (RR 1.13, 95% CI 0.98 to 1.31, $P = 0.094$). Although the sensitivity analysis demonstrated that the consolidated statistics about mid-term complete occlusion were stabilized, the results might be influenced by the high heterogeneity. Subgroup analyses depicted that second-generation hydrogel coils could improve complete occlusion ($P = 0.005$) compare to first-generation coils ($P = 0.450$) when hydrogel coil was detached.

In addition, recurrence was a high-profile and controversial issue among different clinical trials and systematic

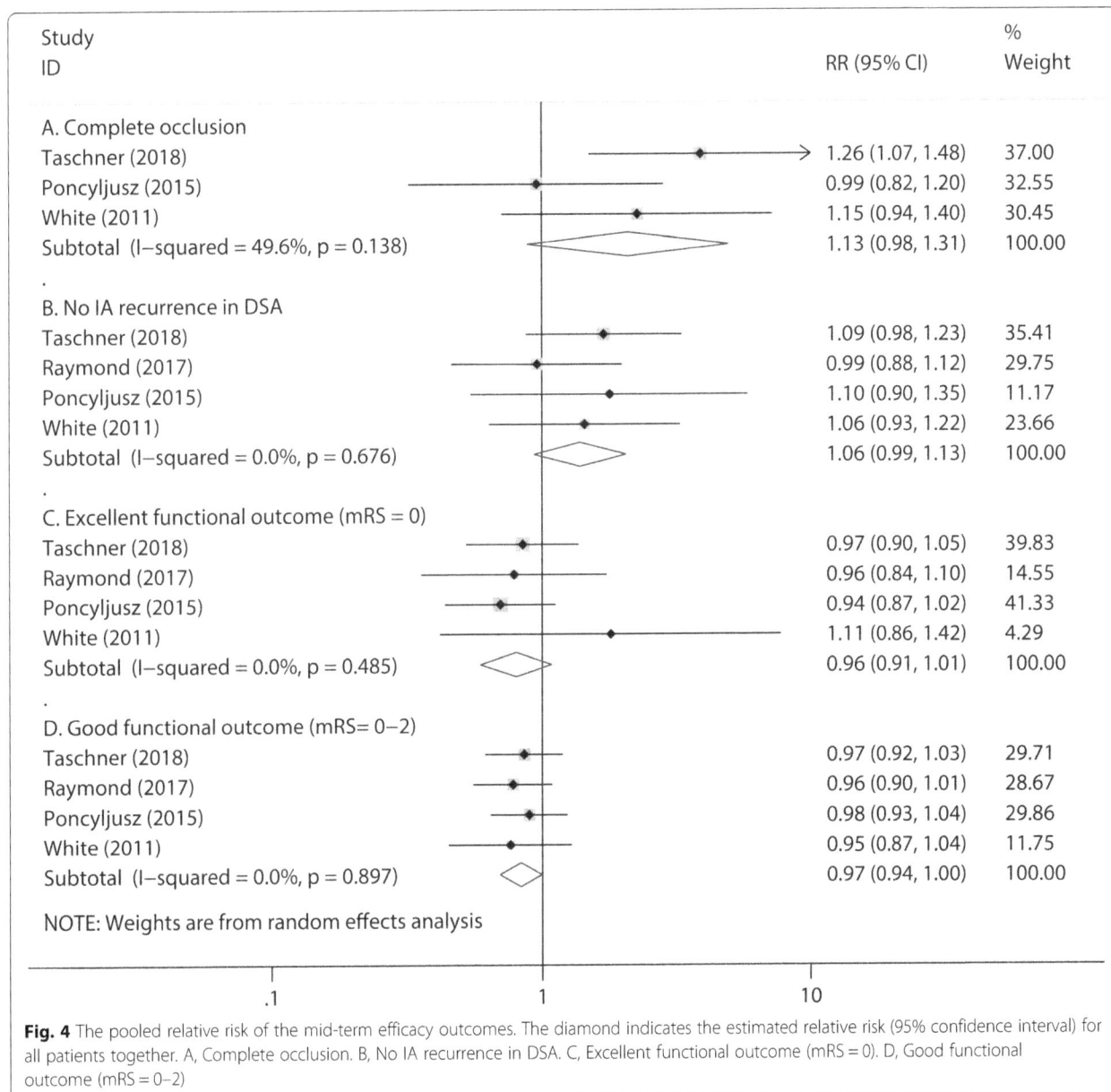

Fig. 4 The pooled relative risk of the mid-term efficacy outcomes. The diamond indicates the estimated relative risk (95% confidence interval) for all patients together. A, Complete occlusion. B, No IA recurrence in DSA. C, Excellent functional outcome (mRS = 0). D, Good functional outcome (mRS = 0–2).

reviews: HELPS (Hydrocoil Endovascular aneurysm occlusion and Packing Study) [25–27], GREAT(German-French Randomized Endovascular Aneurysm Trial) [15, 20] and Serafin's systematic review [4] illustrated that hydrogel coils resulted in a lower rate of recurrence. In contrast, no significant differences by using hydrogel coils in terms of aneurysm recurrence were observed through Poncyljusz's RCT [17] and PRET (Patients prone to Recurrence after Endovascular Treatment) [21, 28, 29]. In our meta-analysis, we pooled 1526 patients from 4 RCTs and drew a conclusion that hydrogel coils showed impacts upon avoiding recurrence (RR 0.78, 95% CI 0.65 to 0.94, $P = 0.008$) against bare platinum coils. Meanwhile, we also found that the number of patients without intracranial aneurysm recurrence in DSA had no distinct difference

for the two groups (RR 1.06, 95% CI 0.99 to 1.13, $P = 0.106$). A hypothesis was established to explain the question that some recurrent patients was not diagnosed with aneurysm recurrence by angiography but through other ways such as CTA, MRA or clinical manifestations [30].

Surprisingly, bare platinum coils group contrarily had an advantage over hydrogel coils group in mid-term patients' good functional outcome, which is defined as the mRS score from 0 to 2. Why did bare platinum coils group have a favorable result of mid-term patients' good functional outcome? Although the statistics revealed that hydrogel coils could prevent intracranial aneurysm patients from mid-term residual aneurysm, recurrence; we suspect that it was the degree of damage at the aneurysm ruptured point and post-operational complications that

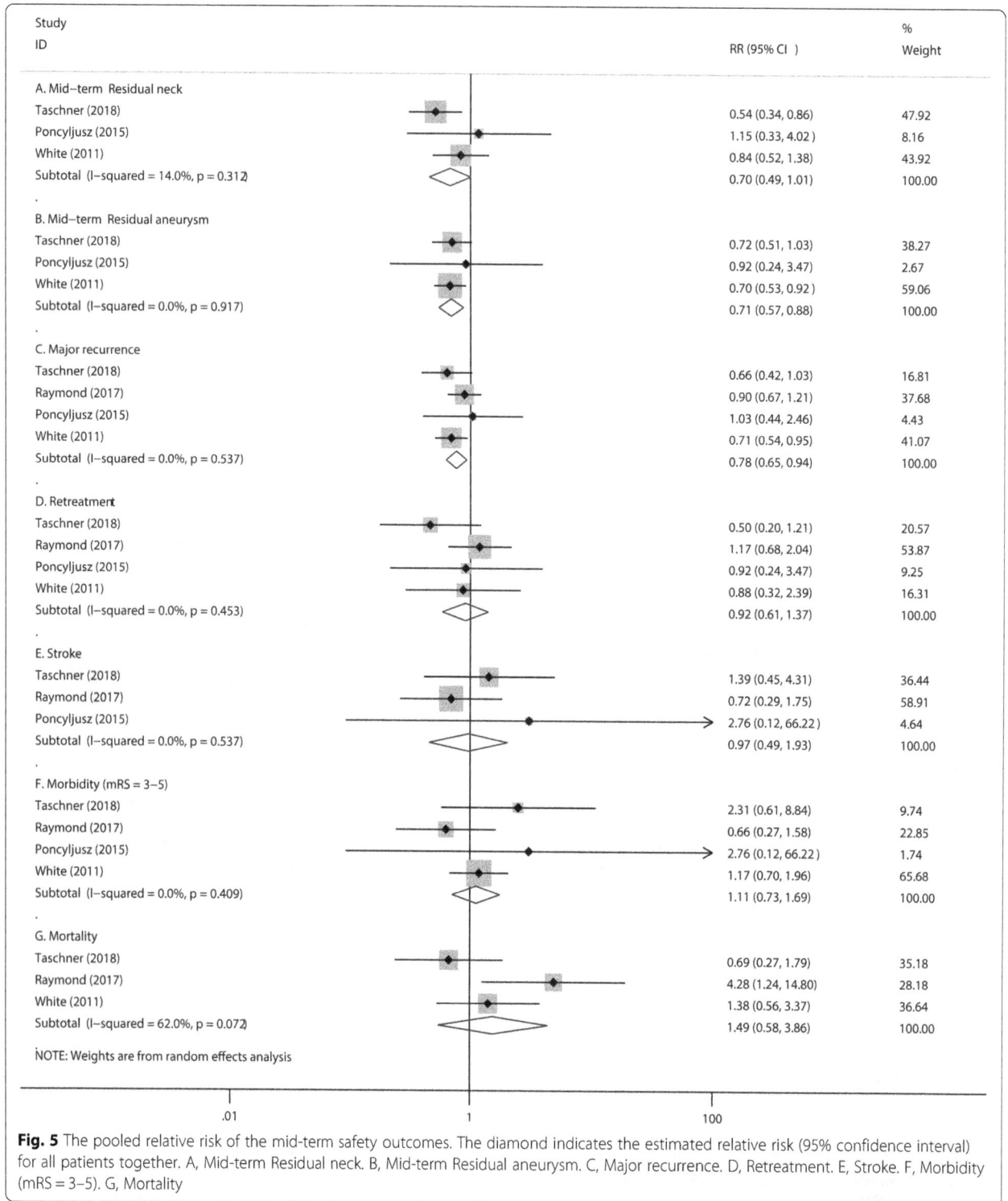

Fig. 5 The pooled relative risk of the mid-term safety outcomes. The diamond indicates the estimated relative risk (95% confidence interval) for all patients together. A, Mid-term Residual neck. B, Mid-term Residual aneurysm. C, Major recurrence. D, Retreatment. E, Stroke. F, Morbidity (mRS = 3–5). G, Mortality

have more influences on the patients' prognosis which could be measured by mRS score [31]. Hence, we performed a subgroup analyses between high ruptured rate subgroup ($N > 30\%$) and low ruptured rate subgroup ($N < 30\%$). We found no significant differences in good functional outcome when we separated high

ruptured rate trials from low ruptured rate trials. Therefore, the favorable outcome of bare platinum coils could be the result of the selection bias of patients in trials and degree of baseline damage patients between hydrogel coils group and bare platinum coils group.

Table 2 Subgroup Analysis of Efficacy and Safety Outcomes

	Efficacy outcomes							
	Complete occlusion		Recurrence in DSA		Excellent functional outcome		Good functional outcome	
	RR (95% CI)	P value	RR (95% CI)	P value	RR (95% CI)	P value	RR (95% CI)	P value
1. Hydrogel coil								
Second generation	1.26 (1.07, 1.48)	0.005	1.09 (0.98, 1.23)	0.119	0.97 (0.90, 1.05)	0.498	0.97 (0.92, 1.03)	0.358
First generation	1.07 (0.90, 1.25)	0.450	1.04 (0.95, 1.13)	0.390	0.97 (0.88, 1.06)	0.482	0.97 (0.93, 1.00)	0.074
2. Ruptured ratio (%)								
$N > 30$	1.21 (1.07, 1.38)	0.002	1.08 (0.99, 1.18)	0.077	1.00 (0.88, 1.12)	0.964	0.97 (0.92, 1.02)	0.187
$N < 30$	0.99 (0.82, 1.20)	0.938	1.02 (0.92, 1.18)	0.684	0.95 (0.88, 1.01)	0.116	0.97 (0.93, 1.01)	0.133
	Safety outcomes							
	Mid-term residual neck		Retreatment		Stroke		Morbidity	
	RR (95% CI)	P value	RR (95% CI)	P value	RR (95% CI)	P value	RR (95% CI)	P value
3. Hydrogel coil								
Second generation	0.54 (0.34, 0.86)	0.010	0.50 (0.20, 1.21)	0.122	1.39 (0.45, 4.31)	0.570	2.31 (0.61, 8.84)	0.220
First generation	0.88 (0.56, 1.39)	0.576	1.08 (0.68, 1.69)	0.752	0.79 (0.34, 1.87)	0.594	1.03 (0.66, 1.60)	0.899
4. Ruptured ratio (%)								
$N > 30$	0.67 (0.43, 1.03)	0.070	0.64 (0.33, 1.24)	0.186	1.39 (0.45, 4.31)	0.570	1.28 (0.79, 2.07)	0.317
$N < 30$	1.15 (0.33, 4.02)	0.827	1.13 (0.68, 1.88)	0.629	0.79 (0.34, 1.87)	0.594	0.73 (0.31, 1.69)	0.461

We were also interested in the reasons of why there were no significant differences in initial retreatment ($P = 0.675$) between the two groups in spite of the fact that bare platinum coils had a distinctly higher rate of recurrence than hydrogel coils ($P = 0.008$). We found that compared with recurrence, the number of retreatment was obviously smaller and it meant only a part of recurrent patients chose or had a chance to retreat. Therefore, we assumed that the small amount of retreatment was not able to get a statistically significant difference under the circumstance that the number of total patients remained relatively large.

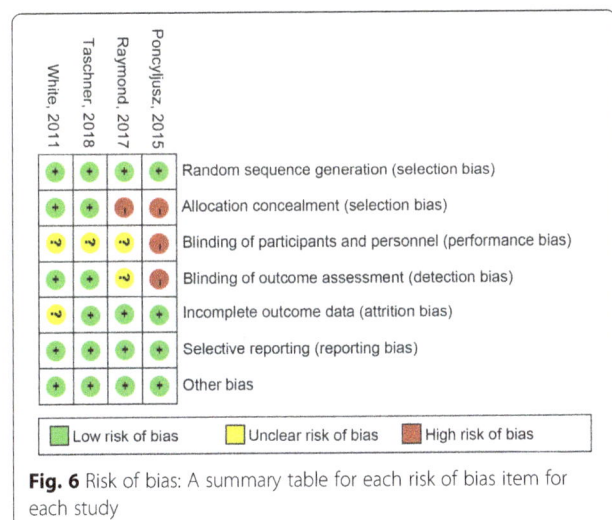

Fig. 6 Risk of bias: A summary table for each risk of bias item for each study

Subgroup analyses indicated that second-generation hydrogel coils could improve complete occlusion and reduce residual aneurysm neck from the results of the mid-term follow-up. We believe it is because that second-generation hydrogel coils were only abundantly employed in GREAT 2018, which could cause the favorable results of hydrogel coils. In the further, when second-generation hydrogel coils are used in more clinical trials, we could get a more reliable outcome of it. The other subgroup analysis found that the high ruptured rate subgroup had a higher probability to get occluded completely. The mechanisms of coils embolization therapy were to form a thrombus in the aneurysm by coils attracting negatively charged blood components (red blood cells, white blood cells and platelets, etc.) to coagulate [32]. Hence, hyperfunction of coagulation system under stress might result in the favorable complete occlusion in high ruptured rate subgroup.

On the basis of our knowledge, it was the first meta-analysis about the comparison between hydrogel coils and bare platinum coils, using evidence solely from RCTs (randomized clinical trials). Previous systematic reviews and meta-analysis were predominantly or entirely based on non-randomized researches [4, 9]. Combining the findings from uncontrolled trials results in a heterogeneous dataset, therefore, these systematic reviews are flawed. Additionally, some systematic reviews and meta-analysis were comprised of not only hydrogel coils but also other bioactive coils [23, 25]. Which resulted in an analysis including mixed types of coil; the outcome of these reviews and meta-analysis inevitable have deviations. In spite of some subgroup analyses about hydrogel coils performed in these research studies [23], the comprehensiveness of the comparison between hydrogel coils and bare platinum coils was insufficient on account of the included trials' quantity [23]. Different from above-mentioned systematic reviews, all patients in our present meta-analysis were intervened by either hydrogel coils or bare platinum coils in randomized trials, which was the best method to divide risk factors equally over the two groups [33]. Limitations of our meta-analysis should be noticed. First, this meta-analysis was performed on the foundation of limited statistics. We only pooled 4 published RCTs [16, 17, 19, 21] with 1526 patients (hydrogel, $n = 767$; bare, $n = 759$) to examine the efficacy and safety of hydrogel coils vs. bare platinum coils for intracranial aneurysm. Additionally, the included RCTs showed heterogeneity in the data of periprocedural mortality ($I^2 = 63.8\%$), mid-term mortality ($I^2 = 62\%$) and mid-term complete occlusion ($I^2 = 49.6\%$). The sensitivity analysis demonstrated that all the consolidated statistics were stabilized, but these disadvantages of the included studies could not be neglected. Lastly, in spite of the patients being randomized in 4 RCTs, the heterogeneous risk factors were still noticeable, and the baseline damage degree or mRS scores between hydrogel coils group and bare platinum coils group might vary patient by patient.

Conclusions

In conclusion, our meta-analysis demonstrated that endovascular treatment for intracranial aneurysms by hydrogel coils had preventive efficacy on mid-term recurrence and residual aneurysm, but didn't show any significant differences in other outcomes. Second-generation hydrogel coils might exhibit potential favorable impacts on mid-term complete occlusion and residual aneurysm neck, and therefore could affect clinical outcome. Based on our findings, we suggest future researchers to consider testing the possible therapeutic effect of second-generation hydrogel coils in patients with intracranial aneurysms.

Abbreviations

CI: Confidence interval; DSA: Digital subtraction angiography; GDC: Guglielmi detachable platinum coils; GREAT: German-French Randomized Endovascular Aneurysm Trial; HELPS: Hydrocoil Endovascular aneurysm occLusion, and Packing Study; HES: Hydrogel embolic system; ISAT: International Subarachnoid Aneurysm Trial; mRS: modified Rankin Scale; PRET: Patients prone to Recurrence after Endovascular Treatment; RCT: Randomized controlled trials; RR: relative risk

Acknowledgements

We thank all the participants for their support of this research. In addition, we are particularly grateful for Taraneh Taheri's assistance in the completion of the language modification process of this article, from the University of Pittsburgh.

Funding

This study and analyses were supported by the National Natural Science Foundation of China (No.81571115). The funding paid staff costs for the design of the study and collection, and interpretation of data and in writing the manuscript.

Authors' contributions

TX, ZC, WL, JX, XS and ZW all made substantial contributions to the study conception and design; analysis and interpretation of data; and drafting and/or critically reviewing the manuscript. TX, ZC and JX was involved in acquisition of data. TX, ZC, WL, JX, XS and ZW all reviewed and approved the final draft of the manuscript. TX, ZC, WL, JX, XS and ZW all agreed to be accountable for all aspects of the work in ensuring that questions related to the accuracy or integrity of any part of the work are appropriately investigated and resolved.

Competing interests

The authors declare that they have no competing interests.

Author details

[1]Department of Neurosurgery & Brain and Nerve Research Laboratory, The First Affiliated Hospital of Soochow University, 188 Shizi Street, Suzhou 215006, China. [2]University of Pittsburgh School of Pharmacy, Pittsburgh, PA 15219, USA. [3]Department of Ophthalmology, The First Affiliated Hospital of Soochow University, Suzhou 215006, Jiangsu Province, China. [4]Department of Neurosurgery, Taicang Affiliated Hospital of Soochow University, Suzhou 215400, Jiangsu Province, China.

References

1. Solenski NJ, Haley EC Jr, Kassell NF, Kongable G, Germanson T, Truskowski L, Torner JC. Medical complications of aneurysmal subarachnoid hemorrhage: a report of the multicenter, cooperative aneurysm study. Participants of the multicenter cooperative aneurysm study. Crit Care Med. 1995;23(6):1007–17.
2. Linn FH, Rinkel GJ, Algra A, van Gijn J. Incidence of subarachnoid hemorrhage: role of region, year, and rate of computed tomography: a meta-analysis. Stroke. 1996;27(4):625–9.
3. Molyneux A, Kerr R, International subarachnoid aneurysm trial collaborative G, Stratton I, Sandercock P, Clarke M, Shrimpton J, Holman R. International subarachnoid aneurysm trial (ISAT) of neurosurgical clipping versus endovascular coiling in 2143 patients with ruptured intracranial aneurysms: a randomized trial. J Stroke Cerebrovasc Dis. 2002;11(6):304–14.
4. Serafin Z, Di Leo G, Palys A, Nowaczewska M, Beuth W, Sardanelli F. Follow-up of cerebral aneurysm embolization with hydrogel embolic system: systematic review and meta-analysis. Eur J Radiol. 2015;84(10):1954–63.
5. Gunnarsson T, Klurfan P, terBrugge KG, Willinsky RA. Treatment of intracranial aneurysms with hydrogel coated expandable coils. Can J Neurol Sci. 2007;34(1):38–46.
6. Bender MT, Wendt H, Monarch T, Lin LM, Jiang B, Huang J, Coon AL, Tamargo RJ, Colby GP. Shifting treatment paradigms for ruptured aneurysms from open surgery to endovascular therapy over 25 years. World neurosurg. 2017;106:919–24.
7. Molyneux AJ, Birks J, Clarke A, Sneade M, Kerr RS. The durability of endovascular coiling versus neurosurgical clipping of ruptured cerebral aneurysms: 18 year follow-up of the UK cohort of the international subarachnoid aneurysm trial (ISAT). Lancet. 2015;385(9969):691–7.
8. Zhang X, Li L, Hong B, Xu Y, Liu Y, Huang Q, Liu J. A systematic review and meta-analysis on economic comparison between endovascular coiling versus neurosurgical clipping for ruptured intracranial aneurysms. World neurosurg. 2018;113:269–75.
9. Rezek I, Mousan G, Wang Z, Murad MH, Kallmes DF. Coil type does not affect angiographic follow-up outcomes of cerebral aneurysm coiling: a systematic review and meta-analysis. AJNR Am J Neuroradiol. 2013;34(9):1769–73.
10. Dabus G, Hacein-Bey L, Varjavand B, Tomalty RD, Han PP, Yerokhin V, Linfante I, Mocco J, Oxley T, Spiotta A, et al. Safety, immediate and mid-term results of the newer generation of hydrogel coils in the treatment of ruptured aneurysms: a multicenter study. J Neurointerv Surg. 2017;9(4):419–24.

11. Zhang X, Tang H, Huang Q, Hong B, Xu Y, Liu J. Total hospital costs (THC) and length of stay (LOS) of endovascular coiling versus neurosurgical clipping for unruptured intracranial aneurysms: a systematic review and meta-analysis. World Neurosurg. 2018;115:393–9.

12. Kang HS, Han MH, Lee TH, Shin YS, Roh HG, Kwon OK, Kwon BJ, Kim SY, Kim SH, Byun HS. Embolization of intracranial aneurysms with hydrogel-coated coils: result of a Korean multicenter trial. Neurosurgery. 2007;61(1):51–8 discussion 58-59.

13. Lanzino G, Kallmes D. Evaluation of the new HydroSoft coil in a canine model of bifurcation aneurysm. J Neurosurg. 2009;111(1):9 discussion 9-10.

14. Ferral H. Hydrogel-coated coils: product description and clinical applications. Semin Interv Radiol. 2015;32(4):343–8.

15. Taschner C, Chapot R, Costalat V, Courtheoux P, Barreau X, Berge J, Pierot L, Kadziolka K, Jean B, Blanc R, et al. GREAT-a randomized aneurysm trial. Design of a randomized controlled multicenter study comparing HydroSoft/HydroFrame and bare platinum coils for endovascular aneurysm treatment. Neuroradiology. 2015;57(6):599–604.

16. White PM, Lewis SC, Gholkar A, Sellar RJ, Nahser H, Cognard C, Forrester L, Wardlaw JM, collaborators Ht. Hydrogel-coated coils versus bare platinum coils for the endovascular treatment of intracranial aneurysms (HELPS): a randomised controlled trial. Lancet. 2011;377(9778):1655–62.

17. Poncyljusz W, Zarzycki A, Zwarzany L, Burke TH. Bare platinum coils vs. HydroCoil in the treatment of unruptured intracranial aneurysms-a single center randomized controlled study. Eur J Radiol. 2015;84(2):261–5.

18. White PM, Lewis SC, Nahser H, Sellar RJ, Goddard T, Gholkar A, Collaboration HT. HydroCoil endovascular aneurysm occlusion and packing study (HELPS trial): procedural safety and operator-assessed efficacy results. AJNR Am J Neuroradiol. 2008;29(2):217–23.

19. Taschner CA, Chapot R, Costalat V, Machi P, Courtheoux P, Barreau X, Berge J, Pierot L, Kadziolka K, Jean B, et al. Second-generation hydrogel coils for the endovascular treatment of intracranial aneurysms: a randomized controlled trial. Stroke. 2018;49(3):667–74.

20. Taschner CA, Chapot R, Costalat V, Machi P, Courtheoux P, Barreau X, Berge J, Pierot L, Kadziolka K, Jean B, et al. GREAT-a randomized controlled trial comparing HydroSoft/HydroFrame and bare platinum coils for endovascular aneurysm treatment: procedural safety and core-lab-assessedangiographic results. Neuroradiology. 2016;58(8):777–86.

21. Raymond J, Klink R, Chagnon M, Barnwell SL, Evans AJ, Mocco J, Hoh BH, Turk AS, Turner RD, Desal H, et al. Hydrogel versus bare platinum coils in patients with large or recurrent aneurysms prone to recurrence after endovascular treatment: a randomized controlled trial. AJNR Am J Neuroradiol. 2017;38(3):432–41.

22. Liberati A, Altman DG, Tetzlaff J, Mulrow C, Gotzsche PC, Ioannidis JP, Clarke M, Devereaux PJ, Kleijnen J, Moher D. The PRISMA statement for reporting systematic reviews and meta-analyses of studies that evaluate healthcare interventions: explanation and elaboration. Bmj. 2009;339:b2700.

23. Broeders JA, Ahmed Ali U, Molyneux AJ, Poncyljusz W, Raymond J, White PM, Steinfort B. Bioactive versus bare platinum coils for the endovascular treatment of intracranial aneurysms: systematic review and meta-analysis of randomized clinical trials. J Neurointerv Surg. 2016;8(9):898–908.

24. Cloft HJ. HydroCoil for endovascular aneurysm occlusion (HEAL) study: periprocedural results. AJNR Am J Neuroradiol. 2006;27(2):289–92.

25. White PM, Raymond J. Endovascular coiling of cerebral aneurysms using "bioactive" or coated-coil technologies: a systematic review of the literature. AJNR Am J Neuroradiol. 2009;30(2):219–26.

26. Brinjikji W, White PM, Nahser H, Wardlaw J, Sellar R, Gholkar A, Cloft HJ, Kallmes DF. HydroCoils are associated with lower angiographic recurrence rates than are bare platinum coils in treatment of "difficult-to-treat" aneurysms: a post hoc subgroup analysis of the HELPS trial. AJNR Am J Neuroradiol. 2015;36(9):1689–94.

27. Brinjikji W, White PM, Nahser H, Wardlaw J, Sellar R, Cloft HJ, Kallmes DF. HydroCoils reduce recurrence rates in recently ruptured medium-sized intracranial aneurysms: a subgroup analysis of the HELPS trial. AJNR Am J Neuroradiol. 2015;36(6):1136–41.

28. Raymond J, Klink R, Chagnon M, Barnwell SL, Evans AJ, Mocco J, Hoh BL, Turk AS, Turner RD, Desal H, et al. Patients prone to recurrence after endovascular treatment: periprocedural results of the PRET randomized trial on large and recurrent aneurysms. AJNR Am J Neuroradiol. 2014;35(9):1667–76.

29. Raymond J, Roy D, White PM, Fiorella D, Chapot R, Bracard S, Kallmes DF, Icone Collaborative G. A randomized trial comparing platinum and hydrogel-coated coils in patients prone to recurrence after endovascular treatment (the PRET trial). Interv Neuroradiol. 2008;14(1):73–83.

30. Fanning NF, Berentei Z, Brennan PR, Thornton J. HydroCoil as an adjuvant to bare platinum coil treatment of 100 cerebral aneurysms. Neuroradiology. 2007;49(2):139–48.

31. Tan H, Huang G, Zhang T, Liu J, Li Z, Wang Z. A retrospective comparison of the influence of surgical clipping and endovascular embolization on recovery of oculomotor nerve palsy in patients with posterior communicating artery aneurysms. Neurosurgery. 2015;76(6):687–94 discussion 694.

32. Brinjikji W, Kallmes DF, Kadirvel R. Mechanisms of healing in coiled intracranial aneurysms: a review of the literature. AJNR Am J Neuroradiol. 2015;36(7):1216–22.

33. Lee S, Kang H. Statistical and methodological considerations for reporting RCTs in medical literature. Korean J Anesthesiol. 2015;68(2):106–15.

20

Neuromyelitis optica spectrum disorders with and without connective tissue disorders

Chun-Sheng Yang[1][*][†]ⓘ, Qiu Xia Zhang[1][†], Sheng Hui Chang[1], Lin Jie Zhang[1], Li Min Li[1], Yuan Qi[1], Jing Wang[1], Zhi Hua Sun[2], Nannan Zhangning[2], Li Yang[1] and Fu-Dong Shi[1,3]

Abstract

Background: Neuromyelitis optica spectrum disorders (NMOSD) often coexist with connective tissue disorders (CTD). The aim of this study was to investigate and compare the features of NMOSD with and without CTD.

Methods: NMOSD patients with ($n = 18$) and without CTD ($n = 39$) were enrolled, and the clinical, laboratory, and magnetic resonance imaging (MRI) features of the two groups were assessed.

Results: Most of the demographic and clinical features examined were similar between NMOSD patients with and without CTD. Serum immunoglobulin G (IgG), percentage of γ-globulin and seropositivity for several other autoantibodies were significantly elevated in NMOSD patients with CTD ($P < 0.05$). NMOSD with CTD was marked by longer spinal cord lesions and a lower frequency of short transverse myelitis (TM) than NMOSD without CTD ($P < 0.05$). NMOSD with CTD also featured more T1 hypointensity and T2 bright spotty lesions (BSLs) on MRI than NMOSD without CTD ($P = 0.001$ and 0.011, respectively). There were no other differences in laboratory, MRI and clinical characteristics between different NMOSD subtypes.

Conclusions: A few characteristics differed between NMOSD with and without CTD. NMOSD patients with CTD had higher serum IgG, longer spinal cord lesions, a lower frequency of short TM and more T1 hypointensity and T2 BSLs on spinal MRI than NMOSD patients without CTD.

Keywords: Neuromyelitis optica, Neuromyelitis optica spectrum disorders, Connective tissue disorders, Autoantibodies, Magnetic resonance imaging

Background

Neuromyelitis optica spectrum disorders (NMOSD) is a severe central nervous system (CNS) demyelinating syndrome, characterized by optic neuritis (ON) and acute myelitis [1]. Immunoglobulin G autoantibodies against aquaporin-4 (AQP4-IgG) play a key role in the pathogenesis and diagnosis of NMOSD. Standardized diagnostic criteria for NMOSD were published in 2015, further stratifying NMOSD based on serologic testing (NMOSD with or without AQP4-IgG). According to these criteria, NMOSD has six core clinical characteristics: ON, acute myelitis, area postrema syndrome, acute brainstem syndrome, acute diencephalic clinical syndrome and symptomatic cerebral syndrome [2].

In addition to AQP4-IgG, antinuclear autoantibodies (ANAs) are also often detectable in patients with NMOSD who do not have clinical evidence of a systemic autoimmune disease [3]. However, an increasing number of reports have revealed that NMOSD often coexists with connective tissue disorders (CTD), particularly systemic lupus erythematosus (SLE) and Sjögren syndrome (SS) [3–5]. Whether there are clinically significant differences in NMOSD with and without CTD remains unclear. In this study, we investigated and compared the demographic, clinical, laboratory, and magnetic resonance imaging (MRI) characteristics of NMOSD with and without CTD.

* Correspondence: cyang01@tmu.edu.cn
[†]Chun-Sheng Yang and Qiu Xia Zhang contributed equally to this work.
[1]Department of Neurology, Tianjin Neurological Institute, Tianjin Medical University General Hospital, No 154 Anshan Road, Heping District, Tianjin 300052, China
Full list of author information is available at the end of the article

Methods

Patients

Through the hospital database, we reviewed the records of all NMOSD patients admitted to Tianjin Medical University General Hospital, Tianjin, China, from December 2014 to December 2017. The mean follow-up time was 5.27 (0.42–19) years. NMOSD was diagnosed according to the 2015 international consensus diagnostic criteria for NMOSD [2], and CTD was diagnosed by rheumatologists according to published criteria and typology guidelines (e.g., SLE [6], SS [7], rheumatoid arthritis (RA) [8], or undifferentiated CTD (UCTD) [9]). Other inclusion criteria were as follows: (a) the serum samples of all the patients were tested for AQP4-IgG, myelin oligodendrocyte glycoprotein immunoglobulin G (MOG-IgG), autoreactive antibodies ((ANAs), extractable nuclear antigen autoantibodies (ENAs), rheumatoid factor (RF), and anti-neutrophil cytoplasmic antibodies (ANCAs)), immunoglobulins, and complement (C); (b) spinal and brain MRI were available before high-dose intravenous methylprednisolone (IVMP) (1.0 g/ d for 3 days) or intravenous immunoglobulin G (IVIG) (0.4 g/kg.d for 5 days); and (c) the time between study inclusion and the last relapse was more than 3 months. We excluded MOG-IgG positive patients, since the pathophysiology of MOG-IgG associated NMOSD is probably different in comparison to AQP4-IgG positive NMOSD. The information of personal accounts and clinical signs, Kurtzke Expanded Disability Status Scale (EDSS) scores, blood and cerebrospinal fluid (CSF) laboratory data, and MRI were recorded in our databank. The EDSS was applied before high-dose IVMP or IVIG during relapse and during the remission period by two neurologists, both certified by Neurostatus for EDSS competency. The database comprised 74 Chinese patients diagnosed with NMOSD during the period. A total of 17 patients were excluded: 10 didn't have adequate data available, and another 7 were MOG-IgG positive. Ultimately, 39 NMOSD patients without CTD and 18 NMOSD patients with CTD were recruited in the cohort.

The study was approved by the Ethics Committee of Tianjin Medical University General Hospital, and written informed consent was obtained from each participant.

Laboratory testing

AQP4-IgG tests, MOG-IgG tests and CSF oligoclonal banding (OCB) were conducted in our clinical neuroimmunological laboratory. AQP4-IgG was detected by a cell-based assay (CBA), which has been described previously [10]. The plasmids were donated by Professor Angela Vincent and Professor David Beeson, Nuffield Department of Clinical Neurosciences, University of Oxford. Tests for autoreactive antibodies (ANAs, ENAs, RF and ANCAs), immunoglobulins, and complement were conducted, along with other serological profiling, in the immunology and clinical laboratory of our hospital.

MRI

MRI was performed using either a 1.5 T or a 3 T magnet from one of two manufacturers: GE (GE Medical Systems, Milwaukee, WI, USA) or Siemens (Siemens AG, Erlangen, Germany). Routine spinal MRI included T1-weighted imaging (T1WI), T2-weighted imaging (T2WI), a sagittal short tau inversion recovery (STIR) sequence, and T1WI with gadolinium enhancement. The T1 signal intensity of the lesion and the appearance of bright spotty lesions (BSLs) on T2 were recorded. 'T1 dark' was defined when the signal intensity of the lesion was similar to that of CSF on the T1WI. BSLs were defined when the signal intensity of the lesion approached that of the surrounding CSF without flow-void effects on the T2WI, as previously described [11, 12]. On axial T2WI, lesion distribution was classified as: 'peripherally- located' or 'centrally- located'. Lesions that were ≥ 50% of the spinal cord area (transverse myelitis, TM) were noted. Short TM (< 3 vertebral segments) was also recorded. The brain MRI protocol included diffusion-weighted images, T1WI, T2WI, fluid-attenuated inversion recovery (FLAIR) imaging, and contrast-enhanced T1WI. The slice thickness of the axial scans was 5 mm. MRI lesions were evaluated independently by two radiologists blinded to the patients' information.

Statistical analysis

Statistical analysis was performed using the Statistical Package for the Social Sciences (SPSS 22.0). All quantitative data in this study were presented as the mean ± standard deviation (SD) or the median and range. We applied the Mann–Whitney U test for quantitative data and the chi-squared test or Fisher's exact test for qualitative data. The relationships between variables were analysed using Spearman's correlation coefficient and partial correlation analysis. P-values of < 0.05 were considered statistically significant.

Results

From 2014 to 2017, a total of 57 patients satisfied the diagnostic criteria for inclusion in this study: 39 NMOSD patients without CTD and 18 with CTD (including 7 with SS, 3 with SLE, 1 with RA, and 7 UCTD). The demographic and clinical features of NMOSD with CTD are summarized in Table 1. Among the 18 patients with CTD, 9 developed CTD before NMOSD (ranging from 2 months to 30 years), and in the other 9 patients, the diagnosis of CTD followed the diagnosis of NMOSD (ranging from 1 month to 5 years). The demographic and clinical features of the patients are summarized in Table 2. Regular therapy was defined as a full dose of

Table 1 Demographic and clinical characteristics of NMOSD with CTD

	SS(7)	UCTD (7)	SLE(3)	RA(1)
Gender, n (% female)	7 (100%)	7 (100%)	3 (100%)	1 (100%)
Age at onset, years	41.29 ± 11.73	39.29 ± 9.07	40.67 ± 11.15	45.0 ± 0
Follow-up duration, years	6.07 ± 4.44	5.54 ± 3.79	2.51 ± 1.96	2.0 ± 0
Annualized relapse rate (ARR)	1.87 ± 2.36	0.92 ± 0.51	1.40 ± 0.45	1.5 ± 0
neuropathic pain, n (%)	3 (30%)	6 (60%)	1 (10%)	0 (0%)
Number of attacks	5.29 ± 2.69	3.71 ± 1.70	3.67 ± 3.06	3.0 ± 0
EDSS at nadir	5.29 ± 2.84	4.21 ± 1.82	6.17 ± 2.36	3.0 ± 0
EDSS at last follow-up	4.07 ± 2.99	2.21 ± 0.57	4.17 ± 2.47	2.0 ± 0
Initial presentation, n (%)				
ON	2 (28.57%)	2 (28.57%)	1 (33.33%)	1 (100%)
Area postrema syndrome	2 (28.57%)	0 (0%)	0 (0%)	0 (0%)
AM	2 (28.57%)	5 (71.43%)	2 (66.67%)	0 (0%)
Others	1 (14.29%)	0 (0%)	0 (0%)	0 (0%)

Abbreviations: NMOSD neuromyelitis optica spectrum disorders, *CTD* connective tissue disorders, *SS* Sjögren syndrome, *UCTD* undifferentiated connective tissue disorders, *SLE* systemic lupus erythematosus, *RA* rheumatoid arthritis, *EDSS* Kurtzke Expanded Disability Status Scale, *ON* optica neuritis, *AM* acute myelitis

Table 2 Demographic and clinical characteristics of NMOSD with and without CTD

	NMOSD (39)	NMOSD with CTD (18)	P
Gender, n (% female)	37 (94.9%)	18 (100%)	0.839
Age at onset, years	39.97 ± 13.82	42.33 ± 11.29	0.530
Follow-up duration, years	5.63 ± 4.63	5.04 ± 3.83	0.641
Annualized relapse rate (ARR)	0.98 ± 0.54	1.40 ± 1.51	0.127
ARR before regular medication	1.58 ± 2.18	1.66 ± 1.44	0.899
ARR after regular medication	0.64 ± 0.79	1.39 ± 1.96	0.100
Number of attacks	3.97 ± 2.07	4.28 ± 2.32	0.623
Neuropathic pain, n (%)	21 (53.8%)	10 (55.6%)	0.904
EDSS at nadir	3.5 (1, 8)	4 (1.5, 8.5)	0.031*
Visual functions	0 (0, 6)	1 (0, 6)	0.139
Pyramidal functions	1 (0, 4)	2 (0, 4)	0.219
Sensory functions	2 (0, 4)	3 (0, 4)	0.007*
Bowel and bladder	0 (0, 5)	3 (0, 5)	0.256
EDSS at last follow-up	2 (1, 8)	2.5 (1.5, 8.5)	0.403
Visual functions	0 (0, 4)	1 (0, 6)	0.111
Pyramidal functions	1 (0, 4)	1 (0, 4)	0.595
Sensory functions	1 (0, 4)	2 (0, 4)	0.063
Bowel and bladder	0 (0, 5)	0 (0, 5)	0.856
Initial presentation, n (%)			
ON	14 (35.9%)	6 (33.3%)	0.850
Area postrema syndrome	8 (20.5%)	2 (11.1%)	0.622
AM	15 (38.5%)	9 (50.0%)	0.412
Others	2 (5.1%)	1 (5.6%)	1.000

Abbreviations: NMOSD neuromyelitis optica spectrum disorders, *CTD* connective tissue disorders, *EDSS* Kurtzke Expanded Disability Status Scale, *ON* optica neuritis, *AM* acute myelitis
*$P < 0.05$

immunosuppressants. NMOSD patients with CTD had higher EDSS scores and more severe sensory disability at nadir than NMOSD patients without CTD ($P < 0.05$). No other significant demographic or clinical features difference was found in between NMOSD patients with and without CTD ($P > 0.05$).

The laboratory features of the patients are summarized in Table 3. CSF white blood cell (WBC) counts, protein,

Table 3 Laboratory features between NMOSD with and without CTD

	NMOSD (39)	NMOSD with CTD (18)	P
CSF Index			
Elevated white cell count ($> 8 \times 10^6$/L), n (%)	5 (12.8%)	5 (27.8%)	0.315
Elevated protein (> 0.4 g/L), n (%)	12 (30.8%)	5 (27.8%)	0.819
OCB, n (%)	1 (2.6%)	1 (5.6%)	1.000
Glu (2.5–4.4 mmol/L)	3.69 ± 1.00	3.19 ± 1.30	0.137
Cl (119-130 mmol/L)	127.25 ± 5.32	126.29 ± 5.41	0.585
Serums Index			
AQP4-Ab, n (%)	29 (74.4%)	12 (66.7%)	0.548
IgG (751–1560 mg/dl)	1161.73 ± 393.18	1696.06 ± 760.54	0.013*
IgA (82-453 mg/dl)	220.90 ± 95.81	372.66 ± 290.69	0.051
IgM (46–304 mg/dl)	114.47 ± 64.61	89.41 ± 35.85	0.144
C3 (79–152 mg/dl)	104.64 ± 67.35	99.29 ± 17.12	0.750
C4 (16–38 mg/dl)	23.20 ± 16.12	22.24 ± 9.92	0.822
CRP (> 0.8 mg/dl), n (%)	4 (10.3%)	6 (33.3%)	0.079
IgE (> 165 IU/ml), n (%)	2 (5.1%)	1 (5.6%)	1.000
ANA (> 1:80), n (%)	22 (56.4%)	17 (94.4%)	0.004*
Anti-dsDNA, n (%)	1 (2.6%)	1 (5.6%)	1.000
Anti-nRNP, n (%)	0 (0.0%)	1 (5.6%)	–
Anti-Sm, n (%)	0 (0.0%)	1 (5.6%)	–
Anti-SSA, n (%)	10 (25.6%)	15 (83.3%)	< 0.001**
Anti-Ro52, n (%)	9 (23.1%)	13 (72.2%)	< 0.001**
Anti-SSB, n (%)	2 (5.1%)	8 (44.4%)	0.001*
Anti-Scl70, n (%)	0 (0.0%)	0 (0.0%)	–
Anti-Jo1, n (%)	0 (0.0%)	0 (0.0%)	–
ACA, n (%)	0 (0.0%)	0 (0.0%)	–
AnuA, n (%)	0 (0.0%)	3 (16.7%)	–
AHA, n (%)	2 (5.1%)	2 (11.1%)	0.792
ARPA, n (%)	0 (0.0%)	0 (0.0%)	–
GPI (> 0.20 mg/L), n (%)	2 (5.1%)	1 (5.6%)	1.000
RF (> 20 IU/ml), n (%)	3 (7.7%)	7 (38.9%)	0.012*
ASO (> 116 IU/ml), n (%)	4 (10.3%)	3 (16.7%)	0.802
globulin (53.8–68.2)	66.91 ± 3.43	63.07 ± 6.61	0.032*
α1 globulin (1.1–3.7%)	2.17 ± 0.52	2.46 ± 1.45	0.328
α2 globulin (8.5–14.5%)	9.05 ± 1.35	8.97 ± 1.40	0.843
βglobulin (8.6–14.8%)	8.92 ± 1.51	8.97 ± 2.22	0.926
γglobulin (9.2–18.2%)	12.95 ± 3.13	16.87 ± 6.35	0.023*

Abbreviations: NMOSD neuromyelitis optica spectrum disorders, *CTD* connective tissue disorders, *CSF* cerebral spinal fluid, *OCB* oligoclonal bands, *Glu* glucose, *Cl* chloride, *C* complements, *CRP* C-reactive protein, *ANA* antinuclear antibodies, *Anti-dsDNA* anti-double stranded DNA antibodies, *Anti-nRNP* antinuclear ribonucleoprotein, *Anti-Sm* anti-Sm antibodies, *Anti-SSA/Ro52/SSB* Anti-SSA/Ro52/SSB antibodies, *Anti-Scl70* anti-topoisomerase I antibodies, *Anti-Jo1* anti-Jo-1 antibodies, *ACA* anti-neutrophil cytoplasmic antibodies, *AnuA* anti-nucleosome antibody, *AHA* anti-histone antibody, *ARPA* anti-ribonucleoprotein antibodies, *GPI* Glucose-6 phosphate isomerase, *RF* rheumatoid factor, *ASO* Anti-streptolysin
**$P < 0.001$, *$P < 0.05$

and chloride (Cl) showed no significant difference between the two groups. The level of serum IgG was significantly higher in NMOSD patients with CTD than those without CTD ($P = 0.013$), and a similar result was found for the percentage of γ-globulin ($P = 0.023$). Furthermore, ANA, anti-SSA/Ro antibodies (anti-SSA), anti-SSB/La antibodies (anti-SSB), anti-Ro52, and RF were significantly higher in NMOSD patients with CTD than in those without CTD ($P < 0.05$). However, there was no difference between the two groups in the positivity rate of AQP4-IgG, OCB, CRP (C-reactive protein), IgE, anti-dsDNA (anti-double stranded DNA antibodies), anti-nRNP (antinuclear ribonucleoprotein), anti-Sm (anti-Sm antibodies), anti-Scl70 (anti-topoisomerase I antibodies), anti-Jo1 (anti-Jo-1 antibodies), ACA (anti-neutrophil cytoplasmic antibodies), AnuA (anti-nucleosome antibody), AHA (anti-histone antibody), ARPA (anti-ribonucleoprotein antibodies), or GPI (Glucose-6 phosphate isomerase). No significant difference was found in the level of IgA, IgM, C3, or C4 between the two groups of patients.

The spinal and brain MRI features of the patients are summarized in Tables 4 and 5, respectively. Representative MRI abnormalities (arrows) in NMOSD patients with CTD are shown in Fig. 1. The length of spinal cord lesions was longer in NMOSD patients with CTD than in NMOSD patients without CTD ($P = 0.018$). There was no significant difference in the frequency of short TM at onset between the two groups. However, the frequency of short TM at the initial manifestation of myelitis was significantly higher in NMOSD patients without CTD than in those with CTD ($P = 0.010$). The frequency of T1 hypointensity and T2 BSLs in acute myelitis was higher in NMOSD patients with CTD than in those without CTD ($P = 0.001$ and 0.011, respectively). No significant difference between the two groups was observed in any of the other MRI features.

Pearson correlation results showed that EDSS scores were positively correlated with group classification (NMOSD with or without CTD) ($r = 0.286$, $P = 0.031$), the length of spinal cord lesions ($r = 0.488$, $P < 0.001$) and T1 hypointensity ($r = 0.362$, $P = 0.006$). EDSS scores showed no correlation with T2 BSLs ($r = 0.172$, $P = 0.202$) or AQP4-IgG positivity status ($r = -0.117$, $P = 0.388$). However, partial correlation results showed that EDSS scores had no correlation with group classification after controlling for lesion length and T1 hypointensity ($r = 0.003$, $P = 0.985$).

Discussion

In the present study, we found that patients with NMOSD and CTD were similar to those without CTD in all tested demographic and clinical features except EDSS scores, especially sensory disability at nadir. Furthermore, most

Table 4 Spinal MRI features between NMOSD with and without CTD

	NMOSD (39)	NMOSD with CTD (18)	P
Sagittal location			
length of lesions (VB)	4.44 ± 2.89	7.56 ± 4.79	0.018*
Short TM at onset, n (%)	7 (17.9%)	1 (5.6%)	0.400
Initial short TM, n (%)	18 (46.2%)	2 (11.1%)	0.010*
Location of spinal lesions, n (%)			
Cervical cord	13 (33.3%)	2 (11.1%)	0.148
Cervico-thoracic cord	16 (41.0%)	10 (55.6%)	0.306
Thoracic cord	10 (25.6%)	6 (33.3%)	0.548
Axial location, n (%)			
Centrally located	38 (97.4%)	18 (100.0%)	1.000
Peripherally located	1 (2.6%)	0 (0.0%)	1.000
enhancement	11 (28.2%)	8 (44.4%)	0.227
Acute phase			
T1 dark, n (%)	17 (43.6%)	16 (88.9%)	0.001*
T2 BSLs, n (%)	14 (35.9%)	13 (72.2%)	0.011*
Chronic phase			
Fragmentation, n (%) or 'bead-like' lesions	25 (64.1%)	8 (44.4%)	0.162
Disappearance, n (%)	9 (23.1%)	7 (38.9%)	0.217
Atrophy, n (%)	5 (12.8%)	3 (16.7%)	1.000

Abbreviations: NMOSD neuromyelitis optica spectrum disorders, *CTD* connective tissue disorders, *VB* vertebral segments, *TM* transverse myelitis, *BSLs* bright spotty lesion
*$P < 0.05$

clinical, laboratory, and MRI features also did not show significant differences between the two groups. However, a number of autoantibodies, CSF indexes, and MRI features differed significantly.

NMOSD patients with CTD had increased amounts of T1 hypointensity and T2 BSLs on spinal MRI in

Table 5 Brain MRI features at onset between NMOSD with and without CTD

	NMOSD (39)	NMOSD with CTD (18)	P
Brain lesions, n (%)	14 (35.9%)	9 (50.0%)	0.313
Brain lobes	5 (12.8%)	5 (27.8%)	0.315
Basal ganglia	0 (0)	3 (16.7%)	–
Hypothalamic and thalamic	1 (2.6%)	0 (0)	–
Callosum	0 (0)	1 (5.6%)	–
Midbrain	1 (2.6%)	1 (5.6%)	1.000
Pons	1 (2.6%)	0 (0)	–
Medulla oblongata	8 (20.5%)	2 (11.1%)	0.622
Area postrema	8 (20.5%)	2 (11.1%)	0.622

Abbreviations: NMOSD neuromyelitis optica spectrum disorders, *CTD* connective tissue disorders

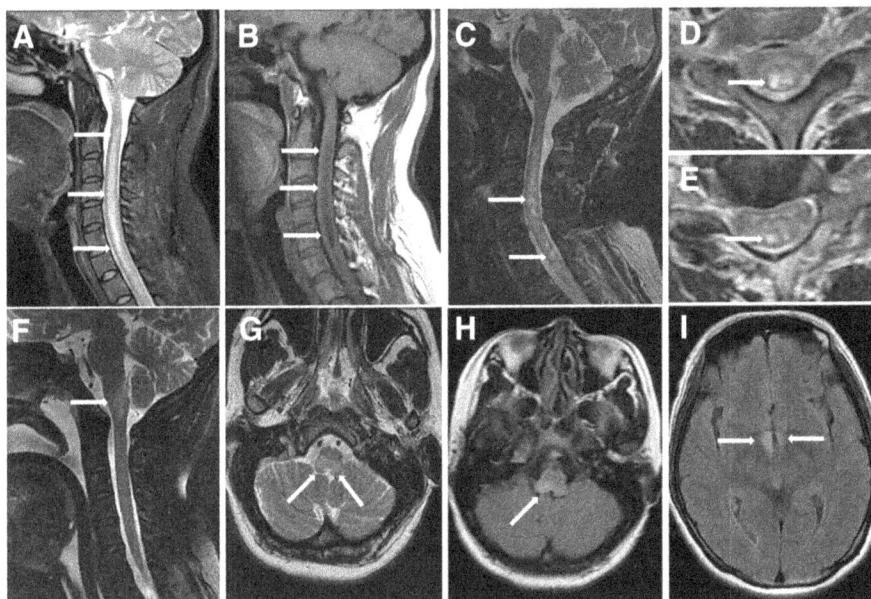

Fig. 1 Representative MRI abnormalities (arrows) in patients with NMOSD with CTD. **a** and **b** are from a 35-year-old woman with NMOSD and SS; (**a**) shows longitudinally extensive transverse myelitis (LETM) lesions on T2WI, and **b** shows 'T1 dark' associated with LETM. **c, d** and **e**, from a 40-year-old woman with NMOSD and SLE, show bright spotty lesions (BSLs) associated with LETM on T2WI. **f**, from a 38-year-old woman with NMOSD and SS, shows an area postrema lesion on T2WI. **g**, A 45-year-old woman with RA, shows a medulla oblongata lesion on T2WI. **h**, from a 39-year-old woman with NMOSD and undifferentiated CTD (UCTD), shows an area postrema lesion on FLAIR imaging. **i**, A 45-year-old woman with NMOSD and UCTD, showed bilateral hypothalamus lesions on the FLAIR imaging

acute myelitis. T1 hypointensity and T2 BSLs probably indicated intense damage of the spinal cord [11, 12]. However, the characteristics of spinal MRI did not show any significant difference between the two groups in the chronic phase. These findings may partially explain the differences in sensory disability and EDSS scores at nadir. Since CTDs can cause peripheral neuropathy leading to sensory deficits, electromyography should be performed to exclude that diagnosis. None of the patients in the present study showed clinical symptoms or signs caused by peripheral neuropathy until the last follow-up, according to their records. Pain is common in NMOSD and can lead to a reduced quality of life [13, 14]. In the present study, neuropathic pain (NP) was defined carefully according to previous reports [13, 15]. Almost half of the patients in both groups complained of NP in the present study, the characteristics and intensity of this pain should be evaluated in the future using previously reported methods [13].

The serum autoantibody AQP4-IgG is highly sensitive and specific for NMOSD [16]. In 2004, Lennon and colleagues reported this autoantibody as a frequent feature of NMOSD; the presence of the antibody was 73% sensitive and 91% specific for clinically defined neuromyelitis optica (NMO) [17]. Since then, many study groups have tested AQP4-IgG in patients with NMO or NMOSD, with the reported frequency varying according to the assay, e.g., immunofluorescence, immunoprecipitation, radioimmunoprecipitation or CBA [18–22]. The new diagnostic criteria for NMOSD recommended CBA for the detection of AQP4-IgG because of its good sensitivity and specificity. Hence, we adopted CBA to detect AQP4-IgG in the present study. The seroprevalence of AQP4-IgG was 74.4% and 66.7% in patients with and without CTD, respectively, with no significant difference. This result was similar to those of Jarius et al. [23], who found that AQP4-IgG seropositivity in patients with CTD and co-existing neurological disorders was restricted to those with NMOSD [23]. This finding strongly suggests that AQP4-IgG was linked to the pathogenesis of NMOSD in those patients.

Although the frequency of ANAs was significantly higher in NMOSD patients with CTD than in those without CTD in our study, the frequency of ANAs in the latter group was more than 50%, which was similar to the frequencies reported in other reports [5, 11, 23–26]. Until now, the exact relationship between NMOSD and CTD has been unknown. A prevailing notion of NMOSD pathogenesis is that it is a complication of CTD manifested predominantly in the CNS. If a complication of CTD were the cause of NMOSD, one would expect that CTD would consistently be diagnosed before the onset of NMOSD. However, of the 18 NMOSD patients with CTD in our study, only 9 developed CTD before NMOSD, and in the other 9, the diagnosis of CTD followed the diagnosis of NMOSD, which was similar to previously reported data [5]. This chronology may support the current hypothesis that NMOSD and CTD can be co-existing conditions that are clinically expressed in patients susceptible to autoimmunity [27]. In the present study, the level of serum IgG and the percentage of γ-globulin were significantly higher in patients with CTD than in those without CTD, which was in agreement with a previous study [28]. Zhang and co-workers also found higher levels of CRP in NMOSD patients with autoimmune diseases than in those without autoimmune diseases. These findings may suggest that NMOSD patients with CTD have an intensified autoimmune response.

Longitudinally extensive transverse myelitis (LETM) lesions on spinal cord MRI are regarded as one of the six core clinical characteristics of NMOSD. The spinal cord lesions of NMOSD patients with CTD were longer than those of NMOSD patients without CTD. An increased frequency of both 'T1 dark' and T2 BSLs was found in NMOSD patients with CTD compared to those without CTD, in contrast to the findings of another study [28]. As previously reported, 'T1 dark' signals on spinal MRI was relatively specific to NMOSD, and were rarely found in MS [11, 12]. This feature may indicates early necrosis and cavity formation caused by intense cord damage. In previous reports, BSLs on axial T2WI were the most distinctive finding of NMO on spinal MRI, with frequencies of 54% and 86.1%, respectively [11, 12]. The pathophysiology of BSLs remains unclear. Compared to BSL-negative patients, BSL-positive patients had a higher frequency of contrast-enhanced lesions. Hence BSLs probably reflect severe damage to the spinal cord, which may destroy the blood-brain barrier (BBB) [11]. These significant differences between the two groups may also indicate that NMOSD patients with CTD are prone to intense autoimmune responses, which is in accordance with the elevated IgG, increased EDSS scores at nadir and intensified sensory disability in these patients compared to those without CTD. CTD-induced tissue damage probably promotes AQP4-IgG-induced pathology. ANAs or other inflammatory mechanisms in CTD may contribute to vascular damage and disruption of the BBB induced by vasculitis, which makes the AQP4-IgG accessible to the CNS and triggers the AQP4-IgG-mediated inflammatory cascade [23, 27]. EDSS scores were positively correlated with group classification (NMOSD and NMOSD with CTD), the length of spinal cord lesions and T1 hypointensity. However, partial correlation results showed that EDSS had no correlation with different groups after adjusting for the length of spinal cord lesions and T1 hypointensity.

Therefore, the elevated EDSS scores in NMOSD patients with CTD may be due to the increased length of spinal cord lesions and frequency of T1 hypointensity. The results may also be influenced by other factors, which we will explore and investigate in the future.

Short TM (< 3 vertebral segments) is considered non-characteristic of NMOSD. In our study, we found that short TM is not uncommon in NMOSD. A short TM episode as an onset symptom was found in 17.9% of NMOSD patients without CTD and 5.6% of those with CTD, which were higher than those published in a previous report [29]. This difference was probably because Flanagan's study included only AQP4-IgG-positive NMOSD cases. The frequency of short TM at the initial manifestation of myelitis was lower in NMOSD patients with CTD than in those without CTD, which may also indicate that NMOSD patients with CTD have a more intense autoimmune response. This finding is also consistent with the elevated levels of IgG and EDSS at nadir in NMOSD patients with CTD. Short TM can be the first presentation of NMOSD, which may delay diagnosis and treatment. Therefore, short TM, especially complicated with 'T1 dark' and/or T2 BSLs, should not exclude consideration of AQP4-IgG and ANAs testing, which may be helpful for avoiding delayed diagnosis and treatment of NMOSD.

Brain MRI in NMOSD is historically thought to be normal or non-specific, especially at the onset of the disease. However, the presence of certain lesions described as specific to NMOSD may be helpful in its diagnosis. Classic NMOSD lesions are those located at sites of high AQP4 expression, such as the periependymal areas, which include the hypothalamus, periaqueductal grey and area postrema [30]. Brain lesions are present in approximately half of patients at presentation [30, 31], and increase in number with disease progression [30, 32]. We investigated brain MRI findings at onset in all patients in the study. The frequency of abnormal brain MRI findings was 35.9% in NMOSD patients without CTD and 50% in those with CTD; these rates were not significantly different. Nearly all of the supratentorial lesions were non-specific and asymptomatic. These lesions were dot-like or patchy, < 3 cm in diameter, and located in the cerebral deep white matter, as previously described [33]. Infratentorial lesions were more common and specific than supratentorial lesions. In our study, patients had a higher frequency of medulla oblongata lesions than pons or midbrain lesions. This result was consistent with previous reports [28, 34–37]. Although the medulla was the most common brainstem lesion location in NMO, only a few patients showed MRI lesions in the area postrema at onset in our study, which was consistent with the findings of our previous study [10], and all but one of the patients were free of apparent hypothalamic lesions at onset. 'Classic-' or 'typical NMO lesions' located at the hypothalamus and area postrema are highly specific to the diagnosis of NMOSD; however, these lesions are seen in only a minority of patients, especially at onset [30, 38, 39].

This study had certain limitations. First, as this study is retrospective, bias is inevitable. Second, all the patients came from a single centre, and were insufficient in number. In the future, we will recruit more NMOSD patients with and without CTD and test the titer of AQP4-IgG, which may lead to a deeper understanding of the significance of CTD in NMOSD.

Conclusions

In conclusion, NMOSD patients with and without CTD were similar in most of the demographic, clinical and laboratory features that we examined. NMOSD patients with CTD have more frequent of T1 hypointensity and T2 BSLs, longer spinal cord lesions on MRI and a lower frequency of short TM than those without CTD.

Abbreviations

ACA: Anti-neutrophil cytoplasmic antibodies; AHA: Anti-histone antibody; AM: Acute myelitis; ANAs: Antinuclear autoantibodies; ANCAs: Anti-neutrophil cytoplasmic antibodies; anti-dsDNA: Anti-double stranded DNA antibodies; anti-Jo1: Anti-Jo-1 antibodies; anti-nRNP: Antinuclear ribonucleoprotein; anti-Scl70: Anti-topoisomerase I antibodies; anti-Sm: Anti-Sm antibodies; anti-SSA: Anti-SSA/Ro antibodies; anti-SSB: Anti-SSB/La antibodies; AnuA: Anti-nucleosome antibody; AQP4-IgG: Immunoglobulin G autoantibodies against aquaporin-4; ARPA: Anti-ribonucleoprotein antibodies; ASO: Anti-streptolysin; BBB: Blood-brain barrier; BSLs: Bright spotty lesions; C: Complement; CBA: Cell-based assay; Cl: Chloride; CNS: Central nervous system; CRP: C-reactive protein; CSF: Cerebrospinal fluid; CTD: Connective tissue disorders; EDSS: Kurtzke Expanded Disability Status Scale; ENAs: Extractable nuclear antigen autoantibodies; FLAIR: Fluid-attenuated inversion recovery; Glu: Glucose; GPI: Glucose-6 phosphate isomerase; IgG: Immunoglobulin G; IVIG: Intravenous immunoglobulin G; IVMP: Intravenous methylprednisolone; LETM: Longitudinally extensive transverse myelitis; MOG-IgG: Myelin oligodendrocyte glycoprotein immunoglobulin G; MRI: Magnetic resonance imaging; NMO: Neuromyelitis optica; NMOSD: Neuromyelitis optica spectrum disorders; NP: Neuropathic pain; OCB: Oligoclonal banding; ON: Optic neuritis; RA: Rheumatoid arthritis; RF: Rheumatoid factor; SD: Standard deviation; SLE: Systemic lupus erythematosus; SPSS: Statistical Package for the Social Sciences; SS: Sjögren syndrome; STIR: Sagittal short tau inversion recovery; T1WI: T1-weighted imaging; T2WI: T2-weighted imaging; TM: Transverse myelitis; UCTD: Undifferentiated connective tissue disorders; VB: Vertebral segments; WBC: White blood cell

Acknowledgements
We thank Drs A. Vincent and D. Beeson for providing plasmids for AQP4, and we thank our patients for participating in this study.

Funding
The study was supported by the National Natural Science Foundation of China (grant number: 81571172) and the Tianjin Research Program of Application Foundation and Advanced Technology (grant number: 15JCYBJC49800).

Authors' contributions
CSY, LY and FDS participated in study design. CSY, QXZ, SHC, LJZ, LML, YQ and JW participated in data collection. ZHS and NNZN participated in MRI analysis. CSY and QXZ participated in statistical analysis. All authors read and approved the final manuscript.

Competing interests
The authors declare that they have no competing interests.

Author details
[1]Department of Neurology, Tianjin Neurological Institute, Tianjin Medical University General Hospital, No 154 Anshan Road, Heping District, Tianjin 300052, China. [2]Department of Radiology, Tianjin Medical University General Hospital, No 154 Anshan Road, Heping District, Tianjin 300052, China. [3]Department of Neurology, Barrow Neurological Institute, St. Joseph's

References
1. Wingerchuk DM, Lennon VA, Pittock SJ, Lucchinetti CF, Weinshenker BG. Revised diagnostic criteria for neuromyelitis optica. Neurology. 2006;66:1485–9.
2. Wingerchuk DM, Banwell B, Bennett JL, et al. International consensus diagnostic criteria for neuromyelitis optica spectrum disorders. Neurology. 2015;85:177–89.
3. Wingerchuk DM, Lennon VA, Lucchinetti CF, Pittock SJ, Weinshenker BG. The spectrum of neuromyelitis optica. Lancet Neurol. 2007;6:805–15.
4. Wang Y, Wu A, Chen X, et al. Comparison of clinical characteristics between neuromyelitis optica spectrum disorders with and without spinal cord atrophy. BMC Neurol. 2014;14:246.
5. Pittock SJ, Lennon VA, de Seze J, et al. Neuromyelitis optica and non organ-specific autoimmunity. Arch Neurol. 2008;65:78–83.
6. Petri M, Orbai AM, Alarcón GS, et al. Derivation and validation of the systemic lupus international collaborating clinics classification criteria for systemic lupus erythematosus. Arthritis Rheum. 2012;64:2677–86.
7. Shiboski SC, Shiboski CH, Criswell L, et al. American College of Rheumatology classification criteria for Sjögren's syndrome: a data-driven, expert consensus approach in the Sjögren's international collaborative clinical Alliance cohort. Arthritis Care Res (Hoboken). 2012;64:475–87.
8. Aletaha D, Neogi T, Silman AJ, et al. 2010 rheumatoid arthritis classification criteria: an American College of Rheumatology/European league against rheumatism collaborative initiative. Arthritis Rheum. 2010;62:2569–81.
9. Mosca M, Tani C, Vagnani S, Carli L, Bombardieri S. The diagnosis and classification of undifferentiated connective tissue diseases. J Autoimmun. 2014;48–49:50–2.
10. Yang C-S, Zhang D-Q, Wang J-H, et al. Clinical features and sera anti-aquaporin 4 antibody positivity in patients with demyelinating disorders of the central nervous system from Tianjin, China. CNS Neurosci Ther. 2014;20:32–9.
11. Yonezu T, Ito S, Mori M, Babb J, Loh J, Shepherd TM. 'Bright spotty lesions' on spinal magnetic resonance imaging differentiate neuromyelitis optica from multiple sclerosis. Mult Scler. 2014;20:331–7.
12. Pekcevik Y, Mitchell CH, Mealy MA, et al. Differentiating neuromyelitis optica from other causes of longitudinally extensive transverse myelitis on spinal magnetic resonance imaging. Mult Scler. 2016;22:302–11.
13. Pellkofer HL, Havla J, Hauer D, et al. The major brain endocannabinoid 2-AG controls neuropathic pain and mechanical hyperalgesia in patients with neuromyelitis optica. PLoS One. 2013;9(8):e71500. https://doi.org/10.1371/journal.pone.0071500 eCollection 2013.
14. Kanamori Y, Nakashima I, Takai Y, et al. Pain in neuromyelitis optica and its effect on quality of life: a cross-sectional study. Neurology. 2011;77:652–8.
15. Bouhassira D, Attal N, Alchaar H, et al. Comparison of pain syndromes associated with nervous or somatic lesions and development of a new neuropathic pain diagnostic questionnaire (DN4). Pain. 2005;114:29–36.
16. Lennon VA, Kryzer TJ, Pittock SJ, Verkman AS, Hinson SR. IgG marker of optic-spinal multiple sclerosis binds to the aquaporin-4 water channel. J Exp Med. 2005;202:473–7.
17. Lennon VA, Wingerchuk DM, Kryzer TJ, et al. A serum autoantibody marker of neuromyelitis optica: distinction from multiple sclerosis. Lancet. 2004;364:2106–12.
18. Marignier R, De Seze J, Durand-Dubief F, et al. NMO-IgG and Devic's neuromyelitis optica: a French experience. Mult Scler. 2008;14:440–5.

19. Jarius S, Franciotta D, Bergamaschi R, et al. NMO-IgG in the diagnosis of neuromyelitis optica. Neurology. 2007;68:1076-7.

20. Takahashi T, Fujihara K, Nakashima I, et al. Antiaquaporin-4 antibody is involved in the pathogenesis of NMO: a study on antibody titre. Brain. 2007;130:1235-43.

21. Waters P, Jarius S, Littleton E, et al. Aquaporin-4 antibodies in neuromyelitis optica and longitudinally-extensive transverse myelitis. Arch Neurol. 2007;65:913-9.

22. Paul F, Jarius S, Aktas O, et al. Antibody to aquaporin 4 in the diagnosis of neuromyelitis optica. PLoS Med. 2007;4:e133.

23. Jarius S, Jacobi C, de Seze J, et al. Frequency and syndrome specificity of antibodies to aquaporin-4 in neurological patients with rheumatic disorders. Mult Scler. 2011;17:1067-73.

24. de Seze J, Stojkovic T, Ferriby D, et al. Devic's neuromyelitis optica: clinical, laboratory, MRI and outcome profile. J Neurol Sci. 2002;197:57-61.

25. Jacob A, McKeon A, Nakashima I, et al. Current concept of neuromyelitis optica (NMO) and NMO spectrum disorders. J Neurol Neurosurg Psychiatry. 2013;84:922-30.

26. Hummers LK, Krishnan C, Casciola-Rosen L, et al. Recurrent transverse myelitis associates with anti-Ro (SSA) autoantibodies. Neurology. 2004; 62:147-9.

27. Wingerchuk DM, Weinshenker BG. The emerging relationship between neuromyelitis optica and systemic rheumatologic autoimmune disease. Mult Scler. 2012;18:5-10.

28. Zhang B, Zhong Y, Wang Y, et al. Neuromyelitis optica spectrum disorders without and with autoimmune diseases. BMC Neurol. 2014;14:162.

29. Flanagan EP, Weinshenker BG, Krecke KN, et al. Short myelitis lesions in aquaporin-4-IgG-positive neuromyelitis optica spectrum disorders. JAMA Neurol. 2015;72:81-7.

30. Pittock SJ, Lennon VA, Krecke K, Wingerchuk DM, Lucchinetti CF, Weinshenker BG. Brain abnormalities in neuromyelitis optica. Arch Neurol. 2006;63:390-6.

31. Kıyat-Atamer A, Ekizoğlu E, Tüzün E, et al. Long-term MRI findings in neuromyelitis optica: seropositive versus seronegative patients. Eur J Neurol. 2013;20:781-7.

32. Cabrera-Gomez JA, Kister I. Conventional brain MRI in neuromyelitis optica. Eur J Neurol. 2012;19:812-9.

33. Kim W, Park MS, Lee SH, et al. Characteristic brain magnetic resonance imaging abnormalities in central nervous system aquaporin-4 autoimmunity. Mult Scler. 2010;16:1229-36.

34. Lu Z, Zhang B, Qiu W, et al. Comparative brain stem lesions on MRI of acute disseminated encephalomyelitis, neuromyelitis optica, and multiple sclerosis. PLoS One. 2011;6:e22766.

35. Downer JJ, Leite MI, Carter R, Palace J, Küker W, Quaghebeur G. Diagnosis of neuromyelitis optica (NMO) spectrum disorders: is MRI obsolete? Neuroradiology. 2012;54:279-85.

36. Asgari N, Skejoe HPB, Lillevang ST, Steenstrup T, Stenager E, Kyvik KO. Modifications of longitudinally extensive transverse myelitis and brainstem lesions in the course of neuromyelitis optica (NMO): a population-based, descriptive study. BMC Neurol. 2013;13:33.

37. Jarius S, Ruprecht K, Wildemann B, et al. Contrasting disease patterns in seropositive and seronegative neuromyelitis optica: a multicentre study of 175 patients. J Neuroinflammation. 2012;9:1-17.

38. Pittock SJ, Weinshenker BG, Lucchinetti CF, Wingerchuk DM, Corboy JR, Lennon VA. Neuromyelitis optica brain lesions localized at sites of high aquaporin 4 expression. Arch Neurol. 2006;63:964-8.

39. Matthews LA, Palace JA. The role of imaging in diagnosing neuromyelitis optica spectrum disorder. Mult Scler Relat Disord. 2013;3:284-93.

21

Low self-reported sports activity before stroke predicts poor one-year-functional outcome after first-ever ischemic stroke in a population-based stroke register

Christian Urbanek[1*], Viola Gokel[2], Anton Safer[3], Heiko Becher[4], Armin J. Grau[1], Florian Buggle[1] and Frederick Palm[1]

Abstract

Background: Physical activity (PA) is associated with lower risk of stroke. We tested the hypothesis that lack of pre-stroke PA is an independent predictor of poor outcome after first-ever ischemic stroke.

Methods: We assessed recent self-reported PA and other potential predictors for loss of functional independence - modified Rankin Scale (mRS) > 2 - one year after first-ever ischemic stroke in 1370 patients registered between 2006 and 2010 in the Ludwigshafen Stroke Study, a population-based stroke registry.

Results: After 1 year, 717 (52.3%) of patients lost their independence including 251 patients (18.3%) who had died. In multivariate logistic regression analysis lack of regular PA prior to stroke (Odds Ratio (OR) 1.7, Confidence Interval (CI) 1.1–2.5), independently predicted poor outcome together with higher age (65–74: OR 1.7; CI 1.1–2.8, 75–84 years: OR 3.3; CI 2.1–5.3; ≥85 years OR 14.5; CI 7.4–28.5), female sex (OR 1.5; CI 1.1–2.1), diabetes mellitus (OR 1.8; CI 1.3–2.5), stroke severity (OR 1.2; CI 1.1–1.2), probable atherothrombotic stroke etiology (OR 1.8; CI 1.1–2.8) and high leukocyte count (> 9.000/mm^3; OR 1.4; CI 1.0–1.9) at admission. Subclassifying unknown stroke etiology, embolic stroke of unknown source (ESUS; $n = 40$, OR 2.2; CI 0.9–5.5) tended to be associated with loss of independence.

Conclusion: In addition to previously reported factors, lack of PA prior to stroke as potential indicator of worse physical condition, high leukocyte count at admission as indicator of the inflammatory response and probable atherothrombotic stroke etiology might be independent predictors for non-functional independence in first-ever ischemic stroke.

Keywords: Stroke, Cerebral infarction, Outcome, Physical activity, Predictors, Risk factors

Background

A high proportion of stroke survivors worldwide require assistance or are fully dependent on caregivers for activities of daily living after stroke [1]. Improved individualized therapy in acute ischemic stroke care, preemptive therapy of risk factors or changes in lifestyle prior to stroke may modify ischemic stroke (IS) outcome. Prediction of functional outcome in patients with IS can support clinicians to improve effective stroke care,

anticipate discharge planning and support patients and family to develop realistic expectations for long-term care provision.

Clinical rating or imaging - based scoring systems like ASTRAL, DRAGON or SEDAN have been published to predict loss of functional independence after IS [2–5]. Age, initial stroke severity, onset to admission time, range of visual fields, level of consciousness, glucose and concentrations of serum neutrophil markers were some predictors for losing functional independence in these studies [6–11]. However, prognostic models had only minor impact on clinical practice. The majority of these scores were based on retrospective analysis of cases from

* Correspondence: christian_urbanek@hotmail.de
[1]Department of Neurology, University of Heidelberg, Städtisches Klinikum Ludwigshafen am Rhein, Bremserstr. 79, 67063 Ludwigshafen, Germany
Full list of author information is available at the end of the article

hospital-based data [3, 12–18]. Few studies have systematically evaluated multiple factors in prospective and unselected data series of consecutive ischemic stroke patients [19–23].

Physical activity (PA) activity before stroke as measured by self-report adds to the risk of poor outcome.

Epidemiologic studies have consistently suggested an association between PA and the risk of stroke [24–27]. PA is recommended to reduce the risk of first-ever and possibly the risk of recurrent stroke [24, 28–30]. Low PA may lower the individual capacity to cope with the metabolic and other stressful sequelae after cerebral ischemia.

The aim of this study was to identify predictors of one-year-functional outcome in patients with first-ever ischemic stroke, using five-year case series data from a prospective, population-based stroke registry. In particular, we tested the hypothesis that lack of self-reported recent PA increases risk of poor functional outcome after IS. Besides the well-established risk-factors, inflammatory parameters such as leukocyte count and fibrinogen were added to our analysis as previous studies showed an effect of a high inflammatory response on stroke outcome [31, 32].

Methods

The "Ludwigshafen Stroke Study" (LuSSt) is a prospective population-based stroke register in Ludwigshafen at Rhine in Germany, that started on January 1st, 2006 [33].

In order to achieve complete case ascertainment, multiple overlapping methods of patient identification were used as described previously [33]. Case ascertainment of hospitalized patients was ensured by collaboration with all hospitals in the city of Ludwigshafen and hospitals in the region. To identify all non-hospitalized stroke patients, general practitioners, specialists in internal medicine, and neurologists practicing in Ludwigshafen were informed about the register before study initiation and were contacted together with nursing and residential homes. All patients treated at "Klinikum Ludwigshafen" were examined by a member of the study team, including an interview based on a structured questionnaire as described previously [34]. We intended to keep the questions as simple as possible for interviews in acutely ill patients. All patients who have been treated outside "Klinikum Ludwigshafen" and gave informed consent, were examined by a member of the study team. In the other patients data were obtained by the attending physician and transmitted to the study center in pseudonymised form. In all patients with informed consent follow-up investigations were performed by telephone 1, 3 and 12 months after stroke utilizing a standardized questionnaire. If patients were unable to provide informations, a next-of-kin was interviewed. In patients

without informed consent, or without response to multiple telephone and letter contact attempts, survival and death information was obtained by the population registration authority. LuSSt has been approved by the ethics committee of the Landesärztekammer Rhineland-Palatinate and by the data protection commissioner of Rhineland-Palatinate.

Stroke was defined according to the definition of the World Health Organization (WHO) [35]. Stroke subtype classification was based on the results of brain imaging, discriminating between IS, intracerebral hemorrhage (ICH), and subarachnoid hemorrhage (SAH). In case brain imaging was unavailable stroke type was defined as undetermined. The present analysis comprises only patients with first-ever ischemic stroke up to December 31st, 2010. Patients with a first ischemic stroke and a history of transient ischemic attack (TIA) were coded as first-ever ischemic stroke according to comparable population-based stroke registries [36]. Patients with recurrent stroke, TIA, SAH and ICH were excluded for present analysis.

Outcome parameters and risk factors

Stroke severity was determined at hospital admission using the National Institute of Health Stroke Scale (NIHSS) [37]. In order to assess functional status prior to stroke and functional outcome after first-ever ischemic stroke, modified Rankin Scale (mRS) was used [38, 39]. MRS is a 7-point scale ranging from 0 (no symptoms) to 6 (death). A score of 2 or less indicates functional independence [40]. Loss of independence in daily life was defined as a mRS > 2 summarizing patients that had survived first 12 months after stroke with significant disabilities, and deceased ones. Cardiovascular risk factors were defined according to current guidelines as described previously [34, 41, 42]. Definitions have already been described earlier [34, 43]. In brief, hypertension was diagnosed if the patient was on antihypertensive medication on admission, if hypertension had been diagnosed before by a physician or if blood pressure was > 140/90 mmHg in two or more measurements > 3 days after stroke. Diabetes mellitus was defined in subjects with fasting blood glucose level above 125 mg/dl in venous blood, present anti-diabetic medication at hospital or known diagnosis of diabetes mellitus. Diagnosis of atrial fibrillation (AF) has been made if permanent or paroxysmal AF was present on ECG or long-term monitoring and additionally, in case of a history of this diagnosis. All in-patients with cholesterol-lowering medication, fasting cholesterol levels > 200 mg/dl or LDL-cholesterol > 140 mg/dl lead to diagnosis of Hypercholesterolemia. We defined current smoking as present daily usage of any kind of tobacco (at least one cigarette, cigar, cigarillo or pipe). We classified history of smoking as smoking for any period of at least 6 months. Patients with previous angina pectoris, myocardial infarction, coronary stenting or coronary artery bypass were selected as subjects with coronary artery disease (CAD) [34]. Patients with medical history of peripheral artery disease (PAD), arterial bypass surgery, stenting vessels of lower limbs and patients with present intermittent claudication or history of intermittent claudication of vascular origin were diagnosed PAD. Alcohol consumption as measured by self-report was coded if > 1 drink per week was consumed on a regular base. Another selection criteria was consumption of alcohol in the past.

We used definition of the German Olympic Sports Association for PA as formerly described: PA as any leisure-time motor activity that had its aim in itself or was performed for no other purpose than to improve or maintain physical fitness [43]. Therefore, all activities such as walking were defined as PA and had been included. However, PA during work, PA on the way to or from employment or activities like gardening were not considered. All subjects were asked whether they had regularly performed sports during the months before stroke [30, 43]. Regular PA was acknowledged as such activity at least once a week.

C-Reactive Protein (CRP) [particle-enhanced immunoturbidimetric assay CRPL3 (cobas®)], fibrinogen (Clauss method on IL Coagulation Systems, Instrumentation Laboratory) and leukocyte count (XE analyserXE-2100; Sysmex) were determined < 48 h after admission.

Medical treatment

Thrombolysis was defined as intravenous application of recombined tissue plasmin activator (rt-PA). During the early years of LuSSt, mechanical recanalisation was not a standard in acute stroke therapy, and therefore not captured in the database. Antiplatetlet treatment included usage of one or more of these drugs: acetylsalicyl acid, clopidogrel, dipyridamol with acetylsalicylic acid and inhibitors of glycopeptide IIb/IIIa.

Classification of stroke etiology

We used a modification of the TOAST (Trial of Org 10,172 in Acute Stroke Treatment) criteria to define etiological subtypes of ischemic stroke [44]. Stroke due to large-artery atherosclerosis, cardioembolism, small-artery occlusion, stroke of other determined cause and stroke of undetermined etiology (except such from two or more competing etiologies) were diagnosed according to the TOAST criteria. In addition, we diagnosed 'probable atherothrombotic stroke' in such patients with stenosis < 50% diameter reduction on duplex sonography, CT-, MR- or digital subtraction angiography and additional brain infarction(s) > 1.5 cm in the absence of any source of cardioembolism. This category is comparable to "athero

thrombotic stroke" in the PERFORM study [45]. In patients with more than one potential cause for stroke, etiology was assigned to the most likely causative mechanism according to the SSS-TOAST classification [46]. Patients with stroke of unknown etiology were analyzed retrospectively, specifically using embolic strokes of undetermined source criteria (ESUS) and reclassified in cryptogenic ESUS, cryptogenic NON-ESUS or stroke of undetermined source (incomplete work-up or concurrent stroke). Classification was performed by experienced neurologists of the study team [47]. Controversial diagnoses were discussed and agreed in study meetings.

Statistical methods

For univariate analyses χ^2-test, t-test with and without log-transformation and the Wilcoxon test were used as appropriate. For multivariate analysis, logistic regression was used. Variables being significant in univariate analyses were included in multivariable logistic regression analysis using the backward elimination procedure. To analyse the influence of early deaths after stroke, we compared our full dataset (Model A) with results after excluding patients who died early within the first 7 days after stroke (Model B). In further analysis, patients with "first ever ischemic stroke of unknown cause" were divided into three groups: "cryptogenic ESUS", "cryptogenic NON-ESUS" and "stroke of undetermined source" (stroke with incomplete work-up or concurrent stroke) (Model C).

All data were analysed using SAS 9.4 software (SAS Institute, North Carolina). All tests were performed for two-sided testing. Level of significance was set to $\alpha = 0.05$ for all tests.

Results

Between January 1st, 2006 and December 31st, 2010, 1547 cases of first-ever ischemic stroke were registered in LuSSt. One-year follow-up information was available for 1370 subjects (88.6%, 677 women and 693 men). Information on mRS prior to stroke was available in 930 patients among whom 63 patients (4.6%) had a mRS > 2. No significant differences between patients with and without follow-up existed regarding age, sex and NIHSS at admission ($p > 0.1$, respectively). Among the 1370 patients, 717 patients (52.3%) had poor outcome with loss of functional independence including 251 (18.3%) patients who had died within the first year.

Clinical characteristics of all patients by one-year functional outcome are shown in Table 1. In univariate analysis, female sex, higher age, higher NIHSS score at admission, stroke etiology, higher leukocyte count, higher fibrinogen level, antiplatelet drugs before stroke, intravenous thrombolysis, arterial hypertension, AF, CAD, hypercholesterolemia, diabetes mellitus, PAD,

Table 1 Baseline characteristics, clinical characteristics and cerebrovascular risk factors by functional-outcome in 1370 patients with first-ever ischemic stroke – *univariate analysis*

Predictor variable (number of missing observations total)	One-year functional outcome			p value
	N (%) [&]Median (lower-upper quartile)			
	Total (n = 1370)	mRS ≤ 2 (n = 653)	mRS > 2 (n = 717)	
Sex (0)				< 0.01
Men	693 (50.6)	385 (59)	308 (43)	
Women	677 (49.4)	268 (41)	409 (57)	
Age (mean ± SD;years) (0)	71.6; ±13	66.1; ±12.3	76.6; ±11.4	< 0.01
Vascular risk factors				
Arterial hypertension (11)				< 0.01
Yes	1195 (87.9)	549 (84.6)	646 (91)	
No	164 (12.1)	100 (15.4)	64 (9)	
Atrial fibrillation (36)				< 0.01
Yes	391 (29.3)	112 (17.6)	279 (39.9)	
No	943 (70.7)	523 (82.4)	420 (60.1)	
Coronary heart disease (46)				< 0.01
Yes	304 (23)	125 (19.7)	179 (25.9)	
No	1020 (77)	509 (80.3)	511 (74.1)	
Hypercholesterolemia (36)				< 0.01
Yes	884 (66.3)	465 (72.5)	419 (60.5)	
No	450 (33.7)	176 (27.5)	274 (39.5)	
Diabetes (20)				< 0.01
Yes	422 (31.3)	167 (25.9)	255 (36.1)	
No	928 (68.7)	477 (74.1)	451 (63.9)	
Peripheral arterial disease (51)				< 0.01
Yes	132 (10)	46 (7.3)	86 (12.6)	
No	1187 (90)	588 (92.7)	599 (87.4)	
Smoking (0)				< 0.01
Yes, actually	305 (22.3)	184 (28.2)	121 (16.9)	
Yes, in the past	394 (28.8)	196 (30)	198 (27.6)	
No	520 (38)	224 (34.3)	296 (41.3)	
Unknown	151 (11)	49 (7.5)	102 (14.2)	
Consumption of alcohol[a] (80)				< 0.01
Yes, actually	504 (39.1)	277 (44.3)	227 (34.1)	
Yes, in the past	38 (2.9)	17 (2.7)	21 (3.2)	
No	665 (51.6)	302 (48.3)	363 (54.6)	
Unknown	83 (6.4)	29 (4.7)	54 (8.1)	
Regular physical activity (0)				< 0.01
Yes	266 (19.4)	187 (28.6)	79 (11)	
No	1104 (80.6)	466 (71.4)	638 (89)	
Clinical characteristics on admission				
NIHSS (33)[b]	3 (2–6)	2 (1–4)	5 (3–11)	< 0.01
TOAST (0)				< 0.01
Probable atherothrombotic	208 (15.2)	98 (15)	110 (15.3)	
Cardioembolic	422 (30.8)	143 (21.9)	279 (39)	

Table 1 Baseline characteristics, clinical characteristics and cerebrovascular risk factors by functional-outcome in 1370 patients with first-ever ischemic stroke – *univariate analysis (Continued)*

Predictor variable (number of missing observations total)	One-year functional outcome			p value
	N (%) &Median (lower-upper quartile)			
	Total (n = 1370)	mRS ≤ 2 (n = 653)	mRS > 2 (n = 717)	
Large-artery atherosclerosis	192 (14)	85 (13)	107 (14.9)	
Small-artery occlusion	369 (27)	237 (36.3)	132 (18.4)	
Other determined	62 (4.5)	28 (4.3)	34 (4.7)	
Unknown	117 (8.5)	62 (9.5)	55 (7.7)	
Leukocytes (47)[b]	8.3 (6.8–10.2)	7.9 (6.6–9.7)	8.6 (7.0–10.7)	< 0.01
Fibrinogen (86)[b]	370 (318–434)	356 (309–412)	386 (329–455)	< 0.01
Antiplatlet drugs (0)				< 0.01
Yes	480 (35)	197 (30.2)	283 (39.5)	
No	890 (65)	456 (69.8)	434 (60.5)	
Lysis therapy (0)				< 0.01
Yes	124 (9.1)	37 (5.7)	87 (12.1)	
No	1246 (90.9)	616 (94.3)	630 (87.9)	
Clinical characteristics at discharge				
NIHSS (109)[b]	2 (1–4)	1 (0–2)	3 (1–7)	< 0.01
mRS (94)				
≤ 2 (0–2)	838 (65.7)	573 (92)	265 (40.6)	< 0.01
> 2 (3–6)	438 (34.3)	50 (8)	388 (59.4)	

Comparisons by X²-test, Student's t-test with and without log-transformation and Wilcoxon test as appropriate

mRS modified Rankin Scale, *N* number, *NIHSS* National Institutes of Health Stroke Scale, *SD* standard deviation, *TOAST* Trial of ORG 10172 in Acute Stroke Treatment; [a] > 1 drink per week; [b] Quartiles

smoking status, alcohol consumption, regular PA prior to stroke and mRS > 2 at discharge were associated with one-year poor functional outcome or loss of independence. Among 117 patients with ischemic stroke of unknown etiology, stroke workup was incomplete in 39 (33.3%) patients, cryptogenic stroke was diagnosed in 60 (51.3%) patients and more than one possible etiology for ischemic stroke was evident in 18 patients (15.4%). Among patients with cryptogenic stroke, ESUS was diagnosed in 40 (66.7%) patients.

In multivariate analysis, lack of regular PA prior to stroke (OR 1.7; CI 1.1–2.5) independently predicted poor outcome together with female sex (OR 1.5; CI 1.1–2.1), higher age (65–74: OR 1.7; CI 1.1–2.8, 75–84 years: OR 3.3; CI 2.1–5.3; ≥85 years OR 14.5; CI 7.4–28.5), higher NIHSS on admission (OR 1.2; CI 1.1–1.2), diabetes mellitus (OR 1.8; CI 1.3–2.5), probable atherothrombotic stroke (OR 1.8; CI 1.1–2.8) mRS > 2 at hospital discharge (OR 8.9; CI 6.0–13.0) and leukocyte count of > 9.000/mm3 (OR 1.4; CI 1.0–1.9);(Table 2, Model A). Threshold that was reported in previous studies [48]. Exclusion of patients who died < 7 days after stroke (Model B) resulted in comparable results.

Subclassifying patients with unknown stroke etiology the diagnosis of cryptogenic ESUS showed a trend towards loss of functional outcome or death (OR 2.2; CI 0.9–5.5) whereas cryptogenic Non-ESUS stroke did not (OR 1.3; CI 0.5–3.7) (Table 2, Model C).

Discussion

In addition to well known predictors of stroke outcome we identified lack of regular PA prior to stroke, high leukocyte count, probable atherothrombotic stroke etiology as independent predictors of poor functional outcome. Stroke severity (measured by NIHSS or mRS), diabetes mellitus and higher age are well established independent predictors for poor stroke outcome [7, 49–53]. Recently published scoring systems also used parameters like arterial hypertension, AF, higher age, sex, blood glucose, level of consciousness, stroke type or severity to predict stroke outcome [3, 7, 54, 55]. Factors like arterial hypertension, AF, CAD, hypercholesterolemia, PAD, smoking status and alcohol consumption were not independent predictors for loss of functional independence in our population. This may partly be explained by too low numbers of subjects in our study, resulting in insufficient statistical power to detect predictors with moderate impact. Moreover, differences between study populations in risk factor control and compliance to medication intake (e.g. oral anticoagulants

Table 2 Results of multivariate logistic regression analysis on 1-year functional outcome after first-ever ischemic stroke. Model A (all observations), Model B (excluding patients that had died early within 0–7 days after hospital admission) and Model C (all observations with subanalysis of the first-ever ischemic stroke "Unknown cause"). Observations with one or more missing variables have been dropped from multivariate analysis. Bold values indicate significance at $p < 0.05$. Adjusted for age, diabetes mellitus and stroke severity

Predictor variable	Model A OR (95% CI)	$n = 1234$ p value	Model B OR (95% CI)	$n = 1230$ p value	Model C OR (95% CI)	$n = 1234$ p value
Sex						
(W vs M)	1.5 (1.1–2.1)	0.01	1.5 (1.1–2.1)	0.01	1.5 (1.1–2.1)	0.01
Age, years (vs 55–64)						
< 55	0.4 (0.2–0.8)	0.01	0.3 (0.2–0.8)	0.01	0.4 (0.2–0.8)	0.01
65–74	1.7 (1.1–2.8)	0.03	1.7 (1.1–2.8)	0.03	1.7 (1.0–2.8)	0.03
75–84	3.3 (2.1–5.3)	< 0.01	3.3 (2.1–5.3)	< 0.01	3.3 (2.0–5.3)	< 0.01
≥ 85	14.5 (7.4–28.5)	< 0.01	14.5 (7.4–28.5)	< 0.01	14.4 (7.4–28.3)	< 0.01
Regular Physical Activity						
(No vs Yes)	1.7 (1.1–2.5)	< 0.01	1.7 (1.1–2.5)	< 0.01	1.7 (1.1–2.5)	< 0.01
Diabetes						
(Yes vs No)	1.8 (1.3–2.5)	< 0.01	1.9 (1.3–2.95)	< 0.01	1.8 (1.3–2.5)	< 0.01
Leukocyte count						
(≥ 9 vs < 9 × 1000/mm³)	1.4 (1.0–1.9)	0.04	1.4 (1.0–1.9)	0.05	1.4 (1.0–1.9)	0.04
TOAST						
(vs Small-artery occlusion)						
Probable atherothrombotic	1.8 (1.1–2.8)	0.02	1.8 (1.0–2.8)	0.02	1.8 (1.1–2.8)	0.02
Cardioembolic	1.4 (0.9–2.1)	0.12	1.4 (0.9–2.1)	0.13	1.4 (0.9–2.1)	0.12
Large-arthery Atherosclerosis	1.4 (0.9–2.3)	0.17	1.4 (0.9–2.3)	0.17	1.4 (0.9–2.3)	0.17
Other determined	2.0 (0.9–4.4)	0.09	2.0 (0.9–4.4)	0.09	2.0 (0.9–4.4)	0.09
Unkown	1.5 (0.8–3.0)	0.21	1.5 (0.8–3.0)	0.21		
Cryptogenic ESUS					2.2 (0.9–5.5)	0.10
Cryptogenic NON-ESUS					1.3 (0.5–3.7)	0.62
Undetermined source					0.9 (0.2–3.8)	0.94
mRS at hospital discharge						
(≥ 3 vs < 3)	8.9 (6.0–13.3)	< 0.01	8.9 (6.0–13.3)	< 0.01	8.9 (6.0–13.4)	< 0.01
NIHSS on admission						
(per point)	1.2 (1.1–1.2)	< 0.01	1.2 (1.1–1.2)	< 0.01	1.2 (1.1–1.2)	< 0.01

ESUS embolic stroke of unknown source, *mRS* modified Rankin Scale, *NON-ESUS* no embolic stroke of unknown source, *N* number, *NIHSS* National Institutes of Health Stroke Scale, *SD* standard deviation, *TOAST* Trial of ORG 10172 in Acute Stroke Treatment;

in AF) may be accountable for variations between studies.

Lack of regular physical activity is a modifiable risk factor for both, ischemic and hemorrhage stroke [56–58]. PA reduces stroke risk by lowering blood pressure, improving lipid and glucose metabolism and endothelial function. Further benefits are reduction of thrombocyte aggregation and blood viscosity [58]. Recently published studies showed endothelial function and atherogenesis to be influenced by PA [59, 60]. Improved physical fitness results in better control of risk factors like hypertension and diabetes mellitus and this could have contributed to the beneficial effect of PA on stroke outcome in our study. Patients who had engaged in regular PA may be in better physical and mental conditions and have more capacity to cope with the sequelae of stroke. An association between prognosis after stroke and previous PA had been reported in few studies so far [56–58]. In the Framingham study there was no reduction for stroke risk beyond a moderate level of physical activity [26]. We therefore used comparable low threshold (≥1 per week) to define regular PA in our study. Physical handicap before stroke was seldom observed (mRS > 2 in only 4.9% of patients) in our patients and did thus, not explain the association between lack of PA and outcome. A strength of our study is higher number of cases and prospective study design compared to other studies. However, our findings should be ascertained by further prospective studies. PA is a modifiable lifestyle risk factor with a major importance in preemptive strategies to prevent strokes and improve mid-term stroke outcome. For future stroke care, PA as a modifiable risk factor should get more focus in stroke research as well as in primary and secondary stroke care. Documenting and focusing on regular PA might have great impact in primary stroke care leading to better stroke outcomes and more functional independence. Being physically active in mid-life increases the odds of being active in old age [61]. However, more research is necessary, e.g. to find out how much PA preceeding first-ever ischemic stroke reduces stroke severity. Visual representation of the overall distribution of mRS 12 months post stroke draws a clear picture of difference by PA activity pre stroke. Even if a part of the difference is attributable to other confounding factors, like NIHSS on admission and mRS at hospital discharge, the cumulative barchart visualizes striking difference of outcomes in favour of PA. In contrast to other studies, we used definition of the German Olympic Sports Association. Registration of leisure-time motor activity only might result in underestimation of physical activity.

Higher leukocyte count was associated with lack of functional independence in our population indicating that the strength of the early inflammatory response heralds poor prognosis independent of clinical stroke severity and factors that are known to contribute to leukocyte counts such as smoking and diabetes mellitus. Infection before ischemia is an established stroke trigger factor which may partly explain the association between leukocyte count and poor prognosis, as well as larger infarct volume which was not investigated in our study [31, 32]. Blood samples were taken within 24 h in the majority of patients; therefore it is unlikely that leukocytosis was due to stroke related infections such as post-stroke pneumonia.

In line with other studies, female sex proved to be an independent predictor for lack of functional independence [7, 62]. Gall et al. hypothesized that females are more vulnerable than men because of differences in chronic diseases, socioeconomic status and medical histories [63]. Females are more likely to suffer from severe strokes [62, 64]. A further reason might be the sex-related differences in muscular strength, or different approaches to handle their disabilities. This difference between sexes may increase in the elderly, because the observed decline in muscle strength with aging is also related to a reduction in PA, normally different between sexes. In people older than 65 years, less than one third of all women performed some PA - compared to men with 47.9%. Elderly women with a higher body mass index have a lower status of PA [65]. Moreover, female patients have a higher risk of walking with a cane [66]. More focus on PA in middle-life could improve level of PA in elderly people [61]. Additionally, more frequent occurrence of depression and lack of social support may increase probability for loss of functional independence in females [7, 55, 67]. However, most authors used univariate analyses and did not adjust for confounders.

Regarding stroke etiology, probable atherothrombotic stroke was an independent predictor for loss of functional independence in our population. The category of stroke of probable atherothrombotic etiology includes patients with distinct signs of non-stenosing arteriosclerosis as a marker of probable atherosclerotic plaques mostly at the orifices of small penetrating arteries, such as lenticulostriate arteries. CAD and PAD, that were associated with loss of functional independence in univariate but not in multivariate analysis are other common atherosclerotic diseases and may have contributed to some degree to the effect of this etiologic subgroup. This group may also include some patients with cardioembolic strokes due to non-detected AF. In contrast to other studies, cardioembolism was not independently associated with poor functional outcome in multivariate analysis. Cardioembolic stroke results in higher stroke severity. Adjustment for NIHSS and mRS at discharge presumeably prompted lack of significance of cardioembolism in our study.

In 117 patients stroke etiology was classified as stroke of unknown origin. Further analysis identified cryptogenic strokes and ESUS as main contributors to this group. Two thirds of patients with cryptogenic strokes were diagnosed as cryptogenic ESUS and tended to be associated with loss of functional independence, a finding that did not reach statistical significance due to small numbers. These cases may partly represent patients with non-detected AF and without any kind of anticoagulation. More effort in detecting AF in patients with ESUS may reduce recurrence of IS and improve functional outcome.

There are strengths and limitations to this study. The data were derived from a population–based stroke register, including both hospitalized and non-hospitalized patients without age-restrictions. Data have been collected prospectively by applying standardized protocols using multiple notification sources widely ensuring complete case ascertainment. Robust quality of case ascertainment is indicated by stable incidence rates over time. A high rate of neuroimaging (98.2%) assures high reliability of first-ever ischemic stroke diagnosis. An intense clinical work-up together with the application of modified TOAST criteria resulted in a low number of patients with undefined stroke causes [48]. This enabled us to study a relatively large cohort of unselected patients, resulting in sufficient statistical power to determine differences in stroke outcome. Our study is characterized by a high rate of follow-up and low rates of missing values (< 5%). Observed early death rates in our study were similar to findings in other population-based stroke registers [36, 68].

Limitations of our current work include the lack of data on the quality of risk factor control and the exploratory character of our results on factors like previous PA without possibility to reanalyze the detected results in a derivation sample. Further statistical limitation is lack of a power as LuSSt is primarily descriptive. Additionally, PA after stroke has not been assessed and an overestimation in amount of sports activity might result in another bias: acquisition of self-reported patients data increase the possibility of a misclassification bias. Distant events are often not precisely recalled, also raising the possibility of recall bias, particularly for sports in early adulthood. In contrast to other studies on physical activity using WHO definition, we used definition of the German Olympic Sports Association. Furthermore, poor outcome had not included standardized patient reported outcome measures like Euro-QOL-5, Frenchay Activities Index, HAD's depression or PROMIS-10 [55, 69–71].

Conclusion

In addition to broadly accepted risk factors for poor functional outcome we found that lack of PA prior to stroke, high leukocyte count at admission and probable atherothrombotic stroke etiology may constitute important independent predictors of loss of functional independence after first-ever ischemic stroke.

Abbreviations

AF: Atrial fibrillation; CAD: Coronary artery disease; CI: Confidence interval; CRP: C-Reactive Protein; ESUS: Embolic stroke of unknown source; ICH: Intracerebral hemorrhage; IS: Ischemic stroke; LuSSt: Ludwigshafen Stroke Study; mRS: Modified Rankin Scale; NIHSS: National Institute of Health Stroke Scale; OR: Odds ratio; PA : Physical activity; PAD: Peripheral artery disease; rt-PA: Recombined tissue plasmin activator; SAH: Subarachnoid hemorrhage; TIA: Transient ischemic attack; WHO: World Health Organization

Acknowledgements

Not applicable

Funding

The Ludwigshafen Stroke Register had received unrestricted funding by Boehringer Ingelheim, Sanofi-Aventis and BASF. Data analysis was supported by a grant from the Deutsche Forschungsgemeinschaft (DFG; GR1102/6 1) Study design, data collection, data analysis and data interpretation were independent from any study sponsor.
LuSSt is part of the German Competence Network Stroke.

Authors' contributions

CU, FP, AJG were responsible for study concept and design. CU and FP were responsible for data acquisition and mainly wrote the manuscript. VG and FB were major contributors in data acquisition. AS and HB mainly contributed to statistical analysis. VG, FB, AS, HB and AJG critically revised the manuscript for important intelectual content. All authors read and approved the final manuscript.

Competing interests

The authors declare that they have no competing interests.

Author details

[1]Department of Neurology, University of Heidelberg, Städtisches Klinikum Ludwigshafen am Rhein, Bremserstr. 79, 67063 Ludwigshafen, Germany. [2]University of Mannheim, Department of Dermatology, Theodor-Kutzer-Ufer 1-3, Mannheim 68167, Germany. [3]University of Heidelberg, Institute of Public Health, Im Neuenheimer Feld 324, Heidelberg, Germany. [4]Institute of Medical Biometry and Epidemiology, University Medical Center Hamburg-Eppendorf, Hamburg, Germany.

References

1. Summers D, Leonard A, Wentworth D, Saver JL, Simpson J, Spilker JA, et al. Comprehensive overview of nursing and interdisciplinary care of the acute ischemic stroke patient: a scientific statement from the American Heart Association. Stroke. 2009;40:2911–44. https://doi.org/10.1161/STROKEAHA. 109.192362.
2. Baek JH, Kim K, Lee Y-B, Park K-H, Park H-M, Shin D-J, et al. Predicting stroke outcome using clinical- versus imaging-based scoring system. J Stroke Cerebrovasc Dis. 2015;24:642–8. https://doi.org/10.1016/j. jstrokecerebrovasdis.2014.10.009.
3. Ntaios G, Faouzi M, Ferrari J, Lang W, Vemmos K, Michel P. An integer-based score to predict functional outcome in acute ischemic stroke: the ASTRAL score. Neurology. 2012;78:1916–22. https://doi.org/10.1212/WNL. 0b013e318259e221.
4. Cooray C, Mazya M, Bottai M, Dorado L, Skoda O, Toni D, et al. External validation of the ASTRAL and DRAGON scores for prediction of functional outcome in stroke. Stroke. 2016;47:1493–9. https://doi.org/10.1161/ STROKEAHA.116.012802.
5. Ntaios G, Gioulekas F, Papavasileiou V, Strbian D, Michel P. ASTRAL, DRAGON and SEDAN scores predict stroke outcome more accurately than physicians. Eur J Neurol. 2016;23:1651–7. https://doi.org/10.1111/ene.13100.
6. Appelros P, Nydevik I, Viitanen M. Poor outcome after first-ever stroke: predictors for death, dependency, and recurrent stroke within the first year. Stroke. 2003;34:122–6. https://doi.org/10.1161/01.STR.0000047852.05842.3C.
7. Weimar C, Ziegler A, Konig IR, Diener H-C. Predicting functional outcome and survival after acute ischemic stroke. J Neurol. 2002;249:888–95. https:// doi.org/10.1007/s00415-002-0755-8.
8. Hankey GJ. Long-term outcome after ischaemic stroke/transient ischaemic attack. Cerebrovasc Dis. 2003;16:14–9. https://doi.org/10.1159/000069936.
9. Phan TG, Clissold BB, Ma H, van Ly J, Srikanth V. Predicting disability after ischemic stroke based on comorbidity index and stroke severity-from the

virtual international stroke trials archive-acute collaboration. Front Neurol. 2017;8:192. https://doi.org/10.3389/fneur.2017.00192.

10. Wouters A, Nysten C, Thijs V, Lemmens R. Prediction of outcome in patients with acute ischemic stroke based on initial severity and improvement in the first 24 h. Front Neurol. 2018;9:308. https://doi.org/10.3389/fneur.2018.00308.

11. Palm F, Pussinen PJ, Safer A, Tervahartiala T, Sorsa T, Urbanek C, et al. Serum matrix metalloproteinase-8, tissue inhibitor of metalloproteinase and myeloperoxidase in ischemic stroke. Atherosclerosis. 2018;271:9–14. https://doi.org/10.1016/j.atherosclerosis.2018.02.012.

12. Kwakkel G, Wagenaar RC, Kollen BJ, Lankhorst GJ. Predicting disability in stroke--a critical review of the literature. Age Ageing. 1996;25:479–89.

13. Counsell C, Dennis M. Systematic review of prognostic models in patients with acute stroke. Cerebrovasc Dis. 2001;12:159–70.

14. Fonarow GC, Pan W, Saver JL, Smith EE, Reeves MJ, Broderick JP, et al. Comparison of 30-day mortality models for profiling hospital performance in acute ischemic stroke with vs without adjustment for stroke severity. JAMA. 2012;308:257–64. https://doi.org/10.1001/jama.2012.7870.

15. Keyhani S, Cheng E, Arling G, Li X, Myers L, Ofner S, et al. Does the inclusion of stroke severity in a 30-day mortality model change standardized mortality rates at veterans affairs hospitals? Circ Cardiovasc Qual Outcomes. 2012;5:508–13. https://doi.org/10.1161/CIRCOUTCOMES.111.962936.

16. Wang W-Y, Sang W-W, Jin D, Yan S-M, Hong Y, Zhang H, Yang X. The prognostic value of the iScore, the PLAN score, and the ASTRAL score in acute ischemic stroke. J Stroke Cerebrovasc Dis. 2017;26:1233–8. https://doi.org/10.1016/j.jstrokecerebrovasdis.2017.01.013.

17. Wang A, Pednekar N, Lehrer R, Todo A, Sahni R, Marks S, Stiefel MF. DRAGON score predicts functional outcomes in acute ischemic stroke patients receiving both intravenous tissue plasminogen activator and endovascular therapy. Surg Neurol Int. 2017;8:149. https://doi.org/10.4103/2152-7806.210993.

18. Flint AC, Kamel H, Rao VA, Cullen SP, Faigeles BS, Smith WS. Validation of the totaled health risks in vascular events (THRIVE) score for outcome prediction in endovascular stroke treatment. Int J Stroke. 2014;9:32–9. https://doi.org/10.1111/j.1747-4949.2012.00872.x.

19. Veerbeek JM, Kwakkel G, van Wegen EEH, JCF K, Heymans MW. Early prediction of outcome of activities of daily living after stroke: a systematic review. Stroke. 2011;42:1482–8. https://doi.org/10.1161/STROKEAHA.110.604090.

20. Rost NS, Bottle A, Lee J-M, Randall M, Middleton S, Shaw L, et al. Stroke severity is a crucial predictor of outcome: an international prospective validation study. J Am Heart Assoc. 2016. https://doi.org/10.1161/JAHA.115.002433.

21. Shen B, Yang X, Sui R-B, Yang B. The prognostic value of the THRIVE score, the iScore score and the ASTRAL score in Chinese patients with acute ischemic stroke. J Stroke Cerebrovasc Dis. 2018. https://doi.org/10.1016/j.jstrokecerebrovasdis.2018.06.011.

22. Forti P, Maioli F, Procaccianti G, Nativio V, Lega M-V, Coveri M, et al. Independent predictors of ischemic stroke in the elderly: prospective data from a stroke unit. Neurology. 2013;80:29–38. https://doi.org/10.1212/WNL.0b013e31827b1a41.

23. Hung K-H, Lai JC-Y, Hsu K-N, Hu C, Chang H-C, Chen C-N, et al. Gender gap and risk factors for poor stroke outcomes: a single hospital-based prospective cohort study. J Stroke Cerebrovasc Dis. 2018;27:2250–8. https://doi.org/10.1016/j.jstrokecerebrovasdis.2018.04.014.

24. Lee CD, Folsom AR, Blair SN. Physical activity and stroke risk: a meta-analysis. Stroke. 2003;34:2475–81. https://doi.org/10.1161/01.STR.0000091843.02517.9D.

25. Autenrieth CS, Evenson KR, Yatsuya H, Shahar E, Baggett C, Rosamond WD. Association between physical activity and risk of stroke subtypes: the atherosclerosis risk in communities study. Neuroepidemiology. 2013;40:109–16. https://doi.org/10.1159/000342151.

26. Kiely DK, Wolf PA, Cupples LA, Beiser AS, Kannel WB. Physical activity and stroke risk: the Framingham study. Am J Epidemiol. 1994;140:608–20.

27. Kubota Y, Iso H, Yamagishi K, Sawada N, Tsugane S. Daily total physical activity and incident stroke: the Japan public health center-based prospective study. Stroke. 2017;48:1730–6. https://doi.org/10.1161/STROKEAHA.117.017560.

28. Gordon NF, Gulanick M, Costa F, Fletcher G, Franklin BA, Roth EJ, Shephard T. Physical activity and exercise recommendations for stroke survivors: an American Heart Association scientific statement from the council on clinical cardiology, subcommittee on exercise, cardiac rehabilitation, and

prevention; the council on cardiovascular nursing; the council on nutrition, physical activity, and metabolism; and the stroke council. Circulation. 2004;109:2031–41. https://doi.org/10.1161/01.CIR.0000126280.65777.A4.

29. Rist PM, Capistrant BD, Mayeda ER, Liu SY, Glymour MM. Physical activity, but not body mass index, predicts less disability before and after stroke. Neurology. 2017;88:1718–26. https://doi.org/10.1212/WNL.0000000000003888.

30. Wannamethee G, Shaper AG. Physical activity and stroke in British middle aged men. BMJ. 1992;304:597–601.

31. Elkind MSV. Infectious burden: a new risk factor and treatment target for atherosclerosis. Infect Disord Drug Targets. 2010;10:84–90.

32. Huang W-Y, Peng T-I, Weng W-C, Chien Y-Y, Wu C-L, Lee M, Chen K-H. Higher leukocyte count is associated with higher risk of 3-year mortality in non-diabetic patients with first-ever ischemic stroke. J Neurol Sci. 2012;316:93–8. https://doi.org/10.1016/j.jns.2012.01.018.

33. Palm F, Urbanek C, Rose S, Buggle F, Bode B, Hennerici MG, et al. Stroke incidence and survival in Ludwigshafen am Rhein, Germany: the Ludwigshafen stroke study (LuSSt). Stroke. 2010;41:1865–70. https://doi.org/10.1161/STROKEAHA.110.592642.

34. Palm F, Urbanek C, Wolf J, Buggle F, Kleemann T, Hennerici MG, et al. Etiology, risk factors and sex differences in ischemic stroke in the Ludwigshafen stroke study, a population-based stroke registry. Cerebrovasc Dis. 2012;33:69–75. https://doi.org/10.1159/000333417.

35. Hatano S. Experience from a multicentre stroke register: a preliminary report. Bull World Health Organ. 1976;54:541–53.

36. Wolfe CD, Giroud M, Kolominsky-Rabas P, Dundas R, Lemesle M, Heuschmann P, Rudd A. Variations in stroke incidence and survival in 3 areas of Europe. European registries of stroke (EROS) collaboration. Stroke. 2000;31:2074–9.

37. Goldstein LB, Bertels C, Davis JN. Interrater reliability of the NIH stroke scale. Arch Neurol. 1989;46:660–2.

38. Rankin J. Cerebral vascular accidents in patients over the age of 60. III. Diagnosis and treatment. Scott Med J. 1957;2:254–68.

39. Savio K, Della Pietra GL, Oddone E, Reggiani M, Leone MA. Reliability of the modified Rankin scale applied by telephone. Neurol Int. 2013;5:e2. https://doi.org/10.4081/ni.2013.e2.

40. Berkhemer OA, Fransen PSS, Beumer D, van den Berg LA, Lingsma HF, Yoo AJ, et al. A randomized trial of intraarterial treatment for acute ischemic stroke. N Engl J Med. 2015;372:11–20. https://doi.org/10.1056/NEJMoa1411587.

41. The sixth report of the Joint National Committee on prevention, detection, evaluation, and treatment of high blood pressure. Arch Intern Med. 1997;157:2413–46.

42. Balkau B. The DECODE study. Diabetes epidemiology: collaborative analysis of diagnostic criteria in Europe. Diabetes Metab. 2000;26:282–6.

43. Grau AJ, Barth C, Geletneky B, Ling P, Palm F, Lichy C, et al. Association between recent sports activity, sports activity in young adulthood, and stroke. Stroke. 2009;40:426–31. https://doi.org/10.1161/STROKEAHA.108.527978.

44. Adams HPJR, Bendixen BH, Kappelle LJ, Biller J, Love BB, Gordon DL, Marsh EE. Classification of subtype of acute ischemic stroke. Definitions for use in a multicenter clinical trial. TOAST. Trial of org 10172 in acute stroke treatment. Stroke. 1993;24:35–41.

45. Hennerici MG, Bots ML, Ford I, Laurent S, Touboul PJ. Rationale, design and population baseline characteristics of the PERFORM vascular project: an ancillary study of the prevention of cerebrovascular and cardiovascular events of ischemic origin with teRutroban in patients with a history oF ischemic strOke or tRansient ischeMic attack (PERFORM) trial. Cardiovasc Drugs Ther. 2010;24:175–80. https://doi.org/10.1007/s10557-010-6231-2.

46. Ay H, Furie KL, Singhal A, Smith WS, Sorensen AG, Koroshetz WJ. An evidence-based causative classification system for acute ischemic stroke. Ann Neurol. 2005;58:688–97. https://doi.org/10.1002/ana.20617.

47. Hart RG, Diener H-C, Coutts SB, Easton JD, Granger CB, O'Donnell MJ, et al. Embolic strokes of undetermined source: the case for a new clinical construct. Lancet Neurol. 2014;13:429–38. https://doi.org/10.1016/S1474-4422(13)70310-7.

48. Palm F, Dos Santos M, Urbanek C, Greulich M, Zimmer K, Safer A, et al. Stroke seasonality associations with subtype, etiology and laboratory results in the Ludwigshafen stroke study (LuSSt). Eur J Epidemiol. 2013;28:373–81. https://doi.org/10.1007/s10654-013-9772-4.

49. Kenmuir CL, Hammer M, Jovin T, Reddy V, Wechsler L, Jadhav A. Predictors of outcome in patients presenting with acute ischemic stroke and mild

stroke scale scores. J Stroke Cerebrovasc Dis. 2015;24:1685–9. https://doi.org/10.1016/j.jstrokecerebrovasdis.2015.03.042.

50. Kaarisalo MM, Raiha I, Sivenius J, Immonen-Raiha P, Lehtonen A, Sarti C, et al. Diabetes worsens the outcome of acute ischemic stroke. Diabetes Res Clin Pract. 2005;69:293–8. https://doi.org/10.1016/j.diabres.2005.02.001.

51. Heuschmann PU, Kolominsky-Rabas PL, Misselwitz B, Hermanek P, Leffmann C, Janzen RWC, et al. Predictors of in-hospital mortality and attributable risks of death after ischemic stroke: the German stroke registers study group. Arch Intern Med. 2004;164:1761–8. https://doi.org/10.1001/archinte.164.16.1761.

52. Jia Q, Zhao X, Wang C, Wang Y, Yan Y, Li H, et al. Diabetes and poor outcomes within 6 months after acute ischemic stroke: the China National Stroke Registry. Stroke. 2011;42:2758–62. https://doi.org/10.1161/STROKEAHA.111.621649.

53. Ullberg T, Zia E, Petersson J, Norrving B. Changes in functional outcome over the first year after stroke: an observational study from the Swedish stroke register. Stroke. 2015;46:389–94. https://doi.org/10.1161/STROKEAHA.114.006538.

54. Bejot Y, Jacquin A, Daubail B, Durier J, Giroud M. Population-based validation of the iScore for predicting mortality and early functional outcome in ischemic stroke patients. Neuroepidemiology. 2013;41:169–73. https://doi.org/10.1159/000354634.

55. Jönsson A-C, Delavaran H, Iwarsson S, Ståhl A, Norrving B, Lindgren A. Functional status and patient-reported outcome 10 years after stroke: the Lund stroke register. Stroke. 2014;45:1784–90. https://doi.org/10.1161/STROKEAHA.114.005164.

56. Armstrong MEG, Green J, Reeves GK, Beral V, Cairns BJ. Frequent physical activity may not reduce vascular disease risk as much as moderate activity: large prospective study of women in the United Kingdom. Circulation. 2015;131:721–9. https://doi.org/10.1161/CIRCULATIONAHA.114.010296.

57. Krarup L-H, Truelsen T, Gluud C, Andersen G, Zeng X, Korv J, et al. Prestroke physical activity is associated with severity and long-term outcome from first-ever stroke. Neurology. 2008;71:1313–8. https://doi.org/10.1212/01.wnl.0000327667.48013.9f.

58. Reimers CD, Knapp G, Reimers AK. Exercise as stroke prophylaxis. Dtsch Arztebl Int. 2009;106:715–21. https://doi.org/10.3238/arztbl.2009.0715.

59. Chin K, Di Zhao TM, Martin SS, Ndumele CE, Florido R, et al. Physical activity, Vitamin D, and incident atherosclerotic cardiovascular disease in Whites and Blacks: the ARIC Study. J Clin Endocrinol Metab. 2017. https://doi.org/10.1210/jc.2016-3743.

60. Mueller UM, Walther C, Adam J, Fikenzer K, Erbs S, Mende M, et al. Endothelial function in children and adolescents is mainly influenced by age, sex and physical activity- an analysis of reactive hyperemic peripheral artery tonometry. Circ J. 2017. https://doi.org/10.1253/circj.CJ-16-0994.

61. Aggio D, Papacosta O, Lennon L, Whincup P, Wannamethee G, Jefferis BJ. Association between physical activity levels in mid-life with physical activity in old age: a 20-year tracking study in a prospective cohort. BMJ Open. 2017;7:e017378. https://doi.org/10.1136/bmjopen-2017-017378.

62. Synhaeve NE, Arntz RM, van Alebeek ME, van Pamelen J, Maaijwee NAM, Rutten-Jacobs LCA, et al. Women have a poorer very long-term functional outcome after stroke among adults aged 18-50 years: the FUTURE study. J Neurol. 2016;263:1099–105. https://doi.org/10.1007/s00415-016-8042-2.

63. Gall SL, Tran PL, Martin K, Blizzard L, Srikanth V. Sex differences in long-term outcomes after stroke: functional outcomes, handicap, and quality of life. Stroke. 2012;43:1982–7. https://doi.org/10.1161/STROKEAHA.111.632547.

64. Mozaffarian D, Benjamin EJ, Go AS, Arnett DK, Blaha MJ, Cushman M, et al. Heart disease and stroke statistics--2015 update: a report from the American Heart Association. Circulation. 2015;131:e29–322. https://doi.org/10.1161/CIR.0000000000000152.

65. Sinaki M, Nwaogwugwu NC, Phillips BE, Mokri MP. Effect of gender, age, and anthropometry on axial and appendicular muscle strength. Am J Phys Med Rehabil. 2001;80:330–8.

66. Paolucci S, Bragoni M, Coiro P, de Angelis D, Fusco FR, Morelli D, et al. Is sex a prognostic factor in stroke rehabilitation? A matched comparison. Stroke. 2006;37:2989–94. https://doi.org/10.1161/01.STR.0000248456.41647.3d.

67. Friberg L, Benson L, Rosenqvist M, Lip GYH. Assessment of female sex as a risk factor in atrial fibrillation in Sweden: nationwide retrospective cohort study. BMJ. 2012;344:e3522. https://doi.org/10.1136/bmj.e3522.

68. Lainay C, Benzenine E, Durier J, Daubail B, Giroud M, Quantin C, Bejot Y. Hospitalization within the first year after stroke: the Dijon stroke registry. Stroke. 2015;46:190–6. https://doi.org/10.1161/STROKEAHA.114.007429.

69. Salinas J, Sprinkhuizen SM, Ackerson T, Bernhardt J, Davie C, George MG, et al. An international standard set of patient-centered outcome measures after stroke. Stroke. 2016;47:180–6. https://doi.org/10.1161/STROKEAHA.115.010898.

70. Revicki DA, Kawata AK, Harnam N, Chen W-H, Hays RD, Cella D. Predicting EuroQol (EQ-5D) scores from the patient-reported outcomes measurement information system (PROMIS) global items and domain item banks in a United States sample. Qual Life Res. 2009;18:783–91. https://doi.org/10.1007/s11136-009-9489-8.

71. Crichton SL, Bray BD, McKevitt C, Rudd AG, Wolfe CDA. Patient outcomes up to 15 years after stroke: survival, disability, quality of life, cognition and mental health. J Neurol Neurosurg Psychiatry. 2016;87:1091–8. https://doi.org/10.1136/jnnp-2016-313361.

22

Neurological signs as early determinants of dementia and predictors of mortality among older adults in Latin America: a 10/66 study using the NEUROEX assessment

Lorenzo Pasquini[1*], Jorge Llibre Guerra[2,3], Martin Prince[4], Kia-Chong Chua[4] and A. Matthew Prina[4]

Abstract

Background: Neurodegenerative processes in the elderly damage the brain, leading to progressive, incapacitating cognitive, behavioral, and motor dysfunctions which culminate in dementia. Fully manifest dementia is likely to be preceded by the presence of neurological signs, which could serve as early determinants of dementia and predictors of mortality. The aims of this study were to assess the construct validity of a neurological battery assessed among older adults living in Latin America, and to test the association of groups of neurological signs with dementia cross-sectionally, and mortality longitudinally.

Methods: The 10/66 Dementia Research Group collected information on neurological symptoms via the NEUROEX assessment in population based surveys of older adults living in low and middle-income countries. Data from 10,856 adults participating in the baseline assessment of the 10/66 study and living in Cuba, Dominican Republic, Peru, Venezuela and Mexico were analysed. Exploratory and confirmatory analysis were used to explore dimensionality of neurological symptoms. Poisson regression analyses were used to link groups of neurological signs with dementia at baseline. Cox hazard regression models were used to explore the predictive validity of neurological signs with mortality at follow up.

Results: Exploratory and confirmatory factor analyses revealed four dimensions of neurological signs, which are associated with lesions of specific brain regions. The identified factors showed consistency with groups of neurological signs such as frontal, cerebellar, extrapyramidal, and more generalized gait disturbance signs. Regression analyses revealed that all groups of neurological signs were positively associated with dementia at baseline and predicted mortality at follow up.

Conclusions: Our findings support the construct and predictive validity of the NEUROEX assessment, linking neurological and gait impairments with dementia at baseline, and with mortality at follow up among older adults living in five Latin American countries.

Keywords: Dementia, Epidemiology, Low and middle-income countries, Mortality, Neurological signs

* Correspondence: lorenzo.pasquini@ucsf.edu
[1]Memory and Aging Center, Department of Neurology, University of California San Francisco, 675 Nelson Rising Lane, San Francisco, CA 94143, USA
Full list of author information is available at the end of the article

Background

As demographic ageing advances, many low and middle-income countries (LMICs) are experiencing a health transition, where non-communicable diseases assume a progressively greater significance. Non-communicable diseases are already the leading cause of death in all world regions apart from sub-Saharan Africa [1]. Given the dynamic interaction of mental health and physical illnesses, neurological and mental disorders need particular attention [2]. Among all mental health disorders, dementia accounts for a large proportion of mortality and years lived-with-disability targeting older adults in LMICs [3, 4]. In neurological disorders such as dementia, early neurological signs are also common in advanced age [5, 6], and are likely to be the result of the ongoing neurodegenerative brain processes taking place several years before first cognitive symptoms appear [7, 8]. Distinct neurological signs are typically anchored on distinct brain regions, and relate to lesions of specific brain structures [9–11]. For example, sequencing tasks and frontal "release" signs are commonly associated with lesions in the frontal lobes as found in frontotemporal and vascular dementia [10, 12]. The inability to perform fast alternating movements– e.g. dysdiadochinesia– is commonly related to lesions of the cerebellum, while symptoms such as tremor and rigidity are indicators of extrapyramidal lesions in the striatopallidonigral system as found in Parkinson's disease [13]. Finally, diffuse disorders of motor function may contribute to impairments of stance and gait.

Notably, a consistent link between several neurological signs, dementia and mortality has been reported in several studies from high income countries [14–19]. Such findings indicate a potential use of neurological symptoms as early determinants of dementia and predictors of mortality among older adults. This may be particular relevant to LMICs, where the older population may experience limited access to advanced diagnostic tools of dementia such as cerebrospinal fluid and neuroimaging biomarkers [7].

The 10/66 Dementia Research Group, a collective of researchers carrying out population-based research into dementia, non-communicable diseases and ageing in LMICs, has started tackling this issue by carrying out population-based surveys using standardised methodology across a large number of LMICs (Cuba, China, Dominican Republic, India, Mexico, Nigeria, Peru, Puerto Rico, & Venezuela). 10/66 refers to the fact that when the group was created in the late 90s, two-thirds (66%) of people with dementia were living in LMICs, and that 10% or less of population-based research had been carried out in those regions. The 10/66 Dementia Research Group included an assessment of neurological symptoms (NEUROEX) as part of population-based surveys investigating dementia and ageing in LMICs [20, 21]. In order to generate evidence about the construct and predictive validity of the NEUROEX assessment, the purposes of this study are to (i) explore the dimensionality of neurological symptoms and their link to groups of neurological signs; (ii) provide evidence for a positive association relating groups of neurological signs with dementia at baseline, and mortality at follow up in older adults living in five Latin American countries.

Methods

Design

Secondary analyses were performed on data from the 10/66 Dementia Research Group surveys of representative samples of older people living in five Latin American countries (urban sites in Cuba, Dominican Republic and Venezuela, and rural and urban sites in Mexico and Peru). Full details of the study protocol can be found elsewhere [20, 21]. Briefly, a cross-sectional one phase survey was carried out in geographically defined catchment areas. All residents aged 65 years and over were included in the survey and an informant was also interviewed. The sample size for each country was between 2000 and 3000 participants. All participants underwent a comprehensive interview, including a structured clinical interview, a physical examination, an assessment of neurological symptoms and an informant interview. The interviews generally took place at the participant's home and were translated in Spanish. Vital status was determined 3–5 years after baseline survey. A detailed account reporting mortality assessment, causes and rates has been provided in previous studies [22]. All studies were approved by local ethical committees and by the King's College London ethical committee.

Measurements

10/66 dementia

Dementia was ascertained according to the Diagnostic and Statistical Manual of Mental Disorders IV (DSM-IV) [23] and the cross-culturally validated 10/66 dementia diagnosis algorithm [24]. For 10/66 dementia diagnosis, a logistic regression model was used to calculate coefficients linked to outputs from a structured clinical mental-state interview [25]. The battery included: a) the Geriatric Mental State [26], b) two cognitive tests; the Community Screening Instrument for Dementia (CSI'D') COGSCORE [27] and the modified CERAD 10 word list learning task with delayed recall [28], and c) informant reports of cognitive and functional decline from the CSI'D' RELSCORE [27]. 10/66 dementia diagnosis has been shown to be highly sensitive and specific and was given to participants scoring above a cut-point of predicted probability for dementia derived from the aforementioned calculated coefficients [24].

Socio-demographical variables and general health indicators

Beside the NEUROEX assessment, socio-demographical and general health indicators were assessed for each country by the interviewers asking participants or a key informant. Socio-demographical variables included gender, educational level, food insecurity (yes no; assessed by the interviewer by asking "have you ever gone hungry because of lack of food?"), income (yes or no; combined measure derived by the interviewer's question asking whether participants received any income, any pension or proxy measure of household income), number of assets and age. General health indicators were assessed by the interviewer if not specified differently and included depression (EURO-D depression scale) [29], care dependence (based on open-ended questions administered by the interviewer to the key informant) [30], having had a stroke diagnosed (yes or no), having had a diagnosis of diabetes (yes or no), hypertension (blood pressure > =140/90 or antihypertensive treatment, assessed by the interviewer) and dementia (yes or no; based on the 10/66 dementia algorithm) [24].

NEUROEX assessment

The NEUROEX assessment was conducted by local trained health workers and health professionals and generally took place within participants' homes and included a brief fully structured neurological assessment with quantifiable measures of lateralising signs, parkinsonism, ataxia, apraxia and primitive "release" reflexes [20] (see Appendix in the Additional file 1 for more details). Based on data completeness, the following NEUROEX items were included in the analyses: vertical gaze; glabellar and pout reflexes; tremor; rigidity; cogwheeling; fist-palm-side sequencing and reciprocal coordination sequencing; fine finger movement; dysdiadochokinesis (speed and coordination); ataxia; bradykinesia; bilateral armswing; gait steps and time needed to walk five metres. Only the presence of bilateral impairments was considered as pathological, since our main interest was to test the link between neurological symptoms and fully manifest dementia or mortality, rather than explore the association to incipient dementia. Bilateral items where dichotomised and testlets were then created to combine these highly correlated bilateral items, which would have likely created multicollinearity issues in further analyses. The only exceptions were for tremor, where items where summed after dichotomisation, and rigidity and cogwheeling, where items where just summed without dichotomisation.

Statistical analyses

All statistical analyses were performed in STATA v.12. We estimated the prevalence of neurological symptoms based on the testlets derived from the NEUROEX assessment battery for each country and across sites. For the only continuous NEUROEX variables used in the analysis, gait steps and time, the median (Q2) and inter-quartile range (Q1-Q3) were reported.

Exploratory and confirmatory factor analysis

In order to avoid circular analysis, the whole dataset was randomly divided in two samples, a smaller one containing 30% of the data, and a bigger one containing 70% of the data. Exploratory factor analysis was used to estimate dimensionality of the selected NEUROEX items on the smaller containing 30% of the data. A four-factor solution principal component analysis was performed on the selected NEUROEX items based on the correlation matrix [31, 32]. Bartlett's test of sphericity, the Kaiser-Meyer-Olkin (KMO) measure of sampling adequacy, Kaiser's criterion, scree tests and Horn's parallel analysis were used as additional criteria to estimate exploratory factor analysis reliability. The cut off used for item loading on a given factor was 0.3. A varimax rotation was carried out and an eigenvalue of one was chosen as initial extraction criterion [33] (see Additional file 1: Supplementary methods).

Based on the output of the exploratory factor analysis across sites, we subsequently tested and compared the goodness-of-fit of a four-factor solution model between sites using confirmatory factor analysis on the second sample containing 70% of the data [33]. All further analyses were performed on this sample. Absolute and relative indices were used to test goodness-of-fit: the Akaike's Information Criterion (AIC) – the lower the AIC value, the better the fit of the model [34]; the Tucker–Lewis Index (TLI) [35] – values greater than 0.80 are considered acceptable; and the root mean square error of approximation (RMSEA) [36] – values between 0.05 to 0.08 indicate reasonable fit for the model.

Factor scores

Individual factor scores were derived from the confirmatory factor analysis across sites via regression analysis. Independent variables in the regression equation were the standardised observed values of the items in the estimated factors. These predictor variables were weighted by regression coefficients, obtained by multiplying the inverse of the observed variable correlation matrix by the matrix of factor loadings. The factor scores were the dependent variables in the regression equation. The computed factor scores were subsequently standardised to a mean of zero with a standard deviation of 1.0 [37]. Factor scores were finally trichotomised based on the empirical distribution of the continuous regression, with half of the standard deviation of 1.0 (0.5 z-value) used as threshold to define three categories reflecting a clinical continuum of respectively neurologically less-impaired (z-values ≤0.0; coded as 0), mildly-impaired (0.0 < z-values ≥0.5; coded as 1) and severely-impaired (0.5 < z-values; coded as 2) subjects. Because of the unusual distribution of factor scores belonging to the latent factor later identified as gait disturbance signs, we carried out additional sensitivity analyses where data binning procedures were applied on these factor scores. One categorisation was based on the 90th percentile resulting in two categories of less-impaired (z-values ≤90th percentile) and impaired (z-values >90th percentile) subjects. A second binning was applied by dividing the factors scores in five bins by steps of 2 z-values resulting in five categories of less-impaired (z-values ≤0.0), mildly-impaired (0.0 < z-values ≥2.0), moderately-impaired (2.0 < z-values ≥4.0), heavily-impaired (4.0 < z-values ≥6.0) and severely-impaired (6.0 < z-values) subjects.

Regression analyses

Poisson regression analyses were used to investigate the relationship between 10/66 dementia and neurological domains. For each latent variable, three types of models were run: a) an unadjusted model with only the factor scores as categorical variables; b) a second model correcting for socio-demographical variables including gender, educational level, food insecurity, income insecurity, number of assets and age as additional covariates in each model; c) a final fully adjusted model including the former variables

and general indicators of health status such as depression (EURO-D depression scale), care dependence, clinically diagnosed stroke, diabetes and hypertension.

Finally, Cox proportional hazard regression analyses were run to predict mortality at follow up from the factor scores [22, 38]. Identical adjustments as in the Poisson regression analysis were carried out. The final models were also adjusted for 10/66 dementia. For the later identified gait disturbance signs, additional sensitivity analyses were carried out by using alternative data binning procedures as explained above. All regression analyses were performed on the dataset across sites.

Results

Socio-demographic characteristics (Table 1) were comparable across countries. Participants tended to be younger in the sample from Venezuela, and to have fewer years of education when coming from Mexico and the Dominican Republic. The number of assets was lower in the Dominican Republic, where participants also experienced the highest food and income insecurity. Participants from Cuba experienced the lowest food and income insecurity. At baseline, 9.5% of participants were diagnosed with 10/66 dementia; 17.0% of participant assessed at baseline died before the follow-up interview.

Table 1 Socio-demographic characteristics by individual countries and over pooled countries

Absolute values (%)	Across sites	Cuba	Dominican Republic	Peru	Venezuela	Mexico
Number of subjects	10,856 (100.0)	2941 (27.1)	2000 (18.5)	1931 (17.8)	1534 (18.1)	2002 (27.1)
Age						
65–69	3230 (29.8)	760 (25.9)	533 (26.4)	554 (28.6)	839 (41.8)	544 (27.1)
70–74	2852 (26.3)	789 (26.9)	520 (25.9)	493 (25.5)	469 (23.6)	581 (29.0)
75–79	2206 (20.3)	639 (21.7)	397 (19.7)	399 (207)	345 (18.4)	426 (21.3)
>79	2555 (23. 6)	749 (25.5)	561 (27.9)	486 (25.2)	308 (16.3)	451 (22.5)
Female	6941 (62.9)	1913 (65.0)	1325 (65.9)	1183 (61.2)	1252 (64.6)	1268 (63.3)
Educational level						
None	1298 (12.0)	75 (2.5)	392 (19.7)	121 (6.3)	156 (8.1)	554 (27.7)
Some, did not complete primary	3217 (29.9)	655 (22.3)	1022 (51.3)	231 (12.0)	445 (23.1)	864 (43.2)
Completed primary	3392 (31.5)	979 (33.3)	370 (18.6)	727 (37.9)	965 (50.1)	351 (17.5)
Completed secondary	1770 (16.4)	728 (24.8)	135 (6.8)	517 (27.0)	266 (13.8)	124 (6.2)
Tertiary	1094 (10.2)	499 (17.0)	73 (3.7)	321 (16.7)	93 (4.8)	108 (5.4)
Number of assets						
0–3 assets	1673 (15.4)	451 (15.4)	643 (32.0)	155 (8.0)	48 (2.4)	376 (18.8)
4–5 assets	4596 (42.4)	876 (29.8)	444 (22.1)	1134 (58.7)	0 (0.0)	844 (42.1)
6 assets	2152 (19.8)	1073 (36.5)	733 (36.5)	181 (9.4)	1298 (66.1)	165 (8.2)
More than 6 assets	2422 (22.3)	536 (18.3)	186 (9.3)	463 (23.9)	619 (31.5)	618 (30.8)
Food insecurity	752 (7.0)	140 (4.8)	240 (12.1)	137 (7.2)	111 (6.0)	124 (6.2)
Income insecurity	4433 (40.8)	527 (17.9)	1400 (69.6)	668 (34.6)	818 (41.6)	1020 (50.9)

Prevalence and distribution of neurological symptoms

There was considerable variation in the prevalence and distribution of neurological symptoms (Table 2). Overall, Cuba had the lowest prevalence of neurological symptoms while the Dominican Republic had the highest. For instance, the prevalence of decreased armswing and bradykinesia was respectively of 14.8% and 13.0% in Cuba and 36.8% and 33.4% in the Dominican Republic. The most common neurological symptoms across sites were the glabellar reflex (29.0%) and first palm side sequencing (34.4%), whereas the least common were cogwheeling (9.9%), dysdiadochokinesia speed (9.3%) and coordination (8.7%).

Exploratory and confirmatory factor analysis

Exploratory factor analysis was performed through a four-factor principal component analysis on randomly selected 30% of the data (see Additional file 1: Table S1). Qualitative and statistical criteria confirmed analysis suitability. All factors together explained 51.0% of the total variance. The loading structure of the dataset across sites classified vertical gaze as not consistently loading on any factor (factor loading threshold < 0.3); armswing, bradykinesia, ataxia, gait speed and steps loaded on factor one (eigenvalue of 2.4) which we interpreted as a gait disturbance sign; fine finger movement, dysdiadochokinesia speed and coordination on factor two (eigenvalue of 2.0) interpreted as a cerebellar sign;; tremor, cogwheeling and rigidity on factor three (eigenvalue of 1.8) interpreted as an extrapyramidal sign; pout and glabellar reflexes, fist palm side sequencing and reciprocal sequencing on factor four (eigenvalue of 1.8) interpreted as a frontal sign. We next tested the goodness-of-fit of the four-factor solution arising from the exploratory factor analysis in both individual countries on 70% of the remaining data. For this purpose, a model derived from the four-factor solution was derived and tested on 70% of the remaining data pooled over countries and at the individual site level using confirmatory factor analysis (see Table 3 and Fig. 1). Importantly, the variable vertical gaze was excluded from further analyses as it did not consistently load on any factor. A schematic illustration of the model used in our confirmatory factor analysis can be seen in Fig. 1.

Across sites, a good fit was found for the variables derived from the NEUROEX assessment in our proposed four-factor model ($\chi^2 = 1072.0.1$; $p < 0.001$; df = 81; AIC = 216,584.0; TLI = 0.94; RMSEA = 0.04). Moderate to high factor loadings were found for all variables on the respective four factors (Table 3 and Fig. 1). Reasonable goodness-of-fit of the model was found as well for individual countries, with RMSEA varying between 0.05 and 0.06 with the highest value found in the Dominican Republic, while TLI varied between 0.91 and 0.95 with the highest value found in Peru and Venezuela and the lowest in the Dominican Republic. Overall moderate to high factor loadings were found across all countries. Measurement invariance analysis over all sites, revealed an acceptable fit of the constrained model (TLI = 0.89; RMSEA = 0.07).

Poisson regression analyses

Poisson regression analyses were run to explore the association between 10/66 dementia at baseline and trichotomised

Table 2 Prevalence of neurological symptoms derived from the NEUROEX assessment by individual country and for pooled countries

NEUROEX Absolute numbers (%)	Across sites	Cuba	Dominican Republic	Peru	Venezuela	Mexico
Glabellar reflex more than 4 taps	3011 (29.0)	1095 (37.3)	367 (18.4)	252 (13.1)	536 (35.2)	761 (38.3)
Pout reflex present	1575 (15.2)	244 (8.0)	382 (19.2)	95 (4.9)	181 (11.9)	673 (33.6)
FPS sequencing unsuccessful after 5 demonstration	3513 (34.4)	750 (26.0)	823 (42.0)	277 (14.5)	431 (28.7)	1232 (62.8)
Reciprocal sequencing unsuccessful after 5 tries	2911 (28.2)	796 (27.2)	385 (19.6)	229 (11.9)	442 (29.6)	1059 (52.9)
Tremor at least one limb	1348 (13.0)	222 (7.8)	224 (11.2)	213 (11.0)	264 (17.4)	425 (21.2)
Cogwheeling at least one limb	832 (9.9)	183 (6.2)	96 (4.8)	221 (11.5)	106 (7.2)	226 (11.3)
Rigidity at least one limb	1549 (15.0)	374 (12.7)	272 (13.7)	278 (14.5)	291 (19.6)	334 (16.7)
Fine finger movement	1214 (11.7)	207 (7.1)	236 (12.0)	184 (9.6)	221 (14.8)	336 (18.3)
Dysdiadochokinesia Speed	970 (9.3)	242 (8.2)	160 (8.1)	231 (12.0)	99 (6.6)	238 (12.0)
Dysdiadochokinesia coordination	910 (8.7)	187 (6.4)	143 (7.3)	168 (8.7)	90 (6.0)	322 (16.1)
Armswing	2160 (21.2)	432 (14.8)	702 (36.8)	276 (14.3)	215 (15.3)	535 (26.7)
Ataxia	1413 (13.9)	234 (8.0)	428 (22.4)	266 (13.8)	125 (8.8)	360 (18.0)
Bradykinesia	1949 (19.1)	382 (13.0)	637 (33.4)	328 (17.0)	178 (12.6)	424 (21.2)
Gait steps Q2 (Q1-Q3) in steps	18 (14–22)	20 (17–24)	20 (18–24)	18 (15–20)	17 (11–20)	12 (10–15)
Gait time Q2 (Q1-Q3) in seconds	14 (10–18)	15 (12–20)	17 (15–23)	14 (10–18)	12 (9–15)	8 (7–11)

FPS fist palm side

Table 3 Confirmatory factor analysis

	NEUROEX items factor loadings	Cuba	Dominican Republic	Peru	Venezuela	Mexico	Across sites
Frontal signs	Pout reflex	0.3	0.5	0.3	0.3	0.5	0.4
	Glabellar reflex	0.3	0.3	0.3	0.3	0.5	0.4
	FPS sequencing	0.6	0.5	0.4	0.5	0.3	0.5
	Reciprocal sequencing	0.5	0.3	0.4	0.4	0.4	0.5
Extrapyramidal signs	Tremor	0.4	0.4	0.5	0.5	0.4	0.5
	Cogwheeling	0.5	0.3	0.6	0.4	0.4	0.5
	Rigidity	0.8	0.4	0.6	0.3	0.3	0.5
Cerebellar signs	Fine finger movement	0.7	0.6	0.7	0.6	0.5	0.6
	Dysdiadochokinesia speed	0.8	0.9	0.7	0.7	0.6	0.7
	Dysdiadochokinesia coordination	0.7	0.8	0.8	0.5	0.7	0.7
Gait disturbance signs	Armswing	0.4	0.6	0.7	0.6	0.6	0.6
	Gait −steps	0.5	0.6	0.3	0.4	0.4	0.3
	Gait −time	0.3	0.5	0.3	0.4	0.4	0.4
	Ataxia	0.7	0.5	0.9	0.7	0.8	0.7
	Bradykinesia	0.9	0.8	0.9	0.9	0.9	0.9
	Goodness of fit						
	χ^2 (81)	531.0	480.5	418.0	323.6	291.0	1072.0
	TLI	0.91	0.90	0.95	0.95	0.93	0.94
	RMSEA	0.05	0.06	0.05	0.05	0.05	0.04
	AIC	58,147.3	40,061.3	51,287.9	35,137.0	41,058.3	216,584.0
	Measurement invariance model	Without constraints	With constraints	Difference			
	χ^2	1942.7	3342.3	χ^2 change	1399.7		
	Df	405	449	df change	44		
	TLI	0.92	0.89	p-value	$p < 0.0001$		
	RMSEA	0.05	0.07				
	AIC	200,452.1	289,429.0				

Confirmatory factor analysis with four-factor solution on 70% of the data, derived from the exploratory factor analysis on randomly selected 30% of the data. Goodness of fit parameters and loading coefficients by country, pooled over countries, and test of measurement invariance over countries. *AIC* Akaike's Information Criterion, *FPS* fist palm side, *RSMA* Root mean square error of approximation, *TLI* Tucker-Lewis index

factor scores respectively reflecting less-impaired, mildly-impaired and severely-impaired levels for the four groups of neurological signs (Table 4). Three models, one unadjusted, one adjusted for socio-demographical variables and one adjusted for socio-demographical variables and general indicators of health status were run separately for each group of neurological signs. In all models, factor scores of latent neurological signs were significantly associated with dementia at baseline. After full adjustment for confounders, the highest prevalence ratios were found for frontal ($PR_{heavily-impaired} = 6.7$ [5.0–8.9]), followed by extrapyramidal ($PR_{heavily-impaired} = 3.3$ [2.5–4.3]), cerebellar ($PR_{heavily-impaired} = 2.9$ [2.9–3.7]), and gait disturbance signs ($PR_{heavily-impaired} = 2.0$ [1.7–2.4]). Prevalence ratios were progressively increased in heavily-impaired subjects compared to mildly-impaired subjects.

Cox proportional hazard regression analyses

Cox proportional hazard regression analyses were run to predict mortality at follow up from trichotomised factor scores, respectively reflecting less-impaired, mildly-impaired and severely-impaired levels for the four neurological signs (Table 5). As for the Poisson regression analysis, adjusted and unadjusted models were run. In all models, factor scores of all latent neurological signs significantly predicted mortality at follow up. Hazard-ratios were progressively increased in heavily-impaired subjects compared to mildly-impaired subjects. For the fully adjusted model, the highest-hazard ratios were found for frontal ($HR_{heavily-impaired} = 1.6$ [1.4–1.8]), followed by extrapyramidal ($HR_{heavily-impaired} = 1.4$ [1.3–1.6]), and cerebellar signs ($HR_{heavily-impaired} = 1.3$ [1.1–1.5]). Gait disturbance signs predicted mortality in the unadjusted model ($HR_{heavily-impaired} = 1.1$ [1.0–1.2]),

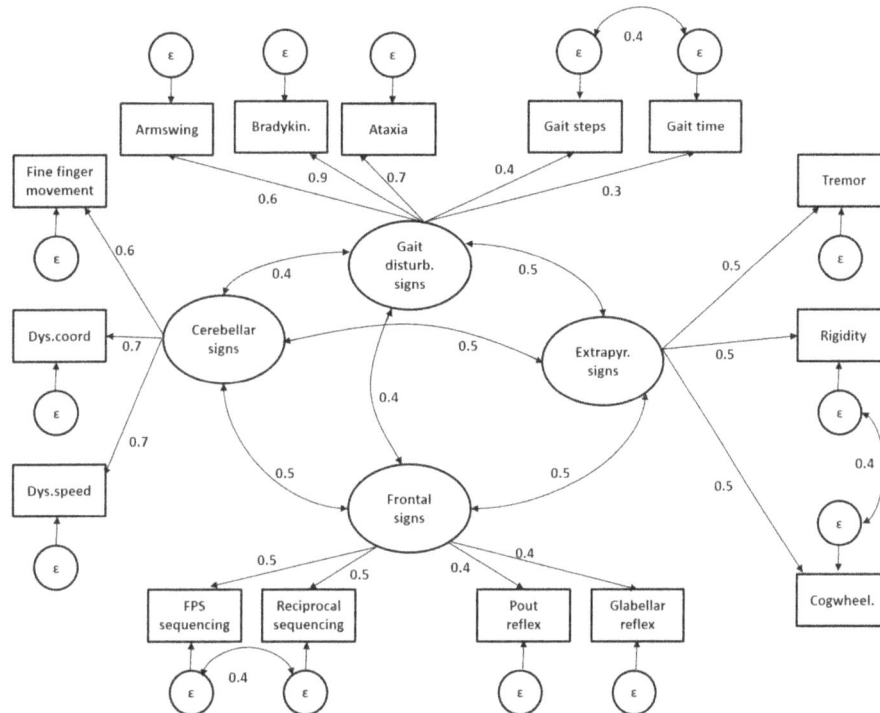

Fig. 1 Schematic representation of the model used for confirmatory factor analysis with corresponding loading coefficients from the analysis pooled across sites. Rectangles reflect observed variables; ovals reflect latent variables and circles error terms of the model (ε). Simple arrows and corresponding values reflect the factor paths and loadings of observed variables to the latent variables and of the error terms to the corresponding observed variable; double arrows and corresponding values reflect covariance between latent variables or error terms. Bradykin. = Bradykinesia; Cogwheel. = Cogwheeling; Dys.coord = Dysdiadochokinesia coordination; Dys.speed = Dysdiadochokinesia speed; ε = Error term; FPS = Fist palm side; Extrapyr. = Extrapyramidal; Gait disturb. = Gait disturbance

but not in the fully adjusted models ($HR_{heavily-impaired}$ = 1.0 [0.9–1.0]). Sensitivity analyses were carried out using distinct data binning on the gait disturbance signs: a) based on the 90th percentile; b) by dividing the factor scores in five bins. The analysis based on the 90th percentile binarisation showed that gait disturbance predicted mortality at follow up in both the unadjusted ($HR_{impaired}$ = 1.3 [1.2–1.4]) and the fully adjusted model ($HR_{impaired}$ = 1.1 [1.1–1.3]). The second sensitivity analysis also revealed that higher gait disturbance predicted mortality at follow up both in the unadjusted ($HR_{heavily-impaired}$ = 1.4 [1.2–1.5]; $HR_{severely-impaired}$ = 1.3 [1.2–1.4]) and fully adjusted model ($HR_{heavily-impaired}$ = 1.1 [1.0–1.2]; $HR_{severely-impaired}$ = 1.1 [1.0–1.2]).

Discussion

In this project, we aimed to investigate the construct and predictive validity of the NEUROEX battery assessing neurological symptoms among older adults in five Latin American countries. Dimensionality estimation of neurological symptoms from the NEUROEX assessment, revealed four groups of neurological signs which are in part anchored on vulnerability of distinct brain regions: frontal, extrapyramidal, cerebellar, and gait disturbance signs. Poisson and Cox regression models provided evidence for

the predictive validity of all groups of signs on dementia and mortality.

Prevalence of neurological symptoms among older adults in LMICs

The prevalence of neurological symptoms was in the range expected from previous works assessing the same question in high income countries [39]. However, variation in prevalence was observed for different sites (see Table 1). Distinct reasons could explain this finding: differences could be caused by diversity in the medical coverage and in the medical service found in the countries examined, as exemplified by Cuba's health care system, which is considered one of the most effective in Latin America [40]. Moreover, the setting and the background of the community health worker could affect the variance found for the prevalence of neurological symptoms across sites (e.g.: training level of the community health worker; medical student versus practitioner).

Exploratory factor analysis and confirmatory factor analysis

A four-factor principal component analysis on 30% randomly selected data consistently loaded neurological symptoms on four latent factors (see results and table in

Table 4 Poisson regression analysis

	Prevalence ratios (PR) with 95% CI		
	Unadjusted model	Adjusted model 1	Adjusted model 2
	PR	PR	PR
Frontal signs			
Mildly-impaired	4.7 (3.8–5.8)	3.9 (3.1–4.9)	3.8 (2.9–4.9)
Heavily-impaired	15.0 (12.1–18.6)	9.5 (7.4–12.1)	6.7 (5.0–8.9)
Extrapyramidal signs			
Mildly-impaired	4.2 (3.4–5.0)	2.9 (2.4–3.6)	2.5 (2.0–3.1)
Heavily-impaired	10.0 (8.1–12.3)	5.4 (4.3–6.9)	3.3 (2.5–4.3)
Cerebellar signs			
Mildly-impaired	4.2 (3.6–5.0)	2.8 (2.4–3.4)	2.4 (2.0–3.0)
Heavily-impaired	8.9 (7.2–10.7)	4.8 (3.9–6.0)	2.9 (2.2–3.7)
Gait disturbance signs			
Mildly-impaired	3.5 (2.3–5.1)	2.5 (1.7–3.7)	2.1 (1.3–3.3)
Heavily-impaired	3.9 (3.3–4.5)	2.3 (1.9–2.7)	2.0 (1.7–2.4)

Multivariate regression analysis of dementia at baseline by four factor scores derived from the NEUROEX assessment at baseline. Prevalence ratios (PR) in the sample pooled across countries (with 95% CI) are shown for an unadjusted model, a model adjusted for socio-demographical variables (adjusted for gender, educational level, food insecurity, income insecurity, number of assets and age; adjusted model 1) and a model adjusted for socio-demographical variables and general indicators of health status (adjusted for gender, educational level, food insecurity, income insecurity, number of assets, age, depression, care dependence, clinically diagnosed stroke, diabetes and hypertension; adjusted model 2)

Table 5 Cox proportional hazard model regression analysis

	Hazard ratios (HR) with 95% CI		
	Unadjusted model	Adjusted model 1	Adjusted model 2
	HR	HR	HR
Frontal signs			
Mildly-impaired	1.2 (1.1–1.2)	1.1 (1.1–1.2)	1.1 (1.1–1.2)
Heavily-impaired	2.1 (2.0–2.3)	1.9 (1.7–2.1)	1.6 (1.4–1.8)
Extrapyramidal signs			
Mildly-impaired	1.3 (1.2–1.3)	1.2 (1.1–1.2)	1.1 (1.1–1.2)
Heavily-impaired	1.9 (1.7–2.1)	1.7 (1.5–1.9)	1.4 (1.3–1.6)
Cerebellar signs			
Mildly-impaired	1.5 (1.4–1.6)	1.4 (1.3–1.5)	1.3 (1.2–1.4)
Heavily-impaired	1.7 (1.5–1.9)	1.6 (1.4–1.7)	1.3 (1.1–1.5)
Gait disturbance signs			
Mildly-impaired	1.1 (1.0–1.3)	1.0 (0.9–1.2)	1.0 (0.8–1.1)
Heavily-impaired	1.1 (1.0–1.2)	1.1 (1.0–1.1)	1.0 (0.9–1.0)

Multivariate prediction analysis of mortality at follow up by four factor scores derived from the NEUROEX assessment at baseline. Hazard ratios (HR) pooled over countries (with 95% CI) are shown for an unadjusted model, a model adjusted for socio-demographical variables (adjusted for gender, educational level and age; adjusted model 1) and a model adjusted for socio-demographical variables and general indicators of health status (adjusted for gender, educational level, age, depression, clinically diagnosed stroke, diabetes, hypertension and dementia; adjusted model 2)

the Additional file 1 on exploratory factor analysis). A subsequent confirmatory factor analysis on the remaining 70% of the data confirmed suitability of four dimensions of neurological sings that can be associated with failure of distinct brain systems showing partial overlap with frontal, extrapyramidal, cerebellar, and gait disturbance signs [9–11]. For example, the pout reflex is a frontal release sign related to impaired inhibitory function of the frontal lobes, and is common in neurodegenerative diseases targeting the frontal lobes, such as frontotemporal lobar degeneration and vascular dementia [10]. Sequencing impairments and related executive dysfunctions are also related to damage of the frontal lobes [41], and are found in distinct dementia types ranging from Alzheimer's disease, to frontotemporal and vascular dementia [41, 42]. Tremor, cogwheeling and rigidity are typical symptoms of extrapyramidal deficits of the striatopallidonigral system as encountered in Parkinson's disease [13]. Difficulties in fine finger movements and dysdiadochinesia are well known impairments related to cerebellar dysfunction as found in multiple system atrophy or multiple sclerosis [12]. However, we advise caution in the interpretation of the findings as neurological symptoms are not exclusive to one specific neurological syndrome and may result from lesions in different brain areas. This inconsistency might result from different aetiologies underlying related neurological signs or by a more distributed failure of several brain structures involved in the manifestation of specific symptoms. For example, a positive glabellar reflex is believed to be caused by a lack of inhibitory function from the frontal lobes, but has been mainly associated with extrapyramidal diseases such as Parkinson's disease [43]. Gait ataxia, commonly considered a cerebellar sign, can also be caused by frontal dysfunctions or disorders of the peripheral nervous system [13], but was associated with the gait disturbance sign in our study. Bradykinesia, which is considered an extrapyramidal sign, consistently loaded on the gait disturbance sign in our study, and may indicate a measurement artifact rather reflecting general slowing of the locomotor system than true bradykinesia. In particular, the latent variable gait disturbance sign might include mixed types of symptoms related to locomotion dysfunction with more complex diffuse contributions – also of non-neurological origin, e.g. arthritis, or impairments of the respiratory and vascular system among others.

Link between neurological signs and dementia at baseline
All neurological signs had high prevalence ratios and were positively associated with dementia at baseline, even after adjustment for socio-demographics factors and general indicators of health status. These results are in line with previous research associating neurological symptoms such as primitive reflexes and parkinsonism with Alzheimer's

disease and other dementias [14, 15, 17]. Notably, in a prospective, longitudinal study of community-dwelling older people who did not have dementia or Parkinson disease at baseline, Louis and colleagues showed that baseline mild extrapyramidal signs can be used as a predictor of incident dementia [17]. In our study, frontal signs had the highest association with dementia, in line with both cross-sectional and longitudinal studies reporting deficits in frontal functioning which are associated with dementia in a variety of conditions ranging from vascular dementia, to Alzheimer' disease, Parkinson's disease dementia, and frontotemporal dementia [44–48] . Our findings support the notion that neurological signs, could be used as non-cognitive, education-independent, and culture-independent determinants of dementia. Importantly, our findings pave the way for a whole new line of research questions, which aim at investigating the predictive validity of neurological signs on longitudinal general health indicators and mental health disorders, including among others hypertension, alcohol abuse, head injury, major depression, Parkinson's disease and distinct dementia subtypes such as Alzheimer's disease, frontotemporal, and vascular dementia.

Link between neurological signs and mortality at follow up
Cox hazard regression models revealed a positive association of neurological signs with mortality at follow up. These results remained statistically significant after adjustment and are in line with other longitudinal studies reporting a robust association of neurological symptoms such as parkinsonism and primitive reflexes with mortality at follow up [15, 16, 18]. In general, our findings are in line with the well-known association between frailty and mortality, particularly in advanced adulthood, suggesting that neurological symptoms might increase vulnerability of older adults and act as frailty and disability indicators increasing the risk of mortality [49, 50]. A level of uncertainty remains for gait disturbance signs, were only modest associations were found with mortality at follow up, as shown by the unadjusted model and the sensitivity analyses. Longitudinal findings from the Sidney Memory and Aging Study revealed a strong association of gait and motor abnormalities with dementia and mortality among older adults [51]. This difference might be caused by a suboptimal trichotomisation of the corresponding factor scores in our study, which may primarily result in the detection of individuals without gait impairments and or by the possibility that gait disturbance signs in our study might reflect symptoms with mixed aetiology rather than specific neurological dysfunctions.

Limitations
Several limitations need to be addressed when interpreting our findings. Fully trained neurologists and psychiatrists assessed the participant in Cuba, medical students performed most of the assessment in Venezuela and Dominican Republic, while in Peru social workers and in Mexico General Practitioners were mainly involved. Although all the interviewers received the same training, we cannot exclude that interobserver variability could influence the differences in prevalence of neurological symptoms across countries. Findings cannot be generalised to higher income countries or to other LMICs, as the study was only conducted in a selected group of Latin American countries. High response rate was achieved by the use of catchment areas but with a general loss of generalisability, as the findings might not be applicable outside these areas and similar districts. Moreover, we did not explore differences between rural and urban areas. Although measurement of invariance across sites was acceptable, our results might be influenced by general methodological issues such as systematic differences in the way in which measures are being administered or coded, in the way in which participants are responding to interviews, and in misclassification of neurological symptoms and clinical diagnoses across sites.

Conclusions
In conclusion, our results support construct and predictive validity of the NEUROEX assessment. Our findings relate neurological symptoms to groups of neurological signs, with dementia at baseline, and with mortality at follow up in older adults living in five Latin American countries. This study informs about the feasibility and utility of including a structured assessment of neurological signs as part of a survey of health and ageing in LMICs, and how this assessment can be used as a research tool to explore determinants of dementia and predictors of mortality [52, 53].

Abbreviations
FPS: First palm side; LMICs: Low and middle-income countries; RMSEA: Root mean square error of approximation; TLI: Tucker–Lewis Index

Acknowledgements
This is a secondary analysis of data collected by the 10/66 Dementia Research Group (DRG) (www.alz.co.uk/10/66-group). The 10/66 DRG is led by M.P. and coordinated by C.P.F. from the Institute of Psychiatry, King's College London. The other principal investigators, responsible for research governance in each site are Juan Llibre Rodriguez (Cuba), Daisy Acosta (Dominican Republic), M.G. (Peru), Aquiles Salas (Venezuela), Ana Luisa Sosa (Mexico), K.S. Jacob (Vellore, India), Joseph D. Williams (Chennai, India) and Yueqin Huang (China). The 10/66 DRG's research has been funded by the Wellcome Trust Health Consequences of Population Change Programme (GR066133 – prevalence phase in Cuba and Brazil; GR08002 – incidence phase in Peru, Mexico, Argentina, Cuba, Dominican Republic, Venezuela and China), the World Health Organization (India, Dominican Republic and China), the US Alzheimer's Association (IIRG-04-1286 – Peru, Mexico and

Argentina), and FONACIT/CDCH/UCV (Venezuela). Matthew Prina was supported by the MRC (MR/K021907/1).

We thank Dr. Carla Sabariego and the Institute for Medical Informatics, Biometry and Epidemiology of the Ludwigs-Maximilians-University Munich for discussion and mentoring, the Rockefeller Foundation for supporting a dissemination meeting at their Bellagio Center, and Alzheimer's Disease International for providing networking and infrastructure support.

Funding
AMP was supported by the MRC (MR/K021907/1). LP was supported by the German Academic Foundation.

Authors' contributions
LP performed all analyses and was primarily involved in writing the manuscript. JLG, MP, KCC, and AMP supervised all statistical analyses and were major contributors in writing the manuscript. All authors read and approved the final manuscript.

Competing interests
The authors declare no commercial or other conflicts of interest.

Author details
[1]Memory and Aging Center, Department of Neurology, University of California San Francisco, 675 Nelson Rising Lane, San Francisco, CA 94143, USA. [2]Global Brain Health Institute, Memory and Aging Center, University of California San Francisco, 675 Nelson Rising Lane, San Francisco, CA 94143, USA. [3]Neurology and Neurosurgery Institute, 139 Calle 29, 10400 Havana, Cuba. [4]King's College London, Health Service and Population Research Department, Centre for Global Mental Health, Institute of Psychiatry, Psychology & Neuroscience, De Crespigny Park, London SE5 8AF, UK.

References
1. Vos T, Barber RM, Bell B, Bertozzi-Villa A, Biryukov S, Bolliger I, Charlson F, Davis A, Degenhardt L, Dicker D. Global, regional, and national incidence, prevalence, and years lived with disability for 301 acute and chronic diseases and injuries in 188 countries, 1990–2013: a systematic analysis for the global burden of disease study 2013. Lancet. 2015;386(9995):743–800.
2. Prince M, Patel V, Saxena S, Maj M, Maselko J, Phillips MR, Rahman A. No health without mental health. Lancet. 2007;370(9590):859–77.
3. Organization WH: The world health report 2001: mental health: new understanding, new hope: World Health Organization; 2001.
4. Prince M, Ali G-C, Guerchet M, Prina AM, Albanese E, Wu Y-T. Recent global trends in the prevalence and incidence of dementia, and survival with dementia. Alzheimers Res Ther. 2016;8(1):23.
5. Broe GA, Akhtar AJ, Andrews GR, Caird FI, Gilmore AJ, McLennan WJ. Neurological disorders in the elderly at home. J Neurol Neurosurg Psychiatry. 1976;39(4):362–6.
6. Broe GA, Jorm AF, Creasey H, Grayson D, Edelbrock D, Waite LM, Bennett H, Cullen JS, Casey B. Impact of chronic systemic and neurological disorders on disability, depression and life satisfaction. Int J Geriatr Psychiatry. 1998; 13(10):667–73.
7. Jack CR Jr, Knopman DS, Jagust WJ, Petersen RC, Weiner MW, Aisen PS, Shaw LM, Vemuri P, Wiste HJ, Weigand SD, et al. Tracking pathophysiological processes in Alzheimer's disease: an updated hypothetical model of dynamic biomarkers. The Lancet Neurology. 2013;12(2):207–16.
8. Bateman RJ, Xiong C, Benzinger TL, Fagan AM, Goate A, Fox NC, Marcus DS, Cairns NJ, Xie X, Blazey TM, et al. Clinical and biomarker changes in dominantly inherited Alzheimer's disease. N Engl J Med. 2012;367(9):795–804.
9. Larner. A dictionary of neurological signs, second edition edn. United States of America: Springer; 2011.
10. Ropper A.H. SMA, Klein J.K: Chapter 1. Approach to the patient with neurologic disease in: Adams and Victor's principles of neurology. 10 edn. McGraw-hill; 2014.
11. Mesulam M: Chapter 1. Behavioral Neuroanatomy: large-scale networks, association cortex, frontal syndromes, the limbic system, and hemispheric specializations. In: Principles of Behavioral and Cognitive Neurology. Second edition edn. Oxford University Press; 2000.
12. Daroff R. JJ, Mazziotta J., Pomeroy S.: Bradley's neurology in clinical practice, 7 edn: Elsevier; 2012.
13. Fahn S JJ, Hallett M: Principles and practice of movement disorders: Elsevier; 2011.
14. Girling DM, Berrios GE. Extrapyramidal signs, primitive reflexes and frontal lobe function in senile dementia of the Alzheimer type. Br J Psychiatry. 1990;157:888–93.
15. Burns A, Jacoby R, Levy R. Neurological signs in Alzheimer's disease. Age Ageing. 1991;20(1):45–51.
16. Bennett DA, Beckett LA, Murray AM, Shannon KM, Goetz CG, Pilgrim DM, Evans DA. Prevalence of parkinsonian signs and associated mortality in a community population of older people. N Engl J Med. 1996;334(2):71–6.
17. Louis ED, Tang MX, Mayeux R. Parkinsonian signs in older people in a community-based study: risk of incident dementia. Arch Neurol. 2004;61(8): 1273–6.
18. Wilson RS, Schneider JA, Beckett LA, Evans DA, Bennett DA. Progression of gait disorder and rigidity and risk of death in older persons. Neurology. 2002;58(12):1815–9.
19. Bakchine S, Lacomblez L, Palisson E, Laurent M, Derouesne C. Relationship between primitive reflexes, extra-pyramidal signs, reflective apraxia and severity of cognitive impairment in dementia of the Alzheimer type. Acta Neurol Scand. 1989;79(1):38–46.
20. Prince M, Ferri CP, Acosta D, Albanese E, Arizaga R, Dewey M, Gavrilova SI, Guerra M, Huang Y, Jacob KS, et al. The protocols for the 10/66 dementia research group population-based research programme. BMC Public Health. 2007;7:165.
21. Prina AM, Acosta D, Acostas I, Guerra M, Huang Y, Jotheeswaran AT, Jimenez-Velazquez IZ, Liu Z, Llibre Rodriguez JJ, Salas A, et al. Cohort profile: the 10/66 study. Int J Epidemiol. 2017; 46(2):406–406.
22. Prince M, Acosta D, Ferri CP, Guerra M, Huang Y, Llibre Rodriguez JJ, Salas A, Sosa AL, Williams JD, Dewey ME, et al. Dementia incidence and mortality in middle-income countries, and associations with indicators of cognitive reserve: a 10/66 dementia research group population-based cohort study. Lancet. 2012;380(9836):50–8.
23. Prince MJ, de Rodriguez JL, Noriega L, Lopez A, Acosta D, Albanese E, Arizaga R, Copeland JR, Dewey M, Ferri CP, et al. The 10/66 dementia research Group's fully operationalised DSM-IV dementia computerized diagnostic algorithm, compared with the 10/66 dementia algorithm and a clinician diagnosis: a population validation study. BMC Public Health. 2008;8:219.
24. Prince M, Acosta D, Chiu H, Scazufca M, Varghese M, Dementia Research G. Dementia diagnosis in developing countries: a cross-cultural validation study. Lancet. 2003;361(9361):909–17.
25. Llibre Rodriguez JJ, Ferri CP, Acosta D, Guerra M, Huang Y, Jacob KS, Krishnamoorthy ES, Salas A, Sosa AL, Acosta I, et al. Prevalence of dementia in Latin America, India, and China: a population-based cross-sectional survey. Lancet. 2008;372(9637):464–74.
26. Copeland JR, Dewey ME, Griffiths-Jones HM. A computerized psychiatric diagnostic system and case nomenclature for elderly subjects: GMS and AGECAT. Psychol Med. 1986;16(1):89–99.
27. Hall KS, Gao S, Emsley CL, Ogunniyi AO, Morgan O, Hendrie HC. Community screening interview for dementia (CSI 'D'); performance in five disparate study sites. Int J Geriatr Psychiatry. 2000;15(6):521–31.
28. Ganguli M, Chandra V, Gilby JE, Ratcliff G, Sharma SD, Pandav R, Seaberg EC, Belle S. Cognitive test performance in a community-based nondemented elderly sample in rural India: the indo-U.S. cross-National Dementia Epidemiology Study. Int Psychogeriatr. 1996;8(4):507–24.
29. Guerra M, Prina AM, Ferri CP, Acosta D, Gallardo S, Huang Y, Jacob KS, Jimenez-Velazquez IZ, Llibre Rodriguez JJ, Liu Z, et al. A comparative cross-cultural study of the prevalence of late life depression in low and middle income countries. J Affect Disord. 2016;190:362–8.
30. Sousa RM, Ferri CP, Acosta D, Guerra M, Huang Y, Jacob K, Jotheeswaran A, Hernandez MA, Liu Z, Pichardo GR, et al. The contribution of chronic diseases to the prevalence of dependence among older people in Latin America, China and India: a 10/66 dementia research group population-based survey. BMC Geriatr. 2010;10:53.

31. Joreskog KG. Latent variable modeling with ordinal variables. Stat Model Latent Variables. 1993:163–71.

32. Joreskog KG. Structural equation modeling with ordinal variables. Inst Math S. 1994;24:297–310.

33. Castro-Costa E, Dewey M, Stewart R, Banerjee S, Huppert F, Mendonca-Lima C, Bula C, Reisches F, Wancata J, Ritchie K, et al. Ascertaining late-life depressive symptoms in Europe: an evaluation of the survey version of the EURO-D scale in 10 nations. The SHARE project. Int J Meth Psych Res. 2008; 17(1):12–29.

34. Anderson DR, Burnham KP, White GC. Comparison of Akaike information criterion and consistent Akaike information criterion for model selection and statistical inference from capture-recapture studies. J Appl Stat. 1998; 25(2):263–82.

35. Tucker LR, Lewis C. Reliability coefficient for maximum likelihood factor-analysis. Psychometrika. 1973;38(1):1–10.

36. Browne: Alternative ways of assessing model fit. Sage Focus Editions 1993, 154:136–136.

37. DiStefano. Undertsanding and using factor scores: considerations for the applied researcher. Pract Assesment Res Eval. 2009;14:1–10.

38. Jotheeswaran AT, Williams JD, Prince MJ. Predictors of mortality among elderly people living in a south Indian urban community; a 10/66 dementia research group prospective population-based cohort study. BMC Public Health. 2010;10:366.

39. Odenheimer G, Funkenstein HH, Beckett L, Chown M, Pilgrim D, Evans D, Albert M. Comparison of neurologic changes in 'successfully aging' persons vs the total aging population. Arch Neurol. 1994;51(6):573–80.

40. Cooper RS, Kennelly JF, Ordunez-Garcia P. Health in Cuba. Int J Epidemiol. 2006;35(4):817–24.

41. Rabinovici GD, Stephens ML, Possin KL: Executive dysfunction. Continuum (Minneap Minn) 2015, 21(3 Behavioral Neurology and Neuropsychiatry):646–659.

42. Viskontas IV, Possin KL, Miller BL. Symptoms of frontotemporal dementia provide insights into orbitofrontal cortex function and social behavior. Ann N Y Acad Sci. 2007;1121:528–45.

43. Masdeu J. C. BJ: localization in clinical neurology, 6th edn: Wolters Kluwer health; 2011.

44. Piccirilli M, D'Alessandro P, Finali G, Piccinin G. Early frontal impairment as a predictor of dementia in Parkinson's disease. Neurology. 1997;48(2):546–7.

45. Hogan DB, Ebly EM. Primitive reflexes and dementia: results from the Canadian study of health and aging. Age Ageing. 1995;24(5):375–81.

46. Vreeling FW, Houx PJ, Jolles J, Verhey FR. Primitive reflexes in Alzheimer's disease and vascular dementia. J Geriatr Psychiatry Neurol. 1995;8(2):111–7.

47. Murphy RR, Abner EL, Jicha GA. Frontal release signs predict future decline in subjects with intact cognition and mild cognitive impairment. Alzheimers Dement. 2015;11(7):P785.

48. Harrington MG, Chiang J, Pogoda JM, Gomez M, Thomas K, Marion SD, Miller KJ, Siddarth P, Yi X, Zhou F, et al. Executive function changes before memory in preclinical Alzheimer's pathology: a prospective, cross-sectional, case control study. PLoS One. 2013;8(11):e79378.

49. Llibre Jde J, Lopez AM, Valhuerdi A, Guerra M, Llibre-Guerra JJ, Sanchez YY, Bosch R, Zayas T, Moreno C. Frailty, dependency and mortality predictors in a cohort of Cuban older adults, 2003-2011. MEDICC Rev. 2014;16(1):24–30.

50. At J, Bryce R, Prina M, Acosta D, Ferri CP, Guerra M, Huang Y, Rodriguez JJ, Salas A, Sosa AL, et al. Frailty and the prediction of dependence and mortality in low- and middle-income countries: a 10/66 population-based cohort study. BMC Med. 2015;13:138.

51. Waite LM, Grayson DA, Piguet O, Creasey H, Bennett HP, Broe GA. Gait slowing as a predictor of incident dementia: 6-year longitudinal data from the Sydney older persons study. J Neurol Sci. 2005;229-230:89–93.

52. Ravindranath V, Dang HM, Goya RG, Mansour H, Nimgaonkar VL, Russell VA, Xin Y. Regional research priorities in brain and nervous system disorders. Nature. 2015;527(7578):S198–206.

53. Baingana F. al'Absi M, Becker AE, Pringle B: global research challenges and opportunities for mental health and substance-use disorders. Nature. 2015; 527(7578):S172–7.

23

Intracranial pressure responsiveness to positive end-expiratory pressure in different respiratory mechanics: a preliminary experimental study in pigs

Han Chen[1]* (iD), Jing Zhou[1], Yi-Qin Lin[1], Jian-Xin Zhou[2] and Rong-Guo Yu[1]

Abstract

Background: Respiratory mechanics affects the effect of positive end-expiratory pressure (PEEP) on intracranial pressure (ICP). Respiratory mechanics of the lung and the chest wall was not differentiated in previous studies. In the present study, we investigated the influence of the following possible determinants of ICP responsiveness to PEEP: chest wall elastance (E_{CW}), lung elastance (E_L), and baseline ICP.

Methods: Eight healthy Bama miniature pigs were studied. The increase of E_L was induced by instillation of hydrochloride, and the increase of E_{CW} was induced by strapping the animals' chest wall and abdomen. A balloon-tipped catheter was placed intracranially for inducing intracranial hypertension. Six experimental conditions were investigated in sequence: 1) *Normal*; 2) *Stiff Chest Wall*; 3) *Lung Injury*; 4) *Lung Injury + Stiff Chest Wall*; 5) *Lung Injury + Stiff Chest Wall + Intracranial Hypertension* and 6) *Lung Injury + Intracranial Hypertension*. PEEP was gradually increased in a 5 cm H_2O interval from 5 to 25 cm H_2O in each condition. Blood pressure, central venous pressure, ICP, airway pressure and esophageal pressure were measured.

Results: Hydrochloride instillation significantly increased E_L in conditions with lung injury. E_{CW} significantly increased in the conditions with chest wall and abdomen strapping (all $p < 0.05$). ICP significantly increased with increments of PEEP in all non-intracranial hypertension conditions ($p < 0.001$). The greatest cumulative increase in ICP was observed in the *Stiff Chest Wall* condition (6 [5.3, 6.8] mm Hg), while the lowest cumulative increase in ICP was observed in the *Lung Injury* condition (2 [1.3, 3.8] mm Hg). ICP significantly decreased when PEEP was increased in the intracranial hypertension conditions ($p < 0.001$). There was no significant difference in cumulative ICP change between the two intracranial hypertension conditions ($p = 0.924$).

Conclusions: Different respiratory mechanics models can be established via hydrochloride induced lung injury and chest wall and abdominal strapping. The effect of PEEP on ICP is determined by respiratory mechanics in pigs with normal ICP. However, the responsiveness of ICP to PEEP is independent of respiratory mechanics when there is intracranial hypertension.

Keywords: Intracranial pressure, Respiratory mechanics, Lung injury, Chest wall, Elastance, Esophageal pressure, Positive end-expiratory pressure

* Correspondence: baojr2@163.com
[1]Surgical Intensive Care Unit, Fujian Provincial Clinical College, Fujian Medical University, No 134, Dongjie Street, Gulou District, Fuzhou 350001, Fujian, China
Full list of author information is available at the end of the article

Background

It has been reported that a significant portion of brain-injured patients can develop pulmonary complications including acute respiratory distress syndrome (ARDS) and neurogenic pulmonary edema [1–5]. Mechanical ventilation is needed in this population, and positive end-expiratory pressure (PEEP) is used to improve oxygenation as well as to recruit and/or prevent alveolar collapse [6–8].

However, there have long been concerns that the use of PEEP in brain-injured patients could cause increase of intracranial pressure (ICP) and deteriorate neurological status, especially in those who are with signs of cerebral edema. Previous studies yielded conflicting results in the effects of PEEP on ICP, with ICP increasing [9–13], not markedly changing [14–16] or even decreasing [17] after the application of PEEP, suggesting a multifactorial mechanism. Several possible determinants for the effect of PEEP on ICP have been proposed, including baseline ICP [11], intracranial compliance [12, 13] and respiratory mechanics [9, 10].

Theoretically, PEEP can increase ICP via elevating intrathoracic pressure and diminishing venous return [18, 19], where the transmission of PEEP into the thoracic cavity depends on the respiratory mechanics. Chapin and colleges reported that increased lung elastance (E_L) and decreased chest wall elastance (E_{CW}) can minimize the effect of PEEP on pleural pressure [20]. Clinical studies have also suggested that the effect of PEEP on ICP is attenuated when respiratory system elastance (E_{RS}) increases. However, E_L and E_{CW} were not differentiated in these studies [9, 10]. For a given increased E_{RS}, it might be attributed to either the increase in E_L due to pulmonary disease (e.g. ARDS), or the increase in E_{CW} due to chest wall impairment (e.g. intra-abdominal hypertension or massive pleural effusion), or both. It has been shown that the E_{CW} to E_{RS} ratio (E_{CW}/E_{RS} ratio) varied from 0.2 to 0.8 in mechanically ventilated patients [21]. Therefore, it is important to clarify the mechanical characteristics of both the lung and the chest wall when investigating the effects of PEEP on ICP.

Although it is known that the decrease of E_{CW}/E_{RS} ratio can attenuate the effect of PEEP to pleural pressure [20], it is still unknown whether it can attenuate the effect of PEEP to ICP. We hypothesized that a greater E_{CW}/E_{RS} ratio would result in a greater ICP responsiveness to increased PEEP. In this preliminary study, we investigated the influence of the following possible determinants of ICP responsiveness to PEEP: the elevated E_{CW}, which increases E_{CW}/E_{RS} ratio; the elevated E_L, which reduces E_{CW}/E_{RS} ratio; and the elevated baseline ICP.

Methods

Animal preparation

Eight healthy, male Bama miniature pigs (weight 10–20 kg, mean 13.6 kg) were studied. All animals received humane care in compliance with the National Institutes of Health guidelines for the care and use of experimental animals and with the approval of the Institutional Review Board of Fujian Provincial Hospital (Approval # KY – 2016010). Animals were purchased from Guangxi University. Animals were fasted preoperatively. Premedication consisted of intramuscular 10 – 20 mg/kg ketamine, followed by an intravenous bolus of 10 mg midazolam. Continuous sedation consisted of intravenous 0.2–1.0 mg/kg/hr midazolam and 0.1–0.2 mcg/kg/hr fentanyl. Maintenance fluid was administrated (lactated Ringer's solution, 5 mL/kg/hr); additional fluids and catecholamine infusions were not allowed. Animals were placed on a heating pad in supine position. Central venous catheter was placed via right internal jugular vein for fluid infusion and central venous pressure (CVP) measurements. Arterial cannula was placed via right femoral artery to measure blood pressure. Tracheotomy was performed and a 5.5–6.5 tracheotomy cuffed tube was placed. Animals were than paralyzed via intravenous infusion of 10 mg vecuronium bromide and mechanically ventilated with a Servo-s ventilator (Maquet, Solna, Sweden). Vecuronium bromide was continuously infused (1 mg/kg/hr) and an additional 5 mg bolus was administrated if there was spontaneous breathing effort, which was determined by a negative deflection in the esophageal pressure (P_{ES}) tracing.

Animals were than turned to right lateral position. A midline, transverse incision was performed along the dorsal surface of the head to expose the underlying skull. One burr hole was created approximately 10 mm left/lateral of midline and 10 mm anterior to the coronal suture. An intraparenchymal ICP monitor catheter (Codman Microsensor, Raynham, MA, USA) was placed through this opening. The distal tip of the catheter was placed in the exposed cortex at a depth of 1 cm. A bedside ICP monitor (Codman ICP Express, Raynham, MA, USA) was connected. Another burr hole was created approximately 10 mm right/lateral of midline and 10 mm anterior to the coronal suture. A balloon-tipped catheter (5 mL, 8Fr Foley) was placed through the hole for inducing intracranial hypertension (IH).

Animals were turned back to supine position. A SmartCath-G esophageal balloon catheter (7003300, CareFusion Co., Yorba Linda, CA, USA) was placed to measure P_{ES}. A positive pressure occlusion test was used to confirm the proper balloon position [22, 23]. P_{ES} and airway pressure (P_{AW}) were measured by two KT 100D-2 pressure transducers (KleisTEK di CosimoMicelli, Italy, range: +/– 100 cm H_2O).

Experimental protocol

Six experimental conditions were investigated in sequence (Fig. 1):

1) *Normal* condition;
2) *Stiff Chest Wall* experimental condition (*CW* condition);
3) *Lung Injury* experimental condition (*L* condition);
4) *Lung Injury + Stiff Chest Wall* experimental condition (*L + CW* condition);
5) *Lung Injury + Stiff Chest Wall + IH* experimental condition (*L + CW + IH* condition);
6) *Lung Injury + IH* experimental condition (*L + IH* condition).

In each condition, PEEP was gradually increased in a 5 cm H_2O interval from 5 to 25 cm H_2O. Animal was ventilated for five minutes after each PEEP increment to allow ICP stabilization. Measurements were taken after the five-minute stabilization (see below). After the last measurement of one condition (25 cmH_2O of PEEP), PEEP was decreased to 5 cmH_2O and the preparation of the next condition was completed under a PEEP setting of 5 cmH_2O. All ventilator settings except PEEP were not changed during the entire experiment. The pig was euthanized in the end of the experiment by overdose pentobarbital injection (100 mg/kg).

The increase of E_{CW} was induced by strapping the animals' chest wall and abdomen with an inelastic, adjustable bellyband. In addition, two pneumatic cuffs were placed between the bellyband and the abdomen as well as the chest wall [24, 25]. The bellyband was adjusted so that inspirations were not hampered when the pneumatic cuffs were not inflated (normal E_{CW}). To increase E_{CW}, the pneumatic cuffs were inflated to a pressure of 20 cm H_2O [24, 25].

The increase of E_L was induced by slowly instillation of 0.1 mol/L hydrochloride (4 mL/kg) down the endotracheal tube via a thin suction catheter placed at the level of the carina. This method has been previously reported as creating an animal model with ARDS-like lung injury including lung inflammation, edema, hemorrhage, and variable lung region aeration [25, 26]. One hour following hydrochloride administration the model was validated by achieving a pulse oxygen saturation ≤ 90%.

IH was induced by inflating the intracranial balloon with saline at a rate of 0.5 mL/min until the ICP was constant between 30 and 40 cm H_2O for > 30 min [26, 27].

Measurements

Mechanical ventilation was set as volume-controlled ventilation with a constant flow, an inspiratory to expiratory ratio of 1:2, a tidal volume (V_T) of 10 mL/kg, a respiratory rate of 20 breaths/min and an inspired oxygen

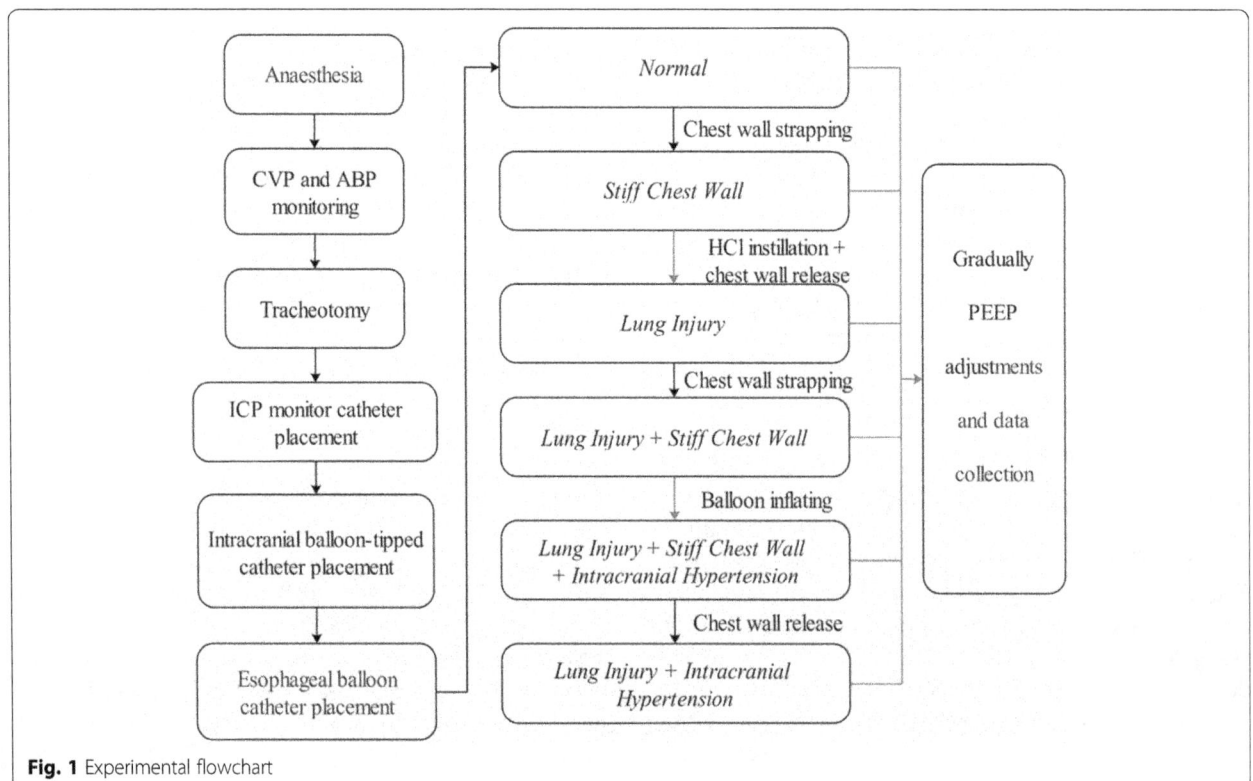

Fig. 1 Experimental flowchart

fraction of 100%. ICP, mean arterial pressure (MAP), cerebral perfusion pressure (CPP, calculated as MAP minus ICP) and CVP were measured. At each tested PEEP level, end-inspiratory and end-expiratory occlusion were performed, each for 3 s. P_{ES} and P_{AW} during the last second of occlusion were recorded. Respiratory mechanics were calculated as follows:

$$E_{RS} = \frac{P_{PLAT} - PEEP_{TOTAL}}{V_T}$$

Where P_{PLAT} and $PEEP_{TOTAL}$ represent P_{AW} at end-inspiratory and end-expiratory occlusion, respectively.

$$E_{CW} = \frac{P_{ES-EI} - P_{ES-EE}}{V_T}$$

Where P_{ES-EI} and P_{ES-EE} are respective P_{ES} determined at end-inspiratory and end-expiratory occlusion.

$$E_L = E_{RS} - E_{CW}$$

Statistical analysis

Continuous variables are presented as the median and inter-quartile range. Data obtained in different experimental conditions were compared by the analysis of variance for repeated measure or Scheirer-Ray-Hare test as appropriate [28]. If significant, a Student's t test or Mann-Whitney U test for paired data with Bonferroni correction for post-hoc multiple comparisons was applied for evaluating the differences between each experimental condition and the others. Spearman's rank-order correlation was used to explore the relationship between ICP and CVP. Significance was established at $p < 0.05$. Analyses were performed with SPSS statistics software (V.23.0 IBM Corporation, New York, USA).

Results
Respiratory mechanics

There were significant differences in all respiratory mechanic parameters except for expiratory V_T among different experimental conditions at baseline PEEP level of 5 cm H_2O (all $p < 0.05$, Table 1). Compared to the *Normal* condition, hydrochloride instillation significantly increased lung driving pressure and E_L in conditions with lung injury (*L*, *L + CW*, *L + CW + IH* and *L + IH* conditions); while P_{ES-EE}, chest wall driving pressure and E_{CW} significantly increased in conditions with chest wall and abdomen strapping (*CW*, *L + CW* and *L + CW + IH* conditions, Table 1).

The highest E_{CW}/E_{RS} ratio was observed in the *CW* condition which was significantly higher than the *Normal* condition ($p = 0.033$, Table 1); while the lowest E_{CW}/E_{RS} ratio was observed in the *L* condition which was significantly lower than the *Normal* condition ($p =$

0.035, Table 1). There was significant difference in E_{CW}/E_{RS} ratio between the two conditions with IH ($p = 0.004$, Table 1). Figure 2 shows data of E_L and E_{CW}, and the E_{CW}/E_{RS} ratio.

Changes of ICP in the non-IH conditions

ICP significantly increased with increments of PEEP in all non-IH conditions ($p < 0.001$, Fig. 3a). The greatest cumulative increase in ICP was observed in the *CW* condition (6 [5.3, 6.8] mm Hg), which was significant higher than the other conditions (p value range: < 0.001 to 0.018). The lowest cumulative increase in ICP was observed in the *L* condition (2 [1.3, 3.8] mm Hg), which was significant lower than the other conditions ($p < 0.001$). There was no significant difference in cumulative ICP change between the *Normal* and the *L + CW* condition (4 [3.0, 4.0] versus 4 [2.3, 4.8] mm Hg, $p > 0.999$, Fig. 3b).

Changes of ICP in the IH conditions

There was no difference in baseline ICP between the two IH conditions. ICP significantly decreased when PEEP was increased ($p < 0.001$, Fig. 3c). There was no significant difference in cumulative ICP change between the *L + CW + IH* and the *L + IH* conditions (– 10 [– 13.5, – 5.5] versus – 9.5 [– 12.5, – 5.3] mm Hg, $p = 0.924$, Fig. 3d). There was no significant difference in ICP change between each PEEP level ($p = 0.389$). Detailed ICP and the change of ICP at each PEEP levels was presented in Table 2.

Changes of hemodynamic parameters

Baseline CVP values were significantly higher in the conditions with chest wall strapping (*CW*, *L + CW* and *L + CW + IH* conditions) than those without chest wall strapping (*Normal*, *L* and *L + IH* conditions, p value range < 0.001 to 0.038, Fig. 4a). CVP significantly increased as increments of PEEP in each condition, with a significant different extent of CVP increase ($p < 0.001$); the increases of CVP in the *L* and the *L + IH* conditions were significantly lower than those in other conditions (p value range 0.001 to 0.020, Fig. 4b). ICP was significantly correlated to CVP in the non-IH conditions ($r = 0.654$, $p < 0.001$); however, ICP and CVP were no longer correlated in the IH conditions ($r = – 0.066$, $p = 0.561$). There was no significant difference in baseline MAP among different conditions ($p = 0.125$, Fig. 4c). MAP significantly decreased when PEEP was increased in each condition, whereas the decrease of MAP in the IH conditions were significantly greater than those in other conditions (p value range 0.007 to 0.025); but no significant difference was observed between the two IH conditions ($p = 0.961$, Fig. 4d). CPP values in the IH conditions were significantly lower than those

Table 1 Respiratory mechanics parameters at 5 cm H_2O of positive end-expiratory pressure in each condition

	Normal	CW	L	L + CW	L + CW + IH	L + IH	p value
V_{TE} (ml)	134 (130.3, 173.8)	136 (131.3, 175)	136 (132.5, 177.5)	138 (131.8, 176)	136.5 (134.5, 175)	136.5 (133.5, 175.8)	> 0.999
P_{PEAK} (cm H_2O)	18.5 (14.5, 21.5)	22 (17.5, 24.5)	23.5 (21.5, 24.8)*	30.5 (24.3, 32.8)*	27 (25.3, 35.8)*	22.5 (19.8, 25.5)	< 0.001
P_{ES-EE} (cm H_2O)	4.1 (4.1, 5.1)	6.8 (5.4, 6.8)*	5.4 (4.1, 6.5)	7.5 (5.4, 10.2)*	6.8 (5.8, 9.2)*	5.4 (4.4, 5.4)	< 0.001
Airway resistance (cm H_2O*s/L)	21.8 (17.5, 23.3)	21.2 (18, 27.8)	26.9 (20.6, 31.3)	34.9 (27.3, 39.5)*	30.4 (22, 42.9)*	23.2 (17.3, 30)	0.007
Airway driving pressure (cm H_2O)	8.8 (6.8, 10.5)	12.2 (9.9, 13.6)*	13.6 (11.2, 13.6)*	19 (12.6, 20.1)*	15.6 (13.9, 22.8)*	12.9 (11.2, 13.6)*	< 0.001
Chest wall driving pressure (cm H_2O)	2.7 (2.7, 4.1)	6.8 (4.4, 6.8)*	2 (1.4, 2.7)	4.8 (2.9, 5.4)*	6.1 (5.4, 6.8) *	2.7 (1.4, 2.7)	< 0.001
Transpulmonary driving pressure (cm H_2O)	4.8 (4.1, 7.8)	5.4 (4.4, 7.8)	10.9 (9.5, 12.2)*	12.2 (9.7, 16.3)*	9.5 (8.5, 17)*	10.9 (8.5, 10.9)*	< 0.001
E_{RS} (cm H_2O/L)	57.1 (48.1, 73.1)	79.3 (72.3, 96.4)	86.8 (77.6, 102.6)*	109.4 (95.4, 149.9)*	114.6 (84.7, 164.4)*	86.8 (78.4, 100)*	< 0.001
E_{CW} (cm H_2O/L)	21.6 (20.3, 23.5)	38.9 (32.5, 49.6)*	13.1 (10.1, 18.6)*	28.1 (22.2, 39.6)*	40.3 (33, 48.1)*	17.6 (10.3, 20.4)	< 0.001
E_L (cm H_2O/L)	37.5 (25.3, 50.2)	39 (31.3, 54.4)	74.2 (63.1, 89.1)*	84.4 (62.3, 112.9)*	70 (52.3, 119.5)*	65.6 (60.8, 85.7)*	0.001
E_{CW}/E_{RS} ratio	0.4 (0.29, 0.48)	0.47 (0.41, 0.61)*	0.16 (0.1, 0.22)*	0.25 (0.21, 0.4)*	0.34 (0.29, 0.42)	0.21 (0.13, 0.27)*	< 0.001

Data are presented as median (interquartile range)

*$p < 0.05$ compared to the *Normal* condition

V_{TE} expiratory tidal volume, P_{PEAK} peak airway pressure, P_{ES-EE} end-expiratory esophageal pressure, E_{RS} respiratory system elastance, E_{CW} chest wall elastance, E_L lung elastance

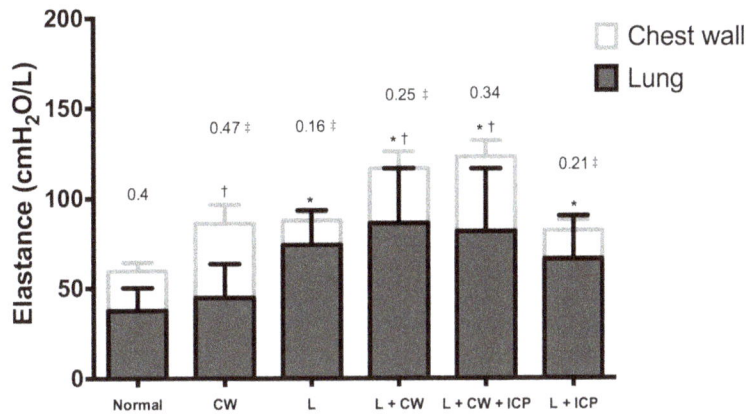

Fig. 2 Stacked histograms of chest wall elastance and lung elastance. *: compared to the *Normal* condition, a significant greater lung elastance (E_L) was observed in the conditions with lung injury. †: compared to the *Normal* condition, a significant greater chest wall elastance (E_{CW}) was observed in the conditions with chest and abdomen strapping. The numbers on the top of each plot are the medians of the ratio of E_{CW} to respiratory system elastance. ‡: $p < 0.05$ compared to the *Normal* condition

in other conditions (p value range < 0.001 to 0.010, Fig. 4e). There was no significant difference in the change of CPP among different conditions ($p = 0.642$, Fig. 4f).

Discussion

The main findings of this preliminary study were:

1) E_L can be increased by hydrochloride induced lung injury, accompanied with a decreased E_{CW}/E_{RS} ratio. In the contrast, E_{CW} can be increased by chest wall and abdominal strapping, accompanied by increased E_{CW}/E_{RS} ratio. 2) In pigs without IH, ICP increases as increasing of PEEP. The extent of ICP increase was determined by respiratory mechanics. The effect of PEEP on ICP was

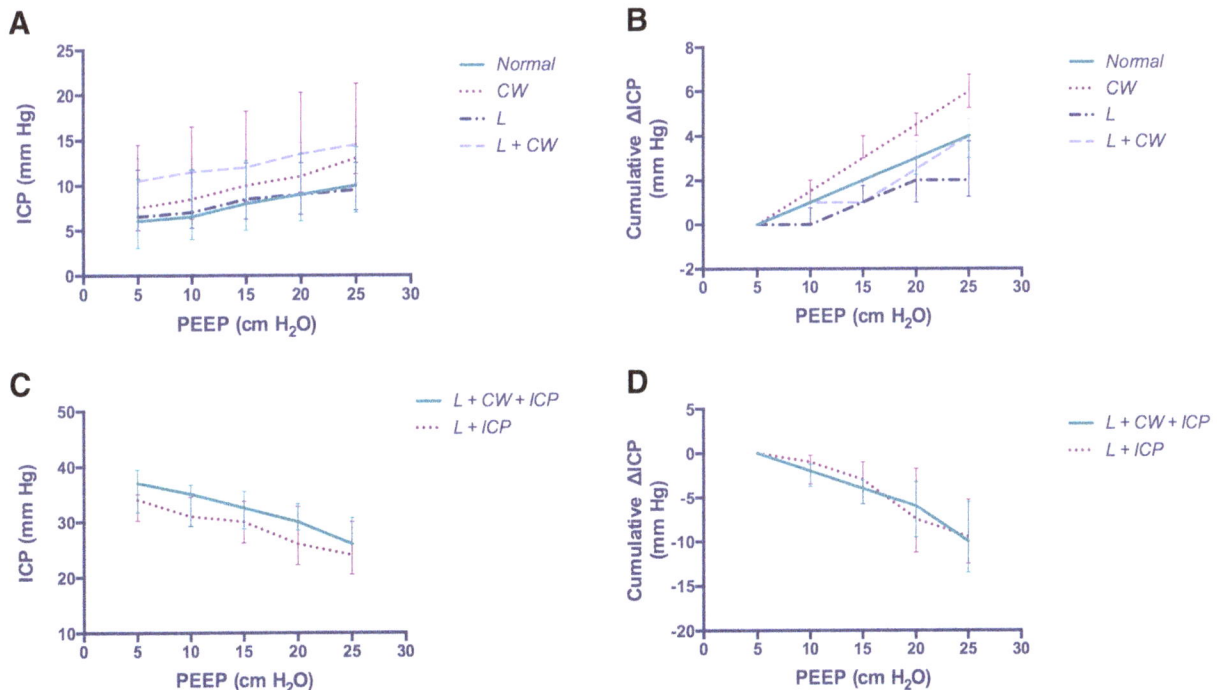

Fig. 3 Changes of intracranial pressure with positive end-expiratory pressure increases. **a** Intracranial pressure (ICP) increased with positive end-expiratory pressure (PEEP) increases in all the conditions without intracranial hypertension (IH). **b** In the conditions without IH, the greatest cumulative change of ICP was observed in the *CW* condition, while the lowest one was observed in the *L* condition (both with statistical significance). **c** ICP decreased with PEEP increases in the conditions without IH. **d** No significant difference was observed in the change of ICP between the two conditions with IH

Table 2 Intracranial pressure and the change of intracranial pressure at each positive end-expiratory pressure level

Condition	PEEP (cm H_2O)	ICP (mm Hg)	ΔICP (mm Hg)	Cumulative ΔICP (mm Hg)
Normal	5	6 (3, 10.8)	–	–
	10	6.5 (4, 11.8)	1 (1, 1)	1 (1, 1)
	15	8 (5, 12.8)	1 (1, 1)	2 (2, 2)
	20	9 (6, 13.5)	1 (1, 1)	3 (2.3, 3)
	25	10 (7, 14.3)	1 (0.3, 1)	4 (3, 4)
CW	5	7.5 (5, 14.5)	–	–
	10	8.5 (6.3, 16.5)	1.5 (1, 2)	1.5 (1, 2)
	15	10 (8.3, 18.3)	2 (1, 2)	3 (3, 4)
	20	11 (9.3, 20.3)	1 (1, 1.8)	4.5 (4, 5)
	25	13 (11.3, 21.3)	1.5 (1, 2)	6 (5.3, 6.8)
L	5	6.5 (5, 11.8)	–	–
	10	7 (5.3, 11.8)	0 (0, 0.8)	0 (0, 0.8)
	15	8.5 (6.3, 12.5)	1 (1, 1)	1 (1, 1.8)
	20	9 (6.8, 12.5)	0.5 (0, 1.8)	2 (1, 3)
	25	9.5 (7.3, 12.5)	0 (0, 1)	2 (1.3, 3.8)
L + CW	5	10.5 (6, 13)	–	–
	10	11.5 (7, 19.8)	1 (0.3, 1)	1 (0.3, 1)
	15	12 (8, 14)	1 (0, 1)	1 (1, 2)
	20	13.5 (9.3, 14.8)	1 (0.3, 2)	2.5 (1.3, 3.8)
	25	14.5 (10.3, 16.5)	1 (1, 1)	4 (2.3, 4.8)
L + CW + IH	5	37 (31.8, 39.5)	–	–
	10	35 (29.3, 36.8)	-2 (−3.8, −1.3)	-2 (−3.8, −1.3)
	15	32.5 (28.8, 35.5)	-2 (−2, −1)	−4 (−5.8, − 3)
	20	30 (28.5, 33.3)	−1.5 (−3.5, 0)	−6 (−9.5, − 3.3)
	25	26 (26, 30.8)	−3.5 (−4, − 1.3)	−10 (− 13.5, − 5.5)
L + IH	5	34 (30.3, 35)	–	–
	10	31 (29.3, 34.5)	−1 (− 3.5, −0.3)	−1 (− 3.5, −0.3)
	15	30 (26.3, 33.8)	− 2 (− 2.8, − 0.3)	− 3 (− 5.8, − 1)
	20	26 (22.3, 32.8)	−2.5 (− 5.5, − 1)	−7.5 (− 11.3, − 1.8)
	25	24 (20.5, 30)	−2 (− 3.5, − 1.3)	−9.5 (− 12.5, − 5.3)

Data are presented as median (interquartile range)

ICP intracranial pressure, *PEEP* positive end-expiratory pressure

enhanced in increased E_{CW} and E_{CW}/E_{RS} ratio condition, whereas the effect of PEEP on ICP was attenuated in increased E_L and thereby reduced E_{CW}/E_{RS} ratio condition. 3) In pigs with IH, however, the increase of PEEP reduced ICP. The difference of respiratory mechanics has nothing to do with the effect of PEEP on ICP under IH conditions.

The Monro-Kellie doctrine suggests that with an intact skull, the combined volume of the brain, the blood and the cerebrospinal fluid is constant and determines the ICP [29]. An increase in volume of single component causes a decrease in volume of remaining one or both of the two components, in a certain degree, to keep ICP remained in a normal range. ICP will increase rapidly once compensation is exhausted. The PEEP-induced increase of pleural pressure may be transmitted to the intracranial cavity directly or may reduce cerebral venous drainage and eventually increase ICP [18, 30], where the pleural pressure serves as an intermediate link from the lung to the cranium.

The transmission of PEEP into the pleural cavity dependents on the respiratory mechanics of the lung and the chest wall. P_{AW} equals the sum of transpulmonary pressure and pleural pressure when the airway resistance

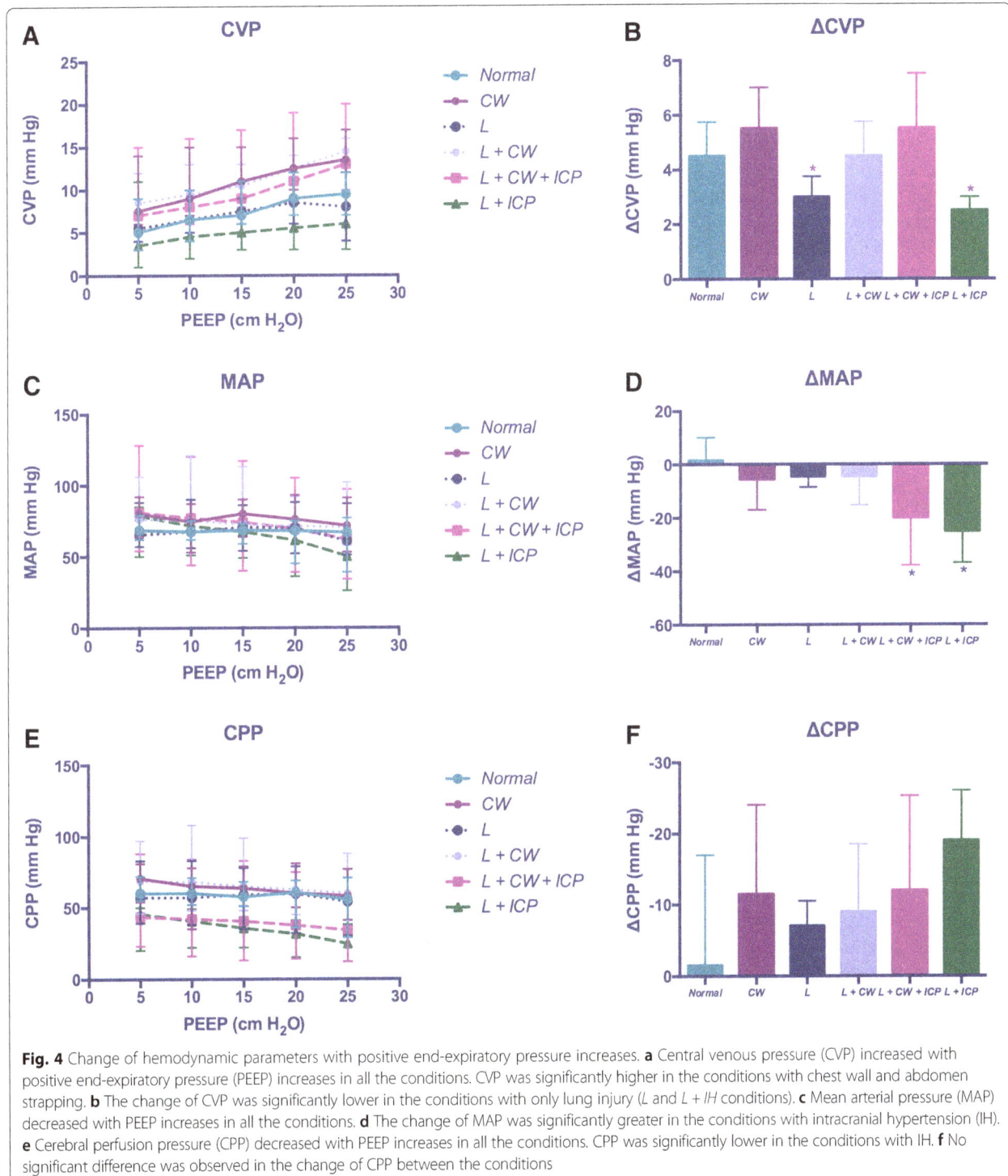

Fig. 4 Change of hemodynamic parameters with positive end-expiratory pressure increases. **a** Central venous pressure (CVP) increased with positive end-expiratory pressure (PEEP) increases in all the conditions. CVP was significantly higher in the conditions with chest wall and abdomen strapping. **b** The change of CVP was significantly lower in the conditions with only lung injury (L and L + IH conditions). **c** Mean arterial pressure (MAP) decreased with PEEP increases in all the conditions. **d** The change of MAP was significantly greater in the conditions with intracranial hypertension (IH). **e** Cerebral perfusion pressure (CPP) decreased with PEEP increases in all the conditions. CPP was significantly lower in the conditions with IH. **f** No significant difference was observed in the change of CPP between the conditions

is nil (i.e. no airflow in the airway). In this situation, the distribution of P_{AW} to pleural cavity depends on the E_{CW}/E_{RS} ratio [21]. In other words, a higher E_{CW}/E_{RS} ratio could lead to a greater impact of PEEP on pleural pressure, which might in turns result in a greater increase of ICP. This was supported by our data: in animals without IH, the effect of PEEP on ICP became

obvious under condition of increased E_{CW}/E_{RS} ratio, but was attenuated under condition of decreased E_{CW}/E_{RS} ratio (Fig. 3a and b).

Surprisingly, however, our data suggested that the increase of PEEP reduces ICP in animals with IH. This might be explained by the change of cerebral blood volume. In our study, an intracranial balloon was inflated to induce IH mimicking that caused by space occupying lesions. The compensatory potential of cerebrospinal fluid was exhausted and thereby the volume in the skull was predominantly determined by the intracranial blood volume in this situation since the brain is almost incompressible and has a relatively constant volume.

An increased cerebral blood volume can be caused by reduced cerebral venous drainage and/or increased arterial perfusion. The application of PEEP can reduce cerebral venous drainage as we discussed above, results in increase of cerebral venous blood volume and elevation of ICP. However, this effect might become less obvious in the IH conditions. In experimental studies conducted in dogs, it was found that the increase of ICP due to PEEP was diminished in the presence of IH, which can be explained by the Starling resistor or waterfall concept [31, 32]. McGuire et al. found a similar phenomenon in a clinical study [11], in which ICP increased in patients with normal baseline ICP but did not significantly change in patients with elevated ICP when a maximal PEEP of 15 cm H_2O was applied. We speculated that the effect of PEEP on ICP from the venous side in IH pigs in the present study might be also diminished. This is supported by our data: ICP was correlated to CVP, which represents the downstream (venous returning) impedance, in the non-IH conditions; however, no such correlationshiop was observed in the IH conditions, which means that the change of ICP was more likely determined by the change of cerebral perfusion in the IH conditions.

The normal brain has several mechanisms for regulating cerebral blood flow and volume, referred as cerebral autoregulation. Under physiological conditions, vessels in the brain can regulate the vascular tone to maintain a constant cerebral blood flow in MAP between 60 and 160 mmHg [33, 34]. However, recent studies suggest an asymmetric dynamic cerebral autoregulatory response that the autoregulatory ability appears to be more effective in buffering increases in MAP and CPP as compared to reductions [35–37]. In the IH conditions in this experiment, MAP and CPP decreased with PEEP increases. In addition, when high PEEP levels were applied, CPP dropped to a low range that was beyond the capacity of autoregulation mechanisms to maintain a constant cerebral blood flow. Therefore, it is reasonable to infer that the cerebral blood flow decreased when PEEP was increased, although we did not measure the actual cerebral blood flow in the present study. The decrease of cerebral blood flow resulted in decrease of cerebral blood volume and eventually resulted in decrease of ICP. Since there was no significant difference in MAP and CPP between the two conditions of IH (although with different respiratory mechanics), no difference was found in the change of ICP.

In the present experiment we provided sedation rather than anesthesia by midazolam and fentanyl infusion. Unlike general anesthesia (inhaled anesthetics or i.v. barbiturates), which is usually considered as a salvage therapy for refractory intracranial hypertension, sedation is more likely to be chosen in the clinical practice (in the ICUs) for intracranial hypertensive patients. Therefore, we used midazolam and fentanyl infusion (to provide sedation) instead of general anesthesia.

Limitations

Due to the nature of a preliminary study, there were many limitations in this study. First, we did not measure/control $PaCO_2$ in this study. Therefore, the influence of $PaCO_2$ on ICP cannot be excluded. Second, animals were not randomized to a certain condition. Instead, we tested all the conditions in sequence in each animal. Third, we used CPP as the indicator of cerebral perfusion. Although strong correlated, CPP does not always reflect cerebral perfusion. Measurement of cerebral blood flow is needed for full understanding of the effects of PEEP in intracranial hemodynamics in future studies.

Conclusions

Different respiratory mechanics models can be established via hydrochloride induced lung injury and chest wall and abdominal strapping. For pigs with normal ICP, the effect of PEEP on ICP becomes more obvious when the E_{CW}/E_{RS} ratio increases, and is attenuated when the ratio decreases. For pigs with IH, the responsiveness of ICP to PEEP is independent of respiratory mechanics and likely depends to a greater extent on the effect of PEEP on hemodynamics.

Abbreviations

ARDS: Acute respiratory distress syndrome; CPP: Cerebral perfusion pressure; CVP: Central venous pressure; E_{CW}: Chest wall elastance; E_L: Lung elastance; E_{RS}: Respiratory system elastance; ICP: Intracranial pressure; IH: Intracranial hypertension; MAP: Mean arterial pressure; P_{AW}: Airway pressure; PEEP: Positive end-expiratory pressure; P_{ES}: Esophageal pressure; P_{ES-EE}: End-expiratory esophageal pressure; P_{ES-EI}: End-inspiratory esophageal pressure; P_{PEAK}: Peak airway pressure; V_{TE}: Expiratory tidal volume

Acknowledgements

We thank Dr. Brian Kavanagh for his valuable suggestions for preparing the manuscript. We thank Jian-Xiang Zhao and Min Li for their technical support in the experiment.

Funding

The study was supported by National Natural Science Foundation of China (Grant No. 81701942) and Fujian Provincial Health and Family Planning Commission Youth Research Project (Grant No. 2017-2-2). The sponsors had no role in the study design, data collection, data analysis, data interpretation or writing of the manuscript.

Authors' contributions

HC, JXZ and RGY participated in the design of the study and drafted the manuscript. HC, JZ, YQL participated in the experiments and data collection. All authors participated in review and revision of the manuscript. All authors read and approved the final manuscript.

Competing interests

The authors declare that they have no competing interests.

Author details

[1]Surgical Intensive Care Unit, Fujian Provincial Clinical College, Fujian Medical University, No 134, Dongjie Street, Gulou District, Fuzhou 350001, Fujian, China. [2]Department of Critical Care Medicine, Beijing Tiantan Hospital, Capital Medical University, Beijing, China.

References

1. Aisiku IP, Yamal JM, Doshi P, Rubin ML, Benoit JS, Hannay J, et al. The incidence of ARDS and associated mortality in severe TBI using the Berlin definition. J Trauma Acute Care Surg. 2016;80:308–12.
2. Quilez ME, Lopez-Aguilar J, Blanch L. Organ crosstalk during acute lung injury, acute respiratory distress syndrome, and mechanical ventilation. Curr Opin Crit Care. 2012;18:23–8.
3. Mascia L. Acute lung injury in patients with severe brain injury: a double hit model. Neurocrit Care. 2009;11:417–26.
4. Hoesch RE, Lin E, Young M, Gottesman RF, Altaweel L, Nyquist PA, et al. Acute lung injury in critical neurological illness. Crit Care Med. 2012;40:587–93.
5. Theodore J, Robin ED. Pathogenesis of neurogenic pulmonary oedema. Lancet. 1975;2:749–51.
6. Ranieri VM, Rubenfeld GD, Thompson BT, Ferguson ND, Caldwell E, Fan E, et al. Acute respiratory distress syndrome: the Berlin definition. JAMA. 2012; 307:2526–33.
7. Tejerina E, Pelosi P, Muriel A, Penuelas O, Sutherasan Y, Frutos-Vivar F, et al. Association between ventilatory settings and development of acute respiratory distress syndrome in mechanically ventilated patients due to brain injury. J Crit Care. 2016.
8. Pelosi P, Ferguson ND, Frutos-Vivar F, Anzueto A, Putensen C, Raymondos K, et al. Management and outcome of mechanically ventilated neurologic patients. Crit Care Med. 2011;39:1482–92.
9. Mascia L, Grasso S, Fiore T, Bruno F, Berardino M, Ducati A. Cerebro-pulmonary interactions during the application of low levels of positive end-expiratory pressure. Intensive Care Med. 2005;31:373–9.
10. Caricato A, Conti G, Della Corte F, Mancino A, Santilli F, Sandroni C, et al. Effects of PEEP on the intracranial system of patients with head injury and subarachnoid hemorrhage: the role of respiratory system compliance. J Trauma. 2005;58:571–6.
11. McGuire G, Crossley D, Richards J, Wong D. Effects of varying levels of positive end-expiratory pressure on intracranial pressure and cerebral perfusion pressure. Crit Care Med. 1997;25:1059–62.
12. Burchiel KJ, Steege TD, Wyler AR. Intracranial pressure changes in brain-injured patients requiring positive end-expiratory pressure ventilation. Neurosurgery. 1981;8:443–9.
13. Apuzzo JL, Wiess MH, Petersons V, Small RB, Kurze T, Heiden JS. Effect of positive end expiratory pressure ventilation on intracranial pressure in man. J Neurosurg. 1977;46:227–32.
14. Cooper KR, Boswell PA, Choi SC. Safe use of PEEP in patients with severe head injury. J Neurosurg. 1985;63:552–5.
15. Frost EA. Effects of positive end-expiratory pressure on intracranial pressure and compliance in brain-injured patients. J Neurosurg. 1977;47:195–200.
16. Koutsoukou A, Perraki H, Raftopoulou A, Koulouris N, Sotiropoulou C, Kotanidou A, et al. Respiratory mechanics in brain-damaged patients. Intensive Care Med. 2006;32:1947–54.
17. Huynh T, Messer M, Sing RF, Miles W, Jacobs DG, Thomason MH. Positive end-expiratory pressure alters intracranial and cerebral perfusion pressure in severe traumatic brain injury. J Trauma. 2002;53:488–92 discussion 92-3.
18. Chang WT, Nyquist PA. Strategies for the use of mechanical ventilation in the neurologic intensive care unit. Neurosurg Clin N Am. 2013;24:407–16.
19. Nyquist P, Stevens RD, Mirski MA. Neurologic injury and mechanical ventilation. Neurocrit Care. 2008;9:400–8.
20. Chapin JC, Downs JB, Douglas ME, Murphy EJ, Ruiz BC. Lung expansion, airway pressure transmission, and positive end-expiratory pressure. Arch Surg. 1979;114:1193–7.
21. Gattinoni L, Chiumello D, Carlesso E, Valenza F. Bench-to-bedside review: chest wall elastance in acute lung injury/acute respiratory distress syndrome patients. Crit Care. 2004;8:350–5.
22. Chen H, Yang YL, Xu M, Shi ZH, He X, Sun XM, et al. Use of the injection test to indicate the oesophageal balloon position in patients without spontaneous breathing: a clinical feasibility study. J Int Med Res. 2017;45:320–31.
23. Chiumello D, Consonni D, Coppola S, Froio S, Crimella F, Colombo A. The occlusion tests and end-expiratory esophageal pressure: measurements and comparison in controlled and assisted ventilation. Ann Intensive Care. 2016;6:13.
24. Hussain SN, Pardy RL. Inspiratory muscle function with restrictive chest wall loading during exercise in normal humans. J Appl Physiol (1985). 1985;58: 2027–32.
25. Staffieri F, Stripoli T, De Monte V, Crovace A, Sacchi M, De Michele M, et al. Physiological effects of an open lung ventilatory strategy titrated on elastance-derived end-inspiratory transpulmonary pressure: study in a pig model. Crit Care Med. 2012;40:2124–31.
26. Davies SW, Leonard KL, Falls RK Jr, Mageau RP, Efird JT, Hollowell JP, et al. Lung protective ventilation (ARDSNet) versus airway pressure release ventilation: ventilatory management in a combined model of acute lung and brain injury. J Trauma Acute Care Surg. 2015;78:240–9 discussion 9-51.
27. Heuer JF, Sauter P, Barwing J, Herrmann P, Crozier TA, Bleckmann A, et al. Effects of high-frequency oscillatory ventilation on systemic and cerebral hemodynamics and tissue oxygenation: an experimental study in pigs. Neurocrit Care. 2012;17:281–92.
28. Scheirer CJ, Ray WS, Hare N. The analysis of ranked data derived from completely randomized factorial designs. Biometrics. 1976;32:429–34.
29. Wilson MH. Monro-Kellie 2.0: the dynamic vascular and venous pathophysiological components of intracranial pressure. J Cereb Blood Flow Metab. 2016;36:1338–50.
30. Koutsoukou A, Katsiari M, Orfanos SE, Kotanidou A, Daganou M, Kyriakopoulou M, et al. Respiratory mechanics in brain injury: a review. World J Crit Care Med. 2016;5:65–73.
31. Luce JM, Huseby JS, Kirk W, Butler J. A Starling resistor regulates cerebral venous outflow in dogs. J Appl Physiol Respir Environ Exerc Physiol. 1982; 53:1496–503.
32. Huseby JS, Luce JM, Cary JM, Pavlin EG, Butler J. Effects of positive end-expiratory pressure on intracranial pressure in dogs with intracranial hypertension. J Neurosurg. 1981;55:704–5.
33. Kinoshita K. Traumatic brain injury: pathophysiology for neurocritical care. J Intensive Care. 2016;4:29.
34. McBryde FD, Malpas SC, Paton JF. Intracranial mechanisms for preserving brain blood flow in health and disease. Acta Physiol (Oxf). 2017;219:274–87.
35. Numan T, Bain AR, Hoiland RL, Smirl JD, Lewis NC, Ainslie PN. Static autoregulation in humans: a review and reanalysis. Med Eng Phys. 2014;36: 1487–95.
36. Schmidt B, Klingelhofer J, Perkes I, Czosnyka M. Cerebral autoregulatory response depends on the direction of change in perfusion pressure. J Neurotrauma. 2009;26:651–6.
37. Aaslid R, Blaha M, Sviri G, Douville CM, Newell DW. Asymmetric dynamic cerebral autoregulatory response to cyclic stimuli. Stroke. 2007;38:1465–9.

24

Is traumatic brain injury a risk factor for neurodegeneration? A meta-analysis of population-based studies

Chi-Hsien Huang[1,2], Chi-Wei Lin[1,2], Yi-Che Lee[2,3], Chih-Yuan Huang[4], Ru-Yi Huang[1,2], Yi-Cheng Tai[5], Kuo-Wei Wang[2,6], San-Nan Yang[2], Yuan-Ting Sun[7] and Hao-kuang Wang[2,6*] (iD)

Abstract

Background: To determine the association of prior traumatic brain injury (TBI) with subsequent diagnosis of neurodegeneration disease.

Methods: All studies from 1980 to 2016 reporting TBI as a risk factor for diagnoses of interest were identified by searching PubMed, Embase, study references, and review articles. The data and study design were assessed by 2 investigators independently. A meta-analysis was performed by RevMan 5.3.

Results: There were 18 studies comprising 3,263,207 patients. Meta-analysis revealed a significant association of prior TBI with subsequent dementia. The pooled odds ratio (OR) for TBI on development of dementia, FTD and TDP-43 associated disease were 1.93 (95% CI 1.47–2.55, $p < 0.001$), 4.44 (95% CI 3.86–5.10, p < 0.001), and 2.97 (95% CI 1.35–6.53, p < 0.001). However, analyses of individual diagnoses found no evidence that the risk of Alzheimer's disease, and Parkinson's disease in individuals with previous TBI compared to those without TBI.

Conclusions: History of TBI is not associated with the development of subsequent neurodegeneration disease. Care must be taken in extrapolating from these results because no suitable criteria define post TBI neurodegenerative processes. Therefore, further research in this area is needed to confirm these questions and uncover the link between TBI and neurodegeneration disease.

Keywords: TBI, Dementia, Neurodegeneration, Meta-analysis

Introduction

Traumatic brain injury (TBI) occurs when an external force injures the brain. Motor vehicle accidents cause most TBIs in young adults, while falls are the leading cause of TBIs in people over 65 years of age [1]. Owing to the increasing use of motor vehicles in developed countries, the incidence of TBI is rapidly growing. TBI is a major cause of death and disabilities—especially in children and young adults—that result in high societal costs [1, 2]. Men sustain TBIs more frequently than women do. These observations suggest that TBIs result in major health and socioeconomic problems throughout the

world. Indeed, the World Health Organization has reported that traffic accidents are the third highest contributor to the global burden of disease and injury [1, 2].

Neurological damage occurs not only at the moment of impact (primary injury) in a TBI, but also it further develops overtime post-impact. Several processes, such as neurotransmitter release, free-radical generation, calcium-mediated damage, gene activation, mitochondrial dysfunction, and inflammatory responses, have been investigated in studies of the secondary injuries that are associated with TBI [3–5]. These mechanisms might occur continuously over patients' lifetimes. Interestingly, a history of TBI has been reported to increase the incidence of Alzheimer disease (AD) [6] and other neurodegenerative conditions, including Parkinson's disease (PD) [7], amyotrophic lateral sclerosis (ALS) [8],

---
* Correspondence: ed101393@gmail.com; ed101393@edah.org.tw
[2]School of Medicine for International Students, I-Shou University, Kaohsiung, Taiwan
[6]Department of Neurosurgery, E-Da Hospital, I-Shou University, No.1, Yida Road, Jiaosu Village, Yanchao District, Kaohsiung City 82445, Taiwan
Full list of author information is available at the end of the article

and frontotemporal dementia (FTD) [5]. However, other studies have yielded contradicting results [9–13].

The goal of our study was to determine whether TBI was associated with an increased risk of neurodegeneration by conducting a systematic review of cohort studies of patients with TBI. In addition, we examined which neurodegenerative process occurred most often.

Methods

Data sources

We conducted systematic literature searches of the association between neurodegeneration and TBI in the Medical Literature Analysis and Retrieval System Online (MEDLINE®)/PubMed (US National Library of Medicine, National Institutes of Health, Bethesda, MD; http://www.ncbi.nlm.nih.gov/pubmed) database and Excerpta Medica Database (EMBASE®, Elsevier, Amsterdam, Netherlands; http://www.elsevier.com/solutions/embase-biomedical-research). We used the following keywords to generate a list of potentially useful studies: ([traumatic brain injury] OR [head injury] OR [brain injury] OR [TBI]) AND ([neurodegeneration] OR [cognitive dysfunction] OR [dementia] OR [alzheimer's disease] OR [AD] OR [parkinson's disease] OR [parkinsonism] OR [frontotemporal dementia] OR [Amyotrophic Lateral Sclerosis]) [14–16]. The search was performed through December 2016. The reference lists in the selected studies, as well as the list of studies

included in earlier meta-analyses on similar topics, were reviewed for additional references. This review considered observational studies, and case series.

Inclusion criteria

We included published articles on the risk of neurodegeneration, including cognitive dysfunction, dementia, AD, PD, FTD, and ALS, among individuals with TBIs compared with the risk of neurodegeneration in individuals in a nonbrain-injured population-based control group. A risk estimate was calculated with the data provided in the article. TBI was not limited in accordance with its severity.

Exclusion criteria

Studies were excluded if (1) they were reviews, case reports, or case series; (2) they only consisted of a follow-up study of a cohort of patients with brain injury with no comparison group; (3) there was a non-population-based control group (i.e., a patient control group); or (4) insufficient information was available to allow for calculations of risk estimates [14–16].

Study selection

The outcomes recorded were neurodegeneration, dementia, PD, and transactive response DNA-binding protein of 43 kDa (TDP-43) aggregation-associated disease. ALS and FTD, which are closely related conditions with overlapping clinical, pathological,

Table 1 Individual for all included studies

Ref	Author, year	Type	TBI+ Neurodegeneration +	TBI+ Neurodegeneration -	TBI- Neurodegeneration +	TBI- Neurodegeneration -
20	Mehta KM, et al. 1999	Dementia (APOE)	11	788	118	5728
21	Luukinen H, et al. 2005		5	3	29	115
22	Sundström A, 2007		25	46	156	316
23	Luukinen H, et al. 2008		11	17	14	92
25	Wang HK, 2012	Dementia	1196	43,729	3499	221,186
26	Gardner RC, et al. 2014		4361	47,438	6610	108,891
27	Nordström P, et al.2014		108	45,141	458	765,915
28	Abner EL, et al. 2014		8	158	31	452
29	Rasmusson DX, et al. 1995	AD	20	1	48	33
30	Nemetz PN, et al. 1999		31	1252	957	2783
31	Barnes DE, et al. 2014		12	1217	1098	186,437
32	Spangenberg S, et al. 2009	Parkinson	87	73,232	8769	2,799,434
33	Lee PC, et al. 2012		42	50	315	704
34	Taylor KM, et al. 2015		69	24	310	206
35	Gardner RC, et al. 2015		891	51,502	1247	112,159
36	Kalkonde YV, 2012	FTD (TDP-43)	8	17	55	474
5	Wang HK, et al. 2015		363	24,222	413	122,512
37	Chen H, et al. 2007	ALS (TDP-43)	24	42	85	213

Table 2 Consensus ACROBAT-NRSI judgments between two reviewers by domain of bias

Component Study	Domain								Overall RoB Bias
	Bias Due to Judgment Confounding	Bias in Selection of Participants	Bias in Measurement of Interventions	Bias Due to Departures from Intended Interventions	Bias in Measurement of Outcomes	Bias in Selection of Reported Results	Bias Due to Missing Data		
Mehta KM, et al. [20]	moderate	moderate	low	low	low	low	low		moderate
Luukinen H, et al. [21]	low	low	low	low	low	low	low		low
Sundström A, [22]	low	low	low	low	low	low	low		low
Luukinen H, et al. [23]	low	low	low	low	low	low	low		low
Wang HK, [25]	low	moderate	low	low	moderate	low	low		low
Gardner RC, et al. [26]	low	moderate	low	low	moderate	low	low		low
Nordström P, et al. [27]	low	moderate	low	low	moderate	low	low		low
Abner EL, et al. [28]	low	moderate	low	low	moderate	low	low		low
Rasmusson DX, et al. [29]	low	low	low	low	low	low	low		low
Nemetz PN, et al. [30]	low	moderate	low	low	moderate	low	low		low
Barnes DE, et al. [31]	low	moderate	low	low	moderate	low	low		low
Spangenberg S, et al. [32]	low	low	low	low	low	low	low		low
Lee PC, et al. [33]	low	low	low	low	low	low	low		low
Taylor KM, et al. [34]	low	low	low	low	low	low	low		low
Gardner RC, et al. [35]	low	moderate	low	low	moderate	low	low		low
Kalkonde YV, [36]	low	low	low	low	low	low	low		low
Wang HK, et al. [5]	low	moderate	low	low	moderate	low	low		low
Chen H, et al. [37]	low	low	low	low	low	low	low		low

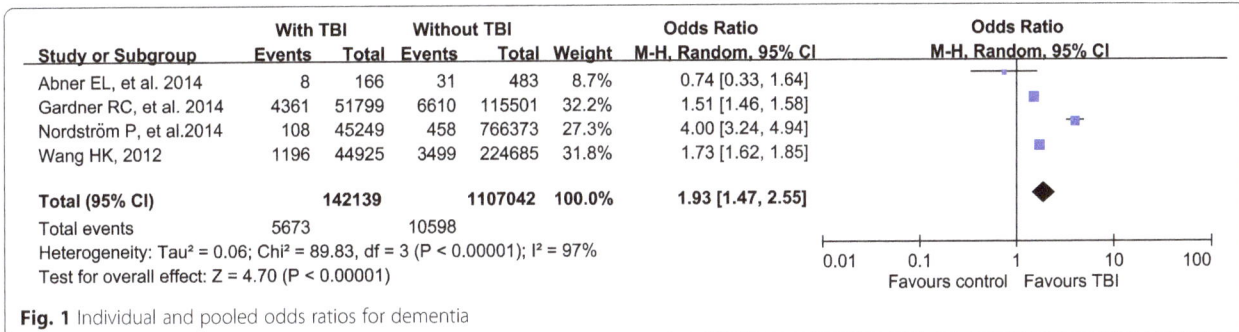

Fig. 1 Individual and pooled odds ratios for dementia

radiological, and genetic characteristics, are characterized by TDP-43 aggregation [17]. Therefore, we defined ALS and FTD as TDP-43-associated diseases. Two authors (H.K. Wang or Y.C. Tai) examined the titles and abstracts of the studies found in the systematic literature search. The entire articles of potentially eligible studies were assessed to determine if the studies met the criteria. The study selection process was performed in accordance with the Preferred Reporting Items for Systematic Reviews and Meta-Analyses (PRISMA) guidelines and documented with a PRISMA flow diagram.

Data analysis

The effects of TBI on the neurodegeneration outcomes were assessed with a random effects model because the designs and patient populations of the observational studies were expected to be heterogeneous. The Odds Ratio (OR) and 95% confidence intervals (CIs) were calculated. Statistical heterogeneity was examined with chi-square and I-squared (I^2) tests of heterogeneity. The data were analyzed with Review Manager (RevMan) Version 5.3 (Copenhagen: The Nordic Cochrane Centre, The Cochrane Collaboration, 2014).

Results

The systematic search

Using the search terms, our literature and reference list searches yielded 1317 references. After examination of

the abstracts and, when indicated, the full texts of the articles, 68 studies were considered potentially relevant [18–37] . Finally, 18 studies met our inclusion criteria and were included in the meta-analysis. The characteristics of the included trials are listed in Table 1. Methodologic qualities of are shown in Table 2.

The subgroup meta-analyses

There was an association between TBI and subsequent dementia (pooled OR = 1.93, 95% CI = 1.47–2.55) (Fig. 1). However, this association does not concur with the apolipoprotein E (APOE) genotype (pooled OR = 1.82, 95% CI = 0.74–4.46) (Fig. 2). The studies associated with AD yielded a pooled OR of 1.03 (95% CI = 0.06–16.33) with heterogeneity (I^2 = 98%, $P < 0.001$) (Fig. 3). The analysis of the risk of TBI that was associated with PD yielded a pooled OR of 1.19 (95% CI = 0.50–2.84) with heterogeneity (I^2 = 98%, P < 0.001) (Fig. 4). The analysis of the risk associated with TDP-43 and FTD yielded a pooled OR of 2.97 (95% CI = 1.35–6.53) and 4.44 (95% CI = 3.86–5.10) (Figs. 5 and 6).

Discussion

Concerns about the relationship between TBI and neurodegeneration have long existed. Our principal finding was that TBI is a potential risk factor for subsequent dementia (1.93, 95% CI = 1.47–2.55), TDP-43 (2.97, 95% CI = 1.35–6.53) and FTD (4.44, 95% CI = 3.86–5.10). However, when we analyzed the associations of the

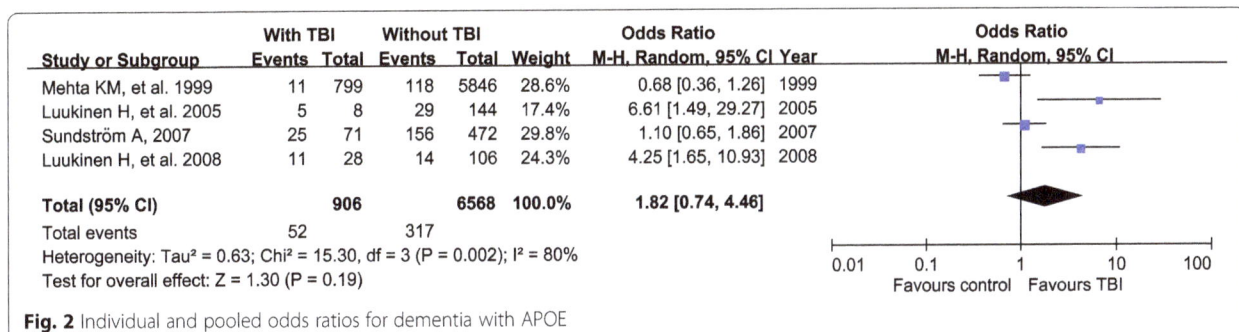

Fig. 2 Individual and pooled odds ratios for dementia with APOE

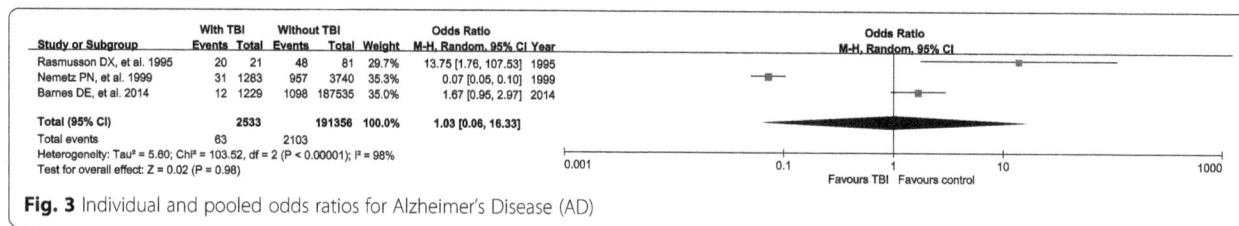

Fig. 3 Individual and pooled odds ratios for Alzheimer's Disease (AD)

incidences of AD, PD, or dementia with APOE genotype, we found that TBI was not a risk.

A common factor between TBI and different neurodegenerative disorders is the abnormal aggregation, accumulation, and/or disposition of proteins in the brain. Patients with TBI have beta-amyloid deposition in their brains, and the pattern of deposition is similar to that observed in patients with AD. Amyloid precursor protein, β-Amyloid precursor protein-cleaving enzyme-1, and presenilin-1, which is a γ-secretase complex protein, serve as sources of amyloid-β peptide deposition after TBI [5, 29–31].

TBI may also exacerbate nigrostriatal dopaminergic degeneration by modulating PD-associated genes. These results suggest that α-synuclein is a pathological link between the chronic effects of TBI and PD symptoms [32–34].

Another mechanism that might link TBI to neurodegeneration is the accumulation of TDP-43 in patients with FTD and ALS [5, 24, 37]. Patients with chronic traumatic encephalopathy (CTE) exhibit widespread TDP-43 proteinopathy in multiple areas of the brain [38]. Some patients also had TDP-43 protein in their spinal cords, and these patients developed a progressive motor neuron disease several years before their deaths [38, 39]. These findings suggest that TDP-43-associated neurodegeneration and head trauma are connected.

The mechanisms underlying the association of TBI and the incidence of neurodegeneration are exceedingly complex. In fact, in TBI, multiple pathologies occur simultaneously. However, systematic analyses of multiple pathologies in individual cases in a large TBI and control population have not been conducted [9–13, 39]. Therefore, a significant association of AD,

PD, and APOE-associated dementia was not observed, and no evidence that head trauma was a risk factor for patients with these disorders was found.

Another noteworthy finding of our study was that AD is not the most common form of neurodegeneration. Several studies have reported that TBI does not affect the development of AD. Whether a single occurrence of moderate-to-severe TBI triggers the development of neurodegeneration remains somewhat controversial [9–13]. In addition, brain injury has been shown to lead to the development of non-AD dementias. However, accurate clinical diagnostic criteria for neurodegeneration that results from TBI do not exist. Therefore, the true risk of neurodegeneration following TBI is hard to define.

Examinations of patients with CTE may help resolve this problem. The symptoms of CTE, which include behavioral disturbances, cognitive dysfunction, and/or motor-related symptoms, generally begin 8–10 years after repetitive mild TBIs are experienced [40–42]. However, the clinical diagnostic criteria for traumatic encephalopathy syndrome have only recently been reported. CTE can be seen after a single moderate or severe TBI while traumatic encephalopathy syndrome exhibits progressive deterioration over time. Therefore, clinical judgment must be used to determine whether the amount of progression is greater than what is expected for the age and comorbidities of the patient [39–42]. Multiple neurodegeneration processes have been used to describe the behavioral disturbances and cognitive dysfunction in patients following TBI owing to the lack of suitable diagnoses. This diagnosis can now be used to define those symptoms.

A major strength of this meta-analysis was the inclusion of a variety of different neurodegenerative outcomes

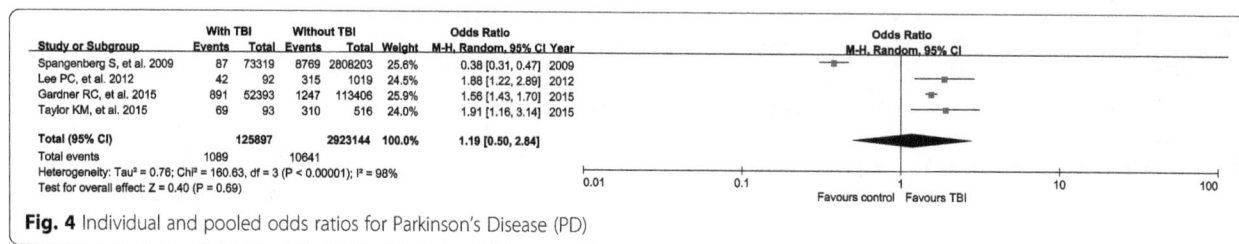

Fig. 4 Individual and pooled odds ratios for Parkinson's Disease (PD)

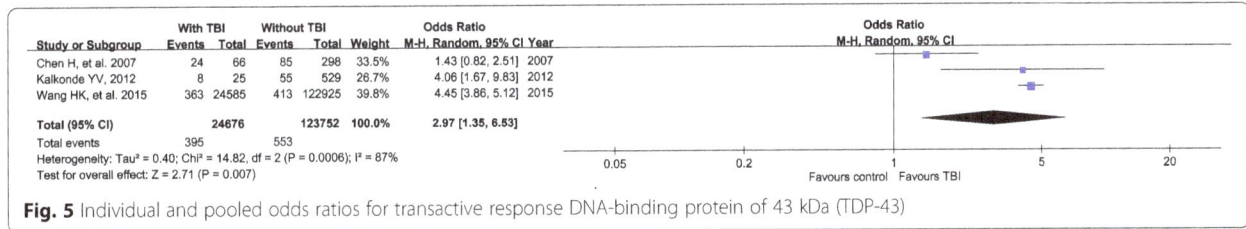

Study or Subgroup	With TBI Events	Total	Without TBI Events	Total	Weight	Odds Ratio M-H, Random, 95% CI	Year
Chen H, et al. 2007	24	66	85	298	33.5%	1.43 [0.82, 2.51]	2007
Kalkonde YV, 2012	8	25	55	529	26.7%	4.06 [1.67, 9.83]	2012
Wang HK, et al. 2015	363	24585	413	122925	39.8%	4.45 [3.86, 5.12]	2015
Total (95% CI)		24676		123752	100.0%	2.97 [1.35, 6.53]	
Total events	395		553				

Heterogeneity: Tau² = 0.40; Chi² = 14.82, df = 2 (P = 0.0006); I² = 87%
Test for overall effect: Z = 2.71 (P = 0.007)

Fig. 5 Individual and pooled odds ratios for transactive response DNA-binding protein of 43 kDa (TDP-43)

rather than a single diagnosis. The literature search was comprehensive because it focused on diagnoses rather than self-reported symptoms, which resulted in a rigorous examination of the topic.

However, several limitations of this meta-analysis warrant consideration. First, the initial severities of the TBIs varied within and across studies. Since our meta-analyses examined only published data, some important parameters, such as sex, alcohol consumption, and comorbidities were missing. Therefore, we were not able to control for these potential confounding factors. Patients with severe TBI had loss of high cortical function and presented in a vegetative state. In our studies, we included only patients who sought treatment for TBI and neurodegeneration disease, but not important parameters indicating clinical severity and imaging information on TBI. Therefore, it is hard to understand the relationship between the severity of TBI and neurodegeneration disease.

Second, we were not able to examine the effects of the locations of the TBIs in this analysis. Some investigators have proposed that temporal and frontal lobe lesions are more likely to be associated with an increased risk of later dementia compared with lesions in other brain regions [5]. In addition, preinjury intelligence and education level are also associated with TBI and dementia. However, the effects of these factors in this study were difficult to determine.

Another limitation was that none of the studies included in this review provided information on genetics [8]. The estimated effect of the apolipoprotein E (APOE) gene 4 on functional outcome might be greatly confounded by such factors, which could thus influence the validity of any meta-analysis that uses unadjusted results. Therefore, future studies on the

relationship between APOE 4 expression and the functional outcome of TBI should consider these important confounding factors. The age may also have an effect on the patients with neurodegeneration diseases. The risk between early-onset and late-onset neurodegeneration diseases maybe different. The patient with young onset neurodegeneration diseases more likely has a genetic or metabolic disease. However, neurodegeneration diseases are far more common in geriatric population, and researches in neurodegeneration disease are focused mainly on old persons. Therefore, it is hard to understand the association between age and neurodegeneration diseases in our study.

Conclusion

Patients with TBI frequently exhibit neurodegeneration. The symptoms of these neurodegenerative processes include behavioral disturbances, cognitive dysfunction, and/or motor-related symptoms. TBI is a potential risk factor only for subsequent dementia, TDP-43, and FTD, but not for AD, PD, or APOE-associated neurodegeneration. The epidemiology and pathology of this association have been difficult to establish. No suitable criteria define these neurodegenerative processes. However, the diagnosis of CTE may help to resolve this problem. Although the evidence suggested that TBI was a risk factor for neurodegeneration, there is limited information on the type, frequency, or amount of trauma that was necessary to induce the neurodegenerative processes. Therefore, further studies in this area are necessary to answer these questions and determine whether the proper management of TBI is effective in reducing the incidence of neurodegeneration.

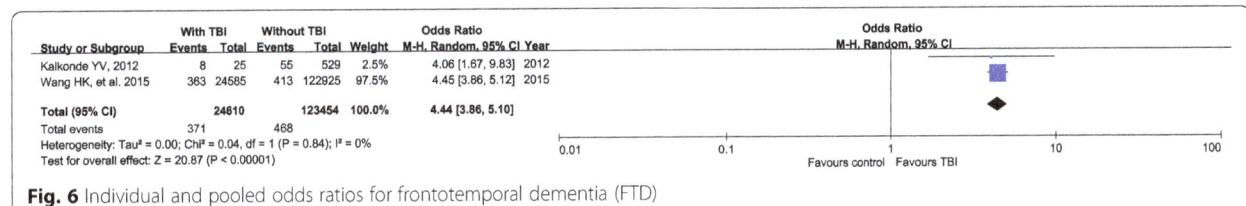

Study or Subgroup	With TBI Events	Total	Without TBI Events	Total	Weight	Odds Ratio M-H, Random, 95% CI	Year
Kalkonde YV, 2012	8	25	55	529	2.5%	4.06 [1.67, 9.83]	2012
Wang HK, et al. 2015	363	24585	413	122925	97.5%	4.45 [3.86, 5.12]	2015
Total (95% CI)		24610		123454	100.0%	4.44 [3.86, 5.10]	
Total events	371		468				

Heterogeneity: Tau² = 0.00; Chi² = 0.04, df = 1 (P = 0.84); I² = 0%
Test for overall effect: Z = 20.87 (P < 0.00001)

Fig. 6 Individual and pooled odds ratios for frontotemporal dementia (FTD)

Abbreviations

AD: Alzheimer disease; ALS: amyotrophic lateral sclerosis; APOE: apolipoprotein E; FTD: frontotemporal dementia (FTD); PD: Parkinson's disease; TBI: traumatic brain injury; TDP-43: transactive response DNA-binding protein of 43 kDa

Acknowledgements

This study was supported by Center for Database Research, E-DA HEALTH-CARE GROUP.

Funding

No funding was received.

Authors' contributions

CHH analyzed the data; CWL analyzed the data; YCL analyzed the data; CYH searched the papers; RYH analyzed the data; YCT examined the titles and abstracts of the studies found in the systematic literature search; KWW searched the papers and analyzed the data; SNY analyzed the data; YTS searched the papers; HKW examined the titles and abstracts of the studies found in the systematic literature search and was a major contributor in writing the manuscript. All authors read and approved the final manuscript.

Competing interests

The authors report no conflict of interest concerning the materials or methods used in this study or the findings specified in this paper.

Author details

[1]Department of Family Medicine, E-Da Hospital, I-Shou University, Kaohsiung, Taiwan. [2]School of Medicine for International Students, I-Shou University, Kaohsiung, Taiwan. [3]Department of Nephrology, E-Da Hospital, I-Shou University, Kaohsiung, Taiwan. [4]Neurosurgical Service, Department of Surgery, National Cheng Kung University Hospital, Tainan, Taiwan. [5]Department of Neurology, E-Da Hospital, I-Shou University, Kaohsiung, Taiwan. [6]Department of Neurosurgery, E-Da Hospital, I-Shou University, No.1, Yida Road, Jiaosu Village, Yanchao District, Kaohsiung City 82445, Taiwan. [7]Department of Neurology, National Cheng Kung University Hospital, College of Medicine, National Cheng Kung University, Tainan, Taiwan.

References

1. Ghajar J. Traumatic brain injury. Lancet. 2000;356(9233):923–9.
2. Risdall JE, Menon DK. Traumatic brain injury. Philos Trans R Soc Lond Ser B Biol Sci. 2011 Jan 27;366(1562):241–50.
3. Ramlackhansingh AF, Brooks DJ, Greenwood RJ, Bose SK, Turkheimer FE, Kinnunen KM, Gentleman S, Heckemann RA, Gunanayagam K, Gelosa G, Sharp DJ. Inflammation after trauma: microglial activation and traumatic brain injury. Ann Neurol. 2011 Sep;70(3):374–83.
4. Masel BE, DeWitt DS. Traumatic brain injury: a disease process, not an event. J Neurotrauma. 2010 Aug;27(8):1529–40. https://doi.org/10.1089/neu.2010.1358.
5. Wang HK, Lee YC, Huang CY, Liliang PC, Lu K, Chen HJ, Li YC, Tsai KJ. Traumatic brain injury causes frontotemporal dementia and TDP-43 proteolysis. Neuroscience. 2015 Aug 6;300:94–103.
6. Fleminger S, Oliver DL, Lovestone S, Rabe-Hesketh S, Giora A. Head injury as a risk factor for Alzheimer's disease: the evidence 10 years on; a partial replication. J Neurol Neurosurg Psychiatry. 2003;74(7):857–62.
7. Rugbjerg K, Ritz B, Korbo L, Martinussen N, Olsen JH. Risk of Parkinson's disease after hospital contact for head injury: population based case-control study. BMJ. 2008;337:a2494.
8. Schmidt S, Kwee LC, Allen KD, Oddone EZ. Association of ALS with head injury, cigarette smoking and APOE genotypes. J Neurol Sci. 2010;291:22e9.
9. Launer LJ, Andersen K, Dewey ME, et al. Rates and risk factors for dementia and Alzheimer's disease: results from EURODEM pooled analyses. EURODEM Incidence Research Group and Work Groups European Studies of Dementia. Neurology. 1999;52:78e84.
10. Fratiglioni L, Ahlbom A, Viitanen M, et al. Risk factors for late-onset Alzheimer's disease: a population-based, case-control study. Ann Neurol. 1993;33:258e66.
11. Williams DB, Annegers JF, Kokmen E, et al. Brain injury and neurologic sequelae: a cohort study of dementia, parkinsonism, and amyotrophic lateral sclerosis. Neurology. 1991;41:1554e7.
12. Levy G, Tang MX, Cote LJ, et al. Do risk factors for Alzheimer's disease predict dementia in Parkinson's disease? An exploratory study. Mov Disord. 2002;17:250e7.
13. Turner MR, Abisgold J, Yeates DG, et al. Head and other physical trauma requiring hospitalisation is not a significant risk factor in the development of ALS. J Neurol Sci. 2010;288:45e8.
14. Barthélemy EJ, Melis M, Gordon E, Ullman JS, Germano IM. Decompressive Craniectomy for severe traumatic brain injury: a systematic review. World Neurosurg. 2016 Apr;88:411–20.
15. Perry DC, Sturm VE, Peterson MJ, Pieper CF, Bullock T, Boeve BF, Miller BL, Guskiewicz KM, Berger MS, Kramer JH, Welsh-Bohmer KA. Association of traumatic brain injury with subsequent neurological and psychiatric disease: a meta-analysis. J Neurosurg. 2015;28:1–16.
16. Zhang BF, Wang J, Liu ZW, Zhao YL, Li DD, Huang TQ, Gu H, Song JN. Meta-analysis of the efficacy and safety of therapeutic hypothermia in children with acute traumatic brain injury. World Neurosurg. 2015;83(4):567–73.
17. Ferrari R, Kapogiannis D, Huey ED, Momeni P. FTD and ALS: a tale of two diseases. Curr Alzheimer Res. 2011;8(3):273–94.
18. Rapoport M, Wolf U, Herrmann N, Kiss A, Shammi P, Reis M, Phillips A, Feinstein A. Traumatic brain injury, apolipoprotein E-epsilon4, and cognition in older adults: a two-year longitudinal study. J Neuropsychiatry Clin Neurosci. 2008 Winter;20(1):68–73.
19. Tanner CM, Goldman SM, Ross GW, Grate SJ. The disease intersection of susceptibility and exposure: chemical exposures and neurodegenerative disease risk. Alzheimers Dement. 2014;10(3 Suppl):S213–25.
20. Mehta KM, Ott A, Kalmijn S, Slooter AJ, van Duijn CM, Hofman A, Breteler MM. Head trauma and risk of dementia and Alzheimer's disease: the Rotterdam study. Neurology. 1999;53(9):1959–62.
21. Luukinen H, Viramo P, Herala M, Kervinen K, Kesäniemi YA, Savola O, Winqvist S, Jokelainen J, Hillbom M. Fall-related brain injuries and the risk of dementia in elderly people: a population-based study. Eur J Neurol. 2005; 12(2):86–92.
22. Sundström A, Nilsson LG, Cruts M, Adolfsson R, Van Broeckhoven C, Nyberg L. Increased risk of dementia following mild head injury for carriers but not for non-carriers of the APOE epsilon4 allele. Int Psychogeriatr. 2007;19(1):159–65.
23. Luukinen H, Jokelainen J, Kervinen K, Kesäniemi YA, Winqvist S, Hillbom M. Risk of dementia associated with the ApoE epsilon4 allele and falls causing head injury without explicit traumatic brain injury. Acta Neurol Scand. 2008; 118(3):153–8.
24. Savica R, Parisi JE, Wold LE, Josephs KA, Ahlskog JE. High school football and risk of neurodegeneration: a community-based study. Mayo Clin Proc. 2012;87(4):335–40.
25. Wang HK, Lin SH, Sung PS, Wu MH, Hung KW, Wang LC, Huang CY, Lu K, Chen HJ, Tsai KJ. Population based study on patients with traumatic brain injury suggests increased risk of dementia. J Neurol Neurosurg Psychiatry. 2012;83(11):1080–5.
26. Gardner RC, Burke JF, Nettiksimmons J, Kaup A, Barnes DE, Yaffe K. Dementia risk after traumatic brain injury vs nonbrain trauma: the role of age and severity. JAMA Neurol. 2014;71(12):1490–7. https://doi.org/10.1001/jamaneurol.2014.2668.
27. Nordström P, Michaëlsson K, Gustafson Y, Nordström A. Traumatic brain injury and young onset dementia: a nationwide cohort study. Ann Neurol. 2014;75(3):374–81.
28. Abner EL, Nelson PT, Schmitt FA, Browning SR, Fardo DW, Wan L, Jicha GA, Cooper GE, Smith CD, Caban-Holt AM, Van Eldik LJ, Kryscio RJ. Self-reported head injury and risk of late-life impairment and AD pathology in an AD center cohort. Dement Geriatr Cogn Disord. 2014;37(5–6):294–306.
29. Rasmusson DX, Brandt J, Martin DB, Folstein MF. Head injury as a risk factor in Alzheimer's disease. Brain Inj. 1995;9(3):213–9.
30. Nemetz PN, Leibson C, Naessens JM, Beard M, Kokmen E, Annegers JF, Kurland LT. Traumatic brain injury and time to onset of Alzheimer's disease: a population-based study. Am J Epidemiol. 1999;149(1):32–40.
31. Barnes DE, Kaup A, Kirby KA, Byers AL, Diaz-Arrastia R, Yaffe K. Traumatic brain injury and risk of dementia in older veterans. Neurology. 2014;83(4): 312–9.
32. Spangenberg S, Hannerz H, Tüchsen F, Mikkelsen KL. A nationwide population study of severe head injury and Parkinson's disease. Parkinsonism Relat Disord. 2009;15(1):12–4.

33. Lee PC, Bordelon Y, Bronstein J, Ritz B. Traumatic brain injury, paraquat exposure, and their relationship to Parkinson disease. Neurology. 2012; 79(20):2061–6.
34. Taylor KM, Saint-Hilaire MH, Sudarsky L, Simon DK, Hersh B, Sparrow D, Hu H, Weisskopf MG. Head injury at early ages is associated with risk of Parkinson's disease. Parkinsonism Relat Disord. 2015.
35. Gardner RC, Burke JF, Nettiksimmons J, Goldman S, Tanner CM, Yaffe K. Traumatic brain injury in later life increases risk for Parkinson disease. Ann Neurol. 2015;77(6):987–95.
36. Kalkonde YV, Jawaid A, Qureshi SU, Shirani P, Wheaton M, Pinto-Patarroyo GP, Schulz PE. Medical and environmental risk factors associated with frontotemporal dementia: a case-control study in a veteran population. Alzheimers Dement. 2012;8(3):204–10.
37. Chen H, Richard M, Sandler DP, Umbach DM, Kamel F. Head injury and amyotrophic lateral sclerosis. Am J Epidemiol. 2007;166(7):810–6.
38. McKee AC, Gavett BE, Stern RA, Nowinski CJ, Cantu RC, Kowall NW, Perl DP, Hedley-Whyte ET, Price B, Sullivan C, Morin P, Lee HS, Kubilus CA, Daneshvar DH, Wulff M, Budson AE. TDP-43 proteinopathy and motor neuron disease in chronic traumatic encephalopathy. J Neuropathol Exp Neurol. 2010;69(9): 918–29.
39. Daneshvar DH, Goldstein LE, Kiernan PT, Stein TD, McKee AC. Post-traumatic neurodegeneration and chronic traumatic encephalopathy. Mol Cell Neurosci. 2015;66(Pt B):81–90.
40. Washington PM, Villapol S, Burns MP. Polypathology and dementia after brain trauma: does brain injury trigger distinct neurodegenerative diseases, or should they be classified together as traumatic encephalopathy? Exp Neurol. 2016;275(Pt 3):381–8.
41. Perrine K, Helcer J, Tsiouris AJ, Pisapia DJ, Stieg P. The Current Status of Research on Chronic Traumatic Encephalopathy. World Neurosurg. 2017.
42. Ojo JO, Mouzon BC, Crawford F. Repetitive head trauma, chronic traumatic encephalopathy and tau: challenges in translating from mice to men. Exp Neurol. 2016 Jan;275(Pt 3):389–404.

25

A phase 3, long-term, open-label safety study of Galcanezumab in patients with migraine

Angelo Camporeale[1], David Kudrow[2,3], Ryan Sides[4], Shufang Wang[4], Annelies Van Dycke[5], Katherine J. Selzler[4] and Virginia L. Stauffer[4*]

Abstract

Background: Galcanezumab, a humanized monoclonal antibody that selectively binds to the calcitonin gene-related peptide, has demonstrated in previous Phase 2 and Phase 3 clinical studies (≤6-month of treatment) a reduction in the number of migraine headache days and improved patients' functioning. This study evaluated the safety and tolerability, as well as the effectiveness of galcanezumab for up to 12 months of treatment in patients with migraine.

Methods: Patients diagnosed with episodic or chronic migraine, 18 to 65 years old, that were not exposed previously to galcanezumab, were randomized to receive galcanezumab 120 mg or 240 mg, administered subcutaneously once monthly for a year. Safety and tolerability were evaluated by frequency of treatment-emergent adverse events (TEAEs), serious adverse events (SAEs), and adverse events (AEs) leading to study discontinuation. Laboratory values, vital signs, electrocardiograms, and suicidality were also analyzed. Additionally, overall change from baseline in the number of monthly migraine headache days, functioning, and disability were assessed.

Results: One hundred thirty five patients were randomized to each galcanezumab dose group. The majority of patients were female (> 80%) and on average were 42 years old with 10.6 migraine headache days per month at baseline. 77.8% of the patients completed the open-label treatment phase, 3.7% of patients experienced an SAE, and 4.8% discontinued due to AEs. TEAEs with a frequency ≥ 10% of patients in either dose group were injection site pain, nasopharyngitis, upper respiratory tract infection, injection site reaction, back pain, and sinusitis. Laboratory values, vital signs, or electrocardiograms did not show anyclinically meaningful differences between galcanezumab dosesOverall mean reduction in monthly migraine headache days over 12 months for the galcanezumab dose groups were 5.6 (120 mg) and 6.5 (240 mg). Level of functioning was improved and headache-related disability was reduced in both dose groups.

Conclusion: Twelve months of treatment with self-administered injections of galcanezumab was safe and associated with a reduction in the number of monthly migraine headache days. Safety and tolerability of the 2 galcanezumab dosing regimens were comparable.

Trial registration: ClinicalTrials.gov as NCT02614287, posted November 15, 2015. These data were previously presented as a poster at the International Headache Congress 2017: PO-01-184, Late-Breaking Abstracts of the 2017 International Headache Congress. (2017). Cephalalgia, 37(1_suppl), 319–374.

Keywords: Migraine, Headache, Galcanezumab, CGRP

---

* Correspondence: vstauffer@lilly.com
[4]Eli Lilly and Company Corporate Center, Indianapolis, IN 46285, USA
Full list of author information is available at the end of the article

Background

In the 2015 Global Burden of Disease study, migraine was reported to be 1 of 8 chronic diseases affecting more than 10% of the world population [1], with higher prevalence among women (17%) than men (6%) [2]. Patients with migraine also have higher lifetime rates of depression, anxiety, panic disorder, sleep disturbances, chronic pain syndromes, musculoskeletal symptoms, ischemic stroke (migraine with aura), and suicide attempts [3–9]. Despite its prevalence, migraine continues to be underdiagnosed and undertreated.

Migraine-specific medications, such as triptans and ergotamines, as well as nonsteroidal anti-inflammatory drugs, are taken acutely to abort the migraine attack. However, for patients with frequent migraine attacks, and for whom abortive treatments are inadequately effective, preventive therapies are recommended [10–12]. It is estimated that approximately 39% of migraine patients would benefit from preventive pharmacotherapy to reduce the frequency of migraine attacks [2], which includes the ability to function at work and school, and interferes with family and social interactions [13].

For patients with chronic migraine, there are two preventive treatments considered as standard of care, onabotulinumtoxinA and topiramate, which are the most frequently prescribed medications for chronic migraine [14, 15]. In the US and Europe the use of beta blockers, calcium channel blockers, anticonvulsants, nonsteroidal anti-inflammatory drugs, and antidepressants as migraine preventive medications are proposed [10, 16, 17]. Although all of these medications are considered preventive treatment for episodic or chronic migraine, none of them were developed specifically to treat migraine, and some are not well tolerated [18].

During migraine attacks, serum concentrations of calcitonin gene-related peptide (CGRP) are significantly elevated in the external jugular vein [19, 20], implicating CGRP in the pathophysiology of migraine. Galcanezumab is a humanized monoclonal antibody that potently and selectively binds to CGRP without blocking the receptor, preventing CGRP-mediated biological effects [21]. In two 12-week Phase 2 [22, 23] and two 6-month Phase 3 [24] clinical studies of patients with episodic migraine, galcanezumab significantly reduced monthly migraine headache days (MHD) compared to placebo. The purpose of this study was to investigate the long-term safety, tolerability, and effectiveness of galcanezumab treatment in patients with migraine.

Methods

This study was a Phase 3, multicenter, randomized, long-term, open-label study to assess the safety of two dosing regimens of galcanezumab, 120 mg/month (with initial loading dose of 240 mg) and 240 mg/month, for the treatment of episodic or chronic migraine. The study protocol was reviewed and approved by appropriate institutional review boards and was conducted according to Good Clinical Practice and the Declaration of Helsinki. Patients provided written informed consent before initiating study procedures. Enrollment began in December 2015 and the last patient completed the study (treatment phase and post-treatment phase) in September 2017. There were 28 clinical sites across 5 countries (United States, Canada, Hungary, Belgium, and France) that participated in the study.

Patient selection

Eligibility for study enrollment was based on the results of migraine history, physical examination, neurological examination, clinical laboratory tests and electrocardiograms (ECGs). Key inclusion criteria were: 18–65 years of age; diagnosis of migraine as defined by the International Headache Society (IHS) International Classification of Headache Disorders (ICHD)-3 beta version [25] a history of at least 1 year of migraine headaches; migraine onset prior to age 50 years; prior to study entry, a history of 4 or more MHD per month on average for the past 3 months and a history of at least 1 headache-free day per month for the past 3 months. Key exclusion criteria were: prior exposure to galcanezumab (or any other CGRP antibody); use of any therapeutic antibody in the past 12 months; current treatment with preventive migraine medication; history of failure to respond to three or more classes of migraine preventive treatments (as defined by the American Academy of Neurology treatment guidelines Level A or Level B evidence [16]); presence of a medical condition that would preclude study participation, including pregnancy, presence of suicidal ideation within the past month, history of substance abuse or dependence in the past year, or recent history of acute cardiovascular events and/or serious cardiovascular risk based on history or ECG findings. Patients were allowed to take acute medications (except opiod and barbituates more than three times per month) for the treatment of migraine during the study, including triptans, ergots, nonsteroidal anti-inflammatory drugs and acetaminophen.

Objectives

The primary objective was to evaluate the long-term safety and tolerability of galcanezumab (120 and 240 mg/month) for up to 1 year of treatment. Assessments included serious adverse events (SAEs), treatment-emergent adverse events (TEAEs), discontinuation rates, vital signs and weight, ECGs, laboratory measures, suicidal ideation and behavior using the Columbia Suicide Severity Rating Scale (C-SSRS) [26], and incidence of treatment-emergent anti-drug antibodies (TE-ADA).

Secondary objectives included the evaluation of efficacy measures to fully assess the longer-term effectiveness of galcanezumab in the prevention of migraine. The evaluation included overall change from baseline in the number of monthly MHD, headache days, responder analysis of ≥30%, ≥50%, ≥75, and 100% reduction in MHD, the percentage of patients who maintained a monthly MHD response, and change from baseline in the number of days acute treatment is taken for migraine or headache. Additional efficacy measures included patient-rated impression of illness improvement, change from baseline in functioning assessed by the Migraine-Specific Quality of Life questionnaire (MSQ) [27] and change from baseline in headache-related disability assessed by the Migraine Disability Assessment (MIDAS) scale [28, 29].

The number of MHD and headache days were reported by patients for the month prior to the study visit. Response rates were based on the reduction in number of MHD reported monthly and overall. Maintenance of response was a post-hoc assessment of patients meeting ≥50% response at any month and subsequently maintaining ≥40% response for at least two months or until the patient's endpoint. This maintenance of response could range from ≥3 months to 12 consecutive months (including initial month of response).

Clinical assessments

The C-SSRS evaluates the occurrence, severity, and frequency of suicide-related thoughts and behaviors during the assessment period. The scale includes suggested questions to solicit the type of information needed to determine if a suicide-related thought or behavior occurred [26].

The Patient Global Impression of Improvement (PGI-I) scale [30] is a patient-rated instrument that measures the improvement of the patient's symptoms. It is a 7-point scale in which a score of 1 indicates that the patient is "very much better," a score of 4 indicates that the patient has experienced "no change," and a score of 7 indicates that the patient is "very much worse."

The MSQ (v2.1) is a self-administered health status instrument that was developed to address physical and emotional limitations of specific concern to individuals suffering from migraine headaches. The instrument consists of 14 items that addresses 3 domains: (1) Role Function-Restrictive (RF-R), (2) Role Function-Preventive, and (3) Emotional Function [27]. The instrument was designed with a 4-week recall period and is considered reliable, valid, and sensitive to change in migraine [27, 31] with a 0 to 100 scale, with higher scores indicating a better health status.

The MIDAS was designed to quantify headache-related disability, recalled over a 3-month period. This instrument consists of five items that reflect the number of days

reported as missing or with reduced productivity at work, home, or social events. The items are weighted in the final scores, with a higher value indicating greater disability [28, 29]. This instrument is considered highly reliable, valid, and is correlated with clinical judgment regarding the need for medical care [28, 29].

Study design

The study was comprised of 3 study periods. Study Period 1 included initial screening procedures and washout of all migraine preventive treatments (3–45 days). In Study Period 2 (open-label treatment period), patients were randomized to treatment with one of two dosing regimens of galcanezumab (120 mg or 240 mg) that were administered subcutaneously once monthly for a total of 12 doses. Patients randomized to galcanezumab 120 mg received an initial loading dose of 240 mg (two injections of 120 mg each), and all subsequent doses were self- or caregiver-administered as a single injection of 120 mg monthly. Those randomized to galcanezumab 240 mg received two injections of 120 mg at each monthly dosing visit. Across the study, there were office visits at Months 1–3, 6, 9, and 12; Months 4, 5, 7, 8, 10, and 11 were telephone visits. Injections were delivered by prefilled syringe or by an investigational autoinjector. Each patient or caregiver received training on the use of the prefilled syringe and autoinjector. Patients were to keep track of their headaches, both migraine and non-migraine, experienced in the past 30 days, as well as the use of medication taken for the acute treatment of a migraine and non-migraine headache. Patients were required to report a migraine headache, headache or use of an acute medication for migraine or headache on a daily basis with a diary or log of their choice, and the daily log was reviewed at each monthly visit and documented in the case report form. Study Period 3 was a 4-month post-treatment period (washout phase), during which patients no longer received study medication, but continued to track headache information and received safety assessments. Patients who discontinued early from the treatment period could enter the post-treatment phase.

Statistical analysis

Safety and effectiveness analyses were conducted on an intent-to-treat (ITT) basis, which included all randomized patients who received at least one dose of study drug. Change from baseline included only those patients who had a baseline and at least one post-baseline assessment.

Continuous variables without repeated measures were analyzed as change from baseline to the last observation carried forward (LOCF) endpoint. Continuous safety and efficacy variables with repeated measures were analyzed using mixed-model repeated measures (MMRM), which included the fixed categorical effects of treatment,

treatment-by-visit interaction, visit, as well as the continuous fixed covariates of baseline and baseline-by-visit interaction. In addition, pooled investigative site was also included in the efficacy analyses.

Categorical variables with repeated measures were summarized and analyzed in a similar manner as mean changes by a categorical, pseudo likelihood-based repeated measures analysis using a generalized linear mixed model (GLIMMIX) procedure in SAS (SAS Enterprise Guide 7.1). Categorical variables without repeated measures were analyzed by Fisher's exact test controlling for pooled investigative site.

The incidence of TE-ADA for each treatment group during the treatment period was summarized. Treatment-emergent ADA positive was defined as a 'not present' baseline ADA result and at least one 'present' post-baseline ADA result with a titer ≥1:20, or a 'present' baseline ADA result and a 'present' post-baseline ADA result with a ≥ 4-fold increase in titer (i.e., baseline titer of 1:10 increasing to ≥1:40 post-baseline).

All statistical tests were conducted at a 2-sided alpha level of 0.05. No adjustments for multiplicity were applied to any safety or effectiveness analyses.

Results

There were 341 patients screened for the study, of whom 270 patients enrolled. Overall completion rate for the treatment phase (Study Period 2) was 77.8% ($N = 210$) (Fig. 1) with a total of 60 patients (22.2%) who discontinued the treatment phase (Study Period 2). There were

236 patients (including some patients who discontinued treatment) who continued into the post-treatment phase (Study Period 3), and of these, 222 patients (94.1%) completed all 4 months.

Baseline demographics and clinical characteristics were similar between the dose groups, except for a statistically significant difference between dose groups in the mean number of MHD and age (Table 1). Patients enrolled in this study were 42 years of age on average, majority were female (83%) with a predominant diagnosis of episodic migraine (79%), and an average of 10.6 monthly MHD. Patients were diagnosed with migraine an average of 20.7 years prior to study enrollment, and a majority of patients (63%) reported prior use migraine preventive treatment, and 18.5% of the patients had one or more cardiovascular disease risk. The most common comorbid conditions (≥10%) were depression (16.7%), seasonal allergy (16.7%), drug hypersensitivity (15.6%), back pain (14.4%), insomnia (14.4%), anxiety (11.5%), and gastroesophageal reflux disease (10.4%). The mean MIDAS total score of 50% indicated very severe headache-related disability [32] and function was restricted, as indicated by the average MSQ RF-R score of 48.

The mean duration of exposure to galcanezumab was 318.5 days and 310.3 days in the 120 mg and 240 mg dose groups, respectively. Of the patients who discontinued the treatment period early, significantly more patients in the galcanezumab 120 mg dose group discontinued compared to the galcanezumab 240 mg dose group ($P = .028$). There were 4 patients who missed an injection at a home dosing

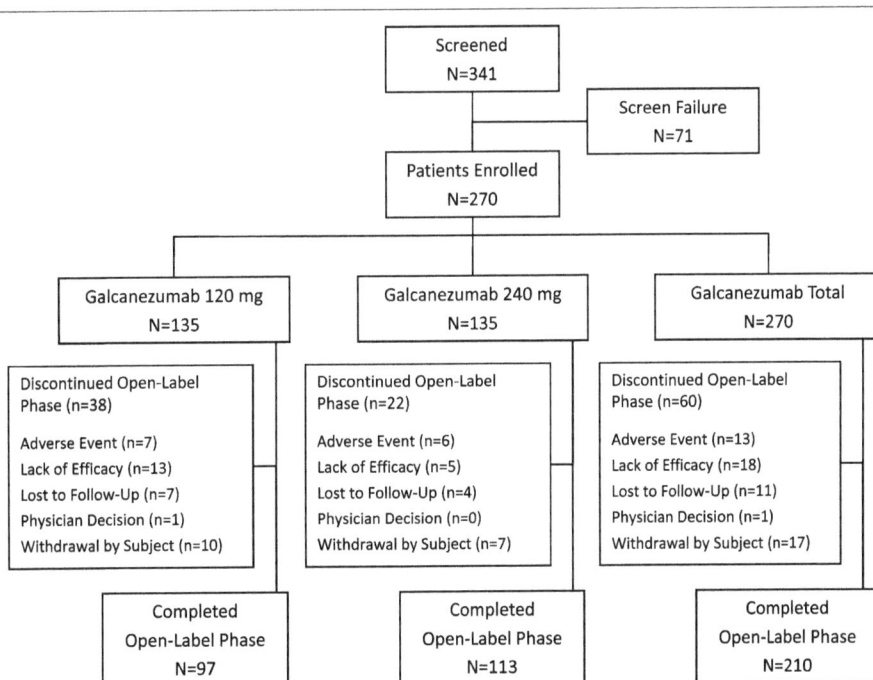

Fig. 1 Patient cohort diagram through the treatment phase of the study

Table 1 Demographics and Clinical Characteristics

	Galcanezumab 120 mg N = 135	Galcanezumab 240 mg N = 135
Age in years, mean (SD)	40.2 (11.7)	43.7 (11.0)*
Female, n (%)	110 (81.5)	113 (83.7)
Body mass index, kg/m², mean (SD)	26.6 (5.4)	27.2 (5.8)
Race, n (%)		
Asian	2 (1.5)	0
Black	6 (4.4)	8 (5.9)
Multiple	23 (17.0)	19 (14.1)
White	103 (76.3)	108 (80.0)
Episodic migraine, n (%)	109 (80.7)	104 (77.0)
Cardiovascular Disease Risk Group, n (%)[a]	22 (17.1)	28 (19.9)
Comorbid conditions, mean (SD)[b]	4.3 (3.2)	4.7 (3.4)
Depression	19 (14.1)	26 (19.3)
Seasonal Allergy	24 (17.8)	21 (15.6)
Drug hypersensitivity	21 (15.6)	21 (15.6)
Back pain	18 (13.3)	21 (15.6)
Insomnia	19 (14.1)	20 (14.8)
Anxiety	15 (11.1)	16 (11.9)
Gastroesophageal reflux disease	12 (8.9)	16 (11.9)
Years since diagnosis, mean (SD)	20.2 (12.4)	21.3 (12.5)
Number of migraine headache days, mean (SD)	9.7 (5.8)	11.4 (6.7)*
Number of headache days, mean (SD)	5.0 (6.8)	6.1 (8.1)
Number of days with acute migraine medication use, mean (SD)	9.8 (6.6)	10.9 (7.2)
Prior preventive treatment, n (%)	81 (60.0)	88 (65.2)
Patient Global Impression - Severity, mean (SD)	4.7 (1.2)	4.7 (1.2)
Migraine Disability Assessment total, mean (SD)	45.8 (42.1)	54.0 (61.2)
Migraine-Specific Questionnaire Role Function-Restrictive domain score, mean (SD)	47.4 (19.2)	47.7 (18.4)

SD standard deviation

[a]Patients with a history or pre-existing condition listed in any of the following MedDRA Standardized Queries: Ischaemic Heart Disease, Hypertension, Cardiac Failure, Cardiomyopathy, Ischaemic CNS Vascular Conditions, Dyslipidaemia, Hyperglycaemia/New Onset Diabetes Mellitus

[b]Most common comorbid conditions (≥10%) are reported. *P < .05

visit, but they did complete the treatment phase, and the mean treatment compliance in this study was 95.8 and 96.9% in the galcanezumab 120 mg and 240 mg dose groups, respectively. There was no between-dose group difference in the percentage of patients who discontinued due to an adverse event (AE) (4.7% vs. 5.0% for galcanezumab 120 mg vs. 240 mg, respectively). In the galcanezumab 120 mg dose group, 2 patients discontinued due to

injection site reaction, and 1 patient each discontinued due to injection site erythema, lethargy, migraine, and suicidal ideation. In the galcanezumab 240 mg dose group, 2 patients discontinued due to injection site reaction, and 1 patient each discontinued due to non-cardiac chest pain, paranoia, rash, tongue discomfort, and vertigo.

All of the 5 patients who discontinued due to an injection site-related TEAE had previous AEs at the injection site prior to discontinuation. Of these 5 patients, 4 patients discontinued after 6 or more self-administration dosing visits. One patient who had a severe injection site reaction discontinued after the tenth dosing visit due to progressive swelling around the site of the injection, with rash and pain that progressed from the previous injection that lasted a few days.

Ten patients reported SAEs, with 3 patients receiving galcanezumab 120 mg and 7 patients receiving galcanezumab 240 mg. Lumbar radiculopathy, migraine, and osteoarthritis occurred in the galcanezumab 120 mg dose group, while uterine leiomyoma embolization, cholecystitis, diverticulum intestinal, intervertebral disc protrusion, non-cardiac chest pain, pain in extremity and pneumonia occurred in the 240 mg dose group. The events of non-cardiac chest pain and migraine led to discontinuation. None of these events was reported by the study investigator to be associated with galcanezumab treatment.

Treatment-emergent AEs that occurred with ≥5% frequency in either dose group are summarized in Table 2.

Table 2 Treatment-emergent adverse events with a ≥ 5% frequency of occurrence in either galcanezumab dose group

Event	Galcanezumab 120 mg N = 129 n (%)	Galcanezumab 240 mg N = 141 n (%)
Patient with ≥1 TEAE	106 (82.2)	121 (85.8)
Injection site pain	22 (17.1)	28 (19.9)
Nasopharyngitis	23 (17.8)	18 (12.8)
Upper respiratory tract infection	9 (7.0)	21 (14.9)
Injection site reaction	15 (11.6)	13 (9.2)
Back pain	12 (9.3)	15 (10.6)
Sinusitis	14 (10.9)	13 (9.2)
Nausea	10 (7.8)	9 (6.4)
Injections site erythema	9 (7.0)	9 (6.4)
Arthralgia	8 (6.2)	8 (5.7)
Influenza	8 (6.2)	8 (5.7)
Dizziness	5 (3.9)	9 (6.4)
Injection site bruising	5 (3.9)	8 (5.7)
Myalgia	8 (6.2)	3 (2.1)
Weight increased	7 (5.4)	4 (2.8)

TEAE treatment-emergent adverse events

There were no statistically significant differences between dose groups in frequency of events

There were no significant differences between dose groups in the frequency of any of these events; however, there was a higher percentage of upper respiratory tract infection events in the galcanezumab 240 mg dose group (14.9%) compared with 120 mg group (7.0%). Most of the TEAEs were reported as mild-to-moderate in severity and there were no deaths. Across both dose groups, the most common (≥10% frequency) events were injection site pain, nasopharyngitis, upper respiratory tract infection, injection site reaction, back pain, and sinusitis. In addition, injection site bruising, injection site hematoma, injection site pruritus, and injection site induration were reported in > 2% in both galcanezumab dose groups combined. There were no SAEs related to injection sites.

There were no clinically meaningful differences in laboratory parameters for either galcanezumab dose or between doses. No TEAE related to a laboratory analyte was reported as an SAE and none led to discontinuation. Elevated liver enzymes (as measured by alanine aminotransferase [ALT] or aspartate aminotransferase [AST] ≥3X upper limit of normal [ULN]; or alkaline phosphatase [ALP] ≥2X ULN; or total bilirubin level [TBL] ≥2X ULN at any time) were reported as TEAEs by 4 patients (galcanezumab 120 mg $N = 3$; galcanezumab 240 mg $N = 1$) and these elevations were not persistent.

Systolic blood pressure mean changes from baseline to each month ranged from − 1.45 to + 0.43 mmHg in the galcanezumab 120 mg group, and from − 1.65 to − 0.27 mmHg in the galcanezumab 240 mg group. Diastolic blood pressure mean changes from baseline to each month ranged from − 0.88 to + 0.87 mmHg in the galcanezumab 120 mg group, and from − 0.81 to + 0.23 mmHg in the galcanezumab 240 mg group. There were statistically significant, but not clinically important, mean increases from baseline in pulse at Months 1, 2, 3, and 9 that were of similar magnitude across both dose groups (range: 2.0 to 3.7 bpm; $P < .01$).

Few patients met criteria for treatment-emergent low systolic blood pressure, diastolic blood pressure, or pulse at any time (Table 3). There were no significant differences between galcanezumab dose groups in the frequencies of patients with treatment-emergent high systolic blood pressure or pulse at any time. There was a statistically significant increase in frequency of treatment-emergent high diastolic blood pressure in the galcanezumab 240 mg dose group compared to the 120 mg dose group ($P = .046$). Four patients had a sustained elevation in diastolic blood pressure (2 patients in each dose group), of whom 2 patients (1 in each dose group) had sustained elevation in systolic blood pressure. However, these were not sustained beyond 2 consecutive visits. A review of the patient-level data revealed that the increased blood pressure findings were transient, isolated events and likely represented

Table 3 Treatment-emergent changes in blood pressure and pulse

Category	Galcanezumab 120 mg		Galcanezumab 240 mg	
	N	n (%)	N	n (%)
Elevated BP and pulse				
Sitting SBP ≥140 mmHg and ≥ 20 mmHg increase from baseline	120	5 (4.2)	124	4 (3.2)
Sitting DBP ≥90 mmHg and ≥ 10 mmHg increase from baseline	116	6 (5.2)	126	16 (12.7)*
Sitting pulse > 100 bpm and ≥ 15 bpm increase from baseline	129	3 (2.3)	139	5 (3.6)
Sustained elevation at 2 consecutive visits				
Sitting SBP	119	1 (0.8)	119	1 (0.8)
Sitting DBP	115	2 (1.7)	121	2 (1.7)
Sitting pulse	128	0	133	3 (2.3)
Potentially clinically significant elevation at anytime				
Sitting SBP ≥180 mmHg and ≥ 20 mmHg increase from baseline	129	0	139	0
Sitting DBP ≥105 mmHg and ≥ 15 mmHg increase from baseline	129	1 (0.8)	138	1 (0.7)

BP blood pressure, *DBP* diastolic blood pressure, *SBP* systolic blood pressure
*$P < .05$

normal variation in blood pressure. Three of these patients did have a TEAE of hypertension. Two patients with high diastolic blood pressure (1 in each dose group) also met the criteria for potentially clinically significant elevations at any time (Table 3).

Across the 12 months of treatment, the mean changes from baseline to LOCF endpoint in weight were small for both galcanezumab dose groups (≤1 kg). Thirteen patients in the galcanezuamb 120 mg dose group and 12 patients in the 240 mg dose group had treatment-emergent weight loss ≥7%; whereas, 17 patients in the 120 mg dose group and 21 patients in the 240 mg dose group had treatment-emergent weight gain ≥7%. Given that the observed categorical weight changes occurred in both directions (weight loss and weight gain), there does not appear to be a clear impact of galcanezumab on weight.

There was a statistically significant mean increase from baseline in temperature of 0.2° F observed in each dose group at a single month (Month 1 for galcanezumab 120 mg [$P < .01$], Month 9 for galcanezumab 240 mg [$P < .05$]). A total of 10 patients overall experienced treatment emergent changes in body temperature. Five patients in the galcanezumab 120 mg dose group and 4 patients in the 240 mg dose group had low body temperatures (<96° F and a decrease of ≥2° F), and 1 patient in the 120 mg group had ≥101 °F and an increase of ≥2° F. Since these changes were temporary and small, they were not considered clinically meaningful.

The percentage of patients with treatment-emergent abnormal changes from baseline in ECG measures were < 5% (Table 4). However, neither galcanezumab dose groups resulted in ECG changes or serious cardiovascular events of concern. There were no discontinuations due to treatment-emergent ECG findings.

Four patients experienced treatment-emergent suicidal ideation based on assessment with the C-SSRS. One of these patients (galcanezumab 120 mg dose) had a history of depression and was discontinued from the study after reporting suicidal ideation. The other 3 patients (galcanezumab 120 mg $N = 2$; 240 mg $N = 1$) had no prior lifetime history of suicidal ideation and continued in the study with no recurrence of suicidal ideation on the C-SSRS. None of the patients had emergence of suicidal behavior during treatment.

Anti-drug antibodies (ADA) were present at baseline in 8 (6.3%) out of 128 patients evaluable for TE-ADA in the galcanezumab 120 mg dose group, and in 12 out of 136 (8.8%) patients in the 240 mg dose group. Patients who developed TE-ADA included 16 (12.4%) patients in the 120 mg dose group and 10 (7.3%) patients in the 240 mg dose group. All of the patients who had TE-ADA also had neutralizing antibodies and the titers were generally low during this phase; the majority of the patients had maximum titers of 1:80 or below. Neutralizing ADA recognize the target-binding sites on galcanezumab and compete with binding to CGRP in vitro; an observable clinical effect requires sufficiently high titers of neutralizing ADA to effectively reduce the activity of galcanezumab in vivo.

Analysis of efficacy measures was a secondary objective in this study. Unless otherwise noted, the difference between galcanezumab 120 mg and 240 mg dose groups was not statistically significant on any efficacy measure.

Compared to baseline, the overall reduction in the number of monthly MHD was 5.6 (95% CI: -6.3, – 5.0) and 6.5 (95% CI: -7.1, – 5.8) for patients treated with galcanezumab 120 mg and 240 mg, respectively (Table 5). Reduction in the mean monthly MHD was apparent as early as the first month and was sustained throughout the treatment period (Fig. 2).

The overall mean reduction from baseline in the number of monthly non-migraine headache days averaged over 12 months was 2.2 and 2.1 in the galcanezumab 120 mg and 240 mg dose groups, respectively (Table 5).

In both galcanezumab dose groups, there were statistically significant within-group reductions from baseline in the number of monthly MHD or headaches with acute medication use at each month ($P < .001$). The overall mean reduction from baseline in number of monthly days with acute medication use for migraines or headaches was 5.1 in both dose groups (Table 5).

Response rate was defined as the mean percentage of patients meeting a pre-specified threshold in the reduction of the number of monthly MHD over Months 1 to 12. The overall response rates at each pre-specified threshold are summarized in Table 5. In each response category, there were more months where patients met that level of response in the galcanezumab 240 mg dose group compared to the galcanezumab 120 mg dose group. Of those patients who had at least a 50% reduction from baseline in the number of monthly MHD, the percentage who continued to maintain at least a 40% reduction over 3 to 12 consecutive months is shown in Fig. 3. In the galcanezumab 120 mg group, maintenance of response ranged from 48.5% (≥6 consecutive months) to 24.2% (up to 12 consecutive months), and in the

Table 4 Change from baseline in electrocardiogram categorical measures

Category	Post Baseline	Galcanezumab 120 mg		Galcanezumab 240 mg	
		N	n (%)	N	n (%)
Heart rate	< 50 bpm and decrease ≥15	117	1 (0.85)	131	1 (0.76)
	> 100 bpm and increase ≥15	119	1 (0.84)	131	0
PR interval	< 120 msec	117	3 (2.56)	127	1 (0.79)
	≥ 220 msec	119	0	130	0
QRS interval	< 60 msec	120	0	131	0
	≥120 msec	118	0	131	1 (0.76)
QTcF	< 330 msec for males, < 340 msec for females	118	0	130	0
	> 450 msec for males; > 470 msec for females	118	2 (1.69)	130	1 (0.77)
	Potentially clinically significant:				
	> 500 msec	118	0	130	0
	Increase > 30 msec	118	2 (1.69)	130	4 (3.08)
	Increase > 60 msec	118	0	130	0

bpm beats per minute, *PR* pulse rate, *QTcF* QT interval adjusted for heart rate using Fridericia's correction

Table 5 Overall change in monthly MHD, non-migraine headache days, and percentage reduction in monthly MHD

	Galcanezumab 120 mg N = 135	Galcanezumab 240 mg N = 135
Overall change from baseline in number of monthly MHD, mean (SD)	−5.6 (0.34)	−6.5 (0.33)
Overall change from baseline in monthly non-migraine headache days, mean (SD)	−2.2 (0.3)	−2.1 (0.3)
Overall change from baseline in number of days with acute medication use, mean (SD)	−5.1 (0.4)	−5.1 (0.4)
Percentage of patients who had ≥30% reduction in MHD	76.1%	80.9%
Percentage of patients who had ≥50% reduction in MHD	65.6%	73.7%
Percentage of patients who had ≥75% reduction in MHD	44.5%	52.5%
Percentage of patients who had 100% reduction in MHD	21.4%	21.8%

MHD migraine headache days, SD standard deviation

240 mg group, maintenance of response ranged from 51.9% (≥6 consecutive months) to 34.8% (up to 12 consecutive months).

Results from the Patient Global Impression of Improvement scale (PGI-I) is summarized in Table 6. In the galcanezumab 120 mg dose group 90 patients completed the PGI-I, and 80% of patients reported that they were "much or very much better" and 4% reported "no change" or "a little worse". In the galcanezumab 240 mg dose group 112 patients completed the PGI-I, and 85% of patients reported that they were "much or very much better" and 8% reported "no change" or "a little worse". There were no patients in either dose group who reported they were "much or very much worse".

Patients in both galcanezumab dose groups had improved functioning, as assessed by the MSQ RF-R domain, with increases from baseline in least squares (LS) mean scores of 31.6 and 33.4 for the 120 mg and 240 mg dose

groups, respectively. Additionally, both galcanezumab dose groups had reduced headache-related disability, as assessed by the MIDAS total score, with LS mean reductions from baseline of − 33.6 and − 32.7 for the 120 mg and 240 mg dose groups, respectively.

Discussion

In this 12-month open-label study of once monthly subcutaneous injections of galcanezumab 120 mg and 240 mg as a preventive treatment for migraine, the safety and effectiveness profile observed was consistent with previous studies: two Phase 2 studies [22, 23], and two Phase 3 studies in patients with episodic migraine [24], and one Phase 3 study in patients with chronic migraine [33].

Tolerability to galcanezumab was demonstrated by the overall high study completion rate, which was 77.8% through all 12 months of treatment. In patients who completed the study, treatment compliance was > 95%

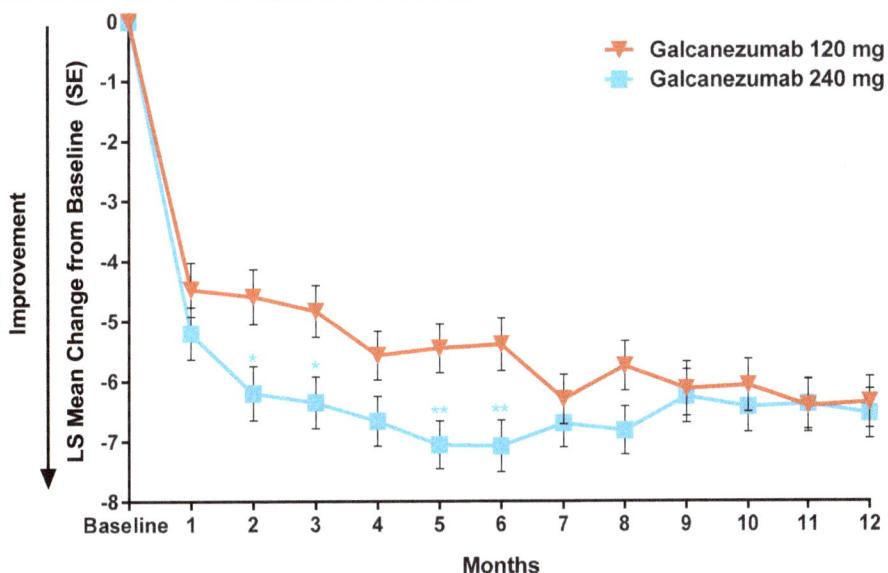

Fig. 2 Overall mean change from baseline in the number of monthly migraine headache days. *P < .05; **P < .01. Overall least squares (LS) mean change from baseline in the number of migraine headache days for patients who were treated with monthly open-label injections of galcanezumab 120 mg or 240 mg

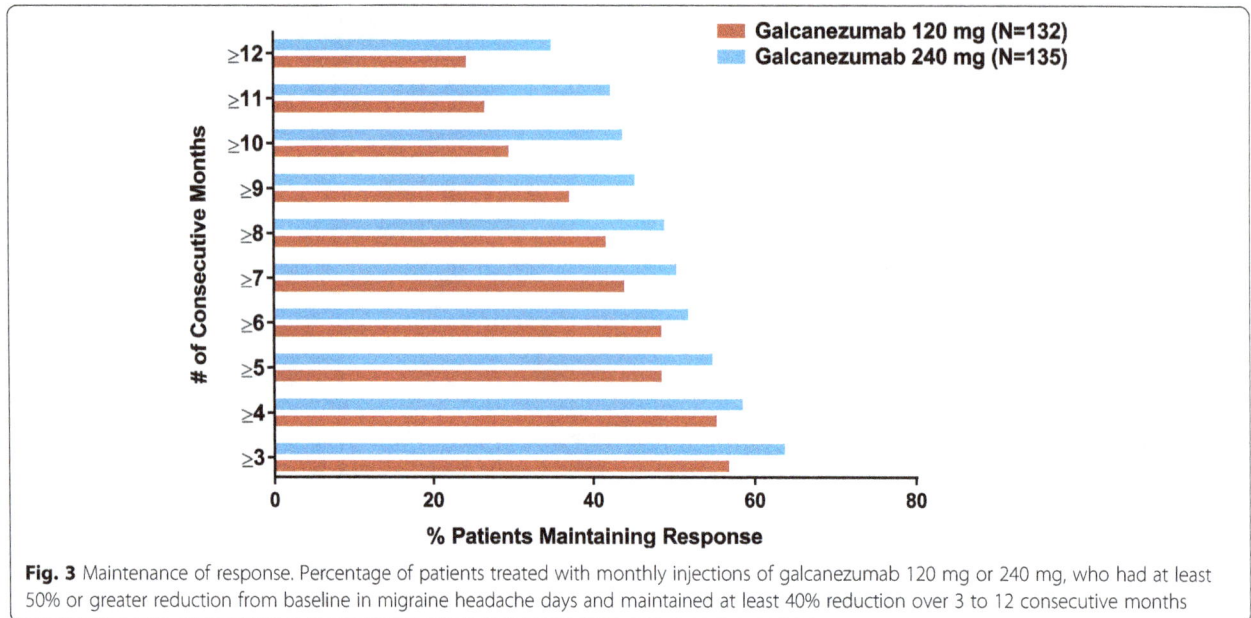

Fig. 3 Maintenance of response. Percentage of patients treated with monthly injections of galcanezumab 120 mg or 240 mg, who had at least 50% or greater reduction from baseline in migraine headache days and maintained at least 40% reduction over 3 to 12 consecutive months

and included at least half of the study visits being self-administered injections at home. Furthermore, the percentage of discontinuations due to AEs was low (< 5% combined doses), and few SAEs occurred (< 4% combined doses, and none considered related to treatment). This is in contrast to long-term treatment with topiramate, which is currently the most prescribed preventive migraine medication, which showed higher rates of study discontinuation and discontinuation due to adverse events [34, 35].

In this study, where patients or caregivers administered subcutaneous injections of galcanezumab, AEs of particular interest were those associated with the injection site. Approximately one-third of the patients experienced an injection site AE, the reason for which 5 patients discontinued. Most of the TEAEs related to

injection sites were mild or moderate in severity and occurred on the day of injection, and the majority were resolved by the next day. Of the 5 patients who discontinued due to an injection site AE, 4 did so after multiple self-administrations. None of the TEAEs appeared to be different between the doses with the exception of the reported AE of upper respiratory tract infection. However, the cluster of events under upper respiratory infections show a similar incidence between the galcanezumab 120 mg dose group (35.7%) and the 240 mg dose group (37.6%). In addition, safety data from the Phase 3, double-blind, placebo-controlled studies for all three treatment groups (galcanezumab 120 mg, galcanezumab 240 mg, and placebo) showed a similar incidence of the AE of the upper respiratory tract infection [36].

Table 6 Improvement in functioning and patient impression of illness improvement

	Galcanezumab 120 mg		Galcanezumab 240 mg	
	N	Mean (SE) or %	N	Mean (SE) or %
MSQ RF-R, mean increase (improvement)	130	31.6 (1.2)	135	33.4 (1.2)
MIDAS total, mean decrease (improvement)	124	−33.6 (2.1)	130	−32.7 (2.0)
Patient Global Impression – Illness Improvement at Month 12	90	–	112	–
Very much better		52.2%		52.7%
Much better		27.8%		32.1%
A little better		15.6%		7.1%
No change		3.3%		7.1%
A little worse		1.1%		0.9%
Much worse		0%		0%
Very much worse		0%		0%

MIDAS Migraine Disability Assessment, *MSQ RF-R* Migraine-Specific Questionnaire Role Function – Restrictive, *SE* standard error

The safety of galcanezumab was supported by generally temporary and minimal changes from baseline in laboratory values, vital signs, ECG parameters, and weight. There were no clinically meaningful differences in laboratory parameters between the galcanezumab doses, based on mean changes from baseline to endpoint, as well as treatment-emergent changes (i.e., treatment-emergent abnormal, low, or high). These findings are supported by safety analyses performed with data pooled from two 6-month and one 3-month, Phase 3, double-blind, placebo-controlled studies [36].

Migraine may be associated with increased risk of suicidal ideation or behavior as reported by several studies [8, 9, 37]. In the current study, nearly 17% of the patients had comorbid depression, but treatment-emergent suicidal behavior was not reported. Four patients reported suicidal ideation as assessed by the C-SSRS. Three of these patients did not have a history of depression, but had a one-time incidence of treatment-emergent suicidal ideation as assessed by the C-SSRS, and all 3 patients continued in the study. One patient discontinued from treatment due to treatment-emergent suicidal ideation.

Immunogenicity is an important topic in therapies using monoclonal antibodies. Of particular interest is the development of ADA and their relevance in contributing to possible allergic drug reactions, neutralization of therapy (possibly reducing efficacy), and potential association with AEs. In this study, there were 26 patients who had TE-ADAs. Of these, only four patients reported one or more hypersensitivity events (specifically, rash and puritis) during the treatment phase and these events were mild-to-moderate in severity and all were resolved by the end of the treatment phase. Future analyses based on integrated safety and efficacy summaries across galcanezumab studies will allow for larger samples sizes, and potentially provide a better understanding of immunogenicity.

Effectiveness of treatment with galcanezumab was demonstrated by both doses on multiple migraine-relevant outcome measures over 12 months of treatment including: reduction in the number of monthly MHD; reduction in the number of days having a non-migraine headache; response rates; maintenance of response; and reduction in the frequency of acute medication use. The findings for the reduction in the number of monthly MHDs and response rates at the 50, 75, and 100% are consistent with findings reported by Ashina et al. 2017 in a 1-year open-label extension study of erenumab, a monoclonal antibody that blocks the CGRP receptor [38]. In addition, over 80% of the patients reported a disease improvement as measured by PGI-I to be "much better" or "very much better". Also, functioning was greatly improved, with changes from baseline in MSQ RF-R scores being three-fold greater than the within-group minimally important difference of 10.9 that

has been determined for this domain [39]. In addition, headache-related disability was reduced from very severe to moderate.

This study is limited by the relatively small sample size, which precludes detection of any rare AE that may occur with long-term galcanezumab treatment. Patients with recent or serious cardiovascular conditions were excluded from participating in galcanezumab clinical studies, therefore caution should be used when treating these patients. In addition, there are limited data from the use of galcanezumab in pregnant women as they were excluded from participating in the galcanezumab studies. Interpretation of the effectiveness outcomes is limited by the open-label study design without comparison to placebo or another active treatment, and while the daily diaries collected the same information (migraine headache, headache, or use of acute medications), the use of a paper diary is a limitation of the study since an electronic diary can provide monitoring of daily entry and minimize recall bias. Nevertheless, the effectiveness results are similar to those of the more rigidly controlled Phase 3 studies. Lastly, in this study, the majority of the patients met criteria for episodic migraine and further assessment of the patients with episodic compared to chronic migraine will be explored in a future publication.

Conclusion

In summary, there were no new safety findings identified during 12 months of treatment with galcanezumab; favorable tolerability was evidenced by low discontinuation rates due to AEs, and TEAEs were transient and predominantly rated as mild or moderate in severity. Furthermore, there were no meaningful differences between galcanezumab doses with respect to measures of safety and tolerability. Although the study design was uncontrolled and open-label, the totality of migraine headache reduction along with improvement in functioning and disability, are considered to be clinically meaningful [39]. Results from this study confirm the long-term effectiveness of galcanezumab in patients with migraine.

Abbreviations

AEs: Adverse events; ALP: Alkaline phosphatase; ALT: Alanine aminotransferase; AST: Aspartate aminotransferase; BP: Blood pressure; bpm: Beats per minute; CGRP: Calcitonin gene-related peptide; C-SSRS: Columbia Suicide Severity Rating Scale; DBP: Diastolic blood pressure; ECGs: Electrocardiograms; GLIMMIX: Generalized linear mixed model; ICHD: International Classification of Headache Disorders; IHS: International Headache Society; ITT: Intent-to-treat; LOCF: Last observation carried forward; LS: Least squares; MHD: Migraine headache days; MIDAS: Migraine Disability Assessment; MMRM: Mixed-model repeated measures; MSQ RF-R: Migraine-Specific Quality of Life questionnaire Role Function – Restrictive; PGI-I: Patient Global Impression of Improvement; PR: Pulse rate; QTcF: QT interval adjusted for heart rate using Fridericia's correction; SAEs: Serious adverse events; SBP: Systolic blood pressure; SD: Standard deviation; SE: Standard error; TBL: Total bilirubin level; TE-ADA: Treatment-emergent anti-drug antibodies; TEAEs: Treatment-emergent adverse events; ULN: Upper limit of normal

Acknowledgements

The authors would like to thank the patients who participated in this trial and the galcanezumab study team. We also thank Jonna Ahl, PhD and Vladimir Skljarevski, MD for their reviews and contributions to this disclosure. The authors especially thank the following study investigators: Michel Vandenheede, MD (Clinique St. Joseph, Liege, Belgium); Annelies Van Dycke, MD (Algemeen Ziekenhuis St Jan Brugge, Brugge, Belgium); Jan Versijpt, MD (Universitair Ziekenhuis Brussel, Brussel, Belgium); Ginette Girard, MD (DIEX Recherche Sherbrooke, Inc., Quebec, Canada); Marek Gawel, MD (Stroyan Research, Ontario, Canada); Farnaz Amoozegar, MD (University of Calgary, Alberta, Canada); Christelle Creác'h, MD (CHU St Etienne Hôpital Nord, Saint Etienne Cedex 2, France); Anne Donnet, MD (Hôpital de la Timone, Marseille Cedex 5, France); Michel Lanteri-Minet, MD (Hôpital de Cimiez, Nice, France); Caroline Roos, MD (Hôpital Lariboisiere, Paris Cedex 10, France); Judit Afra, MD (Orszagos Idegtudomanyi Intezet, Budapest, Hungary); Attila Csanyi, MD (Petz Aladar Megyei Oktato Korhaz, Gyor-Moson-Sopron, Hungary); Csaba Ertsey, MD (SE Neurologiai Klinika, Budapest, Hungary); Maria Satori, MD (Valeomed Kft., Komarom-Esztergom, Hungary); Brian Averell, DO (September 2015 – April 2016) (Wilmington Health Associates, Wilmington, NC, USA); Timothy James Oster, MD (April 2016- June 2016) (Wilmington Health Associates, Wilmington, NC, USA); Mesha McKinney Chadwick, MD (June 2016 – present) (Wilmington Health Associates, Wilmington, NC, USA); Jo H. Jaeger Bonner, MD (Mercy Health Research, St. Louis, MO, USA); John Burch, MD (Blue Ridge Research Center, Roanoke, VA, USA); Erin G. Doty, MD (Jacksonville Center for Clinical Research; Jacksonville, FL, USA); Corey Ericksen, DO (Ericksen Research and Development, Clinton, UT, USA); Shivkumar Hatti, MD (Suburban Research Associates, Media, PA, USA); David B. Kudrow, MD (California Medical Clinic for Headache, Santa Monica, CA, USA); Paula J. Lane, MD (Albuquerque Neuroscience, Inc., Albuquerque, NM, USA); Thomas G. Ledbetter, MD (ClinPoint Trials, LLC, Waxahachie, TX, USA); Hanid Audish, DO (Encompass Clinical Research, Spring Valley, CA, USA); Peter McAllister, MD (New England Institute for Clinical Research, Stamford, CT, USA); Harvey D. Schwartz, MD (Infinity Clinical Research, LLC, Hollywoood, FL, USA); Randal Lee Von Seggern, PharmD (PharmQuest, Greensboro, NC, USA); Elisabeth A. Barranco-Santana, MD (Ponce School of Medicine CAIMED Center, Ponce, Puerto Rico).

Funding

This study was sponsored by Eli Lilly and Company. Eli Lilly and Company designed the study, collected, analyzed, and interpreted the data as well as drafted the manuscript.

Authors' contributions

AC participated in the analyses and interpretation of data. DK participated in the data acquisition and interpretation of the data. SW participated in the study design and performing the statistical analyses. RS participated in the statistical analyses, interpretation of data, and drafting the manuscript. AVD and KJS participated in the interpretation of data. VLS participated in the study design, data acquisition, interpretation of the data, and drafting the manuscript. All authors have revised the manuscript critically for important content and approved the final manuscript.

Ethics approval and consent to participate

This study was reviewed and approved by appropriate institutional review boards and was conducted according to Good Clinical Practice and the Declaration of Helsinki. The ethical review boards included: Commissie Medische Ethiek Universitair Ziekenhuis (Institutes: Clinique St. Joseph, Algemeen Ziekenhuis St Jan Brugge, Universitair Ziekenhuis Brussel; Belgium), IRB Services (Institutes: DIEX Recherche Sherbrooke, Inc., Stroyan Research; Canada), Conjoint Medical Ethics Committee (Institute: University of Calgary, Canada), CPP Sud Mediterannée V (Institutes: CHU St Etienne Hôpital Nord, Hôpital de la Timone, Hôpital de Cimiez, Hôpital Lariboisiere; France), Egeszsegugyi Tudomanyos Tanacs (Institutes: Orszagos Idegtudomanyi Intezet, Petz Aladar Megyei Oktato Korhaz, SE Neurologiai Klinika, Valeomed Kft.; Hungary), Quorum Review, Inc. (Institutes: Wilmington Health Associates, Mercy Health Research, Blue Ridge Research Center, Jacksonville Center for Clinical Research, Ericksen Research and Development, Suburban Research Associates, California Medical Clinic for Headache, Albuquerque Neuroscience, Inc., ClinPoint Trials, LLC, Encompass Clinical Research, New England Institute for Clinical Research, Infinity Clinical Research, LLC, PharmQuest, Ponce School of Medicine CAIMED Center; USA).Patients provided written informed consent before initiating study procedures. The ethics committee approval covers all the sites in each country at the national level.

Competing interests

AC, SW, KJS, and VLS are full-time employees and minor shareholders of Eli Lilly and Company or one of its affiliates. RS was a full-time employee of Eli Lilly and Company at the time the manuscript was submitted. DK has received consultant fees from Eli Lilly, Amgen, Novartis and Alder and has received research support from Eli Lilly, Amgen, Alder, Teva, Allergan, Biohaven, CoLucid, VM Biopharma, and Roche-Genentech. AVD has received speaker fees from UCB, GSK, and Pfizer.

Author details

[1]Eli Lilly Italia, Sesto Fiorentino, Italy. [2]California Medical Clinic for Headache, Santa Monica, CA, USA. [3]UCLA David Geffen School of Medicine, Los Angeles, CA, USA. [4]Eli Lilly and Company Corporate Center, Indianapolis, IN 46285, USA. [5]Neurology Department, AZ Sint-Jan Brugge, Brugge, Belgium.

References

1. GBD 2015 Disease and Injury Incidence and Prevalence Collaborators. Global, regional, and national incidence, prevalence, and years lived with disability for 310 diseases and injuries, 1990–2015: a systematic analysis for the Global Burden of Disease Study 2015. Lancet. 2016;388:1545–602.
2. Lipton RB, Bigal ME, Diamond M, et al. Migraine prevalence, disease burden, and the need for preventive therapy. Neurology. 2007;68:343–9.
3. Buse DC, Rupnow MF, Lipton RB. Assessing and managing all aspects of migraine: migraine attacks, migraine-related functional impairment, common comorbidities, and quality of life. Mayo Clin Proc. 2009;84:422–35.
4. Von Korff M, Crane P, Lane M, et al. Chronic spinal pain and physical-mental comorbidity in the United States: results from the national comorbidity survey replication. Pain. 2005;113:331–9.
5. Ifergane G, Buskila D, Simisesshvely N, Zeev K, Cohen H. Prevalence of fibromyalgia syndrome in migraine patients. Cephalalgia. 2006;26:451–6.
6. Hagen K, Einarsen C, Zwart JA, Svebak S, Bovim G. The co-occurrence of headache and musculoskeletal symptoms amongst 51 050 adults in Norway. Eur J Neurol. 2002;9:527–33.
7. Sacco S, Kurth T. Migraine and the risk for stroke and cardiovascular disease. Curr Cardiol Rep. 2014;16:524.
8. Breslau N, Schultz L, Lipton R, Peterson E, Welch KM. Migraine headaches and suicide attempt. Headache. 2012;52:723–31.
9. Ilgen MA, Kleinberg F, Ignacio RV, et al. Noncancer pain conditions and risk of suicide. JAMA Psychiatry. 2013;70:692–7.
10. Evers S, Áfra J, Frese A, et al. EFNS guideline on the drug treatment of migraine - revised report of an EFNS task force. Eur J Neurol. 2009;16:968–81.
11. Silberstein SD and the US Headache Consortium. Practice parameter: evidence-based guidelines for migraine headache (an evidence-based review). Neurology. 2000;55:754–62.
12. Canadian Headache Society Guideline for Migraine Prophylaxis. A Peer-reviewed supplement to The Canadian Journal of Neurological Sciences. Can J Neurol Sci. 2012;39 Suppl 2:S1–2.
13. Diamond S, Bigal ME, Silberstein S, et al. Patterns of diagnosis and acute and preventive treatment for migraine in the United States: results from the American migraine prevalence and prevention study. Headache. 2007;47:355–63.
14. Silberstein SD. Topiramate in migraine prevention: a 2016 perspective. Headache. 2017;57:165–78.
15. Dodick DW. Migraine. Lancet. 2018;391:1315–30.

16. Silberstein SD, Holland S, Freitag F, et al. Evidence-based guideline update: pharmacologic treatment for episodic migraine prevention in adults. Report of the quality standards Subcommittee of the American Academy of neurology and the American headache society. Neurology. 2012;78:1337–45.

17. Steiner TJ, Paemeleire K, Jensen R, et al. European principles of management of common headache disorders in primary care. J Headache Pain. 2007;8(Suppl 1):S3–47.

18. VanderPluym J, Evans RW, Starling AJ. Long-term use and safety of migraine preventive medications. Headache. 2016;56:1335–43.

19. Goadsby PJ, Edvinsson L, Ekman R. Vasoactive peptide release in the extracerebral circulation of humans during migraine headache. Ann Neurol. 1990;28:183–7.

20. Goadsby PJ, Edvinsson L. The trigeminovascular system and migraine: studies characterizing cerebrovascular and neuropeptide changes seen in humans and cats. Ann Neurol. 1993;33:48–56.

21. Vermeersch S, Benschop RJ, Van Hecken A, et al. Translational pharmacodynamics of calcitonin gene-related peptide monoclonal antibody LY2951742 in a capsaicin-induced dermal blood flow model. J Pharmacol Exp Ther. 2015;354:350–7.

22. Dodick DW, Goadsby PJ, Spierings ELH, et al. Safety and efficacy of LY2951742, a monoclonal antibody to calcitonin gene-related peptide, for the prevention of migraine: a phase 2, randomised, double-blind, placebo-controlled study. Lancet Neurol. 2014;13:885–92.

23. Skljarevski V, Oakes TM, Zhang Q, et al. Effect of different doses of galcanezumab vs placebo for episodic migraine prevention: a randomized clinical trial. JAMA Neurol. 2018;75:187–93.

24. Skljarevski V, Stauffer VL, Zhang Q, et al. Phase 3 Studies (EVOLVE-1 & EVOLVE-2) of Galcanezumab in Episodic Migraine: Results of 6-Month Treatment Phase. Cephalalgia. 2017;37 Suppl 1:339.

25. Headache Classification Committee of the International Headache Society (IHS). ICHD-3 beta. The International Classification of Headache Disorders, 3rd edition (beta version). Cephalalgia. 2013;33:629–808.

26. Posner K, Brown GK, Stanley B, et al. The Columbia-suicide severity rating scale: initial validity and internal consistency findings from three multisite studies with adolescents and adults. Am J Psychiatry. 2011;168:1266–77.

27. Jhingran P, Osterhaus JT, Miller DW, Lee JT, Kirchdoerfer L. Development and validation of the migraine-specific quality of life questionnaire. Headache. 1998;38:295–302.

28. Stewart WF, Lipton RB, Kolodner K, Liberman J, Sawyer J. Reliability of the migraine disability assessment score in a population-based sample of headache sufferers. Cephalalgia. 1999;19:107–14.

29. Stewart WF, Lipton RB, Dowson AJ, Sawyer J. Development and testing of the migraine disability assessment (MIDAS) questionnaire to assess headache-related disability. Neurology. 2001;56(Suppl 1):S20–8.

30. Guy W. ECDEU assessment manual for psychopharmacology. Rockville: National Institute of Mental Health, Psychopharmacology Research Branch. Revised 1976. p 217 -222. https://archive.org/details/ecdeuassessmentm1933guyw. Accessed 11 May 2018

31. Rendas-Baum R, Bloudek LM, Maglinte GA, Varon SF. The psychometric properties of the migraine-specific quality of life questionnaire version 2.1 (MSQ) in chronic migraine patients. Qual Life Res. 2013;22:1123–33.

32. Lipton RB, Stewart WF, Sawyer J, Edmeads JG. Clinical utility of an instrument assessing migraine disability: the migraine disability assessment (MIDAS) questionnaire. Headache. 2001;41:854–61.

33. Detke HC, Wang S, Skljarevski V, et al. A Phase 3 Placebo-Controlled Study of Galcanezumab in Patients with Chronic Migraine: Results from the 3-month Double-Blind Treatment Phase of the REGAIN Study. Cephalalgia. 2017;37 Suppl 1:338.

34. Malessa R, Gendolla A, Steinberg B, et al. Prevention of episodic migraine with topiramate: a prospective 24-week, open-label, flexible-dose clinical trial with optional 24 weeks follow-up in a community setting. Curr Med Res Opin. 2010;26:1119–29.

35. Nelles G, Schmitt L, Humbert T, et al. Prevention of episodic migraines with topiramate: results from a non-interventional study in a general practice setting. J Headache Pain. 2010;11:33–44.

36. Stauffer VL, Wang S, Bangs, M, et al. Phase-3 safety data from studies comparing galcanezumab and placebo in patients with episodic and chronic migraine. Eur J Neurol. 2018;25(Suppl. 2):298.

37. Friedman LE, Zhong QY, Gelaye B, Williams MA, Peterlin BL. Association between migraine and suicidal behaviors: a nationwide study in the USA. Headache. 2018;58:371–80.

38. Ashina M, Dodick D, Goadsby PJ, et al. Erenumab (AMG 334) in episodic migraine: interim analysis of an ongoing open-label study. Neurology. 2017; 89:1237–43.

39. Dodick DW, Turkel CC, DeGryse RE, et al. Assessing clinically meaningful treatment effects in controlled trials: chronic migraine as an example. J Pain. 2015;16:164–75.

26

Validation of the brief international cognitive assessment for multiple sclerosis (BICAMS) in the Portuguese population with multiple sclerosis

Cláudia Sousa[1][*][†] ⓘ, Mariana Rigueiro-Neves[2][†], Telma Miranda[1], Paulo Alegria[3], José Vale[3], Ana Margarida Passos[2], Dawn Langdon[4] and Maria José Sá[1,5]

Abstract

Background: The validation of international cognitive batteries in different multiple sclerosis (MS) populations is essential. Our objective was to obtain normative data for the Portuguese population of the Brief International Cognitive Assessment for Multiple Sclerosis (BICAMS) and assess its reliability.

Methods: The BICAMS was applied to 105 MS patients and 60 age, gender and education matched healthy controls (HC). In order to test its reliability, BICAMS was re-administered in a subset of 25 patients after a 7-month interval.

Results: Most participants were women, with a mean age of 37, 21 years and a mean of 14,08 years of education. The vast majority of the MS patients (92.4%) had the relapsing remitting type, 58.1% were professionally active, mean disease duration was 6.52 years, median EDSS score was 1.5 (range: 0–6.0) and the median MSSS score was 2.01 (IQR range: 3.83). The MS group presented significantly higher scores of anxiety and depression than HC and 47,4% had fatigue. The MS group performed significantly worse than the control group across the three neuropsychological tests, yielding the following values: SDMT: $t(165) = 3.77$, $p = .000$; CVLT-II: $t(165) = 2.98$, $p = .003$; and BVMT-R: $t(165) = 2.94$, $p = .004$. The mean raw scores for Portuguese normative data were as follows: SDMT: 58.68 ± 10.02; CVLT-II: 60.47 ± 10.12; and BVMT-R: 24.68 ± 5.52. Finally, test–retest reliability coefficients for each test were as follows: SDMT: $r = .90$; CVLT-II: $r = .71$; and BVMT-R: $r = .84$.

Conclusions: The Portuguese version of BICAMS here in described is a reliable monitoring instrument for identifying MS patients with cognitive impairment.

Keywords: Multiple sclerosis, Cognitive impairment, BICAMS, Normative values for Portugal

Background

Multiple sclerosis (MS) is a chronic inflammatory demyelinating disease of the central nervous system that can impair any body function, including cognition [1]. Cognitive dysfunction affects 40 to 70% patients [2, 3]. Irrespective of age and gender [3, 4], may occur at all stages of the disease, even at the very early beginning [5,

6] and definitely impacts the lives of MS patients and their families [3, 7, 8].

The characteristic pattern of cognitive impairment in MS has been described early on to include memory, information processing efficiency, executive functioning, attention and processing speed [1]. However, the cognitive domains most likely to be affected in MS are information processing speed and memory, whilst visual processing and executive function are less likely to be impaired and language is largely intact [1, 9–12].

The most frequently used neuropsychological batteries for patients with MS such us, the Brief Repeatable Battery of Neuropsychological tests and the Minimal

* Correspondence: claudia-sousa@sapo.pt

[†]Cláudia Sousa and Mariana Rigueiro-Neves contributed equally to this work.

[1]MS Clinic, Department of Neurology, Centro Hospitalar São João Porto, Alameda Prof. Hernâni Monteiro, 4200 – 319 Porto, Portugal

Full list of author information is available at the end of the article

Assessment of Cognitive Function in MS, require specialized technical and human resources and take a considerable time for evaluation in the daily clinical setting [1, 13]. Recently, the Brief International Cognitive Assessment for MS (BICAMS) was developed and recommended as a validated and standardized international screening test, because it is an easier assessment tool that can be administered by a technician who is not a specialist in neuropsychology and lasts only about 15 min to apply [14, 15]. Besides, the three instruments that compose BICAMS – Symbol Digit Modalities Test (SDMT) [16], California Verbal Learning Test (CVLT-II) [17] and Brief Visuo-spatial Memory Test Revised (BVMT-R) [18] – have previously been shown to have good psychometric properties.

The aims of this study are to describe the normative values of the Portuguese version of the BICAMS with gender, age and education corrections and to test the validity of this battery in a sample of Portuguese patients with MS.

Methods

Participants

A group of 105 patients with MS diagnosed according to the McDonald criteria [19] and a control group of 60 age, gender and education matched healthy subjects (HC), entered this study, and conducted in the period 2015–2016.

The MS patients were consecutively recruited at the MS Clinics from two hospitals located in separate regions of the country, Hospital de São João (Oporto; North) and Hospital Beatriz Ângelo (Loures; South), whereas the HC group was recruited from the community and among relatives and friends of MS patients. All participants were aged between 17 and 69 years and they were fluent in Portuguese as first language.

Exclusion criteria were current or past neurological disorder other than MS, presence of major psychiatric illness, history of learning disability, history of serious head trauma, presence of alcohol or drug abuse, relapse and/or corticosteroid use within 4 weeks preceding the neuropsychological assessment. HC were also required to present scores > 21 on Montreal Cognitive Assessment Portuguese version (MoCA) [20, 21].

The study was approved by the ethical committees of both hospitals. All the participants, from MS group and HC, volunteered to participate in this study, giving written informed consent.

Procedures

An initial demographic interview was conducted. This was based on a common script that included a demographic questionnaire, medical history, drinking and drug habits and present health status. The MS data, such

as type, duration, and degree of disability and severity, as assessed by the Expanded Disability Status Scale (EDSS) [22] score and the Multiple Severity Status Score (MSSS) [23], respectively, were obtained in the clinical protocols.

Then, participants underwent the BICAMS battery [14], which included the oral version of Symbol Digit Modalities Test (SDMT) [16], the learning trials from the California Verbal Learning Test-II (CVLT-II) [17] and the Brief Visuo-spatial Memory Test-Revised learning trials (BVMT-R) [18].

The SDMT [16] examines sustained attention, concentration and processing speed. In the oral version, the participant examines a series of nine meaningless geometric symbols, which are labeled from 1 to 9. Then, during 90 s the participant is instructed to say the corresponding number to each symbol, as rapidly as possible. The test score corresponds to the number of correct responses.

The CVLT-II [17] is a measure of verbal learning and memory. The test begins with the examiner reading a list of 16 words to the patient and then he/she is asked to report as many of the items as possible, in any order. After recall is recorded, the entire list is read again followed by a second attempt at recall. Altogether, there are five learning trials. The outcome measure is the total number of recalled items over the five learning trials.

The BVMT-R [18] is a measure of visuo-spatial learning and memory. The participant is exposed to a matrix of six simple abstract designs for 10 s followed by an unaided recall; we used the form 1 of the original test. After that, the participant is asked to render the designs using paper and pencil, taking as much time as needed for reproduction. The scoring criterion is based on location and accuracy of each design (from 0 to 2, maximum total score for each array 12). The outcome measure of this test corresponds to the total recall score across the three trials.

The validation was conducted per the international standards given by the expert consensus committee [15]. As the first step, the CVLT-II list of words were translated and re-translated from English to Portuguese and vice versa respectively; the other two tests did not require translation due to their nature. In the second step, the test instructions were translated into Portuguese.

In both groups, anxiety and depression symptoms were also measured using the Portuguese version of Hospital Anxiety and Depression Scale (HADS) [24]. In the MS group the level of fatigue was measured with the Modified Fatigue Impact Scale (MFIS) [25–27].

"The participants of both groups were asked to return for a follow-up session to allow for test–retest reliability analyses. A subgroup of 26 patients and 13 HC returned after a mean time of 7 months and all the tests administered in the first session were repeated in the same manner and in the same order."

Well-trained clinical psychologists conducted all sessions and the tests were applied in a standardized way and in a fixed order. The mean time for BICAMS application was 15 min, as described [14, 15].

Statistical analysis

Statistical analysis was performed using the Statistical Package for the Social Sciences (IBM SPSS), version 23.0. Descriptive statistics (e.g., mean, standard deviation, median, interquartile range and percentages) were used for demographic characterization of both groups. Student's t-test for independent samples was used to analyze the differences between groups, at the level of $p < .05$. The values shown in the tables are bilateral p-values. The effect sizes of those differences were calculated using Cohen's d. Spearman's correlations (P) were used to analyze reliability measures and the relationship between BICAMS, HADS and MFIS results. Raw scores were analyzed for the full sample and Z-scores were calculated. Multiple regression analysis was used to produce normative data.

Results
Demographics and MS characteristics

The groups were similar with regard to age (MS group: M = 38.26 years±11.03; HC: M = 36.17 years ±12.01, p = .63), gender (MS group: %Female = 66.7; HC: %Female = 58.3, p = .28) or number of educational years (MS group: M = 13.55 ± 3.71; HC: M = 14.62 ± 3.47, p = .42). With respect to professional status, the majority of subjects were employed, with a much higher proportion of HC than MS, as is usually reported (n = 56, 94.9%; n = 61, 58.1%, respectively). In the MS group, 92,4% (n = 97) of patients had the relapsing remitting type and 3,8% (n = 4) secondary progressive type and 3,8% (n = 4) clinically isolated syndrome. The average disease duration was 6.52 years (SD = 5.95) and the median EDSS score was 1.5 (range: 0–6.0). The MSSS score, calculated in patients from 1 to 30 years of disease duration (n = 95), had a median value of 2.01 (IQR range: 3.83).

Criterion-related validity: Group differences

Means, standard deviations and t test's for independent samples from the three tests are presented in Table 1. The results showed that MS group performed significantly worse than the HC group on all measures.

Cohen's d was analyzed for each neuropsychological test and were satisfactory: SDMT - 0.65 (large); CVLT-II - 0.49 (medium); BVMT-R - 0.45 (medium) [28].

Reliability: Test-retest

The test–retest reliability data obtained in a subgroup of MS patients are presented in Table 2. The test-retest reliability coefficients showed a strong to a very strong and significant effect for all BICAMS tests.

The test-retest results in the HC were not considered in view of the low number of cases.

Regression based-norms

To obtain a regression-based normative model for BICAMS, the distribution of the SDMT, CVLT-II and BVMT-R raw scores was analyzed for the complete sample and the Z scores were calculated. The raw scores were then converted into scaled scores (M = 10 and SD = 3), as presented in Table 3. For each test a multiple regression analysis with a stepwise method using the scaled scores as dependent variable and age, gender and education as predictors was performed. Education was introduced as the number of regular academic school years that the participant successfully completed. As some studies suggest that there is a curvilinear relationship between demographic variables and cognitive function [29], the quadratic term of age and education were also introduced as predictors. These results allow us to detect which variables contributed significantly to explain each of the scaled neuropsychological test scores.

The T-scores corrected for education, age and gender were generated through a procedure suggested by Diehr and colleagues [30]. Therefore, another multiple regression (enter method) with each of the BICAMS test scaled scores as the dependent variable and the significant predictors of each test was performed. The non-standardized predicted values of this equation were saved and a new variable was calculated corresponding to the difference between an individual's actual and predicted scale score (i.e., the residual) divided by the standard deviation of those residuals. These values were then rescaled for a T-score (M = 50 and SD = 10).

Finally, another multiple regression analysis with corrected T-score as the dependent variable was performed to generate each test normative formula for the

Table 1 Group differences on BICAMS measures

	MS (N = 105)	HC (N = 60)	t	P
SDMT	51.77 (11.20)	58.68 (10.02)	3.77	0.000
CVLT-II	55.05 (11.84)	60.47 (10.12)	2.98	0.003
BVMT-R	21.72 (7.27)	24.68 (5.52)	2.94	0.004

Table 2 Test–retest means and correlations for MS group (n = 26)

	Time 1		Time 2		Spearman's correlation	P
	Mean	SD	Mean	SD		
SDMT	50.96	11.56	53.92	13.99	0.90	< 0.001
CVLT-II	57.08	12.75	57.31	17.44	0.71	< 0.001
BVMT-R	22.00	7.43	25.12	6.94	0.84	< 0.001

Table 3 Raw score to scaled score conversions for the BICAMSs tests

Scaled score	SDMT	CVLT-II	BVMT-R
1	–	0–21	–
2	0–20	22–27	1–3
3	21–24	28–33	4–5
4	25–27	34–37	6–8
5	28–33	38–41	9–10
6	34–37	42–44	11–14
7	38–40	45	15
8	41–45	46–49	16–17
9	46–49	50–53	18–20
10	50–53	54–57	21–22
11	54–57	58–60	23–25
12	58–61	61–64	26–27
13	62–65	65–68	28–30
14	66–69	69–72	31–32
15	70–73	73–76	33–34
16	74–76	77–79	–
17	77–78	–	–

Portuguese population. The final formula to calculate the T-scores for each of BICAMS's test are presented below:

$$\textbf{SDMT T score} = 10.511 + \left(0.007^* \text{ age}^2\right)$$
$$+ \left(-0.966^* \text{ years of education}\right)$$
$$+ \left(4.138^* \text{ scaled score}\right)$$

$$\textbf{CVLT–II T score} = 3.195 + \left(0.006^* \text{ age}^2\right)$$
$$+ \left(3.761^* \text{ scaled score}\right)$$

$$\textbf{BVMT–R T score} = -8.004 + \left(0.514^* \text{ age}\right)$$
$$+ \left(3,833^* \text{ scaled score}\right)$$

In determining impairment, the 5th percentile value based on the performance of healthy control sample was calculated for each test. Participants were considered impaired if their score was equal of below the percentile 5th of the control group (results are presented on the Table 4) [31]. Then, using the previously reported criteria of impairment defined by "one or more abnormal

Table 4 The prevalence of cognitive impairment in MS patients according to the 5th percentile value of HC on BICAMS tests

	5th Percentile value for HC on each test	Percentage of MS patients under 5th percentile
SDMT	38	14.3%
CVLT-II	41	9.5%
BVMT-R	12	11.4%

tests" [32, 33], it was found that 24.8% of the MS sample was impaired at baseline.

Analysing the degree of disability assessed by EDSS and cognitive performance, we found significant correlations with all cognitive tests (SDMT: –.497, p = .000; CVLT: –.334, p = .000; BVMT: –.275, p = .005).

Regarding anxiety and depression symptoms, it was found that MS group presented higher scores on these measures than HC, and that these differences were statistically significant: anxiety (MS group: M = 7.85 ± 4.51; HC: M = 6.32 ± 3.00, t = – 2.348; p = .20) and depression (MS group: M = 5.14 ± 3.95; HC: M = 3.18 ± 2.57). Anxiety symptoms were found to be more frequent (n = 56; 53.3%) than depression symptoms (n = 29; 27.6%) in MS patients. In the MS group depression symptoms had a modest significantly negative effect only on CVLT-II results (R – 0.196; p = .45), whereas anxiety was not significantly correlated with any BICAMS test. The assessment with the MFIS scale (n = 95) showed that fatigue was present in 50 MS patients (47,4%) and was significantly correlated with the EDSS score (R – .279; p = .006), and with anxiety (R – .631; p = .0001) and depression symptoms (R – .754; p = .0001). Conversely, fatigue was negatively correlated with SDMT score (R – .266; p = .009); similar results were observed in both MFIS subscales, physical (M = 18.04 ± 9.66; R-.289; p = .005) and cognitive (M = 17.84 ± 10.21; R-.203; p = .049).

Discussion

An international consensus committee of experts recently recommended a short battery of tests for cognitive assessment in MS that allows monitoring of cognition over time and is a fast and reliable instrument that may be administered by healthcare professionals with no specific experience in neuropsychological testing. According to the international standards for validation [15], several validation studies of BICAMS have been carried out in different cultures and languages, with the aim of making this psychometric tool more solid and internationally applicable. Up to now, there exists normative data for populations of several countries, such as Czech Republic [32], Italy [34], Hungary [35], Ireland [36], Brazil [37], Lithuania [38] Argentina [39], Canada [33], Greece [31], Belgium [40], Japan [41] and Turkish [42].

The current study followed the recommendations and standards of the BICAMS consensus committee [14, 15] and is the first to publish the Portuguese normative data for SDMT, CVLT-II and BVMT-R. Our results showed that MS group performed significantly worse than HC group on all measures (SDMT, CVLT-II and BVMT-R), a finding that is in agreement with the other recently published validations. These differences were more marked in the SDMT and CVLT-II than the BVMT-R, and similar results were found by O'Connell and colleagues (2015), Spedo and colleagues (2015) and Vanotti and colleagues (2016). Test-retest reliability in our population fits the recommended international standards for BICAMS validation [14]. Test–retest reliability for raw scores was adequate to excellent for all the three tests in this validation; more than .80 in SDMT and BVMT, replicating prior finds [33, 34]. Yet our results are lower than those of Vanotti and colleagues (2016). In addition we confirmed that the SDMT has particularly high test-retest reliability. We used a wider time span than other authors [37, 40] in order to avoid the learning effect, since at both evaluation times the same forms were applied.

The BICAMS tasks were able to identify cognitive impairment in 24.8% of MS patients using the criteria of impairment defined by one or more abnormal tests. This is a lower value than those found in other studies, which ranged from 47.3 to 58% [31–33, 35, 36]. This result may reflect the characteristics of our MS sample, which were mainly RRMS and rather early cases (mean disease duration 6.5 years) and a correspondingly low level of physical disability, median EDSS 1.5 [31–33, 36]. The lower level of disability in our sample is further supported by our MSSS data [23].

We found a significant correlation between EDSS and cognitive performance in the three tests used, that is, the higher the EDSS score the worse the cognitive test performance.

Regarding anxiety and depression symptoms, we found that the MS group also presented with higher scores on these measures then the HC, fitting the results of other BICAMS validation studies [32, 33, 37]. The Hungarian BICAMS validation reported a negative correlation of fatigue with all BICAMS tests [31]. In our study an association with fatigue was only seen in the SDMT test, possibly reflecting the lower fatigue in our patients as well as the lower physical disability.

This study was some limitations. First, follow-up assessments were done in a low number of cases, especially in the HC group, which is due to the fact that some individuals live far from the Hospital and incur additional personal costs. Another limitation is the fact that effect size for CVLT and BVMT-R although satisfactory, is on the threshold of the effect size classified as medium.

Conclusions

In conclusion, our study provides the Portuguese BICAMS standards for use with MS patients and evidences the strong psychometric properties of the Portuguese BICAMS version. The normative data of the BICAMS for the Portuguese population enables the use of the battery in clinical practice, for longitudinal patient assessments and as an outcome measure of cognitive functioning in clinical trials. Future prospective studies with larger samples of MS patients, with different types of disease evolution, will certainly add valuable information concerning the clinical applicability of the Portuguese BICAMS version.

Abbreviations

BICAMS: Brief International cognitive assessment for multiple sclerosis; BRB-N: Brief repeatable battery of neuropsychological tests; BVMT-R: Brief visuo-spatial memory test – revised; CI: Cognitive impairment; CVLT-II: California verbal learning test – II; EDSS: Expanded disability status scale; HADS: Hospital anxiety and depression scale; HC: Healthy subjects; IBM SPSS: Statistical package for the social sciences; MACFIMS: Minimal assessment of cognitive function in multiple sclerosis; MFIS: Modified fatigue impact scale; MoCa: Montreal cognitive assessment; MS: Multiple sclerosis; MSSS: Multiple severity status score; SDMT: Symbol digit modalities test

Acknowledgements

The authors would like to thank all participants of this study.
An earlier version of this paper was presented at the ECTRIMS-ACTRIMS Meeting, Paris, France, 25–28 October 2017. The abstract of the e-Poster was published in the Multiple Sclerosis Journal (2017): 23: (S3): 680 – 975. http://journals.sagepub.com/doi/10.1177/1352458517731285.

Funding

This work was funded by an unrestricted educational grant from Bayer, which had any role in the study, namely in its design, sample collection, analyses and interpretation of data and in the writing of the manuscript.

Authors' contributions

CS contributed in study concept and design, drafting and revising the manuscript and in the acquisition and interpretation of data. MRN contributed in study concept and design, drafting and revising the manuscript, in the acquisition and interpretation of data and statistical analysis. TM contributed in the acquisition of data and statistical analysis. PA and JV contributed in patient recruitment, acquisition of clinical data and revising the manuscript. AMP contributed in study concept and design, revising the manuscript, in the interpretation of data and statistical analysis. DL contributed in study concept and design and in revising the manuscript. MJS contributed in study concept and design, drafting and revising the manuscript, in the analysis and interpretation of data and study supervision. All authors read and approved the final manuscript.

Competing interests

MJS has received consulting/speaker fees from Bayer, Biogen, CSL Behring, Merck, Novartis, Roche, Sanofi and Teva.
DL has participated in speaker bureau for Bayer, Merck, Almirall, Execemed, TEVA, Roche, Novartis, Biogen, Sanofi; has had consultancy from Novartis, Bayer, Merck, Biogen, TEVA, Sanofi; has had research grants from Bayer, Merck, Novartis, Biogen. All are paid into DL's institution.
The other authors have nothing to disclose regarding this study.

Author details

[1]MS Clinic, Department of Neurology, Centro Hospitalar São João Porto, Alameda Prof. Hernâni Monteiro, 4200 – 319 Porto, Portugal. [2]BRU-IUL, Instituto Universitário de Lisboa (ISCTE-IUL), Lisbon, Portugal. [3]Department of Neurology, Hospital Beatriz Ângelo, Loures, Portugal. [4]Department of Psychology, Royal Holloway, University of London, London, UK. [5]Faculty of Health Sciences, University Fernando Pessoa, Porto, Portugal.

References

1. Rao SM, Leo GJ, Bernardin L, Unverzagt F. Cognitive impairment in multiple sclerosis. I. Frequency, patterns, and prediction. Neurology. 1991;41:685–91.

2. Amato MP, Zipoli V, Portaccio E. Multiple sclerosis-related cognitive changes: a review of cross-sectional and longitudinal studies. J Neurol Sci. 2006;245:1–2.

3. Langdon DW. Cognition in multiple sclerosis. Curr Opin Neurol. 2011;24(3): 244–9.

4. Glanz BI, Holand M, Gauthier SA, Amunwa EL, Liptak Z, Houtchens MK, Sperling RA, Khoury SJ, Guttmann CR, Weiner HL. Cognitive dysfunction in patients with clinically isolated syndromes or newly diagnosed multiple sclerosis. Mult Scler. 2007;13(8):1004–10.

5. Amato MP, Hakiki B, Goretti B, et al. Association of MRI metrics and cognitive impairment in radiologically isolated syndromes. Neurology. 2012; 78:309–14.

6. Zipoli V, Goretti B, Hakiki B, et al. Cognitive impairment predicts conversion to multiple sclerosis in clinically isolated syndromes. Mult Scler. 2010;16:62–7.

7. Kobelt G, Thompson A, Berg J, et al. New insights into the burden and costs of multiple sclerosis in Europe. Mult Scler. 2017;23(8):1123–36.

8. Sá MJ, Kobelt G, Berg J, Capsa D, Dalén J. European Multiple Sclerosis Platform. New insights into the burden and costs of multiple sclerosis in Europe: Results for Portugal. Mult Scler. 2017;23(2-suppl):143–54.

9. Langdon D. Cognitive assessment in MS. Neurodegenerative Disease Management. 2015;5(6s):43–5.

10. Rimkus MC, Steenwijk MD, Barkhof F. Causes, effects and connectivity changes in MS-related cognitive decline. Dement Neuropsychology. 2006; 10(1):2–11.

11. Vanotti S, Caceres FJ. Cognitive and neuropsychiatric disorders among MS patients from Latin America. Multiple Sclerosis: Journal experimental translational clinical. 2017:1–11.

12. Giedraitiene N, Kaubrys G, Kizlaitiene R. Cognition during and after multiple sclerosis relapse as assesses with the brief international cognitive assessment for multiple sclerosis. Sci Rep. 2018;8:8169.

13. Benedict RH, Cookfair D, Gavett R, Gunther M, Munschauer F, Garg N, Weinstock-Guttman B. Validity of the minimal assessment of cognitive function in multiple sclerosis (MACFIMS). J Int Neuropsychol Soc. 2006;12:549–58.

14. Langdon DW, Amato MP, Boringa J, Brochet B, Foley F, Fredrikson S, Hämäläinen P, Hartung HP, Krupp L, Penner IK, Reder AT, Benedict RH. Recommendations for a brief international cognitive assessment for multiple sclerosis (BICAMS). Mult Scler. 2012;18:891–8.

15. Benedict RH, Amato MP, Boringa J, Brochet B, Foley F, Fredrikson S, Hamalainen P, Hartung H, Krupp L, Penner I, Reder AT, Langdon DW. Brief international cognitive assessment for MS (BICAMS): international standard for validation. BMC Neurol. 2012;16:55.

16. Smith A. Symbol digit modalities test: manual. Los Angeles, CA: Western Psychological Services; 1982.

17. Delis DC, Kramer JH, Kaplan E, Ober BA. California verbal learning test, second edition (CVLT-II). San Antonio, TX: Psychological Corporation; 2000.

18. Benedict RHB. The brief visuospatial memory test revised (BVMT-R). Lutz, FL: Psychosocial Assessment Resources Inc.; 1997.

19. Polman CH, Reingold SC, Banwell B, Clanet M, Cohen JA, Filippi M, Wolinsky JS. Diagnostic criteria for multiple sclerosis: 2010 revisions to the McDonald criteria. Ann Neurol. 2011;69(2):292–302.

20. Nasreddine ZS, Phllips NA, Béridian V, Charbonneau S, Whitehead V, Collin I, Cummings JL, Chertkow H. The Montreal cognitive assessment, MoCA: a brief screening tool for mild cognitive impairment. J Am Geriatr Soc. 2005; 53(4):695–9.

21. Freitas S, Simões MR, Alves L, Santana I. Montreal cognitive assessment (MoCA): normative study for the Portuguese population. J Clin Exp Neuropsychol. 2011;33(9):989–96.

22. Kurzke JF. Rating neurologic impairment in multiple sclerosis: an expanded disability status scale (EDSS). Neurology. 1983;33:1444–52.

23. Roxburgh RHSR, Seaman SR, Masterman T, Hensiek AE, et al. Multiple sclerosis severity score using disability and disease duration to rate disease severity. Neurology. 2005;64:1144–51.

24. Silva AM, Vilhena E, Lopes A, Santos E, Gonçalves MA, Pinto C, et al. Depression and anxiety in a Portuguese MS population: association with physical disability and severity of disease. J Neurol Sci. 2011;306:66–70.

25. Fisk JD, Ritvo PG, Haase DA, Marrie TJ, Schlech WF. Measuring the functional impact of fatigue: initial validation of the fatigue impact scale. Clin Infect Dis. 1994;18(Suppl 1):S79–83.

26. Larson RD. Psychometric properties of the modified fatigue impact scale. Int J MS Care. 2013;15(1):15–20.

27. Gomes LR. Validação da versão portuguesa da Escala de Impacto da Fadiga Modificada e da Escala de Severidade da Fadiga na Esclerose Múltipla (Validation of the Portuguese version of the Modified Fatigue Impact Scale and the Fatigue Severity Scale in Multiple Sclerosis). Thesis.Minho University. 2011.

28. Cohen J. Statistical power analysis for the behavioral sciences. New York, NY: Routledge Academic; 1988.

29. Strauss E, Sherman E, Spreen O. A compendium of neuropsychological tests: administration, norms and commentary. 3rd ed. Oxford, UK: University Oxford Press; 2006.

30. Diehr MC, Cherner M, Wolfson TJ, Miller SW, Grant I, Heaton RK, the HIV Neurobehavioral Research Center. The 50 and 100-item short forms of the paced auditory serial addition task (PASAT): demographic corrected norms and comparisons with the full PASAT in normal and clinical samples. J Clin Exp Neuropsychol. 2003;25:571–58.

31. Polychroniadou E, Bakirtzis C, Langdon D, Lagoudaki E, Kesidou E, Theotokis P, et al. Validation of the brief international cognitive assessment for multiple sclerosis (BICAMS) in Greek population with multiple sclerosis. Multiple Sclerosis and Related Disorders. 2016;9:68–72.

32. Dusankova JB, Kalincik T, Havrdova E, Benedict RH. Cross cultural validation of the minimal assessment of cognitive function in multiple sclerosis (MACFIMS) and the brief international cognitive assessment for multiple sclerosis (BICAMS). Clin Neuropsychol. 2012;26(7):1186–200.

33. Walker LA, Osman L, Berard JA, Rees LM, Freedman MS, MacLean H, Cousineau D. Brief international cognitive assessment for multiple sclerosis (BICAMS): Canadian contribution to the international validation project. J Neurol Sci. 2006;362:147–52.

34. Goretti B, Niccolai C, Hakiki B, Sturchio A, Falautano M, Minacapelli E, Amato M. The brief international cognitive assessment for multiple sclerosis (BICAMS): normative values with gender, age and education corrections in the Italian population. BMC Neurol. 2014;14:171.

35. Sandi D, Rudisch T, Füvesi J, Fricska-Nagy Z, Huszka H, Biernacki T, Bencsik K. The Hungarian validation of the brief international cognitive assessment for multiple sclerosis (BICAMS) battery and the correlation of cognitive impairment with fatigue and quality of life. Multiple Sclerosis and Related Disorders. 2015;4:499–504.

36. O'Connell K, Langdon D, Tubridy N, Hutchinson M, McGuigan C. A preliminary validation of the brief international cognitive assessment for multiple sclerosis (BICAMS) tool in an Irish population with multiple sclerosis (MS). Multiple Sclerosis and Related Disorders. 2015; 4:521–5.

37. Spedo CT, Frndak SE, Marques VD, Foss MP, Pereira DA, Carvalho L, Barreira AA. Cross-cultural adaptation, reliability, and validity of the BICAMS in Brazil. Clin Neuropsychol. 2015;29:836–46.

38. Giedraitienė N, Kizlaitienė R, Kaubrys G. The BICAMS battery for assessment of Lithuanian-speaking multiple sclerosis patients: relationship with age, education, disease disability, and duration. Med Sci Monit. 2015;21:3853–9.

39. Vanotti S, Smerbeck A, Benedict RHB, Caceres F. A new assessment tool for patients with multiple sclerosis from Spanish-speaking countries: validation of the Brief International Cognitive Assessment for MS (BICAMS) in Argentina. Neurology. 2015;84(14):Suppl.P5. 201.

40. Costers L, Gielen J, Eelen PL, Schependom JV, Laton J, Remoortel AV, Vanzeir E, Wijmeersch BV, Seeldrayers P, Haelewyck MC, D'Haeseleer M, D'hooghe MB, Langdon D, Nagels G. Does including the full CVLT-II and BVMT-R improve BICAMS? Evidence from a Belgian (Dutch) validation study. Multiple Sclerosis Related Disorders. 2017;18:33–40.

Permissions

All chapters in this book were first published in NEUROLOGY, by BioMed Central; hereby published with permission under the Creative Commons Attribution License or equivalent. Every chapter published in this book has been scrutinized by our experts. Their significance has been extensively debated. The topics covered herein carry significant findings which will fuel the growth of the discipline. They may even be implemented as practical applications or may be referred to as a beginning point for another development.

The contributors of this book come from diverse backgrounds, making this book a truly international effort. This book will bring forth new frontiers with its revolutionizing research information and detailed analysis of the nascent developments around the world.

We would like to thank all the contributing authors for lending their expertise to make the book truly unique. They have played a crucial role in the development of this book. Without their invaluable contributions this book wouldn't have been possible. They have made vital efforts to compile up to date information on the varied aspects of this subject to make this book a valuable addition to the collection of many professionals and students.

This book was conceptualized with the vision of imparting up-to-date information and advanced data in this field. To ensure the same, a matchless editorial board was set up. Every individual on the board went through rigorous rounds of assessment to prove their worth. After which they invested a large part of their time researching and compiling the most relevant data for our readers.

The editorial board has been involved in producing this book since its inception. They have spent rigorous hours researching and exploring the diverse topics which have resulted in the successful publishing of this book. They have passed on their knowledge of decades through this book. To expedite this challenging task, the publisher supported the team at every step. A small team of assistant editors was also appointed to further simplify the editing procedure and attain best results for the readers.

Apart from the editorial board, the designing team has also invested a significant amount of their time in understanding the subject and creating the most relevant covers. They scrutinized every image to scout for the most suitable representation of the subject and create an appropriate cover for the book.

The publishing team has been an ardent support to the editorial, designing and production team. Their endless efforts to recruit the best for this project, has resulted in the accomplishment of this book. They are a veteran in the field of academics and their pool of knowledge is as vast as their experience in printing. Their expertise and guidance has proved useful at every step. Their uncompromising quality standards have made this book an exceptional effort. Their encouragement from time to time has been an inspiration for everyone.

The publisher and the editorial board hope that this book will prove to be a valuable piece of knowledge for researchers, students, practitioners and scholars across the globe.

List of Contributors

Hui Xie, Kang Huo, Rui Liu, Zhi-Jie Jian, Dan Zhu, Li-Hui Zhang, and Guo-Gang Luo
Department of Neurology, The First Affiliated Hospital of Xi'an Jiaotong University, No. 277 Yanta West Road, Xi'an 710061, Shaanxi, China

Qiang Zhang
Department of Neurology, The First Affiliated Hospital of Xi'an Jiaotong University, No. 277 Yanta West Road, Xi'an 710061, Shaanxi, China
Department of Neurology, Shaanxi Provincial People's Hospital, Xi'an 710068, China

Jian Yang and Yi-Tong Bian
Department of Radiology, The First Affiliated Hospital of Xi'an Jiaotong University, Xi'an 710061, China

Guo-Liang Li
Arrhythmia Unit, Department of Cardiovascular Medicine, The First Affiliated Hospital of Xi'an Jiaotong University, Xi'an 710061, China

Hideraldo Luis Souza Cabeça
Departamento de Neurologia, Hospital Ophir Loyola, Belém, PA, Brazil

Luciano Chaves Rocha, Amanda Ferreira Sabbá, Alessandra Mendonça Tomás, Cristovam Wanderley and Picanço Diniz
Laboratório de Investigações em Neurodegeneração e Infecção, Hospital Universitário João de Barros Barreto, Universidade Federal do Pará, Instituto de Ciências Biológicas, Belém, PA, Brazil

Natali Valim Oliver Bento-Torres
Laboratório de Investigações em Neurodegeneração e Infecção, Hospital Universitário João de Barros Barreto, Universidade Federal do Pará, Instituto de Ciências Biológicas, Belém, PA, Brazil
Faculdade de Fisioterapia e Terapia Ocupacional, Instituto de Ciências da Saúde, Universidade Federal do Pará, Belém, PA, Brazil

Daniel Clive Anthony
Laboratory of Experimental Neuropathology, Department of Pharmacology, University of Oxford, Oxford, UK

Keon-Joo Lee
Department of Neurology, Seoul National University Bundang Hospital, Seoul, South Korea

Ji Sung Lee
Clinical Research Center, Asan Medical Center, Seoul, South Korea

Keun-Hwa Jung
Department of Neurology, Seoul National University Hospital, 101, Daehangno, Jongno-gu, Seoul 03080, South Korea

Anca Moțățăianu, Smaranda Maier, Zoltan Bajko and Rodica Bălașa
Department of Neurology, University of Medicine and Pharmacy Târgu Mureș, Gh Marinescu 50, 540136 Târgu Mureș, Romania

Septimiu Voidazan
Department of Epidemiology, University of Medicine and Pharmacy Târgu Mureș, Târgu Mureș, Romania

Adina Stoian
Department of Pathophysiology, University of Medicine and Pharmacy Târgu Mureș, Târgu Mureș, Romania

Klaus Weckbecker
Institute of General Practice and Family Medicine, University of Bonn, Bonn, Germany

Bettina Engel
Institute of General Practice and Family Medicine, University of Bonn, Bonn, Germany
Department of Health Services Research, Division of General Medicine, University of Oldenburg, Oldenburg, Germany

Willy Gomm
German Center for Neurodegenerative Diseases (DZNE), Bonn, Germany

Britta Haenisch
German Center for Neurodegenerative Diseases (DZNE), Bonn, Germany
Federal Institute for Drugs and Medical Devices (BfArM), Kurt-Georg-Kiesinger-Allee 3, D-53175 Bonn, Germany
Center for Translational Medicine, University of Bonn, Bonn, Germany

Wolfgang Maier
German Center for Neurodegenerative Diseases (DZNE), Bonn, Germany

Department of Psychiatry, University of Bonn, Bonn, Germany

Karl Broich
Federal Institute for Drugs and Medical Devices (BfArM), Kurt-Georg-Kiesinger-Allee 3, D-53175 Bonn, Germany

Yiqi Lin, Binyin Li, Huidong Tang, Qun Xu, Yuncheng Wu, Qi Cheng, Chunbo Li, Shifu Xiao, Lu Shen, Weiguo Tang, Hui Yu, Naying He, Huawei Lin, Fuhua Yan, Wenwei Cao, Shilin Yang, Ye Liu, Wei Zhao, Dong Lu, Bin Jiao, Xuewen Xiao, Lin Zhou and Shengdi Chen
Department of Neurology and Institute of Neurology, Rui Jin Hospital affiliated to Shanghai Jiao Tong University School of Medicine, Shanghai 200025, China

Qiuyou Xie, Yan Chen, Yanbin He, Xiaoxiao Ni, Jiechun Zhang and Ronghao Yu
Coma Research Group, Centre for Hyperbaric Oxygen and Neurorehabilitation, Guangzhou General Hospital of Guangzhou Military Command, Guangzhou 510010, China

Jiahui Pan
School of Software, South China Normal University, Guangzhou 510641, China
Center for Brain Computer Interfaces and Brain Information Processing, South China University of Technology, Guangzhou 510640, China

Fei Wang and Yuanqing Li
Center for Brain Computer Interfaces and Brain Information Processing, South China University of Technology, Guangzhou 510640, China

Huan Liao, Xiaoming Rong and Hongxuan Wang
Department of Neurology, Sun Yat-sen Memorial Hospital, Sun Yat-Sen University, No. 107 West Yanjiang Road, Guangzhou 510120, China

Ying Peng
Department of Neurology, Sun Yat-sen Memorial Hospital, Sun Yat-Sen University, No. 107 West Yanjiang Road, Guangzhou 510120, China
Guangdong Provincial Key Laboratory of Malignant Tumor Epigenetics and Gene Regulation, Sun Yat-sen Memorial Hospital, Sun Yat-sen University, Guangzhou, China

Zhuoting Zhu
State Key Laboratory of Ophthalmology, Zhongshan Ophthalmic Center, Sun Yat-sen University, Guangzhou, China

Anthony Traboulsee and David K. B. Li
University of British Columbia, S113-2211 Wesbrook Mall, Vancouver, BC V6T 1Z7, Canada
Mark Cascione
Tampa Neurology Associates, South Tampa Multiple Sclerosis Center, 2919 W. Swann Avenue, Suite 401, South Tampa, FL 33609, USA

Juanzhi Fang
EMD Serono, Inc., One Technology Place, Rockland, MA 02370, USA

Fernando Dangond
EMD Serono, Inc, 45A Middlesex Tpke, Billerica, MA 01821, USA

Aaron Miller
Mount Sinai Hospital, 5 East 98th Street, 1st Floor, New York, NY 10029, USA

Sylvia Kotterba
Klinik für Geriatrie, Klinikum Leer gemeinnützige GmbH, Leer, Germany

Thomas Neusser, Thomas Glaser, Martin Dörner and Markus Schürks
Bayer Vital GmbH, Leverkusen, Germany

Christiane Norenberg
Bayer AG, Wuppertal, Germany

Patrick Bussfeld
Bayer Consumer Care AG, Basel, Switzerland

Marina de Tommaso and Marianna Delussi
Applied Neurophysiology and Pain Unit, Basic Medical Science, Neuroscience and Sensory System-SMBNOS-Department, Policlinico General Hospital, Bari Aldo Moro University, Giovanni XXIII Building, Via Amendola 207 A, 70124 Bari, Italy

Ricardo C. Nogueira, Adriana B. Conforto, Manoel J. Texeira and Edson Bor-Seng-Shu
Neurology Department, School of Medicine, University of São Paulo, São Paulo, SP, Brazil

Angela S. M. Salinet
Neurology Department, School of Medicine, University of São Paulo, São Paulo, SP, Brazil
Biomedical Engineering, Engineering, Modelling and Applied Social Sciences Centre, Federal ABC University, Sao Bernardo do Campo, Sao Paulo, Brazil
Faculty of Physiotherapy, Ibirapuera University, São Paulo, Brazil

Juliana Caldas
Neurology Department, School of Medicine, University of São Paulo, São Paulo, SP, Brazil
Critical Care Unit Hospital São Rafael, Salvador, Brazil

Ronney B. Panerai and Thompson G. Robinson
Department of Cardiovascular Sciences, Cerebral Haemodynamics in Ageing and Stroke Medicine Research Group, University of Leicester, Leicester, UK
NIHR Leicester Biomedical Research Centre, University of Leicester, Leicester, UK

Gang Wang, Hai-Lun Cui, Jun Liu, Qin Xiao, Ying Wang, Jian-Fang Ma, Hai-Yan Zhou, Jing Pan, Yu-Yan Tan and Sheng-Di Chen
Department of Neurology& Institute of Neurology, Ruijin Hospital affiliated to Shanghai Jiaotong University School of Medicine, No.197, Rui Jin Er Road, Shanghai 200025, China

Audny Anke
Department of Rehabilitation, University Hospital of North Norway, Tromsø, Norway
Department of Clinical Medicine, Faculty of Health Sciences, University of Tromsø, The Arctic University of Norway, Tromsø, Norway

Guri Heiberg
Department of Rehabilitation, University Hospital of North Norway, Tromsø, Norway
Department of Clinical Medicine, Faculty of Health Sciences, University of Tromsø, The Arctic University of Norway, Tromsø, Norway
Department of Rehabilitation, University Hospital of North Norway- Harstad, 9480 Harstad, Norway

Cathrine Arntzen and Synne Garder Pedersen
Department of Health and Care Sciences, Faculty of Health Sciences, University of Tromsø The Artic University of Norway, Tromsø, Norway

Oddgeir Friborg
Department of Psychology, Faculty of Health Sciences, University of Tromsø, the Artic University of Norway, Tromsø, Norway

Jørgen Feldbæk Nielsen and Henriette Stabel Holm
Hammel Neurorehabilitation Centre and University Research Clinic, Aarhus University, Aarhus, Denmark

Nicole Steinbüchel von
Universitäty Medicine, Georg-August-University, Göttingen, Germany

Taim A. Muayqil, Mohammed H. Alanazy, H, Fawaz Al-hussain and Bandar N. Aljafen
Division of Neurology, College of Medicine, King Saud Universtiy, Riyadh 11472, Saudi Arabia

Assan M. Almalak, Hussain Khaled Alsalman, Faroq Walid Abdulfattah and Abdullah Ibrahim Aldraihem
College of Medicine, King Saud University, PO Box 7805 (38), Riyadh 11472, Saudi Arabia

Jessica Baggaley
Institute of Neuroscience, Newcastle University, Newcastle upon Tyne NE1 7RU

Anna Purna Basu
Institute of Neuroscience, Newcastle University, Newcastle upon Tyne NE1 7RU, UK
Department of Paediatric Neurology, Newcastle upon Tyne Hospitals NHS Foundation Trust, Newcastle upon Tyne NE7 7DN, UK

Janice Pearse
Therapy Services, Newcastle upon Tyne Hospitals NHS Foundation Trust, Newcastle upon Tyne NE7 7DN, UK

Rose Watson, Denise Howel and Luke Vale
Institute of Health and Society, Newcastle University, Newcastle upon Tyne NE2 4AX, UK

Pat Dulson and Nick Embleton
Newcastle Neonatal Service, Newcastle upon Tyne Hospitals NHS Foundation Trust, Newcastle upon Tyne, UK

Blythe Wright
Human Biosciences, Northumbria University, Newcastle upon Tyne NE1 8ST, UK

Dipayan Mitra
Department of Neuroradiology, Newcastle upon Tyne Hospitals NHS Foundation Trust, Newcastle upon Tyne NE7 7DN, UK

Tim Rapley
Department of Social Work, Education and Community Wellbeing, Northumbria University, Coach Lane Campus West, Newcastle upon Tyne NE7 7XA, UK

Pablo Hervella, Esteban López-Arias, Andrés da Silva-Candal, Tomás Sobrino and Francisco Campos,
Clinical Neurosciences Research Laboratory, Health Research Institute of Santiago de Compostela (IDIS), Santiago de Compostela, Spain

Emilio Rodríguez-Castro, Iria López-Dequit, María Santamaría-Cadavid, Susana Arias-Rivas and Manuel Rodríguez-Yáñez
Clinical Neurosciences Research Laboratory, Health Research Institute of Santiago de Compostela (IDIS), Santiago de Compostela, Spain
Stroke Unit, Department of Neurology, Hospital Clínico Universitario, Santiago de Compostela, Spain

José Manuel Pumar
Clinical Neurosciences Research Laboratory, Health Research Institute of Santiago de Compostela (IDIS), Santiago de Compostela, Spain
Department of Neuroradiology, Hospital Clínico Universitario, Santiago de Compostela, Spain

Ana Estany
Unit of Methodology of the Research, Health Research Institute of Santiago de Compostela (IDIS), Santiago de Compostela, Spain
María Piñeiro-Lamas
Consortium for Biomedical Research in Epidemiology and Public Health, Instituto de Salud Carlos III, Madrid. Health Research Institute of Santiago de Compostela, Santiago de Compostela, Spain

Manuel Portela
Clinical Neurosciences Research Laboratory, Health Research Institute of Santiago de Compostela (IDIS), Santiago de Compostela, Spain
Health Area Management of Santiago de Compostela, Servicio Galego de Saúde, Santiago de Compostela, Spain

Manuel Vázquez-Lima
Emergency Department, Hospital do Salnés, Pontevedra, Vilagarcía de Arousa, Spain

José Castillo and Ramón Iglesias-Rey
Clinical Neurosciences Research Laboratory, Health Research Institute of Santiago de Compostela (IDIS), Santiago de Compostela, Spain
Clinical Neuroscience Research Laboratory (Hospital Clínico Universitario), Rúa Travesa da Choupana, s/n, 15706 Santiago de Compostela, Spain

Shaheen Ahmed and Sven Vanneste
School of Behavioral and Brain Sciences, The University of Texas at Dallas, Richardson, Texas, USA

Mark Plazier
Department of Neurosurgery, University Hospital Antwerp, Antwerp, Belgium

Jan Ost
BRAI3N, Ghent, Belgium

Gaetane Stassijns
Department of physical health hand rehabilitation, University Hospital Antwerp, Edegem, Belgium

Steven Deleye, Sarah Ceyssens and Patrick Dupont
Department of Cognitive Neurology, UZ Leuven, Leuven, Belgium

Sigrid Stroobants
Department of nuclear medicine, University Hospital Antwerp, Edegem, Belgium

Steven Staelens
Molecular Imaging Centre, University of Antwerp, Edegem, Belgium

Dirk De Ridder
Department of Surgical Sciences, Dunedin School of Medicine, University of Otago, Dunedin, New Zealand

Tao Xue, Zhouqing Chen and Zhong Wang
Department of Neurosurgery and Brain and Nerve Research Laboratory, The First Affiliated Hospital of Soochow University, 188 Shizi Street, Suzhou 215006, China

Weiwei Lin
University of Pittsburgh School of Pharmacy, Pittsburgh, PA 15219, USA

Jiayi Xu
Department of Ophthalmology, The First Affiliated Hospital of Soochow University, Suzhou 215006, Jiangsu Province, China

Xuming Shen
Department of Neurosurgery, Taicang Affiliated Hospital of Soochow University, Suzhou 215400, Jiangsu Province, China

Chun-Sheng Yang, Qiu Xia Zhang, Sheng Hui Chang, Lin Jie Zhang, Li Min Li, Yuan Qi, Jing Wang and Li Yang
Department of Neurology, Tianjin Neurological Institute, Tianjin Medical University General Hospital, No 154 Anshan Road, Heping District, Tianjin 300052, China

Fu-Dong Shi
Department of Neurology, Tianjin Neurological Institute, Tianjin Medical University General Hospital, No 154 Anshan Road, Heping District, Tianjin 300052, China
Department of Neurology, Barrow Neurological Institute, St. Joseph's

Zhi Hua Sun and Nannan Zhangning
Department of Radiology, Tianjin Medical University General Hospital, No 154 Anshan Road, Heping District, Tianjin 300052, China

Christian Urbanek, Armin J. Grau, Florian Buggle and Frederick Palm
Department of Neurology, University of Heidelberg, Städtisches Klinikum Ludwigshafen am Rhein, Bremserstr. 79, 67063 Ludwigshafen, Germany

Viola Gokel
University of Mannheim, Department of Dermatology, Theodor-Kutzer-Ufer 1-3, Mannheim 68167, Germany

Anton Safer
University of Heidelberg, Institute of Public Health, Im Neuenheimer Feld 324, Heidelberg, Germany

Heiko Becher
Institute of Medical Biometry and Epidemiology, University Medical Center Hamburg-Eppendorf, Hamburg, Germany

Lorenzo Pasquini
Memory and Aging Center, Department of Neurology, University of California San Francisco, 675 Nelson Rising Lane, San Francisco, CA 94143, USA

Jorge Llibre Guerra
Global Brain Health Institute, Memory and Aging Center, University of California San Francisco, 675 Nelson Rising Lane, San Francisco, CA 94143, USA
Neurology and Neurosurgery Institute, 139 Calle 29, 10400 Havana, Cuba

Martin Prince, Kia-Chong Chua and A. Matthew Prina
King's College London, Health Service and Population Research Department, Centre for Global Mental Health, Institute of Psychiatry, Psychology and Neuroscience, De Crespigny Park, London SE5 8AF, UK

Han Chen, Jing Zhou, Yi-Qin Lin and Rong-Guo Yu
Surgical Intensive Care Unit, Fujian Provincial Clinical College, Fujian Medical University, No 134, Dongjie Street, Gulou District, Fuzhou 350001, Fujian, China

Jian-Xin Zhou
Department of Critical Care Medicine, Beijing Tiantan Hospital, Capital Medical University, Beijing, China

Chi-Hsien Huang, Chi-Wei Lin and Ru-Yi Huang
Department of Family Medicine, E-Da Hospital, I-Shou University, Kaohsiung, Taiwan
School of Medicine for International Students, I-Shou University, Kaohsiung, Taiwan

San-Nan Yang
School of Medicine for International Students, I-Shou University, Kaohsiung, Taiwan

Yi-Che Lee
School of Medicine for International Students, I-Shou University, Kaohsiung, Taiwan
Department of Nephrology, E-Da Hospital, I-Shou University, Kaohsiung, Taiwan

Hao-kuang Wang and Kuo-Wei Wang
School of Medicine for International Students, I-Shou University, Kaohsiung, Taiwan
Department of Neurosurgery, E-Da Hospital, I-Shou University, No.1, Yida Road, Jiaosu Village, Yanchao District, Kaohsiung City 82445, Taiwan

Chih-Yuan Huang
Neurosurgical Service, Department of Surgery, National Cheng Kung University Hospital, Tainan, Taiwan

Yi-Cheng Tai
Department of Neurology, E-Da Hospital, I-Shou University, Kaohsiung, Taiwan

Yuan-Ting Sun
Department of Neurology, National Cheng Kung University Hospital, College of Medicine, National Cheng Kung University, Tainan, Taiwan

Angelo Camporeale
Eli Lilly Italia, Sesto Fiorentino, Italy

David Kudrow
California Medical Clinic for Headache, Santa Monica, CA, USA
UCLA David Geffen School of Medicine, Los Angeles, CA, USA

Ryan Sides, Shufang Wang, Katherine J. Selzler and Virginia L. Stauffer
Eli Lilly and Company Corporate Center, Indianapolis, IN 46285, USA

Annelies Van Dycke
Neurology Department, AZ Sint-Jan Brugge, Brugge, Belgium

Cláudia Sousa, Telma Miranda
MS Clinic, Department of Neurology, Centro Hospitalar São João Porto, Alameda Prof. Hernâni Monteiro, 4200 – 319 Porto, Portugal

Maria José Sá
MS Clinic, Department of Neurology, Centro Hospitalar São João Porto, Alameda Prof. Hernâni Monteiro, 4200 – 319 Porto, Portugal
Faculty of Health Sciences, University Fernando Pessoa, Porto, Portugal

Mariana Rigueiro-Neves and Ana Margarida Passos
BRU-IUL, Instituto Universitário de Lisboa (ISCTE-IUL), Lisbon, Portugal

Paulo Alegria and José Vale
Department of Neurology, Hospital Beatriz Ângelo, Loures, Portugal

Dawn Langdon
Department of Psychology, Royal Holloway, University of London, London, UK

Index